THE ENCYCLOPEDIA OF

HEPATITIS AND OTHER LIVER DISEASES

THE ENCYCLOPEDIA OF

HEPATITIS AND OTHER LIVER DISEASES

James H. Chow, M.D.
Cheryl Chow

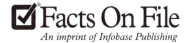

An imprint of Infobase Publishing

Facts On File, Inc.
An imprint of Infobase Publishing
132 West 31st Street
New York NY 10001

Library of Congress Cataloging-in-Publication Data

Chow, James H., 1948–
The encyclopedia of hepatitis and other liver diseases / James H. Chow, Cheryl Chow.
p. cm.
Includes bibliographical references and index.
ISBN 0-8160-5710-9 (hc : alk. paper)
1. Liver—Diseases—Encyclopedias. 2. Hepatitis—Encyclopedias. [DNLM: 1. Hepatitis—Encyclopedias—English. 2. Liver Diseases—Encyclopedias—English. WI 13 C552e 2005] I. Chow, Cheryl, 1952– II. Title.
RC845.C46 2005
616.3′62′003—dc22   2005018489

Facts On File books are available at special discounts when purchased in bulk quantities for businesses, associations, institutions, or sales promotions. Please call our Special Sales Department in New York at (212) 967-8800 or (800) 322-8755.

You can find Facts On File on the World Wide Web at http://www.factsonfile.com

Text and cover design by Cathy Rincon

Printed in the United States of America

VB FOF 10 9 8 7 6 5 4 3 2 1

This book is printed on acid-free paper.

CONTENTS

FOREWORD

The liver is susceptible to numerous disorders that range from mild to advanced, irreversible disease. Because the liver is the largest organ in the body, performing more than 200 different functions, including the processing of nutrients and storing of vitamins and iron, to name just a few, when the liver is injured for any reason, various bodily processes start to go wrong, leading to a variety of syndromes. Thus, liver diseases are wide and varied, encompassing a large number of conditions with different causes.

Liver disease affects millions of people worldwide; overall, it is the seventh-leading cause of mortality in the United States. Hepatitis C alone affects an estimated 4 million people in the United States. Hepatitis C turns into a chronic liver disease for 75 to 80 percent of those who become infected. It is a progressive disease that leads to cirrhosis—irreversible liver scarring—in more than 25 percent of chronic sufferers of hepatitis C. And cirrhosis in turn kills more than 25,000 Americans annually, ranking fourth in the cause of death for people between the ages of 25 and 44.

Worldwide, some 300 million people—representing about 5 percent of the world population—suffer from chronic hepatitis B infection, which is one of the major causes of liver cancer, particularly in developing countries.

Aside from viral hepatitis, common liver diseases include those induced by toxins (most notably alcoholic liver disease, which affects millions of individuals) and autoimmune chronic liver diseases such as autoimmune hepatitis, primarily sclerosing cholangitis, and primary biliary cirrho-

sis. Other types of liver disorders are hereditary diseases. These include hemochromatosis, alpha 1-antitrypsin deficiency, and Wilson's disease. Other liver diseases are cancer of the liver, cystic disease of the liver, and fatty liver. There is some indication that fatty liver, often associated with diabetes and obesity, is on the rise because of an epidemic of vastly overweight people in the United States. (But obesity is not the only factor contributing to fatty liver.) Some liver diseases also occur for as yet unidentifiable causes.

No one is exempt from liver disease, including children. But with children, disorders of the liver mostly have a genetic origin. More than 100 different liver diseases are found in infants and children, some of them fatal; fortunately, most of them are rare.

The economic cost of liver disease amounts to billions of dollars annually when lost productivity is added to the cost of medical care. Quite aside from economics, the impact of liver disease on the daily lives of many individuals and their loved ones is incalculable. It is my hope that this situation can be rectified by a better-informed public and policymakers.

As a clinician with a medical practice spanning more than two decades, I have long recognized the relative indifference or ignorance when it comes to the liver and the myriad diseases that can afflict it. The number of patients with liver disease is increasing. But compared to cardiovascular diseases, there is little awareness of disorders related to the liver—aside from a recent surge of interest in hepatitis C, thanks to a rising number of baby boomers manifesting signs of the infection. It is understandable, though unfortunate, that so many people, distracted by the urgencies of their daily lives, neglect their livers. After all, the liver suffers in silence for many years. More often than not, liver diseases are asymptomatic in the early stages; it is often only after irreparable damage has been done to the liver that any symptoms appear.

I cannot overemphasize the importance of becoming well acquainted with one's liver. Knowledge is power; it helps one lead a healthy lifestyle, and in the event of illness, it provides one the tools to make informed choices regarding medical care. Those currently suffering from any type of liver disease should find out all they can about the condition, or learn as much as possible for the sake of their families or friends who may be so afflicted.

This book was written to fulfill such a need, to provide an easy-to-read reference for patients and their family, friends, employers, and coworkers, who have to live and work with the patients. I have tried to clarify complex and confusing issues, and to write in language that is understandable to the layperson, my target audience for this book. I have also attempted, however, to include enough information that the book may serve as well as a handy guide for health professionals involved in the care of patients with liver disease. The materials have been compiled into an easily accessible, alphabetized format.

Yet this book is not meant to be a comprehensive or exhaustive description of every liver disease, known and unknown, as such an undertaking would require volumes. Nor is the information in this book meant to substitute for proper medical care from an experienced and licensed physician. Readers must understand that specific diagnosis and recommendations for treatment cannot be obtained from a book.

Finally, to anyone suffering from a chronic liver disease, I would like to offer a message of hope. Even for chronic disease for which there is no cure at present, the patient and the physician can often do a lot to extend the time before cirrhosis and its attendant complications develop.

The times between laboratory research and practical application are being continually narrowed, and significant strides have been made in the treatment and management of chronic liver disease. Scientists are making stunning contributions, ranging from an understanding of molecular virology to the genetics of many inherited diseases, allowing new drugs and treatments to be developed. Liver transplantation, the final option for patients with end-stage liver disease, has made such astonishing progress that it is becoming a routine procedure. But we have only just embarked on this incredible journey of hope—hope that every single person may have a healthy, functioning liver.

—James Y. H. Chow, M.D.
Medical Director
Nihon Clinic

ACKNOWLEDGMENTS

From the conception of this book, many people have contributed their assistance and advice.

We would especially like to thank the patients and individuals with liver disease who shared with us their perspective on living with a chronic disease.

Thanks also to the research librarians at the Boulder Public Main Library and Meadows Public Library in Boulder, Colorado.

We are also extremely grateful to our editor, James Chambers, for his patience and dedication in editing our manuscript. And we are indebted to Elizabeth Knappman-Frost of New England Publishing Associates for her kindness.

James Y. H. Chow would like to thank the entire staff at the Nihon Clinic in New York, Atlanta, Chicago, San Diego, and Tokyo, as well as the staff of Noguchi Hideyo Memorial Foundation, New York. Finally, he would like to thank his parents for putting him through college, in particular his mother, without whose encouragement he would never have entered medical school, and this book would never have been written.

Cheryl Chow would especially like to thank several individuals who have been exceptionally helpful in the execution of this book, notably Dr. Marian Furst for her critical review and analysis of the manuscript; Professor Tian Tai Min for his generosity and unflagging support; and James Adams for his critical insight and keen mind. Without them, this book could never have been completed. She would also like to thank Dr. Chen Tsui Chang and Dr. Howard Worman. And she remembers with regret her aunt Wen-fang, for whom medical attention for chronic liver disease came too late. She was the impetus behind the undertaking of this book.

ENTRIES A–Z

acute vs. chronic liver disease   On the surface, the difference between an acute liver disease and a chronic one seems easy to describe. The definitions are simple: an acute illness is one that lasts less than six months; a chronic illness lasts more than six months. In practice, however, it is not always easy to distinguish between the two. A patient with a chronic liver disease may have few or no symptoms for some time, until the disease worsens and symptoms suddenly become apparent. Upon seeing a doctor, such a patient may seem to have a newly contracted illness. Conversely, a patient with an acute illness, such as viral hepatitis, may be misdiagnosed as having a chronic illness, such as CIRRHOSIS, a chronic disease with advanced scarring of liver tissue, because the symptoms are often quite similar. In the case of viral hepatitis, however, the illness and symptoms can resolve completely and the patient recover; whereas cirrhosis is considered to be irreversible, and all that can be done is to keep the disease from progressing and manage the complications that arise.

It is also possible for a person with chronic liver disease to contract an acute liver disease. An individual with chronic HEPATITIS C, for example, may contract HEPATITIS A, and develop sudden, acute symptoms. Similarly, a patient with cirrhosis may develop acute liver disease from a drug overdose. Such cases are examples of an acute illness superimposed over a chronic one.

Acute Liver Disease

Generally speaking, an acute illness is one that occurs suddenly. In some viral infections, for instance, an individual suddenly becomes ill and displays a variety of symptoms, such as chills, fever, and vomiting. Although some viral infections can be serious, even deadly, the infection usually runs

a swift course, and the patient recovers within a few days.

Liver disease can display the same patterns. With acute liver disease, a patient may suddenly display a variety of symptoms and be quite ill. For most such infections—hepatitis A, for example—the illness resolves itself and the patient recovers quickly. There are other possibilities, however. In some instances, acute liver disease can kill the patient by causing a severe type of liver disease known as fulminant liver failure.

Acute liver disease may also turn chronic, though it often depends on the cause of the acute illness. Hepatitis A and HEPATITIS E, for example, never turn chronic; the vast majority of hepatitis C cases, however, do become chronic.

The causes of acute liver disease can vary. Viral infections can often be acute. Drug overdoses can cause acute liver disease as well. An individual who takes an overdose of a drug—even an over-the-counter medication such as acetaminophen (Tylenol)—may contract acute liver disease.

When a patient is suffering from acute liver disease, the goal is to cure the patient and keep the disease from becoming chronic.

Chronic Liver Disease

A chronic condition is one that lingers. The onset is often less clear and more insidious than that of an acute illness. Hepatitis C, for example, usually displays no obvious early symptoms. Most individuals with hepatitis C are not even aware that they have become infected. It is often only decades later that the illness manifests itself. It can last a lifetime unless the individual receives medical treatment, and even then only half the patients manage to eliminate the virus from their bodies. With chronic disease, the goal is to cure the disease if possible, to keep it from becoming worse, or to control the complications that may occur. In the case of liver disease, that means keeping the disease from progressing to cirrhosis, in which the scarring is so extensive that the liver becomes distorted and often develops cancer. If cirrhosis is already present, the goal of treatment is to prevent further deterioration of liver function and to control the complications.

Congenital disorders are chronic. For example, HEMOCHROMATOSIS, WILSON DISEASE, PRIMARY BILIARY CIRRHOSIS, and AUTOIMMUNE HEPATITIS are all congenital and chronic liver diseases.

Some liver diseases can be either acute or chronic. HEPATITIS B, C, and D, for example, can cause either acute or chronic illness. Similarly, years of excessive alcohol consumption will cause chronic ALCOHOLIC LIVER DISEASE, but a person who binge drinks may develop acute FATTY LIVER (steatosis) or hepatitis. Such acute disease resolves if the drinking stops. If the individual continues drinking, however, or engages in binge drinking repeatedly over a span of time, the disease becomes chronic.

advocacy   Patients at risk for or affected by LIVER DISEASE do not have to be passive recipients of the medical care they receive. By exercising their rights as patients, and actively collaborating with their physicians and other health care professionals, they can help assure that the care they receive is as effective as possible.

Patient rights are both an ethical and a legal issue. The American Hospital Association (AHA) first adopted A Patient's Bill of Rights in 1973, to help define the ethical issue, and most U.S. states have enacted laws that define the legal rights of patients. In hospitals that accept Medicare and Medicaid payments, a patient's legal rights are defined by the Patient Self-Determination Act of 1990.

The AHA's original Bill of Rights, as revised in 1992, defined 12 basic rights for patients:

1. the right to considerate and respectful care
2. the right to current and understandable information about diagnosis, treatment, and care, including the right to know the identity of everyone involved in their care
3. the right to make decisions about their care, including refusing a recommended treatment
4. the right to prepare, and have honored, an advance directive, such as a living will or a health care proxy
5. the right to privacy
6. the right to confidentiality
7. the right to review their medical records
8. the right to expect a reasonable response to requests for appropriate care and services
9. the right to be informed of the existence of any business relationships of the hospital that may influence treatment
10. the right to consent to or decline participation in proposed research studies or human experimentation
11. the right to be informed of realistic care options when hospital care is no longer appropriate
12. the right to be informed of hospital policies and procedures regarding patient treatment, care, and responsibilities

Many of those rights have been legally recognized by the states, although there may be differences in their legal application. Some rights defined by the states have been mandated by the federal government in the Patient Self-Determination Act of 1990. The act requires health care providers to give patients, in writing and before treatment, information about their legal rights in medical decisions and advance directives. That requirement, however, applies only to providers that accept Medicare and Medicaid dollars and does not affect state law. Questions about the legal rights of patients in a particular state should be directed to the state's attorney general's office or consumer affairs department.

The impetus behind these philosophical statements and legal regulations is the idea that health care should be a collaboration between the physician and the patient. An effective collaboration, however, requires that patients be well informed, both about the disease they face and about the treatments proposed. By seeking out the information they need, patients can make better decisions about what medical procedures are available to them, and what procedures they may prefer not to receive.

For general information about patients' rights, a local library is a good place to start. Most local libraries have, or can acquire through interlibrary loan, books about how patients may take charge of their medical treatment. Many hospitals have patient advocates on staff, and local medical societies may offer help too. Patients may also find it useful to obtain a copy of the AHA's original Patients' Bill of Rights; the complete text is available on the AHA's Web site. Also available from the AHA Web site is a brochure "The Patient Care Partnership," which replaced the Patient's Bill of Rights in 2002. (The brochure incorporates essentially the same points as the bill but uses language that is less intimidating and easier to understand.)

For more information about the causes and treatment of liver disease, contact the following:

American Hospital Association (AHA)
One North Franklin
Chicago, IL 60606-3421
(312) 422-3000
http://www.aha.org
http://hospitalconnect.com (for health news)

Centers for Disease Control and Prevention (CDC)
1600 Clifton Road
Atlanta, Georgia 30333
(404) 639-3311
Public inquiries: (404) 639-3534/(800) 311-3435
http://www.cdc.gov

National Institutes of Health (NIH)
9000 Rockville Park
Bethesda, MD 20892
http://www.nih.gov

U.S. Department of Health and Human Services
200 Independence Avenue SW
Washington, DC 20201
http://www.os.ddhs.gov

"A patient's bill of rights." *American Hospital Association,* October 1992.
"Federal patient self-determination act final regulations." *Federal Register* 60, no. 123 (June 27, 1995): 33294.

Alagille syndrome Alagille syndrome is an inherited condition in which the BILE DUCTS fail to develop normally in the fetus; this results in a lack of small bile ducts in the LIVER. The lack of small bile ducts slows the release of bile into the small intestine, causing a wide range of symptoms that may include jaundice, heart problems, bone problems, and physical malformations.

BILE, is produced by the liver, consists of bile salts, cholesterol, and waste products from the liver. Bile rids the body of certain waste products and is essential to absorbing fat and the fat-soluble vitamins A, D, E, and K. When the bile flow is obstructed, its constituent products build up in the body, and the body is unable to absorb fat or the fat-soluble vitamins.

Alagille syndrome is associated with mutations in a gene called Jagged 1. The mutation is usually inherited from only one of the parents. A parent with Alagille syndrome has a 50 percent chance of transmitting it to the offspring. The disorder is found in all areas of the world and in all races. It is more often reported in males, but it affects females as well.

Symptoms and Diagnostic Path

The symptoms of Alagille syndrome range from mild to severe, depending on the severity of the bile flow obstruction. Symptoms may not be apparent for the first two or three weeks of life, although jaundice—yellowing of the skin—may be present at birth. Other symptoms, often observed in the first three months of life, are

- severe, unstoppable itching (pruritis). The itching is believed to be caused by the buildup of bile salt in the body.

- loose, pale, or clay-colored stools. Because bile gives feces its color, the lack of fecal color results from insufficient quantities of bile reaching the intestine.

- poor weight gain or poor growth. Bile is essential to digesting fat; a lack of bile means fat is being underabsorbed.

- difficulty with vision, balance, or blood clotting. These characteristics are due to deficiencies in vitamins A, D, E, and K, which require bile acids to be absorbed.

Other symptoms may develop later. Those symptoms include

- persistent jaundice
- growth and development problems in early childhood
- enlarged liver
- hard, whitish nodules in the skin. The nodules are called xanthomas; they are deposits of cholesterol and fat. In young children they usually appear in spots of repeated injury, such as knees and elbows.
- dark yellow or brown urine. The color is due to high levels of BILIRUBIN, a pigment that is one of the constituents of bile.

Because the lack of proper bile flow causes vitamin deficiencies, a child with Alagille syndrome may develop physical malformations typical of such deficiencies, such as a broad forehead, a pointed jaw, and a bulbous nose.

Though Alagille syndrome is associated with rather specific symptoms, not all Alagille sufferers display those symptoms. Consequently, the syndrome is diagnosed through tests and a physical examination. A genetic test to indicate Alagille syndrome is not routinely available.

A physical examination that finds jaundice, itching, cholesterol deposits in the skin, or other hints of reduced bile flow is one indication of Alagille syndrome. Other indications include

- heart murmur
- bone defects
- kidney problems or kidney failure
- physical malformations associated with vitamin deficiency, such as a broad forehead, a long straight nose with a bulbous tip, deeply set eyes, abnormally short fingers, and a small pointed chin
- eye problems; specifically, the thickening of a line called the Schwalbe's line on the surface of the eye

LIVER-FUNCTION TESTS may uncover problems in the biliary system, and a LIVER BIOPSY may be done to find out whether there are enough bile ducts in the liver.

Other tests that may be done include a radioisotope—or "nuclear"—scan. A nuclear scan is a type of imaging test that involves ingesting a minute amount of radioactive material that can be detected by special instruments, producing an image of the internal organs. A bile salt test may also be done to distinguish Alagille syndrome from other conditions that cause liver problems.

Treatment Options and Outlook

There is no cure for Alagille syndrome. Treatment is directed toward preventing complications and managing symptoms, and must be continued in one form or another for the rest of the patient's life.

Because the condition causes fat-soluble vitamin deficiencies, children with Alagille syndrome are often given vitamin A, D, E, and K supplements, and the levels of those vitamins in the system may be monitored.

Infants having trouble absorbing fat may be given formulas that are high in medium-chain triglycerides, which can be absorbed despite the reduced bile flow. The goal is to maximize the absorption of fat and bring the children closer to normal levels of growth and development.

The severe itching (pruritis) associated with Alagille syndrome may be difficult to treat. Antihistamines may be effective for some patients. For severe cases, some doctors may consider trials of bile acid-binding resins such as cholestyramine, which may also help the high cholesterol levels associated with the syndrome. A Kasai portoenterostomy—a surgical procedure that uses a loop of bowel to increase the bile flow to the intestine—has no value for sufferers of Alagille syndrome. Another surgical procedure that has occasionally been tried is a partial external biliary diversion. In this procedure, a connection is made between the gallbladder and the skin to allow bile to be drained externally. While effective for some forms of inherited liver disorder, it is not as effective for sufferers of Alagille syndrome.

One thing that needs to be considered before any invasive procedure is that sufferers of Alagille syndrome may be at an increased risk for bleeding. Spontaneous intercranial bleeding is a recognized complication—and cause of death—in patients with Alagille syndrome. When researchers looked for other sites of bleeding, they concluded that Alagille syndrome patients are at a special risk. They were unable to determine the mechanism involved, but speculated that abnormalities in the Jagged 1 gene may impair the body's hemostatic function—the ability to check bleeding.

Eventually, scarring of the liver and other complications may require LIVER TRANSPLANTATION. The timing of such a procedure, however, should be considered carefully. The temptation to perform a liver transplant sooner rather than later should be resisted. According to a study of Alagille syndrome patients reported in the September 2001 issue of *Gut*, only 11 percent of transplant patients studied showed signs of end-stage liver disease at the time of the procedure, and the post-procedure mortality rate of the rest was 20 percent. Findings like those indicate the need to weigh carefully the expected improvement in quality of life against the chances of a premature death.

The long-term prognosis for sufferers of Alagille syndrome depends upon the severity of the bile flow obstruction and liver scarring, and the severity of other problems that might develop.

The prognosis for children born with jaundice due to a bile flow obstruction is worse than that for people whose symptoms develop later in life, but liver complications are always a possibility for both. Patients must be closely monitored for such complications for life.

Typically, an Alagille syndrome patient experiences decreasing bile flow for a period of several years, followed by some improvement. In general, children with Alagille syndrome have a better outcome than children with other liver disorders at the same age.

Many adults with Alagille syndrome lead normal lives.

Lykavieris, Panayotis, Cecile Crosnier, Catherine Trichet, Michele Meunier-Rotival, and Michelle Hadchouel. "Bleeding tendency in children with Alagille syndrome." *Gut* 49, no. 3 (September 2001): 431.

albumin   Albumin, like prothrombin (blood-clotting factors) and immunoglobulins (antibodies), is a protein that is primarily synthesized in the LIVER. The highest concentration of protein in the blood is albumin—about 65 percent of the protein.

Albumin carries small molecules, such as calcium, in the blood. There is a much higher concentration of albumin in the blood than in the fluid outside the cell, and albumin plays a key role in regulating the fluid balance in the body by maintaining the oncotic pressure of the blood—the amount of blood in the veins and arteries. This pressure helps to keep the fluid from leaking out of blood vessels and into the surrounding tissues. When fluid leaks out into the tissues, it can cause a swelling in the feet and ankles known as edema, one of the symptoms of liver disease. (Not all cases of edema are caused by liver dysfunction.)

When the liver is badly damaged, the liver cells lose their ability to secrete albumin. This occurs quite commonly in chronic liver disease, but not as often in acute liver disease, as it may take weeks or months before the albumin level reflects the liver injury, because of the protein's long half-life.

A low level of albumin is known as hypoalbuminemia. It may indicate that the ability of the liver to synthesize proteins has been diminished.

Although albumin is only one of many proteins synthesized by the liver, checking the albumin level is a popular method of assessing the functioning of the liver and its degree of damage. The laboratory test is a reliable and inexpensive way to determine the protein-building capacity of the liver.

A low albumin level of around 3 g/dl may suggest various liver dysfunctions, such as chronic liver disease with CIRRHOSIS (an advanced and irreversible scarring of the liver) or hepatitis. When albumin levels drop below 2.5 g/dl, edema occurs. A patient with very low albumin levels may need to be considered for LIVER TRANSPLANTATION.

There are also non-liver-related reasons for a low level of albumin. These include the following:

- serious malnutrition

- Crohn's disease

- kidney disease

- intestinal disorders
- extensive burns

alcohol abuse and dependence Alcoholism is an illness marked by physical and psychological dependence on alcoholic beverages. It is a form of addiction, which may be defined as the continued use of a substance despite adverse medical or social consequences. Excessive alcohol consumption has serious emotional and social problems and markedly endangers one's health. Alcohol is especially detrimental to the LIVER, which breaks it down in the body.

Liver disease is one of the most serious medical consequences of long-term alcohol abuse, which is the most common cause of CIRRHOSIS in the Western world. Research shows that for people who already have liver disease, such as patients with chronic HEPATITIS C, even moderate levels of alcohol consumption can be harmful.

Alcohol-related liver disease is widespread worldwide and remains a major cause of mortality. It is a persistent problem. In the United States, half of the population aged 12 or older—an estimated 120 million people—reported being current drinkers of alcohol in SAMHSA's 2002 National Survey on Drug Use & Health (NSDUH; formerly called the National Household Survey on Drug Abuse). About 15.9 million Americans aged 12 or older reported heavy drinking. Data from various sources suggest that some 12.5 million people, or about 15 percent of the U.S. population, are problem drinkers.

Alcohol abuse and dependence rates are higher for men (approximately 5 to 10 percent) than for women (3 to 5 percent) and higher for whites than for blacks. An estimated 55 percent of whites reported current use of alcohol, compared to 39.9 percent for blacks. Despite this lower rate of alcohol use, progression to cirrhosis occurs at a higher rate in blacks than nonblacks.

An individual with an alcoholic parent is more likely to become an alcoholic than someone whose immediate family does not have problems with alcohol abuse. Research suggests that certain genes may predispose a person to developing alcoholism, but so far no single genetic marker clearly associated with susceptibility to alcoholism has been discovered. Many different factors are probably involved in the development of alcoholism.

Symptoms and Diagnostic Path

The *Diagnostic and Statistical Manual of Mental Disorders-IV* (DSM) of the American Psychiatric Association has separate criteria for alcohol dependence and alcohol abuse. Alcohol abuse is defined as alcohol use that leads to significant impairment or persistent problems occurring within a 12-month period. The defining characteristics of alcohol dependence, on the other hand, are the loss of control and failure to abstain from drinking even though the individual is aware of the physical, psychological, or social problems caused or exacerbated by excessive drinking.

To assess correctly whether a patient has alcoholism, the physician needs to screen for alcohol abuse or dependence. One questionnaire widely used by physicians is the CAGE, an acronym for "Cut down on, Annoyed at, Guilty about, and using as Eye-opener." The questionnaire asks:

Have you ever tried to Cut down on your drinking?
Do you ever feel Annoyed at others' concern about your drinking?
Do you ever feel Guilty about your drinking?
Do you ever use alcohol as an Eye-opener in the morning?

Another screening method that is easy for physicians to use is the conjoint screening test. It involves only the following two questions:

In the past year, have you ever drunk (or used drugs) more than you meant to?
Have you felt you wanted or needed to cut down on your drinking (or drug use) in the past year?

If the patient replies in the affirmative to at least one question, this points to an alcohol use disorder. The same test can be used to detect drug or other substance use.

The American Society of Addiction Medicine adopted somewhat different screening standards that are based on the number of drinks ingested per week. An individual is considered to have a problem if he consumes more than 14 drinks per week or more than four drinks per occasion if he is a male. For women, seven drinks per week or more than three drinks per occasion indicates a possible problem. (One drink is defined as a 12-ounce bottle of beer, a five-ounce glass of wine, or a 1 ½ ounce shot of liquor.) For various reasons, such as differences in body weight and hormonal releases, alcohol has a much more detrimental effect on women than on men. Women develop alcoholic liver disease after a shorter period of heavy drinking and at a lower level of drinking than men.

Treatment Options and Outlook

Anyone with alcoholic liver disease must abstain completely from alcohol. Admittedly, this presents quite a challenge, because one of the most salient characteristics of alcohol dependency is the inability to stop drinking. Patients must therefore be encouraged to enter treatment programs and see addiction counselors. In the past, it was believed that a confrontational approach works best, but research now shows that it is best to use a compassionate and empathetic approach. Family members may need to convey honestly their concern and help the patient understand that drinking has become a problem.

One of the best-known support groups for alcoholism is Alcoholics Anonymous (AA). The group offers emotional support and—for individuals who desire such help—personal mentoring from recovering alcoholics who offer a model of abstinence. Some people, however, may not be comfortable with AA's 12-step approach. These people should not give up seeking help; other groups are available offering different models of recovery.

One such resource is SMART Recovery, which offers free face-to-face and online support groups. It uses cognitive techniques to help alcoholics recover. LifeRing is a secular program that offers peer support in a conversational format. Another non-12-step, alternative program is Secular Organizations for Sobriety (SOS, or Save Our Selves). Women for Sobriety is a self-help group that helps women achieve sobriety and sustain ongoing recovery by following a program developed for the group. The reason for having an all-women's group is that many female alcoholics have different concerns than men.

Alcohol-induced disorders are the leading cause of death from liver disease. When the disease progresses to liver failure despite medical treatment and abstinence, liver transplantation may be considered. Because there is a dire shortage of available organs, some controversy exists over giving a new liver to patients with alcohol abuse or dependence problems. Some feel that candidates with non-self-inflicted disease are more deserving and make better surgical risks. Patients with alcohol-induced disease often have severe dysfunction not only in the liver but also in other organs; this decreases the likelihood of a successful outcome. Some also question how compliant these patients might be taking their medications (transplant patients must take anti-rejection drugs for the rest of their lives), observing other aspects of follow-up care, and avoiding renewed alcohol abuse leading to damage in the new liver.

On the other hand, some experts argue that barring patients who have abused alcohol punishes them for an illness over which they have no control. Many patients with alcohol damage have had successful transplants, and some studies show that many of these patients are able to maintain their abstinence after surgery. The key is to assess which patients are likely to abstain from alcohol. A thorough evaluation process to determine eligibility is necessary. Many transplant centers require patients to participate in an alcoholism recovery program, and to maintain a six-month period of complete abstinence from alcohol before accepting anyone as a candidate for transplantation. Each center may have different requirements, so patients are advised to contact the centers directly.

In addition to medical treatment programs, many patients find self-help support groups to be invaluable in their road to recovery. Some groups to contact are listed below:

LifeRing Secular Recovery
Oakland, CA
(510) 763-0779
service@lifering.org

SMART Recovery Central Office
7537 Mentor Avenue, Suite #306
Mentor, OH 44060
(440) 951-5357
Fax: (440) 951-5358
http://www.smartrecovery.org

SOS Clearinghouse
4773 Hollywood Boulevard
Hollywood, CA 90027
(323) 666-4295
http://www.secularsobriety.org
sos@cfiwest.org

Anderson, Kenneth, Louis E. Anderson, and Walter P. Glanze. *Mosby's Medical, Nursing & Allied Health Dictionary.* St. Louis, Mo.: Mosby–Year Book, 1998.

Brown, R. L. "Identification and office management of alcohol and drug disorders." *Addictive Disorders,* 1992, p. 28.

Brown, R. L., T. Leonard, L. A. Saunders, and O. Papasouliotis. "A two-item conjoint screen for alcohol and other drug problems." *Journal of American Board Family Practitioners* 14, no. 2 (March–April 2001): 95–106.

Ewing, J. A. "Detecting alcoholism: The CAGE questionnaire." *Journal of the American Medical Association* 252, no. 14 (October 12, 1984): 1,905–1,907.

alcohol and hepatitis C   An estimated 170 million people worldwide are infected with the hepatitis C virus (HCV), one of the leading causes of liver disease in the United States. Contrary to some common portrayals of HCV, however, only in a minority of those 170 million people will the disease progress to CIRRHOSIS, HEPATOCELLULAR CARCINOMA (HCC), or end-stage liver disease. There is little research to clarify the reasons that some sufferers experience such gloomy outcomes while others do not, but the most important factor is probably alcohol.

Alcohol, a toxic chemical, is metabolized mostly by the liver. When the liver is forced to metabolize large quantities of alcohol over a long period of time, cells in the liver can change—they may swell, scar, or die. Such changes at the cellular level can eventually lead to an ALCOHOLIC LIVER DISEASE such as fat deposits or FATTY LIVER, cirrhosis, or liver failure. After a time, the liver may cease to function properly and have trouble producing materials needed for healthy body functions, making an individual more susceptible to infections and disease. In drinkers, the degree of liver damage correlates generally to the level of alcohol consumption.

It has long been known that habitual alcohol users have higher blood levels of the hepatitis C virus than infrequent drinkers, even when both are infected. Heavy drinkers are about seven times more likely to carry the hepatitis C virus than light drinkers, or those who do not drink at all. About 10 percent of heavy drinkers are infected with HCV, compared to 1.4 percent of the general population, and 30 percent of alcoholics carry HCV antibodies.

Research also indicates that heavy drinkers infected with HCV are at substantially increased risk for developing HCC, and that drinking more than eight drinks per day accelerates the progression of chronic HCV to cirrhosis and HCC, and increases mortality.

Studies of the biochemical mechanisms involved show that alcohol produces its effect on HCV by increasing the activity of a protein called "nuclear factor kappa B," which causes the virus to replicate. Research also indicates that alcohol may interfere with the antiviral activity of interferon alpha, the drug used to treat people with HCV. Other dangers faced by habitual drinkers with HCV include enhanced viral complexity, an increase in the death of liver cells, and iron overload.

The effects of light drinking are less clear. Some studies report that people infected with HCV are at increased risk of developing cirrhosis even at light to moderate levels of drinking. Other studies reveal a similar relationship between HCV and cirrhosis only at heavy drinking levels. Yet other studies have shown that drinking fewer than three drinks per day may increase the risk of cirrhosis, while the effect of more than eight drinks per day is much more than proportionately higher.

The resolution of the question must await further study. To date, research studies on the subject have relied heavily on patients recalling levels of alcohol intake over several decades. Patient recall is unreliable in all cases, and heavy drinkers especially tend either to underestimate seriously their alcohol consumption or to deny completely any excessive drinking. Somewhat more reliable estimates might be obtained by asking patients to recall specific types of drinks consumed rather than alcohol consumption in general. Biopsies of liver tissue can also be of some help in determining the role of alcohol consumption in the progression of HCV, even in people who deny drinking.

The situation is further complicated by the cardiovascular benefits of light drinking. Even though no amount of alcohol is considered completely safe for people with chronic HCV, some researchers are studying the possibility that the cardiovascular benefit of light drinking could outweigh its effect on the progression of liver disease in HCV patients who are also at high risk for developing cardiovascular disease. This is a minority position, however, and individuals with any type of liver dysfunction are urged to abstain from alcohol. The March 2004 issue of *Hepatology* reported just such a conclusion in a study at the University of California at San Francisco. The study, conducted on a cohort of 800 people with chronic HCV, included alcohol consumption data, disease-related data such as HCV GENOTYPE (different strains of the HCV virus) and VIRAL LOAD (the amount of virus circulating in the bloodstream), and results of LIVER BIOPSIES done on each patient to measure fibrosis levels.

The study found no "statistically significant" relationship between alcohol consumption and fibrosis levels until that consumption reached a daily level of 50 grams, or about five drinks. At the same time, however, the study buttressed the connection between alcohol and liver disease, finding that in the study group as a whole the odds of developing fibrosis "increased step-wise even among patients with less than 50 g/day of alcohol consumption."

In short, although alcohol use clearly promotes HCV infection, and some of the biological mechanisms involved are known, specific evidence concerning the relative effects of light drinking versus heavy drinking on HCV remains contradictory.

Also contradictory are the results of studies designed to measure the effects of alcohol consumption on HCV treatment therapies. A 1994 Japanese study, for example, concluded that lifetime alcohol consumption reduces the response to interferon therapy. The study was conducted on Japanese patients, however, so the results may not hold true for other populations. In addition, all the patients studied were being treated with interferon alone. A more recent but similar U.S. study found no effect among a small sample of male veterans being treated with a combination of interferon and ribovirin. Consequently, it is impossible to say definitively that alcohol use interferes with the effectiveness of HCV treatment options. In practice, however, doctors recommend abstinence from alcohol for all patients suffering from liver diseases.

There is no recognized treatment of HCV geared specifically to alcohol drinkers. Although one study suggests that the drug naltrexone, used to help alcoholics avoid relapse, may block the harmful effects of alcohol on HCV infections, the only treatment known to help is abstinence.

Alcohol consumption is a difficult, if not impossible, habit to stop. Although virtually all doctors advise complete abstinence from alcohol as the only completely safe alternative for people infected with chronic HCV, fewer than 50 percent of alcohol drinkers stop their consumption after being diagnosed.

Drinkers who use alcohol only socially may succeed by substituting mineral water or fruit juice at parties and other social functions. Those who use alcohol to relieve stress may be able to learn other, less harmful techniques of stress management, such as yoga, regular exercise, or meditation.

An HCV patient with a severe addiction to alcohol should consult his or her doctor, who can provide information and referrals. Options may include social support programs, such as Alcoholics Anonymous, and detoxification programs designed to monitor and assist in the withdrawal process. Comprehensive detoxification programs can be especially helpful, because they also evaluate the patient's physical and mental health and any psychosocial, occupational, and family stresses. A diagnosis of depression, for example, allows the formulation of a treatment plan designed especially to address that condition.

It is vitally important that drinkers infected with HCV control their habit. Despite statistical uncertainty about some of the details of the alcohol-HCV connection, it is clear that the connection exists, and that it can be deadly. No one with HCV should ever drink to excess; for the problem drinker, even a drop may be too much.

Bain V. G., and others. "A multicentre study of the usefulness of liver biopsy in hepatitis C." *Journal of Viral Hepatitis* 11, no. 4 (July 2004): 375.

Vento, Sandro, and Francesca Cainelli. "Does hepatitis C virus (HCV) infection cause severe liver disease only in people who drink alcohol?" *Lancet Infectious Diseases* 2 (May 1, 2002): 303–309.

alcoholic liver disease The damaging effects of excessive alcohol consumption are widely recognized. Alcohol negatively affects all organs and systems within the body. The LIVER is especially vulnerable, being the body's first line of defense against toxins. It is the liver that metabolizes (breaks down) any ingested alcohol into less toxic by-products, and converts fat-soluble substances into water-soluble substances for elimination. Drinking copious amounts of alcohol over time overtaxes the liver and damages it anatomically. Alcohol not properly metabolized by the liver further compromises health.

Alcohol also reduces the drinker's appetite and decreases the body's ability to absorb nutrients properly. Deficiencies in proteins, calories, or minerals produce less than optimal functioning and may further aggravate injuries to the liver.

Alcoholic liver disease (ALD) is widespread worldwide and remains a major cause of mortality. According to a statement published by the Colorado Center for Digestive Disorders, ALD is the most common liver disease in the United States, and the fourth-leading cause of death among Americans.

Symptoms and Diagnostic Path

Alcoholic liver disease goes through three stages, which may or may not exhibit outward signs. Excessive alcohol consumption results in an accumulation of fat in the liver (alcoholic FATTY LIVER),

and there may also be inflammation of the liver (alcoholic hepatitis). Eventually, the liver can develop scar tissue (alcoholic CIRRHOSIS) that changes its architecture, weakening and compromising its ability to function. It is possible to have all three stages concurrently.

A patient presenting with ALD almost always suffers from ALCOHOL ABUSE AND DEPENDENCE. Such a person needs counseling as well as medical and nutritional support to help abstain from alcohol. The physician should encourage the patient to attend alcohol treatment centers and groups, such as Alcoholics Anonymous (AA). In some cases, the physician may need to discuss treatment options with the family of the patient.

A persistent problem in diagnosing liver disease is that symptoms are often absent or are vague and nonspecific and can be associated with any type of liver disorder, or even problems completely unrelated to the liver. For instance, symptoms such as depression, fatigue, insomnia, or lack of concentration can be due to any number of causes. By the time a person experiences recognizable symptoms, ALD could already have progressed to an advanced stage. On the other hand, the severity of symptoms does not always correlate with the severity of the disease; some people suffer no symptoms even at the end stage. The following symptoms, therefore, are meant only as a general guideline, and their presence or absence should not be the sole basis of identifying ALD:

- abdominal swelling or increased abdominal circumference (from enlarged liver)
- abdominal pain and tenderness
- abnormal blood clotting
- ascites (fluid collection in the abdomen)
- bleeding esophageal varices (varicose veins in the esophagus)
- breast development in males
- depression
- diarrhea
- difficulty paying attention
- dry mouth
- excessive thirst

- fatigue
- fever
- fluctuating mood
- JAUNDICE (yellowing of skin and eyes)
- loss of appetite
- malaise
- mental confusion
- nausea
- unintentional weight gain
- vomiting

Anyone who experiences the following symptoms should go to an emergency room immediately, as they could be signs that he or she is suffering from advanced scarring of the liver (cirrhosis):

vomiting blood or material that looks like coffee grounds
bloody black or tarry bowel movements (melena)

Generally speaking, the longer a person has been drinking, and the greater the amount of alcohol consumed, the greater the likelihood of developing alcoholic liver disease. The higher the alcoholic content of the beverage, the greater the danger.

Excessive use is commonly defined as greater than 75 grams a day for men (about seven ounces of 86-proof liquor, six 12-ounce beers, or 15 ounces of wine), and more than 30 grams for women. In fact, for women, as little as 20 grams of daily alcohol over a course of years may be enough to cause ALD. However, the incidence of alcohol-induced disease varies considerably among people with comparable levels of intake. Various factors, including genetic predisposition, nutritional status, lifestyle choices, and other considerations influence an individual's susceptibility to alcohol-induced disease. What is certain is that there is a significant correlation between the development of ALD and alcohol abuse.

Genetics Genetics plays an important role in the development of ALD. Studies of twins indicate that genes influencing metabolism of alcohol are the most likely ones connected to alcohol-induced liver disease. Therefore, research has centered around the role of the enzymes involved in alcohol metabolism.

Two enzymes are primarily responsible for metabolizing ethanol alcohol: alcohol dehydrogenase and aldehyde dehydrogenase. Alcohol dehydrogenase is responsible for more than 90 percent of ethanol metabolism in the liver, converting alcohol into acetaldehyde, which is highly toxic and is associated with the unpleasant effects of drinking, such as flushing and nausea. Alcohol dehydrogenase determines the rate of acetaldehyde formation, and is therefore regarded as the key player in producing alcohol-induced liver damage, and possibly of alcohol dependency. Individuals with a variation in this enzyme may be more susceptible to developing alcoholism and ALD.

Aldehyde dehydrogenase metabolizes acetaldehyde into acetic acid (vinegar). Individuals with a genetic deficiency or "slow" aldehyde dehydrogenase experience nausea or an uncomfortable reddening of their faces after just a few sips of alcohol. Conversely, some individuals have enzymes that are much more efficient at metabolizing alcohol, and they must drink larger quantities than the average person to feel the same intoxicating effect. Consuming larger quantities of alcohol means that they are at higher risk for ALD.

Gender Men are more likely to become alcoholic than women, but women are more susceptible to the ill effects of alcohol even if they drink less. Women also develop ALD at a younger age than men, and when their cirrhosis is caused by alcohol, they have a shorter life expectancy than men with similar conditions.

One obvious reason that women are more susceptible to the ill effects of alcohol is their lower body weight. Another significant difference is that compared to men many, though not all, women have less of the enzyme alcohol dehydrogenase, which helps to break down alcohol. Hence women are more likely to absorb alcohol that has not been metabolized directly into their bloodstream.

Hormonal differences are also suspected, but the evidence is as yet inconclusive. Other causes for the gender disparity are currently being investigated.

Ethnicity Although many more Caucasians than African Americans are considered chronic alcohol users, cirrhosis of the liver progresses faster among African Americans than Caucasians. Asians are much less likely to suffer from habitual alcohol use and the resulting alcoholic liver disease. One reason for this may be that many people of Asian descent are deficient in the enzyme aldehyde dehydrogenase.

Coinfections Acute and chronic hepatitis B or C accelerates the progression of alcoholic liver disease. Patients infected with the hepatitis C virus (HCV) and who also abuse alcohol are predisposed to more serious liver injury than is caused by alcohol alone. They tend to have earlier onset of ALD, their disease is more severe, and their survival is shorter. HCV infection also greatly increases the risk for liver cancer in patients with alcoholic cirrhosis.

The Veterans Administration Cooperative Studies reported in the September 8, 2003, issue of *Hepatitis Weekly* that patients with cirrhosis and superimposed alcoholic hepatitis have a four-year mortality of greater than 60 percent.

Alcoholic fatty liver The accumulation of fat on the liver is considered to be one of the first signs of alcoholic-induced liver injury. Heavy drinking can result in considerable amounts of fat being deposited within the hepatocytes, the predominant cell types in the liver. (About 90 percent of chronic drinkers have fatty liver.) Even short-term binge drinking can also cause fatty liver (steatosis). People who have indulged in a three-day weekend of binge drinking may have had fatty liver without knowing it, as the condition is usually asymptomatic. Fortunately, the process is benign and reversible, at least initially. No long-term consequences will be suffered if the individual stops drinking alcohol altogether at this stage. If the fatty liver also develops inflammation, the condition is called steatohepatitis, and the prognosis becomes serious.

Alcohol abuse is not the only cause of fatty liver. Other causes include drug use, obesity, starvation, and vitamin A toxicity. It is not easy to differentiate alcohol-induced fatty liver from one that is not caused by alcohol abuse—referred to as nonalcoholic steatohepatitis (NASH). No tests can conclusively determine whether the fatty liver was caused by excessive alcohol consumption.

Alcoholic hepatitis Hepatitis is the medical term for liver inflammation. Indulging in years of excessive drinking can lead to acute and chronic hepatitis. The condition can range from mild, with few or no symptoms, to severe liver dysfunction that can ultimately lead to death. The widespread inflammation of the liver and destruction of cells lead to the distortion of hepatic architecture.

Alcoholic hepatitis is a very severe illness with a very high mortality rate. Up to 50 percent of patients may require hospitalization, and anyone with alcoholic hepatitis has a roughly 50 percent chance for developing cirrhosis within 10 years from the onset of the disease. Studies have shown that approximately two-thirds of individuals who need hospitalization for the treatment of alcoholic hepatitis develop cirrhosis.

Each individual experiences symptoms differently, and sometimes there are none, but the following symptoms are the most common:

- abdominal tenderness
- fatigue
- feeling ill
- low fever
- poor appetite
- spiderlike blood vessels in the skin

In severe cases, alcoholic hepatitis can cause many of the same complications as cirrhosis. These include ascites (abdominal fluid) and encephalopathy (damage to brain tissue leading to altered mental states). Patients can also have multiple organ failure and abnormal electrolytes (substances that regulate body chemistry). The mortality rate for untreated hepatitis is between 20 and 50 percent.

Alcoholics who already have cirrhosis frequently suffer from alcohol-induced hepatitis as well. If the hepatitis is strictly a result of alcohol ingestion, it can be reversed if the person stops drinking completely, although it can take at least six months for the inflammation and other injuries to resolve themselves.

Alcoholic cirrhosis Excessive consumption of alcohol causes chronic inflammation, which, unchecked, can culminate in cirrhosis. In the United States, alcohol is the number-one cause of cirrhosis.

Irreversible scarring occurs as healthy liver cells are replaced by fibrous tissue. This may lead to the development of PORTAL HYPERTENSION, which is akin to high blood pressure within the liver. The liver suffers from the effects of portal hypertension as well as its inability to remove waste products adequately from the bloodstream.

Malnutrition is extremely common with cirrhosis. As the disease progresses, the total body water increases while the total body protein decreases. There is a significant decrease in the levels of serum albumin, a water-soluble protein manufactured by the liver.

Some of the symptoms associated with cirrhosis include the following:

- anorexia
- fatigue
- feeling ill
- loss of libido
- nausea
- vomiting
- weight loss

In many cases there may be no symptoms. Complications of cirrhosis include jaundice, ascites (fluid collection in the abdomen), bleeding esophageal varices (varicose veins in the esophagus), and encephalopathy (confusion and other altered mental states).

The outcome is variable, but anyone with cirrhosis, whatever the cause, is at risk for liver cancer (hepatocellular carcinoma). If the cirrhosis was induced by alcohol, the lifetime risk is approximately 15 percent.

Although alcoholic cirrhosis, unlike alcoholic fatty liver or alcoholic hepatitis, cannot be reversed, the patient who abstains from alcohol can expect a healthier and longer life span than those who continue to drink.

Alcohol and other liver disease   People with liver disorders of any type should refrain from drinking alcohol. Alcohol has been shown to worsen the course of many liver diseases. For example, hepatitis C carriers who abuse alcohol will accelerate the progression to cirrhosis.

Diagnosis   As with other liver disease, there may be few or no clinical signs or symptoms of ALD, or only nonspecific ones. Diagnosis is also complicated because alcohol affects so many organs. Individuals with ALD may, for instance, also have heart problems, inflammation of the pancreas, or neurological dysfunctions. It is not always easy to determine whether a liver disorder is caused by excessive alcohol consumption. A good approach is to use a combination of history, physical exam, laboratory tests, radiological tests when needed, and, frequently, a liver biopsy.

A detailed history of alcohol use is of primary importance in diagnosing people with suspected ALD. Patients tend to deny or underreport drinking, but there are clues that can point to alcohol abuse, such as the presence of other alcohol-associated medical conditions and a history of frequent trauma and emergency room visits. Screening questionnaires can also be used, though they rely on patients answering honestly. A handy questionnaire for the physician to use is one called CAGE, an acronym for "Cut down on, Annoyed at, Guilty about, and using as Eye-opener".

Special attention should be paid to patients at high risk. For instance, women are more susceptible to the negative effects of alcohol and they have a worse prognosis than men if they develop ALD, yet their problems with alcohol are often overlooked because of cultural bias. Patients infected with hepatitis C should also be screened for alcohol use because it is associated with ALD, and magnifies the patient's risk factor.

Physicians should not rule out the possibility that liver abnormalities are due to other, non-alcohol-related causes, or that a patient has them concurrently with ALD.

A complete blood count (CBC) and liver chemistry profile can lend weight to clinical suspicions of ALD, but no tests are completely specific or sensitive for ALD.

There may be blood test abnormalities and mild elevations in aspartate aminotransferase (AST) and/or alanine aminotransferase (ALT) activities with fatty liver. If alcoholic hepatitis is present, AMINOTRANSFERASE TESTS may show mild to moderate elevation of AST relative to ALT activity and alkaline phosphatase. AST and ALT are enzymes normally found in the liver. When the liver is damaged, as with alcoholic liver disease or viral hepatitis, the enzymes are released into the blood, thus elevating serum levels of AST and ALT.

Alkaline phosphatase may be elevated or normal. Bilirubin may be increased or normal. AST activity may be elevated relative to ALT activity in patients with alcoholic hepatitis. But in other forms of hepatitis, ALT and AST activities may be roughly equal.

Imaging can help diagnose fatty liver, and to help rule out biliary obstruction or tumor. But a liver biopsy is necessary to make a diagnosis with certainty. Liver biopsy may also confirm the diagnosis of alcoholic hepatitis and cirrhosis, helps exclude other causes of ALD, and asses the extent of liver damage.

Treatment Options and Outlook

Although research continues for medications and nutritional therapies for use in the treatment of ALD, the most effective form of therapy is abstinence from alcohol.

Because malnutrition is so common when alcohol is consumed excessively, a nutritious diet should be followed. It is not too late to improve one's diet.

Complications of ALD and possible withdrawal symptoms of alcohol should also be addressed. Patients with significant complications of alcoholism (for example, cardiac dysfunction, infection, major alcohol withdrawal syndromes) will benefit from hospitalization.

Specific therapies for acute ALD   Some potential therapies include corticosteroids and pentoxifylline as anti-inflammatory agents for alcoholic hepatitis. Some studies show that corticosteroids can reduce mortality by about 25 percent. It is not known how effective these therapies are when viral hepatitis, cancer, diabetes, and other conditions are also present.

To prevent deficiencies in protein and calories, nutritional therapy may be given aggressively. During acute illnesses, high protein and calorie allowances are usually needed.

Specific therapies for chronic ALD   One study published in *Hepatitis Weekly,* September 8, 2003, states, "lifestyle modifications improve outcomes for those with alcoholic liver disease." Lifestyle modifications include drinking and smoking cessation, and losing weight (when appropriate). Alcohol interferes with intestinal absorption and storage of nutrients, which can cause deficiencies of protein, vitamins, and minerals. Therefore, nutritional support is important on both an inpatient and outpatient basis.

A nutritional approach where patients are placed on a high-calorie, high-carbohydrate diet to reduce protein breakdown in the body appears to be beneficial. Alternative treatments for liver disease may include administration of vitamins, especially B_1, and folic acid. This malnutrition increases the mortality rates of patients with ALD. Supplemental amino acid therapy (administering supplementary amino acid to improve nutritional status), on the other hand, has yielded conflicting results. Some studies found the therapy to be beneficial, while others did not.

When patients are severely depleted of magnesium, potassium, and phosphate, as they are when they are actively drinking, it can precipitate multiorgan system dysfunction. These elements should be replenished promptly.

Liver transplantation   This improves survival in patients with alcoholic cirrhosis. People with end-stage liver disease who are abstinent should be considered for LIVER TRANSPLANTATION.

Prognosis   The critical factor in prognosis is alcohol consumption and hepatic inflammation. Individuals who have stopped drinking before developing cirrhosis can generally expect a reversal of any inflammation or injury of the liver. Patients with either alcoholic fatty liver or alcoholic hepatitis improve their survival when they abstain from alcohol. If, however, patients with alcoholic hepatitis continue to drink, they are at high risk for developing cirrhosis. The degree of hepatic inflammation is another important factor.

Cirrhotic patients who stop drinking improve their chances of survival. For those patients who have already had major complications but continue to drink, the one-year survival rate is less than 50 percent.

Colchicine and other antifibrotic agents may prove beneficial in preventing overall liver-related mortality. But further research is needed before there is conclusive proof that these agents are effective in treating ALD.

The October 11, 1999, edition of *Hepatitis Weekly* reported an effective therapy for alleviating liver injuries. Cytokines (pro-inflammatory molecules) appear to play a role in the signs and symptoms of ALD. According to the study, "Cytokines are not only involved in acute and chronic inflammation, they also facilitate the production of more cytokines, which then results in more tissue injury and inflammation." Researchers are saying that "an effective strategy is to curb the over-production of cytokines while preserving their beneficial effects."

American Association for the Study of Liver Disease, "Alcoholic liver disease may have genetic basis." *Alcoholism & Drug Abuse Weekly* 12, no. 14 (November 13, 2000): 8.

Arteel, G., et al. "Advances in alcoholic liver disease." *Best Practice & Research in Clinical Gastroenterology* 17, no. 4 (2003): 625–647.

Day, C. P., R. Bashir, O. F. W. James, M. Bassendine, D. W. Crabb, H. R. Thomasson, et al. "Investigation of the role of polymorphisms at the alcohol and aldehyde dehydrogenase loci in genetic predisposition to alcohol-related end organ damage." *Hepatology* 15, no. 4 (November 1991): 798–801.

McClain, Craig J., Steven Shedlofsky, Shirish Barve, and Danielle B. Hill. "Cytokines and alcoholic liver disease." *Alcohol Health & Research World* 21, no. 4 (Fall 1997): 317(4).

McCullough, Arthur, M. D., and J. F. Barry Connor, M.D. "Alcoholic Liver Disease, proposed recommendations for the American College of Gastroenterology." *American Journal of Gastroenterology* 93, no. 11 (November 1998): 2,022.

Prijatmoko, D., B. J. Strauss, J. R. Lambert, W. Sievert, D. B. Stroud, M. L. Wahlqvist, B. Katz, J. Colman, P. Jones, and M. G. Korman. "Early detection of protein depletion in alcoholic cirrhosis: role of body composition analysis." *Gastroenterology* 105, no. 6 (December 1993): 1,839–1,845.

Sherman, D. I. N., R. J. Ward, M. Warren-Perry, Roger Williams, T. J. Peters. "Association of restriction fragment length polymorphism in alcohol dehydrogenase 2 gene with alcohol induced liver damage." *British Medical Journal* 307, no. 6916 (November 27, 1993): 1388(3).

Theal, Robert M., and Kendall Scott. "Evaluating asymptomatic patients with abnormal liver function test results." *American Family Physician* 53, no. 6 (May 1, 1996): 2111(9).

alkaline phosphatase (ALP) and gammaglutamyltranspeptidase (GGTP) tests Alkaline phosphatase (ALP or AP) and gammaglutamyltranspeptidase (GGTP or GGT) are two enzymes whose activities are frequently measured in diagnosing LIVER DISEASE. ALP is found throughout the body, while GGTP is found mainly in the liver, especially in the cells that secrete bile and the cells of the bile duct.

Normal levels of ALP are anywhere from 35 to 115 international units per liter (IU/L); for GGTP, from three to 60 IU/L. Different laboratories may use different ranges to define normal. It is important therefore to check the normal reference range printed out next to the results in the lab report.

Alkaline phosphatase and GGTP are sometimes known as cholestatic liver enzymes because high levels of these two enzymes suggest disorders of bile ducts or bile flow, as in acute or chronic (long-term) cholestatic liver disorders. Cholestatic disorders include primary biliary cirrhosis (PBC), primary sclerosing cholangitis (PSC), and intrahepatic cholestasis of pregnancy (ICP).

High concentrations of ALP can be found in the liver, kidney, bile ducts, and intestine, as well as bone and placenta. Disorders involving any of these tissues can cause elevations of ALP in the blood. For instance, large amounts of the enzyme in the blood may be an indication of bone disease, liver disease, or tumor.

Each of the tissues that produce alkaline phosphatase—liver, bone, and so forth—secretes slightly different forms of the enzyme. These variations are called isoenzymes. By measuring the various isoenzyme concentrations, one may identify which specific organ has produced the increased amount of alkaline phosphatase in the blood.

Increased levels of ALP are normal in pregnancy, in periods of growth during childhood and adolescence, and when bones are healing.

Because GGTP is mostly found in the liver, it is more specific for liver disease than is alkaline phosphatase. In almost any liver disease, GGTP is frequently elevated. Unlike ALP, GGTP activity is not influenced by pregnancy or bone growth. GGTP is extremely sensitive, however, and many drugs and alcohol can increase its level.

When GGTP levels alone are elevated, it is difficult to draw any conclusions. It could mean that the patient is suffering from the early stages of bile duct disorders, or has been drinking excessively or using drugs. On the other hand, some healthy individuals with no liver disease or alcohol and drug history may test high for GGTP. Depending on the patient's history, further tests may be indicated.

Hepatitis (liver inflammation), cirrhosis (permanent liver scarring), and other liver diseases that do not primarily affect the bile ducts may cause only modest increases in ALP and GGTP activities. The aminotransferases ALT and AST usually rise higher in contrast when there is a significant degree of liver tissue death (hepatic necrosis), such as in acute viral hepatitis.

allocating organs   Allocation is the process by which organs are distributed to patients waiting for transplants. The process includes policies and guidelines for fairly distributing available organs and tissues.

The allocation system currently used in the United States is managed by the United Network for Organ Sharing (UNOS), a nonprofit organization based in Richmond, Virginia, under contract to the federal government. UNOS maintains a nationwide list of patients waiting to receive organs for transplant. When an organ becomes available, UNOS searches its waiting list and selects potential recipients, looking for a match with the donor. Usually there are many matches, ranked by a combination of medical and logistical criteria. The organ is offered to the transplant surgeon who is caring for the top-ranked candidate.

The current U.S. allocation system traces its roots to 1984. In that year, in response to public demand for an equitable system of distributing organs for transplant, Congress passed the National Organ Transplant Act. The act created the Organ Procurement and Transplantation Network

(OPTN), intended to organize organ transplant centers, procurement organizations, tissue-typing laboratories, patients, and other interested organizations and individuals into a national network that would be able to ensure access to organs for transplant and distribute those organs efficiently. The act also set up a national task force to discuss transplantation issues and make recommendations for further action.

The task force published its report in April 1986, and the Department of Health and Human Services (HHS) awarded a contract for developing and managing the OPTN to UNOS, which has operated the network ever since.

Controversy gathered around the system in the 1990s. Critics charged that the system placed too much emphasis on geographical considerations, and that organs should be offered first to those in greatest need. Other critics were concerned that some organs were being "wasted" by being offered to patients whose conditions had worsened to the point that transplantation had become useless. Some worried that the HHS was not exercising the oversight role assigned to it by the National Transplant Act. In response, the HHS revised the final rule that governs the operation of the OPTN. The revisions to the final rule became effective in late 1999, and included provisions intended to increase HHS oversight, standardize the methods of determining suitable transplant candidates, and decrease reliance on geographical considerations in allocating organs. Today the top-ranked patient is the one most critically in need of an organ, regardless of geographic location.

Organ Matching

The criteria that determine a match between a donated organ and a transplant patient involve a variety of factors that differ somewhat by organ. In general, the organ-matching process looks at

- blood type
- organ size
- geographical proximity of the donor and potential recipient

- amount of time a potential recipient has been waiting for a transplant

Other factors include these:

- urgency of the recipient's medical need for a transplant, which is now given top priority
- degree of immune system match between donor and recipient
- age of recipient

In general, the matching process treats the nationwide list of transplant candidates as a pool of patients. When an organ becomes available, a computer creates a new list consisting of all the patients in the pool who match the available organ, ordered by the degree of match. The organ is then offered to the transplant center of the highest-ranked patient on the list. If the organ is refused for any reason, it is offered to the hospital of the next patient on the list. The process continues until a transplant hospital accepts the organ.

This occurs in five-steps:

1. *The organ becomes available.* When an organ becomes available for transplant, the local organ procurement organization (OPO) that has been managing the donor contacts UNOS and sends medical and genetic data about the organ. That data includes all the items required for a match, such as organ size and condition, donor blood type, and so on.
2. *UNOS generates a list of possible recipients.* Armed with the information from the OPO and a list of all transplant candidates in the country, the UNOS computer generates a list of possible recipients. The computer selects and ranks candidates through a combination of medical and biologic criteria, clinical criteria, and time spent on the waiting list.
3. *The appropriate transplant center is notified.* Either UNOS or, in some cases, the OPO, contacts the transplant center handling the highest-ranked transplant candidate, and offers her or him the organ.

4. *The transplant center considers the offer.* The transplant team gathers and considers the offer of the organ. Among the factors considered are the condition of the organ, the condition of the patient, staff availability, and transportation requirements. By policy, the team has only one hour to decide.
5. *The offer is accepted or refused.* The transplant team either accepts the organ or declines it. If it is declined, it is offered to the transplant center of the next patient on the list.

Getting on the List

To be included on the national waiting list for a transplant, a patient must first obtain a referral from his or her regular physician, then contact a transplantation hospital for an evaluation. There are more than 200 transplant hospitals in the United States, and it is important to learn as much as possible about the available choices. Factors that may help to determine that choice include financial status, health insurance, and geographical location.

Another factor to be considered is hospital policies that the patient may find inconvenient. For example, UNOS policy allows a patient to be listed at more than one transplant center. Individual hospitals, however, may take different views of the practice, and a patient who plans to attempt multiple listings should make sure hospital policy allows it.

The hospital's transplant team will make the final decision as to whether the patient is a good candidate for transplantation. Although UNOS has developed guidelines for some organs, there is no universal set of criteria that the hospital is bound to follow. Each hospital has its own listing criteria.

Once on the list, a patient has no guarantee of how long the wait for an organ will be. Although waiting time and urgency of need are factors in determining organ distribution, what determines the wait is the availability of compatible organs. It is conceivable that a wait could be only a few days, if the patient's need is acute and a compatible organ happens to become available. On average, however, the wait varies from a few months to a few years, due to difficulties in finding a matching organ.

alpha-1-antitrypsin deficiency (AATD) Alpha-1-antitrypsin deficiency (AATD) is an inherited disease that can cause both lung and LIVER damage. An individual suffering from the disease is deficient—or in rare cases, completely lacking—in alpha-1-antitrypsin, a protein that protects the body against the harmful effects of an enzyme released by white blood cells.

Although the disease retains the name alpha-1-antitrypsin, the deficient protein is referred to today as alpha-1-proteinase inhibitor (alpha-1-PI). Alpha-1-PI is made in the liver and released into the bloodstream. Its role is to inhibit the formation of neutrophil elastase, which ingests and kills bacteria in the lungs. If neutrophil elastase is left unchecked, it destroys lung tissue, causing the lungs to lose elasticity. Thus, there is a delicate balance between the destruction and protection of lung tissue, which is disrupted when not enough alpha-1-PI is available to do its job.

The disease most commonly manifests in adults as emphysema (a chronic lung disease) rather than liver dysfunction, though some may suffer from both lung and liver disease. People with AATD are at increased risk for developing liver disease or liver cancer, particularly if they had liver abnormalities as children.

Researchers do not know why some patients with AATD develop progressive LIVER DISEASE while others do not. It is also not completely clear how AATD can cause liver disease, though evidence suggests that it is related to inflammation. In AATD, in addition to being deficient, some alpha-1-PI proteins are abnormal. These abnormal proteins may remain in the liver instead of being secreted into the bloodstream. The accumulation of these abnormal proteins in the liver cells may lead to liver inflammation and damage.

In infants and children, the deficiency of alpha-1-PI usually manifests as liver disease, which may then progress to CIRRHOSIS. Alpha-1-antitrypsin deficiency is the most common genetic disease for which children receive LIVER TRANSPLANTATION. Males, both children and adults, develop liver disease more often than females.

The age of onset, the progression of the illness, the type and severity of symptoms, and the stage at which it is diagnosed vary considerably among individuals, even within the same family. Environmental exposure can make a significant difference, as tobacco smoke and noxious fumes accelerate the development of lung disease.

AATD affects an estimated 100,000 Americans, most commonly Caucasians of northern European descent. People of Asian, African, and American Indian descent are less frequently affected. Not everyone who carries the gene for AATD deficiency manifests the disease.

It is recommended that anyone who has relatives with AATD be tested for the genes.

Alpha-1-antitrypsin deficiency is caused by a mutation on a gene located on chromosome 14. This gene is responsible for the expression of the alpha-1-PL, the protein that is deficient in the disease.

More than 75 different alleles have been identified for the alpha-1-PI. Alleles are genetic variations, alternative forms of a gene that may occur at a given locus. The risk level for developing liver or lung disease depends on how these alleles are present on chromosomes.

Letters are used to identify the different alleles. Their effect on the secretion of alpha-1-PI can be categorized into four groups: normal, deficient, null, and dysfunctional.

"M" is the normal and the most common gene for the key protein, alpha-1-PI. Individuals who carry two copies of the "M" gene have normal levels of the protein.

Some individuals carry a variation that scientists call Z. This is the most significant defect causing AATD. Individuals who inherit an "M" gene from one parent and a Z gene from the other parent are carriers. They may have reduced amounts of the protein (about 60 percent of the normal level), but it is enough to protect them from lung disease. They may still be at increased risk for liver disease, however.

Individuals who have inherited the Z gene from each parent—in other words, they have two Z genes—have only about 15 percent of the normal level of alpha-1-PI, and what they do have is less effective at inhibiting neutrophil elastase.

There are rare individuals who do not produce any alpha-1-PI. They are called the "null-null" type. None of these individuals appears to have liver disease.

The fourth type, also uncommon, is one in which normal levels of alpha-1-PI are present, but the protein is somehow not working as it should.

Symptoms and Diagnostic Path

The age at which patients start to have symptoms varies considerably. Some may fall ill as infants, others as adults by age 30, while still others never develop clinical signs. People with AATD are at risk for early onset, rapidly progressive emphysema. They may experience wheezing and shortness of breath during daily activities, with or without exertion. Patients whose liver dysfunction has progressed to CIRRHOSIS will show symptoms associated with the condition, such as dark bowel movements, skin rash or lesion on the hands or feet, and a swollen abdomen.

The methods of diagnosis are the same for anyone with lung or liver disease, whether or not AATD is the underlying cause. Abnormalities may be observed in liver-function tests. A specific diagnosis can be made by measuring the amount of alpha-1-PI in the blood. If the level is deficient, genetic tests are available to determine directly which abnormal forms of the gene are present.

Alpha-1-antitrypsin deficiency in infants and children The link between AATD and liver disease in children was first noted 30 years ago. In infants and children, alpha-1-antitrypsin deficiency is the most common genetic cause of liver disease. AATD may account for idiopathic (of unknown origin) neonatal hepatitis in 15 to 30 percent of cases.

The most frequent sign of AATD within the first four months of life is conjugated hyperbilirubinemia. In this condition the bloodstream contains excessive amounts of bilirubin, a by-product of the breakdown of old red blood cells.

Cholestatic jaundice is a yellowing of the skin and eyes caused by a buildup of bile, a digestive fluid that the liver secretes. A newborn or child with cholestatic jaundice, a swollen abdomen, and poor appetite should be tested for AATD.

Treatment Options and Outlook

Patients with emphysema may be treated with replacement, or augmentation, therapy that raises the alpha-1-PI level in the blood through an infusion. Liver conditions, however, cannot be treated by replacing alpha-1-PI in the blood. The only replacement therapy available is liver transplantation. The new liver will produce normal, functional alpha-1-PI, and relieve any symptoms of liver disease.

A liver transplant must be ruled out, however, if the individual also has emphysema. The patient must first be treated for emphysema, and encouraged to avoid any forms of pollution, cigarette smoke, and other environmental toxins.

Some doctors recommend that AATD patients stay away from alcohol (good advice for anyone with a liver condition), get vaccinations for hepatitis A and B, and prevent exposure to HEPATITIS C.

The prognosis for most infants with liver disease is poor, but if they get a successful liver transplant, the long-term outlook is excellent.

Fortunately, most infants will not show signs of deficiency and symptoms may not develop until early childhood or adolescence. Even individuals with two abnormal Z genes for alpha-1-PI (they are the most susceptible to AATD) will not actually develop liver disease during infancy. When they do become ill, symptoms can range from mild to severe; it is difficult to predict the course of illness in an individual child. Within one family, one child may show no signs, while its siblings are seriously affected.

Screening Since 1987, tests have been available to find out whether the baby in the womb has the genetic mutation responsible for AATD. Whether parents ought to screen or not remains a controversial subject. The decision presents a moral dilemma to families who know that they carry the gene. Not every child will inherit the mutant gene (the odds depend on the particular genetic combination of the parents), and not all those who carry the gene will manifest the disease. Families who discover that they have the genetic constitution for the disease often feel isolated, but there are many organizations, Web sites, and groups for AATD to which they can turn for support.

American Family Physician 40, no. 3 (September 1989): 223(6).

Bosworth, Michelle Queneau. "Alpha-1 antitrypsin." *The Gale Encyclopedia of Genetic Disorders.* Farmington Hills, Mich.: Thomson Gale, 2001.

Dawkins, P. A., L. J. Dowson, P. J. Guest, and R. A. Stock-
ley. "Predictors of mortality in alpha-1-antitrypsin
deficiency." *Thorax* 58, no. 2 (December 2003): 1,020–
1,026.

alpha-fetoprotein (AFP) blood test The alpha-
fetoprotein (AFP) blood test is the most widely
used biochemical blood test for LIVER CANCER. The
test measures the amount of AFP in the blood,
which acts as a marker for tumors.

AFP is a substance produced by the immature
liver cells of a fetus. Levels begin to decrease soon
after birth, and reach adult levels by the end of the
first year. AFP has no known function in adults,
but its level in the blood can indicate any of several
conditions.

The normal level of AFP in males and nonpregnant females is 20 nanograms (ng) per milliliter (ml) of blood. Pregnant females typically
have higher levels, from 24 to 124 ng/ml.

Levels considered abnormally low are seen
only during pregnancy, and may indicate either
an inaccurate estimate of the age of the fetus or a
fetus with Down's syndrome. An abnormally high
level during pregnancy may mean that the fetus
has neural tube defects. A neural tube defect is an
abnormal fetal brain or spinal cord, caused by a
folic acid deficiency.

In males and nonpregnant females, mildly
high to moderately high levels of AFP are often
seen in patients with chronic hepatitis or other
LIVER DISEASES. Excessively high levels of AFP—
greater than 500 ng/ml—are seen only in the
following:

- people who have hepatocellular carcinoma
  (HCC)

- people who have germ cell tumors (cancer of the
  testes or ovaries)

- people who have metastatic cancer in the liver
  (cancer that originated in some other organ)

The AFP test is one of the tumor markers. It is
indicative, but not diagnostic, of cancer. Its sensitivity is about 60 percent; that is, about 60 percent
of patients with HCC have elevated levels of AFP,
and the AFP level can loosely correlate to the size
of the tumor. The test, in fact, is often used as a
marker of a patient's response to treatment. An
elevated level of AFP, for example, is expected to
fall to normal in a patient whose tumor has been
surgically removed (called a resection).

Since 40 percent of patients with HCC do not
have elevated levels of AFP, a normal result does
not by itself exclude the possibility of cancer. Nor
does an elevated level necessarily mean that HCC
is present. High levels of AFP can sometimes also
be caused by benign disease. However, patients
with both CIRRHOSIS and elevated AFP levels are at
a substantially increased risk for developing HCC,
and will most likely develop it eventually. Elevated
levels in a cirrhotic patient may, in fact, indicate an
undiscovered HCC.

Because the AFP is not highly sensitive, some
researchers are exploring alternative tests. Alternatives being explored include DES-GAMMA-
CARBOXYPROTHROMBIN (DCP), a variant of the
gamma-glutamyltransferase enzymes, and variants of other enzymes such as alpha-L-fucosidase,
which are produced by normal liver cells. (Enzymes
are proteins that speed up biochemical reactions.)
It is hoped that such tests, when used in conjunction with AFP, can help diagnose more cases of
HCC earlier than with AFP alone. Those alternative
tests, however, are currently research tools, and are
not widely available yet.

alternative treatment for liver disease See
COMPLEMENTARY AND ALTERNATIVE MEDICINE in
APPENDIX I.

aminotransferase tests Aminotransferases (or
transaminases) are enzymes produced by the
LIVER. Enzymes are proteins that catalyze, or facilitate, certain chemical reactions in cells. There
are two aminotransferases, also known as transaminases, which are the most useful markers for
liver injury and inflammation. They are aspartate
aminotransferase (AST) and alanine aminotransferase (ALT). These enzymes help the liver metab-

olize amino acids and make proteins. When the liver is damaged, AST and ALT may leak into the bloodstream.

An older name for AST is serum glutamic oxaloacetic transaminase (SGOT). AST is released into the bloodstream when a certain organ or body tissue is affected by injury or disease, and the cells are destroyed. Because the enzyme is found particularly in the heart as well as the liver, the AST test was also used to diagnose heart attacks (myocardial infarction), but it has been replaced today by more accurate tests.

AST is also found in other organs and body tissues such as the pancreas, spleen, lung, red blood cells, skeletal muscles, and brain tissue. That means that an elevated AST level is not specific for LIVER DISEASE. When combined with other tests, however, it can be useful in the monitoring of and the diagnosis of various liver disorders.

ALT was formerly called serum glutamic pyruvic transaminase (SGPT). Because ALT is primarily found in the liver, it is more sensitive and specific than AST for liver inflammation and cell necrosis. A high level of ALT almost always indicates a problem with the liver. As with AST, however, the severity of liver damage does not correspond to higher ALT levels.

The normal range of AST on blood work tests is generally 0 to 40 international units per liter (IU/L); for ALT, the normal range is approximately 0 to 45 IU/L. Different laboratories may have different ranges depending on the equipment used. It should also be noted that some healthy individuals may have somewhat elevated AST or ALT levels. Conversely, it is possible for individuals suffering from a liver disease—even advanced cases—to test in the normal range for AST and ALT. This is why additional tests are needed to get a clearer assessment of what is occurring within the liver.

Elevated AST and/or ALT levels may indicate that there has been trauma to the liver or other organs. But as mentioned above, not every liver disease raises enzyme levels, and the level of elevation does not always correlate with the degree of damage. For instance, an individual with only a mild case of liver disease may show a very high reading, while someone with severe damage to the liver may have only a slight elevation, or even test normal. Therefore, it does not mean that a score of 400 on an aminotransferase test is twice as bad as 200.

The amount of aminotransferase in the bloodstream may be a better indicator of how much of the liver has been damaged—in other words, the number of liver cells that are dead (liver necrosis). Sometimes elevations of the two enzymes are caused by muscle injury rather than liver damage. A simple blood test called creatine phosphokinase (CPK or CK) can show whether the raised enzyme level was caused by a muscle problem.

The time of day that a blood sample is drawn may also affect the reading. In general, aminotransferase levels tend to be higher in the morning and afternoon than evening. The level of enzyme elevation also depends in part on the length of time after the injury. Levels peak after several hours, then drop down and may return to normal in a few days, though sometimes they may remain elevated.

Acute hepatitis (liver inflammation) can cause a marked elevation in aminotransferase levels. Other liver diseases responsible for an elevation include AUTOIMMUNE HEPATITIS, ALCOHOLIC LIVER DISEASE, FATTY LIVER, drug and herbal toxicity, liver tumors, genetic liver diseases, and heart failure.

AST and ALT tests are usually given together. When the readings for both tests are compared, they may provide important clues to the nature of the liver disease. For example, within a certain range of values, the AST/ALT ratio of greater than 1 (2:1 or greater) might indicate that the patient suffers from alcoholic liver disease, but if the ratio is less than 1, the disease may be a nonalcoholic one.

A blood sample will be taken for analysis. The blood is usually drawn from the vein in the patient's elbow. A few patients may become dizzy temporarily from having their blood drawn, but there is little to no risk involved in the test.

It is advisable to stop taking drugs that may affect the test. Certain medications can raise or lower the AST level, including trifuloperazine (antipsychotic drug) and metronidazole (antibiotic). In general avoid antihypertensives (for lowering blood pressure), anticoagulants (blood-thinning drugs), medications that lower cholesterol levels, and contraceptives. The patient should also cut back on strenuous activities temporarily, because exercise can also elevate AST.

angiography   Angiography is the study of the blood vessels using an X-ray or similar device. It is used to detect abnormalities in blood vessels throughout the circulatory system and in some organs.

The procedure is commonly used to identify atherosclerosis (plaque deposits on the inside walls of arteries), to diagnose heart disease, to evaluate kidney function and detect kidney cysts or tumors, to detect aneurysms (an abnormal bulge in an artery) and other conditions in the brain, and to diagnose problems with the retina.

In treatment of the LIVER, angiography is typically used to do the following:

- help distinguish between noncancerous lesions and hepatocellular carcinoma

- help distinguish between primary cancer and metastatic cancer (cancer that has spread to the liver from other parts of the body)

- assess damage to the organ resulting from trauma of the type typically suffered in automobile accidents

- evaluate a liver's vascular structure prior to a resection for tumor treatment or living-donor transplantation

Procedure

The conventional method of obtaining information about the structure of blood vessels has been a procedure known as catheter angiography. In catheter angiography, a catheter—a long, hollow tube—is passed through an artery to the area of interest, and used to inject a contrast enhancer that allows X-rays of the area to show the vascular structure more clearly.

Catheter angiography is gradually being replaced by noninvasive methods of obtaining the same information. Computed tomography (CT) and magnetic resonance imaging (MRI) scans can often obtain images that rival the clarity of images obtained through catheter angiography. That replacement process is likely to continue as new CT and MRI technology and techniques are developed, but the more conventional method is still the standard, and in many situations gives results superior to those of the newer technologies. Catheter angiography is still widely used in evaluating patients for surgery, angioplasty, or stent placement.

Catheter angiography   Catheter angiography is an X-ray. The catheter is necessary to deliver a contrast dye to the area being x-rayed so the blood vessels show more clearly in the resulting pictures.

The dye is injected through a procedure called an arterial puncture. The puncture is usually made in the groin, the armpit, the inside of the elbow, or the neck. First, a small incision is made in the skin and a needle containing an inner wire called a stylet is inserted into the artery. When the artery has been punctured, the stylet is removed and replaced with another long wire called a guide wire.

Using a fluoroscopic screen that displays a view of the patient's vascular system, the radiologist or surgeon feeds the guide wire through the outer needle and into the artery until it reaches the area that requires study. Once the guide wire is in position, the needle is removed and a catheter is slid over the wire until it, too, reaches the area of study. Then the guide wire is removed and the catheter is left in place so it can be used to inject the dye.

The dye may be injected by hand, with a syringe, or it may be injected using an automatic injector connected to the catheter. The advantage of an automatic injector is that it can propel a large volume of dye to the site very quickly.

Throughout the dye injection procedure, X-ray or fluoroscopic pictures are taken using automatic film changers or computer storage devices. The high pressure of arterial blood flow quickly dissipates the dye through the patient's system, so pictures must be taken in rapid succession. The patient may be asked to change position several times, in order to capture views of the area from different angles, and additional dye injections may be required.

When the X-rays are complete, the catheter is removed. Pressure is applied to the site of the incision with a sandbag or other weight to allow the blood to clot and the arterial puncture to reseal itself. A pressure bandage is then applied.

CT and MR angiography CT angiography (CTA) and MR angiography (MRA) are noninvasive methods of conducting blood vessel studies. A CTA procedure is performed using a spiral— also called helical—CT scanner and a contrast enhancer similar to the dye used in a conventional catheter procedure. MRA procedures can give reasonably clear images without an enhancer, depending on the area being studied, but enhancers are commonly given with those procedures as well. The enhancer given with an MRA, however, is fundamentally different from that used with catheter and CT procedures, and is generally associated with fewer and less severe side effects.

The procedures themselves are essentially similar to other CT and MR imaging procedures, and involve the same general preparation and recovery parameters.

Risks and Complications

Because catheter angiography is an invasive procedure, its risks are somewhat greater, and potentially more serious, than those associated with either CTA or MRA. Internal bleeding or hemorrhage is possible, and as with any invasive procedure infection of the puncture site is a risk.

A catheter procedure can also trigger a stroke or heart attack if blood clots form or the catheter dislodges plaque from the interior surface of a blood vessel. In pulmonary (lung) and coronary (heart) angiography, a catheter can irritate the heart and cause arrhythmias, but that is not a risk with liver studies.

Both catheter angiography and CTA involve exposure to radiation, and for that reason are not recommended for pregnant women. In both procedures the exposure is slight, although multiple catheter procedures performed within a short period have been known to cause skin necrosis (death of skin cells) in some patients. That risk can be minimized by careful monitoring and documentation of cumulative radiation doses.

In both CT and catheter angiography, there is a risk of reaction to the contrast medium used.

Symptoms of allergic reactions include swelling, difficulty breathing, heart failure, or a sudden drop in blood pressure. If the patient is aware of the allergy, steroids can be administered before the test to counteract the reaction. Since the contrast enhancers are eliminated in urine, they can also injure the kidneys and may worsen existing kidney disease. The contrast enhancers used in MRA procedures are associated with reactions that are both less frequent and less severe.

Catheter angiography is not usually a good choice for patients with impaired kidney function, especially those who also have diabetes. Patients who have had allergic reactions to X-ray contrast materials in the past are at risk for reaction to the contrast materials used in catheter angiography, and it is a bad choice for patients who have a tendency to bleed excessively.

The limitations of CTA are similar to those of any procedure using CT imagery. Images of blood vessels can be fuzzy if the patient moves during the exam or if the heart is not functioning normally. Blocked blood vessels may make the images hard to interpret, and CTA images of small, twisted arteries or vessels in organs that move rapidly may be unreliable. A patient who is breast feeding should consult with the radiologist. And because CTA exposes patients to X-rays, pregnant women, especially those in the first three months, should not have the procedure.

Similarly, the limitations of MRA are the same as those of any other MR procedure. MRA does not image calcium well, and in that respect is inferior to CTA. Because of the strong magnetic field generated by MR equipment, MRA must be avoided in any patient with metal implants that may not be securely anchored. The procedure is particularly dangerous if the patient has pacemakers, metallic ear implants, implanted neurostimulators, and metallic objects in the eye. Other situations that may present dangers to the patient include the possible presence of bullet fragments or the presence of a port for delivering insulin or chemotherapy.

In addition, the clarity of MRA images does not yet match that of catheter angiography. MR images of small blood vessels, for example, can be inadequate for diagnosis and treatment planning, and MR images may not adequately differentiate between arteries and veins.

antibody See ANTIGEN; HEPATITIS B; HEPATITIS C TREATMENT; IMMUNE SYSTEM.

antigen An antigen is any substance that the body recognizes as foreign. It triggers an immune response, causing the body to create antibodies against the antigen. An antigen may be formed within the body or it may be a foreign substance from the environment. Examples of antigens within the body are bacterial toxins and tissue cells; antigens from the environment may be chemicals, viruses, bacteria, and so forth.

applying for disability See FINANCING HEALTH CARE in APPENDIX I.

artificial and bio-artificial livers LIVER TRANSPLANTATION offers hope for the thousands of patients suffering from end-stage LIVER DISEASE. Improved surgical techniques enable more people to receive a segment of liver tissue from living donors. The number of people receiving liver transplants increases each year. But even so, with more people needing a new liver because of chronic liver disease or acute LIVER FAILURE, the demand continues to grow, far outstripping the number of available organs. Many patients, nearly 1,000 of them children and teenagers, die while waiting for an organ. To keep these patients alive until a graft becomes available or until the patient's own liver recovers, researchers have been trying to create liver-assist devices.

These machines that temporarily assist the liver are called "artificial livers," or liver dialysis. Like the kidney dialysis machine, these devices can support a diseased or damaged liver that cannot function properly. Creating such a machine for the liver, however, is far more challenging because the liver is so complex and has so many varied functions, that it is difficult to duplicate them artificially. Scientists and engineers have tried for more

than 40 years to create liver-assist devices, but they have met with limited success. Efforts have been hampered by uncertainty as to which functions of the liver were absolutely essential in keeping patients alive and by the daunting challenge of removing toxins and waste particles from the blood while leaving behind the valuable components. Blood carries many beneficial substances, such as proteins, antibodies, and vitamins, whose removal could harm the patient.

Recent years have seen a number of innovative developments with support systems designed to duplicate at least some of the liver's functions. Basically, they all work by circulating the patient's blood outside the body through filters that remove waste products that the diseased liver fails to filter out. The systems differ in the kinds of filters they use. The artificial (mechanical) system uses various filtering mechanisms such as charcoal or resins that absorb the waste products. The bio-artificial system uses liver cells (hepatocytes) from a living animal, typically a pig, or a human donor. The bio-artificial type may also attempt to duplicate other functions of the liver besides filtration, particularly synthesizing various chemical compounds.

By temporarily taking over some of the functions of a failing liver, the liver-assist devices buy time for the patient with acute liver failure who may otherwise die while waiting for a suitable organ. Time is critical when the liver fails. Patients in fulminant hepatic failure may not be able to survive even a short wait for donor organs. Some may not last more than a day or two, but it can take a week or so for a donor liver to arrive. The machines that can provide temporary support can be lifesavers for such patients.

When a liver is failing, the toxins are no longer broken down and cleared out. They stay in the blood, increase pressure in the brain, and damage important systems such as nerve function. The artificial and bio-artificial livers can filter out the toxins and protect the patient's brain and other organs until a suitable graft becomes available. Being the only organ that can regenerate itself, the liver can sometimes recover its functions after rest and appropriate medical treatment. However, a liver that is badly scarred cannot regenerate itself. If the liver recovers, it saves the patient the cost and risk of transplantation; and should a transplant become necessary, the artificial (or bio-artificial) liver may also provide support to a patient until the new organ can begin functioning adequately.

Bio-artificial Livers

Attention has turned in recent years to bio-artificial livers that include liver cells (hepatocytes) from animal or human sources largely because of improved technology and medical advances in isolating liver cell cultures. Most of these devices use liver cells from porcine sources to filter the blood because pig livers are similar in function to human livers. But baboon and rabbit cells have also been used. One concern with using animal cells is that viruses from the animals can be passed to the human patient.

Researchers at the University of Minnesota worked to minimize this possibility by making sure the patient's blood never touched the pig cells they used in the dialysis. At the same time, the pig cells, which were suspended in a collagen gel inside the hollow fibers of the dialysis cartridge, remained more vital because they were protected from the patient's immune defenses. The patient's blood cells are kept from touching the pig cells because they are too big to pass through the fibers. However, the smaller molecules of the toxins in the blood easily diffuse through the fibers and into the enclosed gel where the pig cells destroy them.

Another researcher also succeeded in shielding the patient's blood from the animal cells that were used as filters. The Alin bio-artificial liver designed by Kenneth Matsumura of Berkeley's Alin Foundation used rabbit liver cells to purify blood. To prevent the passage of viruses from the animal cells to the patient's blood, a semipermeable synthetic membrane separates the rabbit cells from the patient's blood. It also prevents the body from forming an immune response that could reject the animal cells.

Because of concerns about the safety of using animal cells, other researchers have been experimenting with liver cells isolated from human cadavers. The first human cell–based bio-artificial liver system was designed to increase the liver's ability to regenerate and recover. VitaGen Incorporated

of California created the ELAD (Extracorporeal Liver Assist Device) system. Using "immortalized" human liver cells, the device not only removes waste products and toxins from the blood, it also produces beneficial proteins. For this, a line of human liver cells that can replicate and function is created using genetic engineering techniques. This gives doctors access to a renewable source of cells without immune-system side effects. Cartridges inside the device contain a cultured human cell line that is supposed to replicate some of the vital functions of a healthy liver. These cartridges can be changed every few hours, ensuring continuous usage.

One problem with using human liver cells is that they are in short supply. They do not survive after thawing, and it is difficult to store them in liquid nitrogen, as with other types of cells. To circumvent that, Scottish scientists developed a technique that allows them to freeze layers of liver cells attached to membranes. Doing so allows them to supply cells for use in bio-artificial livers.

Albumin Dialysis

Beginning in 1998, the University of Michigan Health System began to test an albumin dialysis called a molecular adsorbent recirculation system (MARS) for the treatment of acute liver failure. The device attempts to replicate the function of the liver by using human albumin to remove toxins from the body while sparing helpful compounds. Albumin is a sticky carrier protein that grabs harmful substances in the blood and takes them to the liver to be neutralized. MARS works by using human albumin to clean the blood. The device pumps the blood out of the body and into a plastic tube. Inside it is a membrane coated with albumin. Toxins in the patient's blood are attracted to the albumin on the membrane and bind to it. The dialysis solution on the other side of the membrane also contains albumin. The blood, cleaned of the toxins, is returned to the patient's body. Beneficial substances remain in the patient's blood. The albumin dialysis appears to be able to reduce blood toxins and also reverse coma and shock.

Speaking at the Fourth International Symposium on Albumin Dialysis in Liver Disease in

Rostock, Germany, in August 2002, Robert Bartlett, M.D., noted that the limitation of bio-artificial livers is that it is difficult to grow liver cells quickly and safely. Bartlett is head of the extracorporeal life support team at the University of Michigan Medical Center. "Filtering devices, on the other hand, have also failed to give consistent results and have often taken the 'good' out of the blood with the 'bad'." Bartlett believed that using human albumin avoided these shortcomings.

In the future, liver-assist devices might become a standard treatment for liver failure in much the same way that kidney dialysis is for kidney failure. Patients may be able to live longer outside the hospital and allow their blood to be cleansed by a "liver dialysis" several times a week.

Currently, the artificial livers are limited in scope. They have succeeded only in clearing toxins from the bloodstream, and cannot yet perform many of the other vital functions of a liver. Researchers are now working on next-generation artificial livers that can perform some of these functions.

Another development of potential benefit is the research into stem cells as an infinite supply of liver cells for bio-artificial livers, or potentially as replacement cells for those that have died from injury or disease. Stem cells are master cells in the body that have the ability to develop into any type of cell.

Gavin, Kara. "Artificial liver trials show progress, as transplant candidates wait: University of Michigan expert describes promise of albumin dialysis approach." University of Michigan Health System. Available online. URL: http://www.med.umich.edu/opm/newspage/2002/artificialliver.htm. Accessed on September 5, 2002.

Jones, Susan K. B. "When the liver fails: Systems that support or temporarily replace the liver's functions can buy time for patients awaiting liver transplant." *Registered Nurse* 66, no. 11 (November 2003): 32(6).

Mayo Clinic. "Mayo Clinic liver specialists testing new machine that serves as a bridge to transplant for those with severe liver disease." Available online. URL: http://www.sciencedaily.com/releases/2000/01/000124074352.htm. Accessed on January 24, 2000.

Northwestern University, Media Relations. "Clinical trial of 'artificial liver' uses albumin dialysis." July 31, 2001. Available online. http://www.northwestern. edu/univ-relations/media_relations/releases/july/liver.html. Updated on July 3, 2002.

University of Chicago Medical Center. "Trial begins for first artificial liver device using human cells." Available online. URL: http://www.sciencedaily.com/releases/1999/04/990406044124.htm. Accessed on April 6, 2002.

University of Pittsburgh Medical Center. "Artificial liver being tested at University of Pittsburgh used successfully in two patients so far—one patient is first ever to be supported with device before a multivisceral transplant." Available online. URL: http://newsbureau.upmc.com/TX/ArtificialLiverTesting.htm. Accessed on February 3, 2003.

University of Minnesota. "University of Minnesota bio-artificial liver ready for human application." Available online. URL: http://newsbureau.upmc.com/TX/ArtificialLiverTesting.htm. Accessed on April 15, 2002.

ascites Ascites is a massive accumulation of fluid in the abdominal cavity. It is a common complication of CIRRHOSIS (irreversible scarring of the LIVER), and may signal a significant worsening of the prognosis. More than 50 percent of patients develop ascites within 10 years of first being diagnosed with cirrhosis.

Ascites may have a number of causes. It is most commonly associated with liver disease—more than 75 percent of patients with ascites have cirrhosis—but it is also seen in people with cancer (10 percent), heart disease (3 percent), tuberculosis (2 percent), or pancreatitis (inflammation of the pancreas, 1 percent). Other, more rare conditions, such as malnutrition, may also cause ascites.

The precise mechanisms that cause the fluid accumulation are not completely understood. It is associated with liver disease because ascites is often a result of PORTAL HYPERTENSION, an increase in blood pressure in the system of veins that drain blood from the intestines into the liver. The increased pressure is commonly a result of damage to the liver or to the lymph system that takes excess fluid away from the liver. Low levels of ALBUMIN and other proteins in the blood can also contribute to ascites by reducing the force that holds plasma in the blood vessels. Other mechanisms that can result in ascites include fluid retention caused by kidney damage or kidney disease, and leakage from the capillaries due to inflammation or infection.

Symptoms and Diagnostic Path

Depending on the amount of fluid involved, ascites may present no symptoms at all or dangles symptoms that are profoundly noticeable. Common symptoms include abdominal pain or discomfort, often a feeling of fullness after eating only small amounts of food, changes in bowel function, difficulty in breathing or walking, lower back pain, and fatigue. As fluid accumulates, the abdomen may enlarge and become distended. It is not uncommon for patients first to seek medical attention because they can no longer fit into a dress or a pair of pants—yet they have not gained weight.

Diagnosis begins with a medical history and a physical exam. An initial diagnosis can often be made by tapping on the abdomen and listening to the sound generated. In one such test, called the shifting dullness test, the examiner has the patient lie on the back on an examining table and taps on, or percusses, various areas of the abdomen until a dull sound is heard. The location is marked with a pen, and the patient lies on his or her side for one minute. Then the test is repeated. If the dull sound recurs in a different area, ascites is suspected.

Other tests that may be conducted include imaging techniques such as a computed tomography (CT) scan. Such techniques may reveal relatively mild fluid accumulations to which percussive tests are not sensitive.

Diagnosing the cause can be somewhat more problematical. If the cause is not obvious from other sources, the examiner will probably perform a procedure called paracentesis. Paracentesis involves inserting a needle into the body cavity to withdraw the fluid. In the case of ascites, paracentesis is both a treatment and a diagnostic tool. In the diagnostic phase, small amounts of the fluid are withdrawn to check for infection and to analyze the contents for clues to the cause of the fluid accumulation. It is particularly important to isolate the cause in cirrhotic patients; non-cirrhotic causes such as cancer, tuberculosis, and pancreatitis occur with greater frequency in patients with liver disease.

Infected fluid indicates a condition known as spontaneous bacterial peritonitis (SBP), a condition that requires hospitalization and treatment with intravenous antibiotics.

Treatment Options and Outlook

Mild ascites can be treated by putting the patient on a low-sodium diet and restricting fluids to about one liter a day. That is effective in only about 20 percent of patients, however, and diuretics (water pills) are often added to dietary restrictions. Diuretics are effective in about 90 percent of patients. When such medical treatment proves ineffective, the patient is said to have "refractory" ascites.

Refractory ascites can be managed by large-volume paracentesis. This is the same procedure as that used in diagnosis, but it withdraws large volumes of accumulated fluid to relieve symptoms. If the fluid is not infected, as much as four to six liters can be safely removed every two weeks. If the fluid reaccumulates, however, and requires repeated paracentesis over a long period of time, a TRANSVENOUS INTRAHEPATIC PORTOSYSTEMIC SHUNT (TIPS) may be considered. The TIPS procedure installs a shunt (an alternative pathway) between the portal veins and hepatic veins inside the liver. The shunt decreases the amount of ascitic fluid by relieving the pressure in the portal veins. Originally developed as a means of controlling bleeding from esophageal and gastric varices (swollen veins), TIPS is now often used to control refractory ascites.

Although TIPS relieves symptoms and makes ascites easier to manage, it has no effect at all on the liver itself. Even with a shunt in place, liver disease progresses as usual, and patient survival remains unaffected. Consequently, a patient with refractory ascites caused by liver disease must inevitably be evaluated for a possible LIVER TRANSPLANTATION.

Moore, K. P., et al. "The management of ascites in cirrhosis: Report on the Consensus Conference of the International Ascites Club." *Hepatology* 38, no. 1 (July 2003): 258–266.

aspartate aminotransferase test (AST)   See LIVER-FUNCTION TESTS.

asymptomatic carriers See HEPATITIS B; HEPATITIS C; HEPATITIS C TREATMENT.

autoimmune hepatitis (AIH) The immune system's job is to protect the body by defending it against foreign invaders. To fight "enemies" like viruses and bacteria, the body secretes white blood cells that attack these invaders. Sometimes, however, a glitch occurs, causing the immune system to become hypervigilant; it becomes intolerant, so to speak, of the body's own cells, targeting them for attack as if they were foreign substances.

Such a condition is known as an autoimmune disease, and it can affect tissues, joints, and muscles. Some examples of autoimmune disorders are rheumatoid arthritis, systemic lupus erythematosus (SLE, an inflammatory connective tissue disease), and Celiac sprue (wheat intolerance). When the liver bears the brunt of the body's onslaught against itself, it results in a condition known as autoimmune hepatitis (AIH). The liver becomes inflamed, and its cells start to die. The illness is chronic and progressive and, if left untreated, can lead to CIRRHOSIS and ultimately, LIVER FAILURE.

Among patients with chronic liver disease in the United States, 11 to 23 percent have autoimmune hepatitis.

AIH was known by different names in the past, including chronic active hepatitis and lupoid hepatitis, because an association was believed to exist between the illness and systemic lupus erythematosus (SLE), an inflammatory connective tissue disease. Today we know that there is no direct link between SLE and autoimmune hepatitis, and the term lupoid hepatitis has been discarded.

AIH is found predominantly in women; in men, it usually affects older age groups. However, AIH can and does occur in males and females of all ages. It can coexist with other liver diseases, such as viral hepatitis, but AIH itself is not contagious.

The cause of the disease is unknown. It is not the result of chronic viral infection, alcohol consumption, or exposure to medications or chemicals that are toxic to the liver. Some individuals seem to be genetically susceptible to developing the illness. Researchers speculate that AIH may be triggered when these people are exposed to certain viruses or drugs. Factors associated with the development of AIH include viral infections such as HEPATITIS A and Epstein-Barr, and medications like minocycline, a broad spectrum tetracycline antibiotic.

The search for the genetic roots of AIH is centered mostly on chromosome 6. Certain genetic markers can be predictive of the general age of onset, as well as the course and prognosis of the illness. These markers are known as HLA-DR3 and HLA-DR4. HLA stands for human leukocyte ANTIGEN. These special antigens are located on chromosomes that may play a role in predisposing people to certain diseases. HLA-DR3 and HLA-DR4 are located on chromosome 6. People with AIH who have HLA-DR3 tend to develop the illness at a comparatively younger age; their disease is also more aggressive and less responsive to medical treatment. In contrast, patients who have HLA-DR4 are relatively older; their disease is less aggressive and responds better to therapy. Yet not everyone suffering from AIH has these genetic markers.

Symptoms and Diagnostic Path
Like any case of hepatitis, AIH presents with symptoms that can range from mild to severe. Some people may have no symptoms but have abnormal results on liver-function tests.

Fatigue is probably one of the most common symptoms. An acute case of AIH—such as occurs in approximately one-third of patients—is frequently accompanied by fever, JAUNDICE, and a tender liver. Other possible symptoms include the following:

- abdominal discomfort
- chest pain
- diarrhea
- edema
- enlarged liver
- itching
- joint pain
- skin rashes (including acne)
- weight loss

In advanced stages of the disease, there may be abdominal fluid buildup (ascites) or mental confusion (encephalopathy). Women's menstrual periods may also stop.

In clinical practice, autoimmune hepatitis is classified into three subtypes, types 1, 2, and 3. The classification is based on the presence of autoantibody markers. Autoantibodies are those that attack the body's own cells and tissues instead of battling foreign invaders like bacteria and viruses—as antibodies would do in a healthy immune system.

The diagnostic autoantibodies for type 1 AIH are antinuclear antibodies (ANA) and smooth-muscle autoantibodies (ASMA); for type 2, they are anti-LKM (as well as P-450 IID6); and for type 3, they are anti-LKM.

Type 1, the "classic" AIH, is by far the most common one in North America, seen in up to 70 to 80 percent of patients. Of these, 78 percent are women. Type 2 progresses to cirrhosis more frequently during therapy than type 1 disease and in general has a poorer prognosis. Type 2 and Type 3 are not commonly seen in the United States.

Type 3 has not yet been firmly established as a distinct subgroup. It may be a variant rather than a separate condition. Antibodies to liver-pancreas (anti-LP) are better markers for type 3 but are not exclusive to the type.

In North America, 11 to 23 percent of patients with chronic liver disease have autoimmune hepatitis. AIH is most common among white people of northern European ancestry in whom a high frequency of both HLA-DR3 and HLA-DR4 markers are seen. By contrast, the Japanese population has a much higher frequency of HLA-DR4 markers than HLA-DR3s.

According to a study published in 2003 in *Revista de Investigacion Clinica* by Garcia-Leiva and colleagues, ANA is the only antibody present in 13 percent of AIH cases, while ASMA is the only antibody present in 33 percent of cases. The autoantigen has been identified (P-450 IID6) in Type 2 AIH, but not in the other types. Autoantigens are normal bodily constituents that evoke an immune response, causing the body to produce autoantibodies.

The clinical picture of AIH can be quite similar to that of acute viral hepatitis. Indeed, it may resemble many other liver diseases. This means that symptoms alone are not a reliable guide to diagnosis.

If the patient is young and has no common risk factors for liver disease—alcoholic, drug, metabolic, conditions or a possible exposure to viruses—AIH should be suspected.

Laboratory tests Tests to be done include a complete blood count (CBC), blood-clotting parameters (relating to the blood's ability to clot), liver-function tests (see below), and hepatitis serologies that test for viral hepatitis.

These tests will help to eliminate other causes of liver disease, including viral hepatitis (A, B, C, D, E), alcohol-induced liver disease, nonalcoholic steatohepatitis (NASH), HEMOCHROMATOSIS, and a metabolic disorder called WILSON'S DISEASE.

One highly critical test that should be done early in the evaluation is the antinuclear antibody (ANA) test that screens for many autoantibodies associated with various autoimmune or rheumatic disease. Patients with autoimmune hepatitis often—though not always—test positive for these autoantibodies. Type 1 is characterized by positive test results for ASMA and/or ANA. Type 2 shows positive for anti-LKM antibody, and type 3 for anti-SLA antibody.

It is possible to test positive even when the individual is healthy; positive tests may also indicate illnesses that are not AIH or other autoimmune diseases.

Liver-function tests Liver-function tests may show somewhat elevated serum ALT and AST activities, while alkaline phosphatase and gamma-glutamyltranspeptidase may be mildly elevated. Abnormal findings, with or without symptoms, should prompt more tests for a definitive diagnosis.

Radiologic studies Imaging studies such as ultrasound and computed axial tomography (CAT scan) are not helpful in obtaining a definitive diagnosis of AIH. But they may confirm the presence of cirrhosis, and also help rule out the presence of liver cancer. (Fortunately, primary liver cancer is rare in AIH.)

Liver biopsy A LIVER BIOPSY is in order if AIH is suspected. It is an important tool that can tell the specialist whether the tissue samples are suggestive of AIH or not and, along with other findings, can confirm the diagnosis. It can also show the extent of liver damage (such as cirrhosis) and exclude other causes of liver dysfunction.

Treatment Options and Outlook

An early diagnosis is important for best treatment results. A successful treatment can avoid or slow the progression of AIH, stopping it from damaging the liver further, and may in some cases reverse the damage already done.

Depending on their condition, patients without any symptoms may not need to undertake therapy; however, they should be closely monitored for progression of the disease, and repeat biopsies should be performed at approximately five-year intervals.

The main therapy is medicine to suppress an overactive immune system. Most commonly, the patient is given a combination of a corticosteroid (prednisone) and azathioprine (Imuran). Both drugs have anti-inflammatory properties and suppress the immune system. Sometimes prednisone alone is prescribed, but the preferred treatment is to take it with azathioprine. The combination can lower the dose of prednisone needed and significantly decrease drug-related side effects.

Treatment typically starts with a high dose of the drug(s); these are tapered over six to 24 months as the disease is controlled.

Most people will need to continue the medication for years; one out of three patients will be able to discontinue the medication after about two years of starting treatment. Some people will have to take a maintenance or low-dose medication for the rest of their lives.

Patients who have stopped treatment should carefully monitor their health because if the disease returns—as it can for some people within three years of stopping treatment—it may be more severe than before. Any recurrence of symptoms should immediately be reported to the doctor.

Obviously, there are no vaccinations for autoimmune disease. But it is advisable for a patient with autoimmune hepatitis to be vaccinated against hepatitis A (HAV) and B (HBV) if the patient does not have immunity or is not already infected. A patient can become very ill if a viral hepatitis is superimposed on an existing condition of autoimmune hepatitis.

Even at high doses taken over a period of a year, the majority of patients do not experience any significant side effects from the medication. Most side effects can be managed by lowering the dos-age; however, one out of 10 patients may develop debilitating side effects.

Prednisone can induce psychological problems such as mood swings, depression, and insomnia. The medication can also worsen some medical conditions such as diabetes, high blood pressure, and osteoporosis (thinning of the bones); patients may also develop fluid retention, headache, cataracts, and menstrual irregularities.

There are various ways to manage potential side effects. For example, to offset the dangers of osteoporosis, women should take calcium (1,200 milligrams a day) and vitamin D (1,000 international units a day), exercise regularly, and receive a bone density test every one to two years.

Patients taking prednisone on a long-term basis are advised to get regular eye exams because they run the risk of developing cataracts.

With azathioprine, some side effects are nausea, diarrhea, rash and itching, mouth sores, bone marrow depression (which lowers the red and white blood cell count), and, rarely, inflammation of the pancreas (pancreatitis), which can cause abdominal pain. Women of childbearing age should note that azathioprine has been shown to cause birth defects. The medication should therefore not be given to pregnant women or women who are planning on becoming pregnant in the near future. People who have cancer are also advised against taking azathioprine.

Some patients may not be able to tolerate prednisone. If that is the case, budesonide, which is associated with fewer side effects, may be an alternative.

For reasons that are unclear, about 10 percent of patients do not respond to conventional therapy. Patients for whom steroid treatments are not effective may try other medications that are commonly used to prevent transplant rejection, such as cyclosporine or tacrolimus (FK-506).

A study conducted at California's Cedars-Sinai Medical Center showed that cyclosporine can induce remission of AIH in people who do not respond to corticosteroids.

Similarly, researchers in Iran at Tehran University of Medical Sciences concluded that cyclosporine is safe and effective. The study further suggested that it was beneficial even in patients newly diagnosed with AIH, and who have not tried other treatments.

The prognosis is generally good for patients whose illness was caught and treated before the development of cirrhosis. The life expectancy of patients in clinical remission is not appreciably different from that for the general population. However, most people with severe AIH who do not get treatment will die within 10 years of onset of the disease.

Sometimes, even when patients respond to treatment, the disease may progress to irreversible scarring of the liver, cirrhosis. Despite the presence of cirrhosis, however, therapy clearly improves survival rate. Although one of the complications of cirrhosis is primary liver cancer, cirrhosis rarely develops into cancer in AIH patients.

If the disease progresses to liver failure, LIVER TRANSPLANTATION is a viable option. AIH patients who receive a liver transplant generally do very well, with an excellent long-term outlook. The survival rate after five years is approximately 90 percent, and AIH rarely recurs. Even if it does, it can usually be managed by adjusting the dosages of the immunosuppressive drugs for AIH.

Having autoimmune hepatitis does not increase the odds of becoming infected with the hepatitis C virus (HCV). But it is possible to suffer from both diseases, and when the two coexist, treatment becomes complicated. That is because prednisone, the medication of choice for AIH, increases the replication of HCV. On the other hand, INTERFERON, the treatment for HCV, can have seriously adverse consequences for anyone with AIH. The question then becomes, What disease should be treated?

The answer in most cases is to target whatever disease dominates. To find out which one that is, it is necessary to find out how many autoantibodies there are in the patient's blood—in other words, the autoantibody titers. A titer is a measurement of the amount of antibodies found in the patient's blood and serum. In general, patients with autoimmune hepatitis have titers of 1:160 for ASMA and 1:320 for ANA. In contrast, patients with chronic viral hepatitis may have titers in the range of 1:80 or less. These ratios are general guidelines; only

hepatologists (liver specialists) can correctly interpret the tests for a given patient.

If there is a question about the diagnosis, the safer bet is to treat the AIH with steroids. Steroids appear to be much less dangerous than beginning treatment with interferon.

Fernandes, N. F. "Cyclosporine therapy in patients with steroid resistant autoimmune hepatitis." *American Journal of Gastroenterology* 94, no. 1 (January 1999): 241–248.

Garcia-Leiva, J., A. Rios-Vaca, and A. Torre-Delgadillo. "Antibodies and pathophysiology of autoimmune hepatitis." *Revista de Investigacion Clinica* 55, no. 5 (2003): 577–582.

Malekzadeh, R. "Cyclosporin A is a promising alternative to corticosteroids in autoimmune hepatitis." *Digestive Diseases and Sciences* 46, no. 6 (2001): 1,321–1,327.

autoimmune liver disorders Normally, the immune system works to defend the body. In an autoimmune disease, the immune system fails to recognize the body's own cells, tissues, and organs, and it attacks them as if they were invading microbes. The body cannot distinguish properly between proteins that it makes and potentially harmful proteins from infectious agents or toxins, so that white blood cells produce antibodies against the tissue or cells of the body. More than 80 serious, chronic illnesses, each affecting the body in different ways, are recognized to be autoimmune conditions. For example, in diabetes mellitus type 1 (formerly known as juvenile-onset diabetes), the insulin-producing cells of the pancreas are permanently damaged; in rheumatoid arthritis, the joints become stiff and swell up.

The LIVER suffers from autoimmune attack in the following three diseases: AUTOIMMUNE HEPATITIS (AIH), PRIMARY SCLEROSING CHOLANGITIS (PSC), and PRIMARY BILIARY CIRRHOSIS (PBC). Significant amounts of time and resources have been spent studying the immune system and pathways of inflammation, and doctors know that inflammation plays a large role in each of these diseases, and it should be controlled. The exact causes of these diseases are unknown; however, it is assumed that an autoimmune disease is responsible. The courses of these diseases are unpredictable; doctors cannot foresee what will happen to a patient. Therefore, the patient needs to be monitored closely. Immunosuppressive medications may help in some cases.

Symptoms and Diagnostic Path

Autoimmune liver disorders used to be considered very rare, and they were poorly recognized and understood. In recent years they are being identified more frequently with better diagnostic methods. Still, it is not easy to differentiate among the three liver diseases in the beginning, as the symptoms are quite similar and often misleading. The symptoms vary widely, even within the same disease, and the severity ranges from mild to disabling. All three disorders lead to CIRRHOSIS of the liver. The autoimmune liver disorders may be differentiated with liver biopsies: the tissue looks quite different under the microscope.

Autoimmune diseases are not contagious, and one cannot catch them like the flu or other infectious diseases. Rather, a gene or cluster of genes seems to influence a person's susceptibility to a disease, as these diseases seem to run in certain families. It appears that the inherited set of abnormal genes is expressed in different ways among individual family members. That means, for example, that one person may have rheumatoid arthritis, while a family member or a cousin may come down with Crohn's disease, a gastrointestinal disorder. This suggests that environmental and other factors may also influence the type of autoimmune disease that a person contracts.

At least 75 percent of autoimmune sufferers are women, usually of childbearing age. Autoimmune diseases are the fourth-largest cause of disability among women in the United States. The reasons for this are not yet understood, although researchers suspect that hormones play a role. Some autoimmune illnesses worsen during pregnancy, others improve, and some occur more frequently after menopause.

auxiliary liver transplantation   This is a transplant that augments the patient's own LIVER to help it function. In this operation a small portion of a healthy liver is added to the patient's diseased liver, which is not removed, as it would be in a regular transplant. Part of the donor liver, usually the left or right lobe, is transplanted just beneath or next to the patient's own liver, which remains in its original location.

Procedure

This type of transplantation is usually performed in people with potentially reversible LIVER FAILURE, as in drug reactions or a major injury to the liver, or any type of end-stage LIVER DISEASE in which it would not be harmful to leave the patient's diseased liver. The grafted organ can assist the patient's own diseased liver until it has regained its functions. In many cases a complete regeneration of the patient's own liver is possible. When the native liver has recovered, the graft can be removed or allowed to atrophy by discontinuing the immunosuppressive medication, which keeps the body from rejecting the transplanted organ. The operation can also be performed on a patient with chronic irreversible liver failure, but so far there has been limited clinical experience and the success rate is uncertain. This procedure is not suited for patients with liver cancer, infection in the liver, or a diseased bile duct.

Risks and complications   These transplantations began in the 1980s, but some of the technical difficulties of the operation have not yet been completely ironed out. Surgeons still find it a challenge to divide proportionately the portal vein blood flow between the two livers.

Outlook and lifestyle modifications   Nonetheless, auxiliary transplantations will continue to be carried out, in part because of the chronic organ shortage. Since only part of a liver is needed, the graft can come from a living donor or the smaller part of a liver from a deceased donor. The rest of the liver can be given to another recipient, as is done in a SPLIT-LIVER TRANSPLANTATION. It can be a lifesaver for patients who cannot obtain a whole liver for a transplant.

Also, should the transplanted liver fail to function or be rejected, severely infected, or damaged, the native liver can still function. Yet another advantage is that patients can avoid the need for lifelong immunosuppressive medication, which not only increases the risk of infection but can also be potentially toxic. At the very least, patients are able to reduce their medication dosage considerably.

The auxiliary transplant is particularly suitable for children born with a congenital metabolic disorder in which the liver is unable to excrete the bile that accumulates in the blood (Crigler-Najjar syndrome). Except for that one defect, the liver functions normally; therefore, it can do well when a portion of a healthy liver assists it. But if nothing is done to correct the defect within the first year of life, this disorder is fatal.

benign liver tumors Tumors—tissue cells growing at an abnormal rate—can be either cancerous (malignant) or noncancerous (benign). Many types of benign tumors grow in the LIVER. The three most common are hemangioma, hepatic adenomas, and focal nodular hyperplasia (FNH). Unlike malignant liver tumors, benign liver tumors are always confined to the liver; they do not spread to other parts of the body.

Symptoms and Diagnostic Path

Hemangiomas of the liver are relatively common. They are identified in at least 1 percent of autopsies, and are estimated to occur in up to 7 percent of the adult population. Their occurrence is more common in women, but it can be found in men as well, and in any age group.

Hemangiomas are a mass of dilated blood vessels in the liver. They are usually small, and their presence is usually not associated with any symptoms, but if the tumor is large enough, there may be some discomfort. In rare cases they can grow larger than 10 centimeters in diameter, but they do not turn malignant.

No specific treatment is required, unless the tumor is extremely large or is causing significant symptoms, in which case surgery is an option. Surgery may also be required for infants with large hemangiomas to prevent clotting and heart failure.

Hepatic adenoma is much more rare than hemangioma. It occurs mostly in women, especially those of childbearing age. It is a proliferation of liver cells, usually single but sometimes multiple. Only rarely are there more than five lesions. This type of tumor varies in size, but is usually greater than five centimeters in diameter at diagnosis. Sometimes the tumor can be massive.

The incidence of adenomas has increased in the last few decades, probably due to the increased use of oral contraceptives and high-dose hormone replacement therapy, as these tumors are associated with the use of estrogens.

Adenomas sometimes enlarge in women taking estrogen or during pregnancy. Discontinuing birth control pills or hormone therapy will stop the tumors from enlarging. Women on oral contraceptive pills and/or hormone therapy should have their liver function checked every year.

Although it is rare for adenomas to develop into cancer, they carry the risk of bleeding within the tumors and into the abdominal cavity. There is also the possibility that the tumors will rupture. If the tumor is large, surgery is usually advisable to confirm diagnosis and to prevent the tumor from rupturing.

People afflicted with glycogen storage type-1A disease, a rare liver disease of abnormal sugar metabolism, tend to have multiple adenomas and a higher incidence of the tumor rupturing and of progressing to malignancy. Such patients are often referred for LIVER TRANSPLANTATION.

Focal nodular hyperplasia (FNH) is a proliferation of liver cells around an abnormal artery of the liver. FNH is more common among women than men. Estrogen most likely does not cause the development of FNH, but pregnancy and the use of birth control pills may cause an existing tumor to grow larger.

Compared to the adenoma, FNH tends to be smaller, is less likely to be multiple, and carries little risk of rupture or hemorrhage. The FNH has never been reported to progress to malignancy. It is not commonly associated with symptoms, but in some cases if the tumor is very large, the patient may feel abdominal pain.

Most benign tumors are found incidentally, during a physical examination, an abdominal surgery for a different reason, or an imaging study of the liver, such as an ultrasound, magnetic resonance imaging (MRI), or computed tomography (CT) scan. No blood tests can determine whether a tumor is benign, and doctors may be uncertain as to the nature of the tumor. Moreover, it is not always easy to distinguish among hemangioma, FNH, and adenoma. But a reliable diagnosis is necessary for making the decision whether to perform surgery.

Diagnosis can be made through the patient's medical history and a variety of radiological studies. If the sonogram indicates that the tumor mass is larger than 2.5 centimeters, then a tagged red blood cell (RBC) scan is ordered to confirm that the tumor is a hemangioma. If the sonogram indicates that the mass is smaller than 2.5 centimeters, then an MRI is usually enough to diagnose the mass as being hemangioma. If a liver biopsy is indicated, a smaller needle should be used, as there is an increased risk of bleeding due to an abundance of blood vessels in many tumors.

Reddy, K. Rajender, M.D., and Eugene R. Schiff, M.D. "Approach to a liver mass." *Seminars in Liver Disease* 13, no. 4 (1993): 127–138.

Weimann, Arved, et al. "Benign liver tumors: differential diagnosis and indications for surgery." *World Journal of Surgery* 21, no. 9 (November 1997): 983–991.

bile   Bile is a yellowish green fluid that the LIVER produces continuously and releases into the small intestine to help digest and absorb fats. An adult produces about 400 to 800 milliliters of bile daily. Many waste products and toxins are also eliminated from the body by secretion into the bile. The GALLBLADDER stores bile and squirts it into the small intestine when the body is ready to digest fat.

The bile is composed primarily of water, electrolytes (including sodium, potassium, and calcium), protein, cholesterol, a pigment called BILIRUBIN cholesterol, bile salts, and bile acids, which are essential for digestion.

bile ducts   Small tubes called bile ducts in the LIVER merge with successively larger ducts until they form a hepatic (liver) duct that emerges from the liver. The liver is connected to the GALLBLADDER, which is a small, saclike organ underneath the liver, by a tube called the cystic duct. The hepatic duct merges with this cystic duct to form the common bile duct that empties into the small intestine.

The liver secretes a yellowish green fluid called BILE to aid in the digestion and absorption of fats. Bile ducts collect the bile and transport it to the gallbladder, whose main function is to store and concentrate bile. When fatty food enters the digestive system, the gallbladder squirts bile into the small intestine through the bile ducts.

Obstructions in the bile ducts from tumors, gallstones, or other causes can lead to liver disease, such as CHOLESTASIS, which is an impairment of bile flow, or cholangitis, bacterial infections of the bile ducts.

biliary atresia   Biliary atresia is a disease of the LIVER and BILE DUCTS that results in a severely decreased bile flow in infants. The liver produces BILE, a liquid made up of cholesterol, waste products, and bile salts. Bile salts are necessary for the digestion of fat. The BILIARY SYSTEM, a network of tubular structures and tiny ducts, carries the bile salts to the small intestine to aid in the digestive process. It also removes waste products by letting the bile drain from the liver into the intestines.

In biliary atresia, there is a closure or disappearance of this biliary system. As a result, bile is blocked from flowing to the GALLBLADDER and becomes trapped inside the liver. This damages the liver, causing scarring to the liver cells, which may result in CIRRHOSIS—a permanent scarring of the tissues—and, unless properly treated, LIVER FAILURE.

The biliary ductal system inside the liver (interhepatic) or outside the liver (extrahepatic) may be affected. Most commonly, the ducts outside the liver are affected.

Biliary atresia is generally regarded as a congenital disease, that is, the baby is born with the condition. The bile ducts may have failed to develop normally during pregnancy. (But the condition is not caused by anything the mother did during her pregnancy.) Recent research suggests that a viral infection damages the bile ducts in susceptible infants after birth. The body's own immune system may also be responsible for the progressive damage that takes place.

About 10 to 25 percent of cases have other associated congenital defects. These most commonly involve the heart, blood vessels, abdomen, and genitourinary tract.

Children with ALAGILLE SYNDROME may have bone and heart valve problems and abnormal pigmentation in the eyes. Alagille syndrome is a rare, inherited disorder characterized by biliary atresia and a decreased number of smaller bile ducts within the liver.

Biliary atresia is a rare disease, occurring only in newborns, in about 1 in 15,000 live births. It affects slightly more girls than boys. Asians and African Americans are affected somewhat more frequently than Caucasians. There are no known genetic links.

Symptoms and Diagnostic Path

Biliary atresia may be suspected in an infant born at term who appears normal at birth but develops JAUNDICE (a yellowing of the skin and eyes) between two and three weeks or later. Other possible symptoms include these:

- clay-colored stools
- floating stools
- dark urine
- swollen abdomen
- enlarged liver
- enlarged spleen
- weight loss
- slow or absent weight gain
- slow growth
- irritability

The doctor will check for these signs and symptoms. The following tests can help diagnose biliary atresia:

- blood tests showing liver-function abnormalities such as elevated BILIRUBIN

- abdominal X-ray to look for an enlarged liver and spleen

- abdominal ultrasound to detect an absent or tiny gallbladder

- HIDA scan (a special radioactive dye that acts like bilirubin injected into the infant's vein to determine bile flow)

- LIVER BIOPSY in which a special needle is used to take a small piece of liver to view under the microscope to see whether there are features typical of an obstruction to the biliary system. If the biopsy suggests biliary atresia, then a surgical exploration of the abdomen may be necessary for a definitive diagnosis.

- If the gallbladder is present, a cholangiogram is performed to determine whether the ducts are blocked. A dye is injected through the gallbladder, and an X-ray is taken to see whether the dye flows normally into the intestine and the liver. If the dye flows the way it should, and biliary atresia is ruled out, another liver biopsy with a bigger tissue sample is taken.

Treatment Options and Outlook

Biliary atresia cannot be effectively treated with medication. Only surgical interventions prolong survival and add to quality of life. These are the Kasai procedure and liver transplant. The first choice of treatment is the Kasai procedure. In this procedure, an open duct is created so that bile can pass from the liver into the intestine. The malformed bile duct outside the liver is removed and a new duct is created using a piece of the baby's intestine.

Early diagnosis is critical to the success of this operation. Ideally, the infants should be operated on before 10 to 12 weeks of age, before severe liver damage has occurred. When caught early enough, the procedure may reestablish bile flow in roughly 60 to 85 percent of infants. But after three months, the operation is much less successful.

Of the successful cases, Kasai procedure can restore bile drainage in about 50 percent of the patients, and in some 30 percent of patients there will be complete drainage and a return to normal bilirubin. The success rate depends on the extent of the liver damage and on the experience of the surgical team.

About 20 percent of the infants will not be helped. Usually this is because the blocked bile ducts are inside the liver (intrahepatic) as well as outside it (extrahepatic). In these cases, the only option is a liver transplant.

After the operation, the infant is closely monitored for resumption of bowel activity. The most common complication is a bacterial infection. Signs include unexplained fever, increased jaundice, or lighter stools. Other complications include irreversible cirrhosis, failure of the Kasai procedure, and liver failure.

If left untreated, most babies will die within one year of diagnosis. The Kasai procedure, which is the first choice of treatment, enables babies to grow and to enjoy several years of fairly good health.

The four-year survival rate in babies who have had the Kasai procedure is about 40 percent. If the procedure has been successful in bringing the bilirubin level back to normal, the children may live well into adulthood. But in most cases, a liver transplant will ultimately be required because slow, progressive damage to the liver will continue if bile flow has been only partly restored. Eighty-five percent of patients will need a liver transplant before the age of 20, and nearly half will require transplantation before age five.

With reduced bile flow, there may be poor growth and malnutrition. The child may also require extra calories because children with liver disease have faster metabolism than healthy children. To maximize growth, the child should be given a well-balanced diet and vitamin supplements; medium-chain triglyceride (MCT) oil, an easily digested form of dietary fat, may be added to foods or infant formulas.

biliary system　The biliary system is the system of organs and ducts that carries BILE through the body. The function of the biliary system is to drain waste products from the LIVER into the duodenum—the first section of the small intestine—and to aid in digestion by controlling the release of bile.

Bile is a greenish yellow fluid secreted by the liver to carry away waste and to break down fats during digestion. Bile consists of waste products, cholesterol, and bile salts. It is bile salts that help to break down fat. Bile, which is flushed from the body in feces, is what gives feces their characteristic brown color.

Bile secreted by liver cells is carried to the duodenum by a system of ducts. About half the bile goes directly to the duodenum; the other half is stored in the GALLBLADDER, a pear-shaped organ directly below the liver. When food is eaten, the gallbladder contracts and releases stored bile into its cystic duct, which joins with the liver's common hepatic duct to form the common bile duct. The common bile duct carries the bile to the duodenum.

bilirubin　Bilirubin is a pigment that is a useless and toxic by-product of the breakdown of old red blood cells. It is generated in large quantities. The protein hemoglobin, which carries oxygen to all the tissues of the body, is contained in red blood cells, and is broken down into "heme" and "globin." Heme is then converted to bilirubin and carried to the liver. Bilirubin is extremely insoluble in water; it is chemically converted in the liver by a process called conjugation to make it more water-soluble so that it can be excreted into the BILE. Almost all of the conjugated bilirubin is secreted into the bile; a small amount may leak out of the liver and back into the bloodstream. Most of the bilirubin in the blood is unconjugated.

Bilirubin gives bile its characteristic yellowish color. Bile is stored in the GALLBLADDER or transported to the small intestine to help digest food. Once in the intestines, bilirubin is further metabolized by intestinal bacteria into urobilins and passed into the feces, contributing to their color. Bilirubin itself has no function in digestion.

Red blood cells have a life span of only 90 to 120 days. Most of the time the body produces enough red blood cells to replace the ones that die, so that the amount of bilirubin released remains relatively constant. If the red blood cells are destroyed at an abnormally high rate (hemolysis), or if the liver is damaged and fails to keep up its task of eliminating bilirubin, the blood bilirubin level becomes elevated. In a healthy individual, the total bilirubin concentration is usually under 1 milligram (mg) per deciliter (dl). When the bilirubin concentration is higher than about 2.5 mg per dl, the skin and whites of the eyes turn yellow, a condition called JAUNDICE. It is one of the symptoms of liver disease, though other illnesses can also cause jaundice.

Measurements of blood bilirubin concentration are taken to screen for liver or gallbladder disease, or to monitor the progression of the disease. Laboratories usually report values for direct and total bilirubin. Direct bilirubin represents the amount of conjugated bilirubin in the blood. Total bilirubin is equal to the amount of unconjugated (indirect) bilirubin and conjugated (direct) bilirubin.

biological therapies Biological therapy is a relatively new type of treatment that is intended to repair, stimulate, or restore the body's IMMUNE SYSTEM responses. It can be used to fight various diseases, including cancer and autoimmune diseases such as rheumatoid arthritis and Crohn's disease. It can also help control side effects of other treatments, such as cancer chemotherapy. Other names for the therapy are immunotherapy, biotherapy, or biological response modifier therapy. The materials used are made either in the body or in a laboratory.

The immune system includes the spleen, lymph nodes, tonsils, bone marrow, and white blood cells. When the system works properly, it attacks and destroys foreign and disease cells. At the cellular level, the immune system fights disease, including cancer, in several ways, and white blood cells play important roles in the process. Two types of white blood cells are monocytes and lymphocytes; lymphocytes include B cells, T cells, and natural killer cells.

Biological therapy is different from standard chemotherapy. Chemotherapy attacks cancer cells directly with anticancer drugs, while biological therapy boosts the immune system itself to battle more effectively against cancer. Researchers do not fully understand the ways in which biological therapy works, but they believe this type of treatment can slow or stop cancer cell growth, help the immune system destroy cancer cells, and prevent cancer from metastasizing, or spreading, to other parts of the body.

Cells in the immune system secrete two types of proteins: cytokines and antibodies. Cytokines play a role in communication between cells. Lymphokines, interferons, interleukins, and colony-stimulating factors are types of cytokines. Cytotoxic (anticancer) cytokines are released by a type of T cell called a cytotoxic T cell. These cytokines may attack cancer cells directly. Antibodies bind with, or latch onto, foreign substances called antigens, similar to the way a key fits into a lock.

Several types of biological therapies are currently in use. Nonspecific immunomodulating agents improve the immune response in a general way. Biological response modifiers (BRMs) are produced by the body in small quantities for specific responses to infection and disease. Modern laboratory methods can produce BRMs in large quantities.

Biological therapy may be used alone or in combination with other cancer treatments, such as surgery, chemotherapy, and radiation treatments, depending on the type of cancer, the stage of its development, and what other treatments have already been tried. It may be administered as pills, injections, or intravenously, either at home or in a clinic or hospital. The treatment schedules are variable, ranging from daily to monthly or even less frequently.

Nonspecific Immunomodulating Agents

Nonspecific immunomodulating agents may target specific immune system cells. For example, they may trigger increased production of cytokines or immunoglobulins. Bacillus Calmette-Guerin (BCG) is used to treat bladder tumors and bladder cancer. A solution containing BCG is placed in the bladder and stays there for about two hours. It may also be useful for treating other types of cancer. Levamisole has been used with fluorouracil (5–FU) chemotherapy in the treatment of stage III (Dukes' C) colon cancer following surgery. Levamisole may act to restore depressed immune function.

Biological Response Modifiers

Biological response modifiers are antibodies, cytokines, and other immune system substances produced in the laboratory. They include interferons, interleukins, colony-stimulating factors, monoclonal antibodies, and vaccines. BRMs help the body fight a disease in several different ways:

- stop, control, or slow down processes that permit cancer growth
- make cancer cells more recognizable to the immune system, which increases the system's ability to destroy the cancer cells
- increase the ability of immune system cells, such as T cells, NK cells, and macrophages, to kill foreign and cancer cells
- change the growth patterns of cancer cells so they behave more like healthy cells
- prevent or reverse the processes that change normal and precancerous cells into cancerous cells
- improve the body's ability to repair or replace normal cells damaged or destroyed by other forms of treatment, such as chemotherapy or radiation
- prevent cancer cells from spreading to other parts of the body

Some BRMs are already considered to be standard treatments for certain diseases and certain types of cancer, while others are still being tested in laboratory and clinical trials. BRMs may be prescribed for use by themselves or in combination with each other. They may also be combined with other treatments, such as radiation therapy and chemotherapy.

Interferons (IFN)

Interferons are cytokines that occur naturally in the body. There are three major types: interferon alpha, interferon beta, and interferon gamma. Interferons may stimulate natural killer cells, T cells, and macrophages to boost the immune system's function, particularly against cancer. Interferons may also slow the growth of cancer cells or promote their development into cells with more normal behavior.

Interferons were the first cytokines produced in laboratories for use in treating cancer. Interferon alpha has been approved by the U.S. Food

and Drug Administration (FDA) for the treatment of chronic hepatitis B and HEPATITIS B, as well as some types of cancer, including hairy cell leukemia, melanoma, chronic myeloid leukemia, and AIDS-related Kaposi's sarcoma. Interferons have been used to treat liver cancers.

Clinical research is looking at combinations of interferon alpha and other BRMs and interferon alpha with chemotherapy to treat a number of cancers.

Interleukins (IL)

Interleukins are another type of cytokines that occur naturally in the body, and they can also be made in the laboratory. The most widely studied interleukin for cancer treatment is interleukin-2 (IL 2, or aldesleukin). IL-2 stimulates the growth and activity of lymphocytes and other immune cells. The FDA has approved IL-2 for the treatment of metastatic kidney cancer and metastatic melanoma. Research is continuing on the use of interleukins to treat other forms of cancer.

Colony-Stimulating Factors (CSFs)

Colony-stimulating factors, also called hematopoietic growth factors, stimulate bone marrow stem cells to divide and form new blood cells—white blood cells, platelets, and red blood cells. CSFs do not usually affect tumor cells directly. CSFs have been used to treat liver cancers.

Chemotherapy drugs can limit the body's ability to make blood cells. As a result, chemotherapy patients are at increased risk of developing infections, anemia, and bleeding. CSFs may be prescribed to increase blood cell production and counteract these effects of chemotherapy. Increased blood cell production allows the use of larger chemotherapy doses without the need for transfusion with blood products. Thus, CSFs are used in combination with high-dose chemotherapy for cancer treatments.

Examples of CSFs used for cancer treatments include the following:

- G-CSF (filgrastim) and GM-CSF (sargramostim) can increase the number of marrow stem cells and white blood cells. They can decrease the risk of infection in patients receiving chemotherapy, and they are also used to prepare patients for stem cell and bone marrow transplants.

- Erythropoietin can increase the number of red blood cells and reduce the need for red blood cell transfusions in patients receiving chemotherapy.

- Oprelvekin can increase the number of platelets and reduce the need for platelet transfusions in patients receiving chemotherapy.

CSFs are being studied for treatment of some types of cancer, including leukemia, melanoma, lung cancer, and metastatic colorectal cancer, which most frequently spreads to the LIVER.

Monoclonal Antibodies (MOABs)

Monoclonal antibodies (MOABs) are produced in a laboratory by a single type of cell and are specific for a particular ANTIGEN. Research is focused on creating MOABs specific to antigens found on the surfaces of cancer cells. Typically, human cancer cells are injected into mice, and the animals' immune systems then make antibodies to the cancer cells. The mouse cells that make the antibodies are then isolated and fused with other laboratory-grown cells to form hybrid cells, called hybridomas. The hybridomas are then cultured to produce large quantities of pure antibodies.

MOABs may be used in cancer treatment in a number of ways:

- increase a patient's immune response to a specific type of cancer

- act against cell growth factors and interfere with the growth of cancer cells

- combined at a molecular level with anticancer drugs, radioisotopes (radioactive substances), other BRMs, or other toxins to deliver these poisons directly to a tumor

- destroy cancer cells in bone marrow that has been removed from a patient in preparation for a bone marrow transplant

- combined with radioisotopes, may be used to diagnose certain cancers, such as colorectal, ovarian, and prostate cancers

The FDA has approved Rituxan (rituximab) for the treatment of B-cell non-Hodgkin's lymphoma that has returned after a period of improvement or has not responded to chemotherapy. It has also approved Herceptin (trastuzumab) to treat metastatic breast cancer in patients with tumors that produce excess amounts of a protein called HER–2. Other MOABs are being tested for treatment of lymphomas, leukemias, colorectal cancer, lung cancer, brain tumors, prostate cancer, and other types of cancer.

Cancer Vaccines

Vaccines have been used for many years to prevent infectious diseases, such as measles, mumps, and tetanus. They include weakened forms of antigens that are present on the surface of the infectious agent. When they are introduced into a person's body, the body's immune cells produce more plasma cells, which make antibodies for the particular antigen in the vaccine. More T cells are also produced that recognize the infectious agent. These T cells remain, and the immune system is prepared to respond quickly if the infectious agent enters the body again.

Vaccines are under development for treating cancer. These vaccines are being given to people who already have the disease, but they work in a similar way to conventional vaccines. Tumor cells are obtained from another person with the same disease, perhaps cultured in the laboratory, and then weakened, such as by exposure to radiation. They are then given to the patient, and the patient's immune system reacts to them and produces antibodies that attack the patient's tumor cells. If a cancer vaccine is given when the tumor is small, it may eliminate the cancer.

Vaccines have been studied for use in treating many types of cancer, including melanoma, lymphomas, and cancers of the kidney, breast, ovary, prostate, colon, and rectum. Researchers are also investigating ways that cancer vaccines can be used in combination with other BRMs.

Side Effects

Like many medications, biological therapies can cause side effects, which vary widely from patient to patient and also depend on the particular type of treatment. Some common side effects are as follows:

- a rash or swelling at the site where the BRM is injected
- flu-like symptoms, including fever, chills, nausea, vomiting, loss of appetite, diarrhea, fatigue, bone pain, and muscle aches. These symptoms are often associated with interferons, interleukins, and cancer vaccines.
- bruising and bleeding easily
- fatigue and weakness
- lowered blood pressure
- swelling, particularly with interleukins
- allergic reactions, which can be serious, particularly with MOABs
- new antibody production, which can interfere with the targeting of the patient's cancer

The side effects can be severe, and hospitalization may be required for all or part of the treatment. However, the side effects are generally of limited duration and should subside after treatment ends. Because biological therapies are relatively new, long-term side effects are not well known.

Research

A great deal of research is underway to isolate specific cells of the immune system and their chemical products, and also to understand how immune system cells exchange messages. Researchers are learning how to manipulate cells and cellular products in the laboratory to target their activity and control their effects. Each component and step of the immune response is a potential target for development of a new therapy.

For information about recent research, contact the following:

National Institutes of Health
MEDLINEplus Web site
http://www.nlm.nih.gov/medlineplus/druginformation.html

For information about ongoing clinical trials involving biological therapies, contact the following:

National Cancer Institute's Cancer Information Service
http://www.cancer.gov/clinical trials

National Cancer Institute's CancerTrials
http://www.cancernet.nci.nih.gov/clinicaltrials

biopsy See LIVER BIOPSY.

bleeding See BLEEDING VARICES; COAGULOPATHY.

bleeding varices (bleeding blood vessels) A varix is a type of varicose vein that occurs within the body. Bleeding varices (plural of varix) are swollen, engorged blood vessels that rupture and bleed. They are usually found in the lower esophagus (the tube that runs from the mouth to the stomach) or the upper part of the stomach; called esophageal varices, they are the most likely to rupture and bleed. Bleeding from varices is one of the most common and serious complications of PORTAL HYPERTENSION. Portal hypertension is an increase in the pressure within the portal vein (the vein that carries blood from the digestive organs to the LIVER) due to blockage of blood flow throughout the liver from disease. This increased pressure in the portal vein causes the development of varices within the esophagus and stomach.

Patients with portal hypertension can also suffer from varices in the rectum. Although rectal varices are a significant source of lower digestive tract bleeding, the etiology and the pathology are still controversial, and adequate treatment protocol has yet to be established. When rectal varices bleed, they may often be mistaken for bleeding from hemorrhoids. But these are two very different conditions requiring different approaches, and it is important to differentiate between them.

CIRRHOSIS from hepatitis and excessive consumption of alcohol is the most common cause of bleeding varices. Patients with portal hypertension often have cirrhosis—advanced scarring of the liver, generally regarded as irreversible. As the liver tries to heal itself of injury caused by hepatitis or other liver disorders, scar tissue develops. The scar tissue impedes the flow of blood through the liver. Between 20 and 70 percent of people with cirrhosis develop varices. It is estimated that one in 10,000 people have bleeding varices. Bleeding of esophageal varices is estimated to occur about one-third of the time.

Symptoms and Diagnostic Path

A patient vomiting massive amounts of blood experiences a life-or-death emergency, and he or she should be hospitalized immediately. If bleeding from the varices is severe, a patient may go into shock from the loss of blood. A person in a state of shock is extremely pale, the breathing is rapid and shallow, the blood pressure is low, and the pulse is rapid and weak. Without immediate intervention, death may result.

The following are symptoms of variceal bleeding:

- nausea
- vomiting of bright red blood (hematemesis)
- black, tarry stools
- vomit that has a coffee ground appearance
- blood in the vomit
- decreased urine output
- ascites (abdominal swelling caused by fluid accumulation)
- encephalopathy (mental confusion caused by poor liver function)
- excessive thirst
- low blood pressure
- shock (in severe cases)

Bleeding varices are suspected if a patient has the above symptoms and cirrhosis or a history of excessive alcohol consumption. The diagnosis can be confirmed by X-ray studies, laboratory tests, and a specialized type of endoscopy called esophagogastroduodenoscopy (EGD). This is a simple procedure in which a thin, flexible tube called a fiberoptic endoscope is inserted into the patient's mouth to locate the sites of the bleeding in the esophagus, stomach, and upper duode-

num. The patient is given intravenous conscious sedation.

Treatment Options and Outlook

Acute bleeding must be stopped immediately, or the patient will die. An emergency endoscopy is performed to diagnose and treat the bleeding. Physicians can perform a schlerotherapy or rubber-band ligation. Schlerotherapy (also known as esophageal schlerotherapy) involves injecting clotting agents directly into the dilated blood vessels. In rubber-band ligation (also known as variceal ligation), the bleeding treatments varices are tied off (ligated) with miniature rubber bands to stop the bleeding. Both appear to be highly effective for bleeding esophageal varices.

Once acute bleeding is stopped, to decrease the incidence of re-bleeding, patients may be placed on beta-blockers such as propranolol (Inderal), which decrease portal blood flow and hence the risk of bleeding from varices. Other commonly used drugs include octreotide and vasopressin. Doctors often prescribe beta-blockers as a prophylactic (preventive) measure to keep the varices from bleeding in the first place. Endoscopic and drug therapies may sometimes be combined.

If endoscopic and pharmacologic therapies fail to work, balloon compression may be employed as an emergency measure. A tube is inserted into the esophagus and inflated with air to produce pressure against the bleeding veins. This helps to stop the bleeding.

If none of the above measures work, a shunt operation that joins the portal vein to systemic circulation may be considered, though its role has diminished since the advent of schlerotherapy. This procedure joins the portal vein to the inferior vena cava, the largest vein in the human body, which travels through the abdomen and returns to the heart. By allowing some portal blood to bypass the liver, it reduces pressure in the portal system. A major complication of this procedure is that it may worsen HEPATIC ENCEPHALOPATHY (mental confusion)—one of the symptoms of portal hypertension and variceal bleeding—by diverting a large portion of the blood away from the liver, which is then prevented from detoxifying the blood. A further danger is that it may also accelerate the progression of the patient's underlying liver disorder.

Distal splenorenal shunt (DSRS) is another type of surgical shunt. It attempts to reduce pressure in the varices and control bleeding by connecting the splenic vein, which carries blood away from the spleen, to the vein leading to the kidney. This allows the blood to continue flowing into the liver through the portal vein. The theory is that doing so will reduce the incidence of encephalopathy and the rate of progression of liver disease, as compared to PSS. However, some studies have cast doubt on this assumption. Moreover, despite a significant reduction in the incidence of re-bleeding, only nonalcoholic patients with cirrhosis gained any survival advantage.

Overall, these surgical shunts may control variceal bleeding, but they do not prolong survival. Additionally, doctors are reluctant to perform any operations that may in the future interfere with LIVER TRANSPLANTATION, should that ever become an option.

The transvenous intrahepatic portosystemic shunt (see TIPS) procedure is a less invasive, alternative procedure to redirect the blood flow. A stent—a hollow, tubular device—is placed in the middle of the liver to connect the portal veins with the hepatic veins that leave the liver and drain to the heart. This lowers the portal vein pressure and prevents bleeding. TIPS can be routinely created in most patients. As with other shunts, TIPS may also worsen hepatic encephalopathy. On the other hand, TIPS can be lifesaving and may be used as a bridge to transplantation in selected cases. It is important to identify potential candidates for transplantation early on. Patients with end-stage liver disease may ultimately have to be evaluated for liver transplantation.

The prognosis is related to the underlying liver disease; but regardless, once the varices rupture and bleed, the prognosis is very poor. Some 30 to 50 percent of patients will die within six weeks of their first episode of bleeding varices. Of the patients who survive, 47 to 84 percent will experience recurrent bleeding, and 70 percent will die during the first year or two.

Risk Factors and Preventive Measures

Various prophylactic measures, such as endoscopic treatments (sclerotherapy and variceal ligation), the use of pharmacological drugs (beta-blockers), and surgical shunts have been attempted to prevent the first episode of variceal hemorrhage and thereby increase the survival rate. The effectiveness of these preventive measures has not been substantiated by studies, however, and it is not yet clear whether they in fact confer survival benefit.

At present, the surest means to prevent the development of bleeding varices is to eliminate the risk factors, such as HEPATITIS B and C. Excessive alcohol consumption is another major cause of cirrhosis—and subsequently, bleeding varices—that can be eliminated.

Johnson, Paul A. "Bleeding varices." *Gale Encyclopedia of Medicine.* Farmington Hills, Mich.: Thomson Gale, 2001.

Kubetin, Sally Koch. "Acute bleeding varices (clinical capsules)." *Internal Medicine News,* 35, no. 9 (May 1, 2002): 27.

Shudo, R., Y. Yazaki, S. Sakurai, H. Uenishi, H. Yamada, and K. Sugawara. "Clinical study comparing bleeding and nonbleeding rectal varices." *Endoscopy* 34, no. 3 (March 2002): 189–194.

Budd-Chiari syndrome (BCS) Budd-Chiari syndrome is a rare disorder in which the circulation of blood in the LIVER becomes obstructed as a result of blood clotting in the hepatic veins, the major veins that flow out of the liver. Both small and large hepatic veins can be obstructed.

The liver, the largest organ in the body, carries out many vital functions in the body that are processed through blood flowing in and out of the liver. If the blood cannot circulate freely in the liver, serious problems can result. Other names for this condition are Chiari's syndrome and Rokitansky's disease.

As blood flow is obstructed in the veins due to blood clots, the blood pressure builds up in the veins. This in turn leads to the enlargement of the liver.

The most common cause of Budd-Chiari syndrome worldwide, and especially in Asia, is the formation of an abnormal web of membranes that obstructs blood flow in the veins that lead out of the liver. This is a relatively rare problem in the United States, however. The origin of these membranous webs is still a matter of controversy. Many investigators assumed that the condition is congenital, but some of the evidence seems to suggest otherwise.

In the United States, the most common cause is blood disorders such as sickle-cell disease and polycythemia rubra vera, a condition in which the number of red blood cells increases, making the blood too thick and more likely to clot. Cancers such as some forms of liver cancer can also increase the likelihood of blood clotting.

Other causes of BCS may include those below:

- inherited predisposition to clotting (thrombosis)
- inflammation of a vein (phlebitis) and other chronic inflammatory diseases
- certain chronic infections
- injury to the abdomen
- pregnancy
- high-dose estrogen use (oral contraceptives)
- tumors

Researchers have recognized for some time that underlying conditions contribute to the development of a blood clot (thrombosis) of the two major veins in the liver (hepatic vein and the hepatic portal vein). In the majority of cases, though, thrombosis of the hepatic vein was not associated with any recognized disorder, and it was considered to be idiopathic (of no known origin). But according to the *British Medical Journal* published in January 26, 1991, thanks to the improvements in laboratory technology, it has recently become clear that the majority of cases are associated with a disorder that results in an abnormal production of bone marrow cells (myeloproliferative disorders).

Symptoms and Diagnostic Path

Most patients seek out their physicians within three months of the onset of symptoms. They may have an acute or chronic disease.

The most common symptom is the accumulation of fluid in the abdomen (ASCITES). As blood flow is obstructed in the veins due to blood clots, the blood pressure builds up in the veins. This can cause fluid in the form of blood plasma to leak through the walls of the veins. Some 70 to 90 percent of patients have this symptom.

The high blood pressure in the veins can also lead to the enlargement of the liver (hepatomegaly). This may cause the area around the liver—the upper right-hand portion of the abdomen—to be tender or painful. Also, about half of the patients may have a spleen that has become abnormally enlarged (splenomegaly). Although some patients may be jaundiced (have a yellow tint to the skin and eyes), this is a rare symptom.

Blood tests may show some abnormality, but lab results and clinical manifestations are nonspecific, with no obvious pattern of abnormalities. A physical examination will often show an enlarged liver.

Often physicians first suspect that cirrhosis is the cause of the symptoms. In the case of Budd-Chiari syndrome, an analysis of the ascitic fluid (the accumulated fluid in the abdomen) may show a high protein concentration. A liver biopsy can reveal a characteristic appearance that is easily identifiable as Budd-Chiari syndrome. It can also determine the extent of fibrosis (scar tissue).

Other useful diagnostic tools are various imaging techniques that help form pictures of the veins in the liver. These are magnetic resonance imaging (MRI) scanning and computed tomography (CT) scanning. One useful imaging technique is ultrasonography (ultrasound scan) using the Doppler effect—a shift in the frequency of waves such as sound and light—to show visually the movement and flow of blood and its regulation. The ultrasound scan may show an abnormal pattern of the veins in the liver, as well as other abnormalities.

A definitive test to indicate whether a vein is clotted is a procedure called hepatic vein catheterization. A narrow tube called a catheter is inserted into the vein in the liver. Next a dye is injected through the tube. An X ray is then taken to determine whether there is clotting.

Treatment Options and Outlook

A sudden onset of clotting in the veins of the liver can generally be effectively dealt with by using anticlotting drugs such as urokinase. But they do not seem to work if the clots are already well established. In many cases, unfortunately, medical therapy alone is effective in the short-term only, and mainly to alleviate symptoms. If medication is the only support given, the mortality rate after two years is as high as 85 to 90 percent.

Most patients with BCS will likely require surgery to reroute blood flow around the clotted vein into a large vein called the vena cava. Other surgical techniques are also available, depending on the patient's condition. Surgery can make long-term survival possible if performed before permanent liver damage has set in.

If there is extensive scarring of the liver, or the liver functions continue to deteriorate, a LIVER TRANSPLANTATION may be necessary. However, certain conditions may preclude such an operation. After transplantation, the five-year survival rates, which are roughly 70 percent, are slightly lower than that of other liver disease.

Other surgical procedures have varying degrees of success. Perhaps the most promising therapy is transjugular intrahepatic portosystemic shunt (TIPS), which lowers the blood pressure within the veins draining into the liver by shunting blood away. This can lessen the fluid buildup in the abdomen and lower the risk of bleeding from the fragile veins. TIPS is not a major surgery. It is a minimally invasive procedure performed through a small nick in the skin.

Boughton, B. J. "Hepatic and portal vein thrombosis: Closely associated with chronic myeloproliferative disorders." *British Medical Journal* 302, no. 6770 (January 26, 1991): 192(2).

Mancuso, A., A. Watkinson, J. Tibballs, D. Patch, and A. K. Burroughs. "Budd-Chiari syndrome with portal, splenic, and superior mesenteric vein thrombosis treated with TIPS: Who dares wins." *Gut* 52, no. 3 (March 2003): 438(1).

C

cancer risk factors The exact causes of primary liver cancer—malignancies originating in the liver—are not fully understood, though there are probably multiple influences rather than one single cause.

Researchers have identified certain risk factors closely associated with the most common type of primary liver cancer, HEPATOCELLULAR CARCINOMA (HCC). Many of these risk factors can be reduced or eliminated through lifestyle changes. For instance, individuals can take precautions against becoming infected with viral hepatitis, avoid alcohol and tobacco, and lead a healthier life in general. People with hereditary liver disease or suffering from chronic HEPATITIS B or HEPATITIS C might consider regular screening tests for cancer. It is encouraging to know that in many ways, hepatocellular carcinoma is preventable.

Three risk factors in particular stand out. One is CIRRHOSIS, severe scarring of the liver, which can be linked to HCC in about 60 to 80 percent of cases. A patient with cirrhosis may be 40 times more likely than a person with a healthy liver to develop HCC.

The other two factors strongly associated with HCC are chronic hepatitis B and hepatitis C. In recent years, there has been an increase in the number of hepatitis C cases around the world, which will unfortunately lead to a predictable surge in liver cancer, even in the United States, where HCC is relatively rare.

Chronic hepatitis B and hepatitis C are the primary reasons that people living in developing countries have a far higher risk of acquiring cancer than do residents of industrialized countries. Although chronic hepatitis B is relatively rare in countries like the United States, it is quite widespread in some areas of Asia and Africa. An additional reason for the higher incidence of liver cancer in these parts of the world is exposure to a cancer-causing agent (carcinogen) called aflatoxin, a substance produced by a mold that grows on peanuts and other nuts, as well as grains, such as rice, stored under humid conditions.

Aflatoxin is frequently found in the soil in Africa, China, and Southeast Asia. In these regions, food is often contaminated by aflatoxin, and exposure to this substance is common. By contrast, exposure to aflatoxin is virtually unheard of in the United States, where the rate of liver cancer is quite low.

People who have the following characteristics have a heightened chance for developing primary liver cancer:

- cirrhosis: The risk for developing cancer exists regardless of what disease caused the cirrhosis. However, some diseases may present a higher risk of cancer, for example, if a person infected with chronic hepatitis B progresses to cirrhosis, there is a greater chance of cancer developing.

- chronic hepatitis B (HBV): Hepatitis is often found among intravenous (injection) drug users. Close to 25 percent of patients with primary liver cancer in the United States are infected with chronic hepatitis B; throughout the rest of the world, as many as 80 percent of patients may show signs of hepatitis B.

- chronic hepatitis C (HCV): In Japan and some Western countries, an exposure to hepatitis C is more closely associated with primary liver cancer than hepatitis B, which is relatively rare in developed countries.

- age: The incidence of liver cancer starts to increase around age 45, and those over age 60 are at much higher risk.

- male gender: Men are eight times more likely than women to get liver cancer.

- carcinogens: Aflatoxin. Studies have found that aflatoxin tends to produce genetic mutations in p53, a major gene that normally prevents the development of hepatocellular carcinomas or other cancers. About half the patients with hepatocellular carcinoma have been found to have a mutation in gene p53.

- thorotrast: Exposure to this contrast dye that was used for X-rays of the liver for a period after World War II has been associated with an increased risk of development of angiosarcoma. This is a tumor in the cells that line the blood vessels in the liver.

- vinyl chloride monomers: Exposure to this substance, which was used in manufacturing plastics, can also cause angiosarcoma. This is relatively rare, being limited to people who work in the plastic industry with vinyl chloride monomer.

- alcohol: Alcohol is probably not carcinogenic, but it is a well-established fact that excessive alcohol consumption can lead to liver damage and cause cirrhosis, which is the number-one risk factor for the development of primary liver cancer. Alcohol is especially deadly when combined with existing liver inflammation, such as chronic hepatitis B or chronic hepatitis C, and significantly increases the odds of developing cirrhosis.

- metabolic liver diseases: A number of inherited diseases that cause metabolic errors may lead to cirrhosis of the liver, which may then eventually be complicated by the development of hepatocellular carcinoma. These include ALPHA-1-ANTITRYPSIN DEFICIENCY, an inherited deficiency of an important protein synthesized in the liver. It can cause lung and LIVER DISEASE and liver inflammation leading to cirrhosis and the development of cancer.

Another example is hereditary HEMOCHROMATOSIS, an iron overload disorder that often develops into cirrhosis. It is the most common metabolic disorder among Caucasians of northern European extraction. As the result of a genetic mutation, the body inappropriately takes in excessive amounts of iron from the diet and stores it mainly in hepatocytes, major liver cells. Eventually, the excess iron damages the cell and its genetic material, and this can lead to the development of cirrhosis. About half the patients who have hemochromatosis and cirrhosis may end up dying from hepatocellular carcinoma.

A third related disorder is type 1 hereditary tyrosinemia, which can cause severe liver damage in infants and young children. Most of them will develop hepatocellular carcinoma by age three or four. LIVER TRANSPLANTATION is generally the best option for these patients.

Although some other metabolic diseases such as WILSON'S DISEASE (too much copper accumulating in the liver and other organs) and glycogen storage disorder (characterized by an abnormal accumulation of glycogen in tissues) can result in cirrhosis and hepatocellular carcinoma, such an occurrence is quite rare.

- oral estrogens for birth control: The long-term use of oral contraceptives containing the hormone estrogen is often associated with the development of adenomas, benign liver tumors. Sometimes a benign tumor can turn cancerous. However, analysis did not show that such a development increased mortality. Oral contraceptives therefore are regarded as a lesser factor in the development of hepatocellular carcinoma.

- smoking: Cigarette smoking may or may not be a causal factor for hepatocellular carcinoma. Some researchers believe that tobacco use can raise the risk level, but more studies are needed to clarify the connection.

- obesity: Although obesity is not an important predictor for patients who have hepatitis B, hepatitis C, and AUTOIMMUNE HEPATITIS, it has been linked to the growth of HCC in patients with cirrhosis caused by alcohol abuse, or whose cause is unknown (cryptogenic). Beyond that, obesity is an important factor in the development of non-alcoholic fatty liver disease (NAFLD), which has been implicated as a factor in the development of HCC.

Evans, Jeff. "Hepatocellular carcinoma risk." *Internal Medicine News* 36, no. 8 (April 15, 2003): 33(1).

Tai, D. I., C. H. Chen, T. T. Chang, et al. "Eight-year nationwide survival analysis in relatives of patients with hepatocellular carcinoma: Role of viral infection." *Journal of Gastroenterology and Hepatology Aims and Scopes* 17 (2002): 682–689.

Nair, S., A. Mason, and J. Eason, et al. "Is obesity an independent risk factor for hepatocellular carcinoma in cirrhosis?" *Hepatology* 36 (2002): 150–155.

cancer staging   "Staging" a cancer is a process that classifies it by severity to help establish an accurate prognosis and determine treatment options. The stage of a cancer is not the only determinant of treatment, but it is an important element.

Cancer begins when cells divide uncontrollably, eventually forming a visible mass, or tumor. Cells from that original mass can break off and travel to other parts of the body. The original mass is called the primary tumor. The process by which cells break off and travel elsewhere is called metastasis. After metastasis has occurred, the cancer is still referred to by the type of primary tumor, but qualified as metastatic. Breast cancer that has spread to the bones, for example, is not bone cancer; it is metastatic breast cancer.

The cancer grade is a characterization of how the cancer cells look under the microscope. Grades are generally numbered from one to four, with four indicating the most abnormal looking and aggressively behaving cells.

In general, staging systems classify the severity of cancers based on the size of the primary tumor and how far the cancer has spread. Where grade looks specifically at the behavior of the cancer cells, stage is more of an overall characterization based on clinical data. Not all cancers use the same classification system, and some cancers—most notably certain types of leukemia—do not use a formal classification system because they are simply not amenable to the staging process.

The determination of stage does not happen all at once. When cancer is first diagnosed, the stage assigned to it is presumed, based on initial tests. The type and extent of the cancer, and hence its actual stage, may not be precisely known until after the primary tumor has been surgically removed and samples of the tissue have been examined.

Patients wishing to research the stage of a diagnosed cancer must know the medical name of the cancer, the stage that has been initially assigned it, and the grade, if relevant. For some types of cancer, it may be necessary, or at least helpful, to be aware of other prognostic and diagnostic information as well. The physician will be able to explain the different stages of a particular cancer.

Staging Systems

Most cancers are staged using either the Roman numeral system, devised by the International Union Against Cancer (Union Internationale Contre le Cancer—UICC) or the T/N/M system.

The UICC system classifies cancer as Stage I, Stage II, Stage III, or Stage IV, depending on the extent of the cancer in the body. Each type of cancer has its own specific definition of what each stage involves, but in general the stages can be summarized as follows:

- Stage I is a "local" cancer that has been diagnosed early and has not spread.
- Stage II is a cancer that has spread to surrounding tissues but has not spread beyond the location of origin.
- Stage III is a "regional" cancer that has spread to the lymph nodes near the location of origin.
- Stage IV is a cancer that has metastasized (spread to other parts of the body).

For some cancers that require additional categories, the Roman numeral system may be extended to include substages, such as Stage II-B. In general, the higher the stage indication, the worse the prognosis. The prognosis, however, is influenced by a number of other factors as well. Two patients with Stage II cancers may or may not have similar prognoses, depending on factors such as medical histories.

The T/N/M system classifies a cancer according to three specific criteria, and assigns a number to each criterion to indicate a level of severity. A typical T/N/M classification, for example, looks like this: T1, N0, M0.

The T portion of the classification is the primary tumor indicator. It is usually numbered zero to four, with zero indicating a tumor that has not yet spread to the surrounding tissue and four indicating a large tumor that has probably invaded other organs.

The N portion classifies the involvement of the lymph nodes that drain the area surrounding the primary tumor. (It does not indicate the involvement of other lymph nodes for the simple reason that if distant nodes are involved, the cancer has metastasized.) Like the T portion, the N portion is usually numbered from zero through four, with zero indicating no lymph node involvement and four indicating extensive involvement.

The M portion indicates whether the cancer has metastasized. M0 indicates that it has not; M1, that it has.

As in the Roman numeral classification system, the specific meanings of the classifications differ with the type of cancer being described. For some cancers the numbering is extended to include indicators such as "X" or "is," to define additional categories.

For some types of cancer, both systems are used. For those cancers, the stages indicated by the Roman numerals are actually defined in terms of the T/N/M system. As an example, imagine an adrenocortical tumor (a tumor of the adrenal glands, located above the kidneys) that is greater than five centimeters but has not invaded surrounding tissue, has no lymph node involvement, and has not metastasized. The staging system for adrenocortical cancer defines that tumor as a T2, N0, M0 tumor, which is characterized as a Stage II cancer.

The T/N/M system is suitable only for cancers that form solid tumors. Cancers that do not form distinct tumors, such as leukemia, sometimes use the Roman numeral system but define the stages based on factors other than tumor characteristics, such as blood count, bone marrow involvement, or symptomatology.

Yet another staging system indicates severity by using the letters A through D, though it is otherwise similar to the Roman numeral system. Called the Duke system, it is often used to stage prostate and colon cancers.

Liver Cancer Staging

Liver cancer is staged using a combination of the UICC and T/N/M systems and currently defines the following six stages:

- Stage I (T1, N0, M0) denotes a single tumor with no invasion of the vascular (blood vessel) system, no involvement of regional lymph nodes, and no metastasis.

- Stage II (T2, N0, M0) denotes a single tumor with vascular invasion, or multiple tumors with none larger than five centimeters.

- Stage IIIA (T3, N0, M0) denotes multiple tumors larger than five centimeters, or a tumor involving a major branch of the portal or hepatic vein.

- Stage IIIB (T4, N0, M0) denotes one or more tumors with direct invasion of adjacent organs other than the gallbladder, or with perforation of the visceral peritoneum. (The peritoneum is a membrane that lines the wall of the abdominal cavity and encloses the soft organs, or viscera, in the cavity.)

- Stage IIIC (any T, N1, M0) denotes a cancer that has invaded the vascular system but has not metastasized.

- Stage IV (any T, any N, M1) denotes a cancer that has metastasized.

Liver cancer staging is unusual in that, in addition to staging information, the cancer is often categorized by whether it may be curable by surgery. There are four classifications to that end: localized resectable, localized unresectable, advanced, and recurrent.

In a localized resectable cancer, the cancer is localized to one area of the liver—a Stage I, II, or IIIA cancer—and the remaining portion of the organ is healthy. This category of liver cancer is operable by resecting (removing) the diseased portion.

A localized unresectable cancer is one in which the cancer is localized, but a resection is not possible. There are many reasons a resection might be impossible. If the unaffected portion of the liver is damaged, for example, as by CIRRHOSIS, a resection may not leave enough tissue for normal liver function. A tumor in close proximity to a junction between the liver and a major vein or artery, or between the liver and the bile duct system, may also be inoperable.

An advanced liver cancer is one that has spread throughout the liver or spread to other organs or to the lymph nodes. Liver cancers in this category are seldom resectable.

In a recurrent liver cancer, the cancer was treated, either through surgical removal or other means, but returned, either in the liver and/or in other organs.

Staging of Metastatic Tumors

There is no standardized system for classifying liver cancer that originated in other parts of the body. The prognosis and survival rates for these types of cancer are based on the staging of the primary tumor. Any tumor that has spread to the liver from elsewhere is usually classed as a Stage IV cancer, implying a well-advanced disease. Once a tumor has metastasized, it is unlikely that a resection will effect a cure: metastasis usually implies diffusion throughout the body, and therefore, the cancer is impossible to remove surgically.

In fact, that is not always the case. Some cancers that spread to the liver may lend themselves to resection. For those cancers, once the primary tumor has been removed and the liver is the sole focus of the remaining cancer, resection of the portion containing the metastatic deposits, called a metasectomy, may be able to effect a cure.

The best-studied cancer in that regard is colorectal carcinoma (a tumor involving both the colon and the rectum). In general, the survival rate for a colorectal tumor that has spread to the liver is less than two years. In patients who have only a single lesion in the liver, however, the three-year survival rate is 14 to 20 percent, while it is zero percent for patients with more extensive liver involvement. And for patients who are able to undergo a metasectomy, the five-year survival rate increases from zero percent to 25 to 30 percent.

A number of variables are involved in determining survivability and recurrence of disease in patients with colorectal cancer that has spread to the liver. It is affected by the stage of the primary

tumor when it was first discovered, by the amount of time elapsed between the discovery of the primary tumor and the discovery of the metastasis (more than one year is better), and by the number of liver nodules (fewer than four usually implies a better prognosis). A single liver lesion discovered at the same time as the colorectal tumor may actually have a worse prognosis than two or three larger lesions discovered three to five years later. There is no reliable way to stage a tumor in that situation.

For other types of cancer that have spread to the liver, data are likewise insufficient to stage the liver involvement. The general guideline for those cases, however, is that if the liver involvement is resectable, then resection is the treatment of choice because it impacts the natural history of the disease.

Greene, Frederick L., et al. "Liver (including intrahepatic bile ducts)." In *American Joint Committee on Cancer (AJCC) Cancer Staging Manual, 131–138*. 6th ed. New York: Springer, 2002.

cardiac cirrhosis   Liver dysfunction can occur as a complication of acute or chronic congestive heart failure in which the heart is unable to maintain an adequate circulation of blood, or to pump out the blood that is returned to it through the veins. Like other organs, the LIVER is dependent on the heart for its supply of blood. When circulation becomes impaired, the blood can back up in the liver. With the passage of time, this causes an increase in fibrous tissue (tissue that resembles fibers) within the liver, and sometimes permanent scarring. This condition is called cardiac cirrhosis. Cardiac cirrhosis can also result from cardiac fibrosis (an increase in fibrous tissue within the heart) and chronic myocarditis, an inflammation of the middle muscular layer of the heart wall called the myocardium.

Other names for the disease are congestive hepatopathy (an abnormal or diseased state of the liver) and chronic passive liver congestion. They are probably more accurate than the term *cardiac cirrhosis*; the condition does not always fill all the strict clinical criteria for cirrhosis, but it is the one that is conventionally used.

Symptoms and Diagnostic Path

Signs and symptoms are mainly those related to congestive heart failure, such as edema (fluid retention) of the lower extremities and weight gain, pigmentation of the lower extremities, and excessive urination at night (nocturia). Other symptoms are suggestive also of liver dysfunction, such as abdominal distention, abdominal pain in the upper-right quadrant, weight loss (anorexia), nausea, and vomiting.

Complications of chronic cholestasis (obstruction or failure of bile flow) are fatigue, generalized itching of the body (pruritus), fat in the stools (steatorrhea), fat-soluble vitamin deficiency (vitamins A, D, E, and K), and thinning of bones (osteoporosis).

Cardiac cirrhosis is not easy to diagnose. First, the condition needs to be distinguished from ischemic hepatitis, or SHOCK LIVER. Ischemic hepatitis is caused by lack of oxygen delivery to liver cells due to obstruction of the inflow of arterial blood. Massive liver cell death may result. Cardiac cirrhosis usually arises from right-sided heart failure, and ischemic hepatitis from left-sided failure.

Liver-function tests typically show elevated serum transaminases and serum bilirubin.

Cardiac cirrhosis rarely occurs today. Exact numbers are hard to obtain because the disease is usually subclinical (not detectable by the usual clinical tests) and often undiagnosed. Even when autopsies are performed, it is rare to find true cases of cardiac cirrhosis.

No data are available in regard to the gender or age of sufferers. Since more men suffer from congestive heart failure than women, however, the same is likely true for cardiac cirrhosis. It is also assumed that, just as congestive heart failure increases with age, the prevalence of cardiac cirrhosis rises with age.

Treatment Options and Outlook

Treatment is directed towards the heart disease; once the underlying heart problem is controlled, the liver function should also normalize, and cirrhosis can be prevented from further developing.

The overall prognosis for cardiac cirrhosis is unknown. Mostly, the outcome depends on the patient's underlying cardiac disease. Cases associated with cardiac cirrhosis tend to be advanced and chronic.

Naschita, Jonathan E., et al. "Heart diseases affecting the liver and liver diseases affecting the heart." *American Heart Journal* 140, no. 1 (July 2000): 111–120.

chemoembolization Chemoembolization is a minimally invasive procedure during which chemotherapy drugs are placed in an artery adjacent to the tumor, then a material is placed in the artery to block blood flow into the tumor. The word *chemoembolization* is taken from "chemo" in *chemotherapy*, and *embolization*, a procedure in which an artery is deliberately blocked to prevent blood flow to tissue supplied by the artery. Chemoembolization is sometimes called TACE, for transarterial chemoembolization.

Chemoembolization provides an additional approach to treating liver tumors that do not respond to traditional chemotherapy (the use of drugs to treat tumors), and also are not treatable with surgery or a liver transplant. Tumors cannot be surgically removed if they are widespread or diffuse, or in multiple locations. It has been reported that only 10 to 15 percent of patients with diffuse tumors are eligible for surgical removal or liver transplant, and that chemotherapy is generally not effective for treatment of these tumors. According to Dr. Jeff Geschwind, M.D., of the Johns Hopkins Hospital in Baltimore, Maryland, "Chemoembolization is the treatment of choice for widespread or diffuse tumors, as well as for tumors in multiple locations that cannot be surgically removed."

Chemoembolization allows much larger doses (20–200 times) of chemotherapy drugs to be delivered to the tumor than can be delivered with traditional systemic administration of the drugs. By preventing or inhibiting the blood supply to the tumor, the embolization accomplishes two purposes. First, it enables the drugs to remain localized where they are needed, and second, it starves the tumor of nutrients necessary for its growth. Although most of the drug delivered to the liver stays there, some systemic effects are often observed when the drug reaches to other parts of the body.

In general, primary liver cancers get their blood exclusively from the hepatic artery, and so this artery is blocked in chemoembolization. The rest of the liver can function with the blood it receives from the portal vein after the chemoembolization. The hepatic artery is almost always accessible percutaneously (through the skin) via catheterization, or insertion of a hollow tube through the aorta and into the hepatic artery.

Procedure

Before receiving a chemoembolization treatment, the patient usually has a number of tests to aid the doctors and staff in planning and administering the treatment. Preliminary tests may include liver-function blood tests and imaging of the tumor and surrounding tissue. The imaging may be with a CAT (computerized axial tomography or computed tomography) scan that provides X-ray images of the liver and surrounding tissues, or with an MRI (magnetic resonance imaging) scan that creates images based on the magnetic properties of the tissue, emphasizing soft tissues and the presence of blood vessels. The images will help ensure that the portal vein in the liver is not blocked, that there is no CIRRHOSIS (scarring) of liver, and that the bile ducts are not blocked. Any of these conditions may indicate that the procedure should not be performed.

Although chemoembolization is a minimally invasive procedure, preparation is similar to that for other surgical procedures. The patient must not consume any food or drink after dinner the night before. Typically, the patient checks into the hospital early in the morning. An intravenous (IV) line is placed into the patient's arm, and the patient is given antibiotics and other medications, along with large amounts of liquid, through the IV line. The patient is then taken to the room where the procedure will be performed.

The chemoembolization treatment takes two to three hours and is usually performed by a radiologist in a special treatment room, depending on the particular type of embolic agent and chemotherapy drug(s) used. A hollow needle is used to insert a small diameter tube, called a catheter, into the patient's femoral artery, located in the groin. The radiologist then guides the catheter up through the aorta and into the hepatic artery, which supplies blood to the tumor. After the catheter is positioned, a contrast material is injected, and X-rays are taken of the tiny blood vessels. The X-rays may be administered in realtime, with fluoroscopy. The radiologist then injects a high dose of chemotherapy agents mixed with an oil-like medium. The oil droplets transport chemotherapy drugs to the tumor.

The radiologist may inject additional contrast material to visualize the blood vessels leading into the tumor, then inject an embolizing material until blood flow stops through the vessels leading to the tumor. Examples of embolizing materials include gel foam, collagen, and small metal coils.

With the blood supply blocked, the chemotherapy drugs are trapped within the tumor, and tumor cells are prevented from rejecting the chemotherapy. As the drugs take effect, tumor tissue breaks down, and, one hopes, the tumor cells die.

After the procedure, the patient is returned to a hospital room, where he or she must lie flat in bed for at least six hours. The patient receives more IV fluids. A sandbag may be placed over the groin to compress the area where the catheter was inserted into the femoral artery. Nurses check for signs of bleeding from the puncture site and also check the pulse in the foot to make sure the femoral artery is not blocked.

Most patients are discharged the next day, although longer hospitalization may be necessary in some cases. Patients should expect to spend one or two additional days in bed to improve blood flow to the liver.

The doctor will request periodic follow-up CT or MRI imaging studies at intervals of perhaps six to 12 weeks to monitor any tumor shrinkage or growth, as well as to look for new tumors.

Chemoembolization treatments may be repeated many times over a period of months to years, depending on the patient's status.

Risks and Complications

Immediately after the chemembolization treatment, it is normal for patients to experience pain, fever, poor appetite, and nausea for several hours to several days. During the first few days, the tumor breaks down, and this can sometimes cause pain or a high fever. Usually, the fever and discomfort decrease within the first week after treatment. However, temperatures up to 101°F may last for one to two weeks after treatment. The poor appetite may result in weight loss. Laxatives can help eliminate waste products normally handled by the liver, but loose stools may result. Many patients experience extreme fatigue for up to three to four weeks while the liver recovers.

If the patient notices any sudden changes in the degree of pain or fever, or if it persists beyond the first week after treatment, or if there are any unusual changes, the physician should be consulted immediately.

The chemotherapeutic agents administered to the tumor in the liver do get distributed throughout the body, causing the usual effects from systemic chemotherapy administration. Regional side effects, such as gallbladder inflammation (cholecystitis), intestinal and stomach ulcers, and inflammation of the pancreas (pancreatitis) may result. LIVER FAILURE may occur in patients with advanced cirrhosis.

Longer term, liver function should improve after the procedure, and with it, the patient's quality of life.

The risks from chemoembolization are much lower than those of surgery and liver transplants. The most common complications are infection and abscess of the tumor, which occurs in fewer than 3 percent of cases, and liver failure resulting in death, which takes place in fewer than 1 percent of cases. Another risk is that the embolus, or arterial block, may lodge in the wrong place, depriving healthy tissue of blood.

Outlook and Lifestyle Modification

Chemembolization appears to shrink tumors, but it does not cure cancer of the liver cells—HEPATOCELLULAR CARCINOMA (HCC). Liver function should improve after the procedure, and with it the patient's quality of life. Long-term survival may be improved only slightly, but in some patients it may lower the stage of the cancer enough to create the option of surgery.

Early studies of the effectiveness of chemoembolization were conducted with critically ill patients. One study reported that about 30 percent of primary hepatocellular carcinoma patients responded to systemic chemotherapy, while 50 to 75 percent of patients responded to chemoemblization. Some of the chemoembolization patients had previously failed to respond to systemic chemotherapy. Another study described in *Cancer Weekly*, March 8, 1993, looked at critically ill patients with primary or metastatic liver cancers and a life expectancy of two to three months. The average survival with treatment was eight months, and some patients survived for 29 months. In addition, four children were treated. Each of the four had a tumor size decrease of at least 50 percent and three survived for at least six to 18 months. The fourth child died from metastatic lung cancer.

Later research studied the effects of treatments on patients who were less critically ill. For example, the May 22, 1995, issue of *Cancer Biotechnology Weekly*, reported a study in which patients with inoperable liver cancer but not severe liver disease were treated with cisplatin and lipiodol. In this study, the chemoembolilzation attempted to decrease arterial flow without causing total obstruction of the hepatic artery. Chemoembolization decreased the tumor size in more than half the patients, but this benefit was offset by decreased liver function, particularly in patients with cirrhosis. Japanese studies showed that although chemoembolization does not cure hepatocellular carcinoma, the procedure can shrink tumors enough to lower the stage of the cancer and may create the option of surgery for some patients. These studies reported that chemoembolization works best in patients with relatively good liver function.

Another study that appeared in the May 18, 2002, issue of *The Lancet* studied less critically ill patients in three treatment groups: conservative treatment, gelfoam embolization, and chemotherapy with the drugs doxorubicin and lipiodol plus gelfoam embolization. Arterial embolization was performed in the embolization and chemoembolization groups at zero, two, and six months, and then every six months for as long as the patients met the criteria for inclusion in the study and agreed to continue to participate. The chemotherapy was administered prior to embolization. The accompanying table summarizes the survival results.

Group	Conservative treatment	Embolization	Chemotherapy plus embolization
survival after 1 year	63%	75%	82%
survival after 2 years	27%	50%	63%
survival after 3 years	17%	29%	29%
mean time until death	14.5 months	21.7 months	21.2 months

The researchers concluded that chemoembolization significantly improved the likelihood of longer survival for carefully selected patients when compared to the control group. It also significantly lowered the probability of portal vein invasion by the tumors, and fewer deaths were attributed to tumor progression in the group receiving chemoembolization treatments than in the control group.

In June 2003, researchers Guo et al. reported that for primary liver cancer (a tumor that started in the liver) that cannot be operated on, chemoembolization is the most effective way of reducing the size of the tumor. In Asia, it has become the most popular treatment, but it cannot cure the disease, and additional therapy is needed to kill any remaining tumor cells. For example, in one case, a patient was successfully treated with chemoembolization followed by radiation treatment. The purpose of the radiation treatment was to kill any cancer remaining after the chemoembolization.

Another recent study described in *Cancer Weekly*, July 15, 2003, reported that the benefits of chemembolization treatments last an average of 10 to 14 months. Although expected survival averages about six months, with other treatments chemoembolization can allow patients to live up to three years longer with a sustained quality of life.

Bennington, Linda, K. "Chemoembolization." *Gale Encyclopedia of Cancer.* Farmington Hills, Mich.: Thomson Gale, 2001.

"Chemoembolization helps patients live longer." *Cancer Weekly,* July 15, 2003, p. 88.

Llovet, Josep M., et al. "Arterial embolisation or chemoembolisation versus symptomatic treatment in patients with unresectable hepatocellular carcinoma: a randomised controlled trial." *Lancet* 359, no. 9319 (May 18, 2002): 1,734.

Pentecost, Michael J., and George P. Teitelbaum. "Chemoembolization in the treatment of hepatic malignancy." *Western Journal of Medicine* 156, no. 3 (March 1992): 301(1).

"Primary liver cancer treated successfully by chemoembolization and radiotherapy." *Gastroenterology Week,* June 2, 2003, p. 21 (cites Guo et al., *Hepatogastroenterol* [2003]: 50(50); 519–522).

Trinchet, Jean-Claude, et al. "Lipiodol chemoembolization and conservative treatment for unresealable hepatocellular carcinoma." *New England Journal of Medicine* 332, no. 19 (May 11, 1995): 1,256–1,261.

Vogelzang, Robert, M.D., et al. "Treatment injects cancer-fighting drugs directly into tumor (chemoembolization)." *Cancer Weekly* (March 8, 1993): 3(2).

chemotherapy Chemotherapy is treatment with anticancer (cytotoxic) drugs that attempts to kill cancer cells while minimizing damage to normal tissue. Usually the drugs are injected into a vein (intravenously) or into a muscle (intramuscular injection), or just under the skin (subcutaneous injection); but sometimes they are given by mouth, as tablets or capsules. Also, the drugs are sometimes injected through a catheter (a thin, flexible tube used for medical purposes) into a large blood vessel, such as a large vein in the chest.

Chemotherapy aims to accomplish three different goals:

- to destroy all the cancer cells so that the patient is free of cancer.
- to keep the cancer from coming back after a patient has received surgery or radiation therapy. Chemotherapy can kill microscopic cancer cells in the body that are too small to see and that the surgeon might have missed.

- to shrink a cancer and to keep it from growing. Sometimes a cure may not be possible. In such a case, the chemotherapy is designed to reduce the number of cancer cells, thereby diminishing any symptoms from the cancer and prolonging life while at the same time improving quality of life.

Systemic and Regional Chemotherapy

Broadly, there are two ways to administer chemotherapy, systemically or regionally. In systemic treatment, the drugs are injected into the body and carried through the bloodstream to most of the patient's body. Regional chemotherapy involves the implantation of a pump containing chemotherapy drugs under the skin. Through the mechanism of the pump, the drugs are delivered directly to the site of the tumor.

Systemic chemotherapy is usually administered to patients in cycles, with a treatment period followed by a recovery period. Although a short hospital stay may be required, chemotherapy treatments are often done on an outpatient basis. The advantage of systemic chemotherapy is that it exposes tumors anywhere in the body to anticancer drugs. Thus, it can be used in cases where the cancer has metastasized—spread from the original site of tumor growth—to different parts of the body. The drawback is that the drugs also affect healthy cells, and side effects can be quite severe.

Regional chemotherapy generally requires a patient to go back to the hospital about once a month on a schedule set by the doctor to have the pump refilled with drugs. The advantage of this method is that it targets the tumor directly, and minimizes the exposure of healthy cells to the drugs. Regional chemotherapy is often used when the tumor is found in only one location.

LIVER CANCER may be treated with either systemic or regional chemotherapy. Both types may also be combined for a more potent treatment.

When Chemotherapy Is Given

Chemotherapy can be combined with surgical treatment called LIVER RESECTION. In a procedure called neoadjuvant therapy, doctors may use chemotherapy first to shrink a tumor if it is too large or in a location that is difficult to reach.

Chemotherapy can also be given after an operation to destroy any microscopic cancer cells that may have been left behind and reduce the risk of the cancer growing back. This treatment is known as adjuvant therapy.

In some cases, chemotherapy is administered at the same time as radiotherapy. This is called chemoradiotherapy. Chemotherapy may also be combined with other types of therapies, such as biological therapies, hormone therapy, and cryoablation, to name just a few.

Chemotherapy Drugs

There are more than 50 different kinds of chemotherapy drugs that work to keep cancer cells from reproducing. The drugs may be given alone, or several drugs may be combined, selected for their different effects.

The drugs have a greater impact on cells that divide quickly, such as cancer cells, and treatments are based on this selectivity. However, other types of healthy cells also divide quickly, particularly blood cells and the cells that line the digestive tract. Therefore, chemotherapy drugs can and often do affect other parts of the body.

Because their blood cells are affected, chemotherapy patients may have difficulty combating infections, bruise easily, and have less energy than normal. Fatigue and nausea are among the most common side effects. Patients are often advised to take precautions to avoid infections and cuts, and also to avoid medications, such as aspirin and ibuprofen, that can cause bleeding. Frequent hand washing and staying away from crowds is recommended when treatment is in progress.

The doctor should be notified immediately if any signs of bleeding develop. These may include the following:

- bleeding gums
- blood in the stools
- bruising easily
- coughing up blood
- vaginal spotting

If the chemotherapy drugs affect the cells that line the digestive tract, the symptoms include loss of appetite, nausea, vomiting, and mouth sores. It may be helpful to eat small but balanced meals at frequent intervals. Medications are also available for treating these problems.

Additional side effects are common from chemotherapy. There may be hair loss, with hair either thinning or falling out entirely. Fertility may decrease, either temporarily or permanently. The drugs may also be toxic to the liver and damage small hepatic veins that exit the liver.

cholangiocarcinoma (CCC) Cholangiocarcinoma is cancer of the BILE DUCTS. This relatively rare type of cancer begins in the cells lining the bile ducts within the LIVER. The bile ducts drain BILE, a greenish yellow fluid, to the upper part of the small intestine (duodenum). Many waste products, such as cholesterol and BILIRUBIN—the by-product of the breakdown of red blood cells— are excreted into the bile. Eventually, the bile is eliminated from the body via the stool. If these tumors develop at the point where the left and right hepatic (liver) ducts meet, they are known as Klatskin tumors.

Other names for CCC include intrahepatic cholangiocarcinoma, peripheral cholangiocarcinoma, cholangiocellular carcinoma, and cholangiolar carcinoma.

Cholangiocarcinoma is classified as a primary liver cancer. It is the second-most common type of primary liver cancer, after hepatocellular carcinoma (HCC). Every year, 3,000 to 5,000 people in the United States develop CCC, accounting for about 10 to 20 percent of all cases of primary LIVER CANCER. Unlike HCC, which predominates in developing countries, CCC is more evenly distributed throughout the world.

Twice as many men as women get cholangiocarcinoma, but when women develop primary cancer, a higher percentage of them develop HCC than do men: 29 percent of women, compared with 19 percent of men. Thus, a woman who develops primary cancer is more likely to have CCC than HCC. For both sexes, the risk of getting cholangiocarcinoma increases with age.

Symptoms and Diagnostic Path

About 80 percent of patients feel pain in the right upper abdomen. Palpation of the area may reveal an enlarged liver or a liver mass if the tumors are large. Other symptoms include loss of appetite and weight loss. If cancer has spread to other areas of the abdominal cavity, fluid may accumulate in the abdomen (ascites).

The tumors tend to be in the small bile ducts within the liver, and do not obstruct the larger ducts, so the flow of bile is normal unless the tumors are quite large. The level of bilirubin— bile pigmentation—is normal. But if the tumors develop and grow in the bile ducts outside of the liver, they can obstruct the bile flow, causing a buildup of bilirubin within the body. This can lead to jaundice, a yellowing of the skin and eyes.

Diagnosis cannot of course be made on the basis of symptoms alone. A complete diagnostic work-up is necessary. When the cancer is identified, the doctor will also attempt to determine whether surgical removal of the tumors is possible.

Treatment Options and Outlook

The only treatment that can cure cholangiocarcinoma is complete surgical removal of the tumors. Unfortunately, CCC is aggressive and quite often spreads elsewhere in the liver, as well as beyond the liver, which means that most patients will not be candidates for surgery. Common sites for the cancer to spread are the lymph nodes around the liver, the abdominal cavity, and the lungs. If the cancer has already spread to the lymph nodes or other organs, then surgery cannot help the patient live longer. Only if the cancer is limited to a part of the liver that can be safely removed can surgery have a chance of succeeding.

Patients whose tumors are large and who are experiencing debilitating symptoms may receive surgery to remove some of the tumors. This procedure is called debulking; it is meant only to alleviate symptoms in cases where complete surgical removal of tumors is not possible.

Chemotherapy and radiation therapy, or a combination of them, may also be attempted if surgery is not an option. But their success rates are not very high. About 10 to 20 percent of patients may experience a decrease in the size of the tumors, or the tumors may at least stabilize. But no studies prove that these therapies can extend the patient's life.

The five-year survival rate for patients who undergo successful surgery of their cancer is between 20 to 40 percent. Patients can expect to be free of tumors. Many of the patients who die do so because of a recurrence of CCC. For patients who are inoperable because the cancer cells have spread, the life expectancy is roughly six months.

Cholangiocarcinoma and Liver Transplantation

If patients have tumors confined to the liver but the tumors cannot be safely removed with surgery because not enough liver tissue will remain for the liver to function, they may be considered for liver transplantation. However, most patients with CCC are not good candidates for LIVER TRANSPLANTATION.

Some transplant centers have begun experimental programs with carefully selected patients. These patients are first given a combination of radiation and chemotherapy before receiving a liver graft. Early results seem encouraging, but more studies will have to be done before any conclusions can be drawn.

Risk Factors and Preventive Measures

Unlike HEPATOCELLULAR CARCINOMA, which is mostly associated with CIRRHOSIS and viral hepatitis, the vast majority of people who develop cholangiocarcinoma have no known risk factors. Risk factors, when they are present, are different than for HCC. They are mostly related to diseases of the bile duct. These include the following:

- PRIMARY SCLEROSING CHOLANGITIS: progressive scarring and obstruction of the bile ducts

- choledochal cysts: a rare congenital disorder in which there are cysts in the bile ducts

- bile duct stones: a rare condition in the United States

People with inflammatory disease of the bowel, such as ulcerative colitis, also tend to be more likely to develop cholangiocarcinomas. In addition, exposure to certain toxins, also extremely rare, increases the likelihood of developing cholangiocarcinoma. These are Thorotrast, a contrast dye used in the 1930s and 1940s to image the liver, and dioxin (Agent Orange). LIVER FLUKE, a parasite, is also believed to cause many cases of cholangiocarcinoma in Asia and Africa.

Cameron, J. L., H. A. Pitt, M. J. Zinner, S. L. Kaufman, and J. Coleman. "Management of proximal cholangiocarcinomas by surgical resection and radiotherapy." *American Journal of Surgery* 159, no. 1 (January 1990): 91–97.

cholestasis   When there is impairment of the flow of BILE, secreted by the LIVER into the intestine, the result is a relatively rare disorder called cholestasis. The liver continuously produces bile, which is essential in breaking down fats. Bile is composed of acids, salts, fats (lipids), and BILIRUBIN, which gives bile its greenish yellow color. If there is a blockage in the liver or in the BILE DUCTS, the bile flow becomes stagnant, with the result that bile salts, bilirubin, and lipids accumulate in the bloodstream instead of being eliminated completely. The cause of the obstruction may originate within the liver (intrahepatic) or outside it (extrahepatic).

Intrahepatic cholestasis is most frequently a result of viral hepatitis, which can impair the body's ability to eliminate bile. Other LIVER DISEASE that produce inflammation of the bile ducts, such as primary biliary CIRRHOSIS and PRIMARY SCLEROSING CHOLANGITIS, can also induce cholestasis.

Other causes include bacterial abscess, generalized infection (sepsis), malignant tumor of the lymphoid tissue (lymphoma), intravenous feeding (total parenteral nutrition), tuberculosis, alcohol-induced liver disease, cancer that has spread from other parts of the body, and the effects of hormonal changes during pregnancy.

In rare cases, chronic cholestasis is attributable to a congenital (existing at birth) disorder of the bile ducts within the liver, called Caroli's syndrome.

Medications may induce cholestasis as a direct result of their toxic effect on the liver, or due to what doctors call idiosyncratic reactions—the unique and unpredictable manner in which an individual reacts to a certain medication. Cholestasis can also be the result of a complication of chemotherapy.

Generally speaking, the greater the amount of medication taken, the more severe the symptoms are. (Allergic reactions are not related to the drug dosage.) When drugs are the cause of cholestasis, symptoms usually develop shortly after treatment begins, follow a predictable pattern, and often cause liver damage. In idiosyncratic reactions, the course of the illness is often unpredictable.

Phenothiazine-derivative drugs, often used in the treatment of schizophrenia, have been implicated in the development of cholestasis. These drugs may cause sudden fever and inflammation, but symptoms generally disappear as soon as the drugs are discontinued. Antidepressants are also known to induce cholestasis in some patients. These include selective serotonin reuptake inhibitor (SSRI) antidepressants such as citalopram (Cipramil), as well as tricyclic (TCA) antidepressants like amitriptyline (Elavil) and imipramine (Tofranil).

Other medications that have been associated with cholestasis include those below:

anticonvulsant and analgesic	carbamazepine (Tegretol)
antihypertensives	captopril (Capoten) ranitidine (Zantac)
immunosuppressant	azathioprine (Imuran)
cardiac rhythm and irregularities	quinidine sulfate (Quinidex)
gout	allopurinol (Zyloprim)
rheumatoid arthritis	sulindac (Clinoril, Saldac)

Cholestasis is the second most common cause of JAUNDICE during pregnancy. The main symptom, however—and sometimes the only symptom—is itching all over the body (pruritus), which can sometimes be quite severe.

Cholestasis occurs as the bile ducts become more sensitive to estrogen because of hormonal changes associated with pregnancy. (Sometimes taking oral contraceptives has a similar effect.) It often develops during the second and third trimester of pregnancy. The incidence is between 10 to 100 cases per 10,000 pregnancies. Genetic factors seem to predispose women to cholestasis of pregnancy. Women who have a history of developing cholestasis during pregnancy are also prone to this condition when taking oral contraceptives, and vice versa.

According to a study published in the May 2003 issue of the journal *Gut,* the Chilean population appears to experience an exceptionally high incidence (16 percent) of cholestasis of pregnancy, as do the Araucanian Indians of Chile (28 percent).

Studies suggest that the condition may lead to increased incidence of fetal distress and premature birth. In most cases cholestasis resolves soon after delivery; in rare cases it leads to cirrhosis and death.

Extrahepatic cholestasis is most often the result of a stone in the common bile duct through which bile travels from the GALLBLADDER to the small intestine. Less frequent causes are a narrowing (stricture) of the common duct, cancer of a bile duct, cysts, cancer of the pancreas, inflammation of the pancreas (pancreatitis), and tumor on a nearby organ.

Symptoms and Diagnostic Path

Pruritus is a prominent feature of cholestasis. The cause for this itching, which can range from mild to severe, is not entirely understood yet. Other characteristic symptoms of cholestasis include these:

- jaundice (excess bilirubin deposit in the skin leading to a yellow discoloration)
- dark urine (excess bilirubin excreted by the kidney)
- pale, clay-colored stools (lack of bilirubin in the intestine)
- too much fat in the stools (inability to digest fats)
- tendency to bleed easily (poor absorption of vitamin K, needed for blood clotting)

Other symptoms, such as abdominal pain or vomiting, depend on the underlying cause of cholestasis. Some drug-induced cholestasis may cause rashes or fever.

Diagnosis depends on physical examination, laboratory analysis, and a detailed medical history.

It is essential to determine whether the cause is within or outside the liver. A history of drug or alcohol use, an enlarged spleen (splenomegaly), and abdominal swelling (ascites) suggest that the obstruction exists inside the liver. Symptoms that suggest a cause outside the liver include intermittent pain in the upper right side of the abdomen, sometimes also pain in the right shoulder, and pain or rigidity in the gallbladder or pancreas.

In patients with cholestasis, the blood levels of an enzyme called alkaline phosphatase (ALP) are typically more than three times greater than normal. If test results are abnormal, ultrasound may be performed to determine obstruction. Computed tomography scans (CT) and magnetic resonance imaging (MRI) will provide more detailed information.

If none of these procedures is sufficient to make a diagnosis, the physician may do one of the following procedures:

- endoscopic retrograde cholangiopancreatography (ERCP): a flexible viewing tube highlights the position of any obstruction using a dye and X-ray
- direct cholangiography: taking an X-ray map of the bile ducts
- percutaneous transhepatic cholangiography: identifying obstructions through contrast dye and X-ray images

Treatment Options and Outlook

There are various ways of treating the blockage depending on the underlying cause. Sometimes surgery may be needed to remove the obstructions or widen the affected ducts. If a particular drug is the suspected cause of the condition, discontinuing its use usually restores normal liver function. In the case of acute hepatitis, cholestasis usually disappears once the hepatitis has run its course.

Various medications are available to relieve the itching associated with cholestasis.

Antibacterial drugs and other medications may be prescribed to cleanse the system of toxic compounds. The patient may have to restrict the amount of fat in the diet if fat digestion is a problem. In all cases alcohol must be avoided.

Prognosis depends on the underlying condition. In most cases, once the cause of cholestasis is controlled, symptoms disappear. Drug-induced cholestasis usually resolves itself after medication is discontinued but, in some instances, may lead to liver failure. If the bile-duct obstruction is chronic, it may lead to cirrhosis.

Elferink, R. Oude. "Genetic aspects of bile secretion disorders." *Gut* 52, no. 5 (May 2003): 42(7).
Savander, M., et al. "Genetic evidence of heterogeneity in intrahepatic cholestasis of pregnancy." *Journal of Medical Genetics* 40, no. 8 (August 2003): 640(1).

chronic liver disorders See ACUTE VS. CHRONIC LIVER DISORDERS.

cirrhosis Cirrhosis of the LIVER is a long-term disease that represents the end stage of a chronic liver injury. In cirrhosis, healthy liver cells are permanently destroyed and are replaced by fibrous scar tissues that block the flow of blood through the organ and disrupt the liver's many important functions. The extensive scarring causes the liver to shrink and atrophy or to become enlarged. Although a healthy liver is smooth, a cirrhotic liver becomes rock hard and nodular, or lumpy. The nodules form when scar tissue encapsulates islands of liver tissue. In addition to changing the structure of the liver and the blood vessels that nourish it, the disease also causes liver cell death until, eventually, there are not enough cells left for the liver to function.

Although cirrhosis is not always fatal, it is estimated to kill about 26,000 people each year. In the United States, it is the seventh most common cause of death; in adults between the ages of 45 to 65, cirrhosis is the third most common cause of death. Cirrhosis is twice as common in men as in women. More than half of all malnourished chronic alcoholics have cirrhosis.

The disease has many causes. It may progress slowly, so it may be many years before the patient is aware that he or she has developed any scarring of the liver. At the present time, the liver damage and scarring are irreversible and cannot be healed.

It is hoped that the extensive research being done may lead to a treatment that can reverse the scarring. Although no treatments are available to cure cirrhosis, symptoms can be lessened and controlled, and some therapies can slow down or halt the disease's progress.

The word *cirrhosis* combines the Greek words *kirrho,* meaning "orange" or "tawny," with *osis,* which means "condition." The World Health Organization (WHO) defines cirrhosis as a process characterized by fibrosis (scarring) that changes the architecture of the normal liver into one that has structurally abnormal nodules, or lumps. Under this definition, cirrhosis is different from other types of liver diseases that have either the fibrosis or the abnormal nodular formation, but not both.

Cirrhosis is classified into two basic types, micronodular and macronodular. In micronodular cirrhosis, the nodules are uniform in size and very small, fewer than three millimeters in diameter. In macronodular cirrhosis, the nodules are greater than three millimeters in diameter and more variable in size. Mixed cirrhosis combines micronodular and macronodular cirrhosis. However, this classification system is not always useful, because there can be considerable variations and overlap in sizes. Furthermore, micronodular cirrhosis frequently develops into macronodular cirrhosis.

Cirrhosis has many causes, including infectious and hereditary diseases. In some cases, the cause is unknown. Whenever liver inflammation and injury last for decades, there is a chance that cirrhosis will develop. The most common causes are as follows:

- long-term ALCOHOL ABUSE AND DEPENDENCE
- viral hepatitis B, C, D, G (Hepatitis D can infect only people already infected with HEPATITIS B.)
- genetic HEMOCHROMATOSIS (iron overload)
- WILSON'S DISEASE (copper overload)
- ALPHA-1-ANTITRYPSIN DEFICIENCY (lack of a specific liver enzyme)
- cystic fibrosis (disorder of certain glands)
- glycogen storage disease (inability to convert sugars to energy)

- galactosemia (absence of a milk-digesting enzyme)
- biliary obstruction
- PRIMARY BILIARY CIRRHOSIS
- PRIMARY SCLEROSING CHOLANGITIS
- childhood biliary disease, such as BILIARY ATRESIA
- BUDD-CHIARI SYNDROME
- severe right-sided heart failure (congestive heart failure)
- AUTOIMMUNE HEPATITIS
- FATTY LIVER and nonalcoholic steatohepatitis (NASH)
- other infections such as syphilis and schistosomiasis (parasitic infection)
- excessive intake of vitamins, such as vitamin A
- certain medications, such as methotrexate (anticancer drug), isoniazid (tuberculosis treatment), and others
- certain harmful herbs
- toxins

A diagnosis of cirrhosis does not automatically mean that the individual has problems with alcohol. Hepatitis B seems to be the most common cause of cirrhosis worldwide, but it is less common in the United States and the rest of the Western world. In the United States, long-term alcohol abuse and chronic HEPATITIS C are the most common culprits. When people die from hepatitis C, it is often due to the development of liver fibrosis (scarring), which then leads to cirrhosis and its complications.

Not all liver disease causes cirrhosis. For example, with most acute liver diseases, such as HEPATITIS A, the patient recovers in a few weeks or months, too soon to lead to extensive scarring.

Symptoms and Diagnostic Path
Regardless of the underlying disease that causes cirrhosis, the signs and symptoms usually result from the loss of functioning liver cells or organ swelling due to scarring. Patients may feel quite normal and have vague symptoms. If an individual has few or no symptoms, the cirrhosis is often called compensated. If the cirrhosis remains at this stage, then

the individual can usually expect to live a normal life span. If the disease progresses and develops complications, such as jaundice or encephalopathy, then it is considered to be decompensated.

Early symptoms of cirrhosis include those below:

- fever
- nausea
- loss of appetite
- vomiting
- loss of libido
- weight loss

Later symptoms of cirrhosis include these:

- black or bloody stools
- bleeding and bruising easily
- jaundice (yellowing of skin and eyes)
- dark urine
- diarrhea
- encephalopathy (mental impairment and confusion)
- spider veins (small blood vessels that resemble a spiderweb)
- swelling of the abdomen (ascites)
- swelling of feet and legs (edema)
- testicular atrophy
- uncontrollable itching
- vomiting blood

On occasion a physical exam will tell the doctor that cirrhosis is present. He or she may be able to feel the area above the liver in the upper right abdomen and detect that the liver is hard and bumpy, not soft and smooth. Percussion (drumming) of the area will produce different sounds than if the liver is healthy. The size of the liver may be normal, or it may be reduced or enlarged. The spleen may also be enlarged to compensate for the liver's decreased ability to function.

Laboratory blood and urine tests and the patient's medical history may further corroborate a suspicion of cirrhosis. Blood tests called LIVER-FUNCTION TESTS may show abnormalities: the ALBUMIN level may be low; or cholesterol may be abnormally low since the liver synthesizes cholesterol; and PROTHROMBIN TIME—the speed at which blood clots form—may be prolonged.

When complications of cirrhosis are present, and the patient has been chronically ill and has a history of liver disease, it is a relatively easy matter to deduce what the patient is suffering from. But in the early stages of the disease, cirrhosis may be clinically silent—there may be no signs or symptoms. In that case, a diagnosis of cirrhosis usually requires a LIVER BIOPSY, which provides the most definitive and complete information about the liver on a cellular level and remains the gold standard for the diagnosis of cirrhosis.

The doctor may want to look at ultrasound, computerized axial tomography (CAT) scan, and/or magnetic resonance imaging (MRI) images of the liver to check for signs of disease. Although some telltale signs can suggest cirrhosis, radiological studies are not a substitute for a biopsy, though the doctor may use radiological studies instead of a biopsy for patients unable to undergo biopsy, for instance, if they have a high risk of bleeding.

The doctor should try to find out what caused the cirrhosis to select the most appropriate treatment. However, in about 10 out of every 100 patients, the cause of cirrhosis is "cryptogenic"—of unknown origin.

The severity of cirrhosis is often classified using the Childs-Pugh classification system. The classification is based on tests that measure albumin (a major protein found in the blood), bilirubin (bile pigment), and prothrombin time. It is useful in determining prognosis, the potential for variceal bleeding, and whether the risk of surgery may be higher than for the general population.

Childs class A disease is the mildest form of cirrhosis. There are no serious problems yet at this point, and if the patient needs surgery for any reason, he or she should be able to undergo it with general anesthesia with little risk.

Childs class B and C, on the other hand, indicate that the cirrhosis has already injured the liver considerably. At this advanced stage of the disease, the prognosis is poorer than for Childs class A. Complications may occur, if they have not already.

Anesthesia and surgical procedures represent significant risks for patients with either of these classifications.

Because the liver performs the greatest number of functions of all the organs (except for the brain), a liver disease such as advanced cirrhosis can affect the body in many ways. The following are some of the common problems, or complications, that can potentially occur because of cirrhosis:

Fluid retention. The liver synthesizes the protein albumin, which plays a major role in regulating fluid balance within the body. When the liver is diseased and loses its ability to make enough albumin, fluid may leak out of blood vessels and into the surrounding tissues, causing water to accumulate in the legs (edema) and the abdomen (ASCITES). Ascites is a potentially life-threatening condition. Patients with this condition may need to be evaluated for LIVER TRANSPLANTATION. Kidney problems also contribute to fluid retention. When the liver, a major filtering organ, is diseased, it strains the kidneys, another filtering organ. Subtle alterations in kidney function lead to hormonal changes that, in turn, can cause the formation of ascites and edema.

Kidney failure. A type of kidney failure, known as HEPATORENAL SYNDROME, is seen only in patients with advanced liver disease, such as severe end-stage cirrhosis of the liver. With this syndrome, the kidneys themselves are normal, and there is no other apparent cause of renal failure.

Bruising and bleeding. When the liver has trouble producing blood-clotting factors, the patient will bruise or bleed easily. The palms may also become reddish and blotchy.

Portal hypertension. In a healthy patient, the portal vein carries blood from the intestines and spleen to the liver. Cirrhosis slows the normal blood flow through the vein, causing a condition known as PORTAL HYPERTENSION, or increased pressure inside the portal vein. The scarring of the liver may also obstruct the blood vessels to and from it, causing blood to back up in the blood vessels. This condition is like high blood pressure of the liver, and it may also result in ascites, a condition with massive accumulation of fluid in the abdomen, as mentioned above.

Bleeding varices. When blood circulation through the liver is impeded, the blood flow through the portal vein slows, and blood backs up in the portal vein. As the pressure increases, blood backs up farther into blood vessels in the stomach and esophagus (the tube leading from the mouth to the stomach), and these vessels become enlarged and distended. These distensions, called varices, are essentially varicose veins inside the body. These blood vessels have very thin walls, and the increased pressure inside them is likely to make them burst, particularly in the upper stomach and esophagus. When the varices rupture, they can bleed massively, and immediate medical attention is required.

Congestive gastropathy. Milder bleeding may occur because of hemorrhaging veins in the esophagus. This condition is called congestive gastropathy or portal hypertensive gastropathy. The portal veins carry blood from the stomach and spleen to the liver. When the pressure in these portal veins increases, it may cause congestion in the lining of the stomach, leading to obvious or subtle blood loss. The bleeding often manifests as upper intestinal bleeding. The stools may turn black.

Insulin resistance and type 2 diabetes. Insulin is a hormone produced by the pancreas to enable cells to use blood glucose (sugar) for energy. Cirrhosis causes resistance to insulin, so the cells are unable to use insulin properly. To compensate, the pancreas produces more insulin. Eventually type 2 diabetes develops.

Encephalopathy. This is a state of mental impairment and confusion. In mild cases, the patient may experience short-term memory loss, a change in sleeping patterns, or irritability. The cause is not completely understood, and a number of different factors may be involved. It is believed that this condition is related to the liver's increasing inability to clear toxins, particularly ammonia, from the body. A buildup of ammonia, a by-product of protein metabolism, in the brain can lead to mental disturbances. In severe cases, the patient may go into a coma. ENCEPHALOPATHY is a sign of liver failure, and the patient may be considered for liver transplantation.

Liver cancer. Anyone with cirrhosis is potentially at risk for developing LIVER CANCER, also known as HEPATOCELLULAR CARCINONMA (HCC), a type of primary liver cancer—a tumor that grows within the liver tissue. Cirrhotic patients do not always develop liver cancer. The risk depends partly on the cause of cirrhosis. For instance, people whose cirrhosis is a result of AUTOIMMUNE HEPATITIS, nonalcoholic steatohepatitis (or FATTY LIVER), or Wilson's disease will rarely get liver cancer. An individual's risk for developing liver cancer is greatest if the cirrhosis was caused by chronic hepatitis B or C. Cirrhotic patients should be monitored for the development of liver cancer by a blood test called ALPHA-FETOPROTEIN (AFP) several times a year.

Treatment Options and Outlook

The goals of treatment for cirrhosis are to cure or reduce the condition causing the illness, to prevent or delay disease progression, and to prevent or treat complications. As mentioned above, treatment depends in part on the cause of cirrhosis. Most of the therapies focus on treating the various symptoms and complications (if any) of cirrhosis. Some of the treatments that may be attempted are described in the following paragraphs.

Reducing water retention. The doctor may prescribe diuretics to increase fluid excretion. He or she may also perform paracentesis, using a needle to remove extra fluid from the abdomen. Patients may be required to limit their fluid and salt intake.

Controlling variceal bleeding. Variceal bleeding often leads to death in cirrhotic patients. To stop the bleeding, the doctor may inject the varices with a clotting agent or perform an esophageal balloon tamponade, where a tube is put into the esophagus and stomach. Alternatively, a rubber-band ligation, which compresses the varices to stop the bleeding, may be performed. Beta-blockers may be prescribed for patients who can tolerate them.

Removing blood from the stomach. Gastric lavage, in which a tube is inserted through the nose and down into the stomach, may be used to remove blood from the stomach.

Eliminating alcohol consumption. Patients with liver disease should not drink alcohol. Alcohol abuse is one of the most common causes of liver disease.

Controlling encephalopathy. The doctor may prescribe the drug lactulose (Cephulac) to reduce the buildup of ammonia. Patients may be put on a low-protein diet. Vegetable and dairy proteins may be better tolerated than meat. To prevent malnourishment, the patient may be given additional fruits and fats if they are tolerated. Some doctors may use some special formulas for these patients.

General nutrition. Patients who are not at risk for encephalopathy may need a high-calorie diet with moderate amounts of protein and a multivitamin and mineral supplement. Patients who experience nausea and vomiting may be prescribed tube feeding or a liquid diet. When they can eat again, they can try eating small, frequent meals. They may keep a food diary to keep track of what they have eaten, when and how much, and how they felt afterward. This is useful in identifying which foods are hard to digest. If a patient suddenly gains more than five pounds, he or she should immediately notify the doctor.

Liver transplantation. If the liver becomes extremely damaged and is unable to function, a liver transplant may be necessary to save the patient's life. Liver transplant is considered a standard treatment today, and survival rates have improved recently because of drugs that are better able to keep the immune system from rejecting the donated organ.

Alternative treatments. Some patients may want to consider alternative treatments. Patients interested in alternative treatments should discuss them with their doctors and obtain referrals to practitioners if possible.

The prognosis for a patient with cirrhosis varies, depending on the cause of the disease, gender, and other considerations. The degree of liver injury may also be related to the nutritional status of the patient. Unless the underlying cause of the cirrhosis is corrected, scarring of the liver will progress, ultimately leading to liver failure. Patients who receive a Childs class C classification may survive fewer than 12 months without a liver transplant.

Further damage to the liver can be prevented by abstaining from alcohol, proper attention to dietary concerns, getting enough rest, and remaining free of infection. Patients who do not have hepatitis A or C might consider vaccinations against them.

The success of liver transplantation and many new advances in the management of cirrhosis complications, such as portal hypertension, have improved the longevity and quality of life of patients with cirrhosis. Some cirrhotic patients are able to lead long, productive lives by adhering to a plan of treatment carefully designed for them. Meanwhile, new researches are being conducted that can further improve the odds for survival.

Risk Factors and Preventive Measures

Living a healthy lifestyle is the best way to prevent chronic liver disease, which develops into cirrhosis. Studies indicate that poor nutrition increases the risk of developing cirrhosis, so people should strive to eat good, well-balanced meals. Because alcohol abuse is the leading cause of cirrhosis in the United States, the best way to prevent cirrhosis from developing in the first place is to abstain from alcohol; those not addicted to alcohol should limit their intake.

To circumvent the other major cause of cirrhosis, viral hepatitis, care should be taken to avoid getting infected. Since sharing needles is a cause of infection, recreational drug use, especially the intravenous use of drugs, should be avoided. Safe sex can also reduce the chance of infection, because sexual intercourse is another mode of transmission for viral hepatitis.

Research Trends

Many new developments are being made in the treatment of liver diseases, and these new developments herald targeted treatments. A new, non-invasive test caught 70 to 80 percent of early-stage cirrhosis in a test group. The test requires only a small blood sample, and it detects changes in the levels of sugars produced by the liver. With further development, this test may be less expensive and safer than a biopsy, and it may make it easier to catch cirrhosis at an early stage before much of the liver has been damaged and complications have set in. This should significantly improve the prognosis for cirrhosis patients.

New research is also developing a better understanding of how fibrosis develops. Until now, the scarring that occurs in cirrhosis was always deemed to be irreversible. However, new data from clinical and laboratory-based research are suggesting that antifibrotic treatments that may reverse scarring may be developed in the next decade.

It is commonly thought that interleukin-6 (IL-6), a chemical substance secreted by immune system cells, is a contributing factor to liver fibrosis or cirrhosis. But a recent study suggests that it may instead help in the recovery of the liver. Researchers are now working to see whether they can use IL-6 to halt the disease process in patients.

Scientists are also investigating gene-therapy technologies to prevent liver failure. Two independent teams of researchers have reported that using gene therapy to alter liver cells and increase their life span may be the key to treating cirrhosis and other chronic disease.

Caregaro, Lorenza, Franca Alberino, Piero Amodio, Carlo Merkel, Massimo Bolognesi, and Paolo Angeli. "Malnutrition in alcoholic and virus-related cirrhosis." *American Journal of Clinical Nutrition* 63, no. 4 (April 1996): 602.

Cerrato, Paul L. "When your patient has liver disease." *RN* 55, no. 3 (March 1992): 77.

Gines, P., E. Quintero, V. Arroyo, J. Teres, M. Bruguera, A. Rimola, J. Caballeria, J. Rodes, and C. Rozman. "Compensated cirrhosis: Natural history and prognostic factors." *Hepatology* 7, no. 1 (January–February 1987): 122–128.

Haggerty, Maureen. "Cirrhosis." *Gale Encyclopedia of Medicine,* ed. 1 (1999): Farmington Hills, Mich.: Thomson Gale, 724.

"Immune system process could halt progress of cirrhosis." *Immunotherapy Weekly,* April 26, 1999.

Iredale, John P. "Cirrhosis: New research provides a basis for rational and targeted treatments." *British Medical Journal* 327, no. 7407 (July 19, 2003): 143(5).

Mullan, Zoe. "Gene therapy may halt end-stage liver failure." *Lancet* 355, no. 9204 (February 19, 2000): 630.

"New liver test less invasive than biopsy." National Institutes of Health. Available online. URL: http://www.nlm.nih.gov/medlineplus/news/fullstory_16442.html. Accessed on March 9, 2004.

"Nutritional assessment and liver cirrhosis." *Nutrition Research Newsletter* 20, no. 11 (November 2001): 2(2).

Pugh, R. N. H., I. M. Murray-Lyon, J. L. Dawson, et al. "Transection of the oesophagus for bleeding oesophageal varices." *British Journal of Surgery* 60, no. 8 (1973).

Sadovsky, Richard. "Preventing initial bleeding in cirrhosis-induced varices." *American Family Physician* 67, no. 3 (February 1, 2003): 609.

cirrhosis and cancer CIRRHOSIS is the number-one cause of HEPATOCELLULAR CARCINOMA (HCC), the most common type of cancer that starts in the LIVER. Cirrhosis is characterized by dense, fibrous scar tissues and distorted architecture of the liver. Once the liver starts developing cirrhosis, its unique and often lifesaving capacity to regenerate works against it. When the liver becomes injured, the hepatocytes—liver cells—attempt to divide and restore liver mass. But the scar tissue prevents the liver cells from forming new normal cells and instead the cells become nodules. During its unsuccessful attempt to regenerate, the cells may start to divide uncontrollably and become cancerous. Studies show that 60 to 80 percent of all patients with LIVER CANCER have cirrhosis. The presence of cirrhosis makes it riskier—often impossible—to remove cancerous cells surgically.

Many chronic liver diseases lead to cirrhosis. For instance, patients with chronic HEPATITIS B and HEPATITIS C have chronic inflammation and scarring of the liver, which can then lead to an even greater scarring that is the characteristic of cirrhosis. Similarly, alcoholic liver disease, which can injure the liver and cause inflammation, often leads to cirrhosis. It is estimated that approximately 15 percent of alcoholics will develop cirrhosis.

Chronic LIVER DISEASE can be a long and insidious condition. Sometimes it progresses slowly, so that it may be years before liver cancer develops. Autopsy results of people with cirrhosis show that up to 28 percent of them died without knowing they had cancer in their liver.

It is also possible to develop hepatocellular carcinoma without having cirrhosis. This is particularly true of patients with chronic hepatitis B. They may have HCC without first developing cirrhosis.

The cause of cirrhosis appears to influence the likelihood that an individual will get HCC. Chronic hepatitis B carriers have a lifetime risk up to 200 times that of the general population. In contrast, cirrhosis associated with PRIMARY BILIARY CIRRHOSIS has a very low risk of HCC.

A combination of other risk factors with cirrhosis increases the chance of developing HCC. For instance, patients who have cirrhosis caused by alcohol abuse are more vulnerable to developing liver cancer if they are 55 years or older and are also carriers of chronic hepatitis C.

coagulopathy Coagulopathy is a disease that affects the coagulation of blood. In a healthy body, the blood clots and becomes viscous or jellylike to stop bleeding and prevent blood loss in the case of an injury. The LIVER produces most of the various plasma proteins known as blood clotting or coagulation factors that interact with other chemicals to stop bleeding. When the liver is diseased, it is unable to produce enough of the coagulation factors, and the process is impaired. Bleeding problems can range from mild to severe.

Causes of coagulopathy include rare inherited disorders, vitamin K deficiency, severe LIVER DISEASE, and the side effects of certain drugs.

Coagulopathy is often present in the case of CIRRHOSIS of the liver, and virtually all patients with end-stage liver disease will suffer from some form of coagulopathy.

Treatment depends on the specific disorder. This may include replacement of the various blood-clotting factors or transfusion of fresh frozen plasma. If CHOLESTASIS (reduced or absent bile flow) is the cause, the administration of vitamin K may correct it. If cirrhosis is present, the liver is too damaged to synthesize the vitamin.

coinfection See SUPERINFECTION AND COINFECTION.

complete blood count (CBC) The complete blood count (CBC) is a panel of tests given both routinely and to monitor the effects of certain drug and radiation therapies. A CBC provides counts of red blood cells, white blood cells, and platelets. Red blood cells contain hemoglobin, a protein that carries oxygen to tissues throughout the body. White blood cells fight off foreign invaders from the body and play an important role in the immune response. Platelets stick to the linings of broken blood vessels to help stop bleeding.

The CBC is a broad screening test that helps to determine general health status. Although it is not particularly useful in the specific diagnosis of LIVER DISEASE, the physician may order a CBC, together with a battery of other tests, to build a detailed clinical picture of the liver's health status. Certain abnormalities may flag the doctor's attention. A low red blood cell count indicates that the patient is anemic, a condition that can occur in people with chronic liver diseases, especially CIRRHOSIS and malignant liver tumors. Normal red cell counts are usually associated with benign liver tumors. A low white cell count can occur in people with cirrhosis. Conversely, a high white blood cell count can indicate the presence of inflammatory liver diseases, such as viral or alcoholic hepatitis.

confusion   See HEPATIC ENCEPHALOPATHY.

cryosurgery   Extreme temperatures can kill both cancer cells and normal cells. In cryosurgery, liver tumor cells are frozen with super-cold liquid nitrogen (or sometimes argon gas) and in the process destroyed. Cryosurgery is possible both for primary LIVER CANCER—where the tumor remains in the liver—and for metastatic cancer that has spread to the liver from another site.

Cryosurgery (also called cryotherapy, or cryoablation) is an alternative surgery for patients who cannot have their tumor removed in the traditional manner due to their age or other medical conditions.

Although cryosurgery was available for many years, only in recent years has cryosurgery come to be used for the removal of LIVER TUMORS. This was thanks to technical improvements in cryotherapy as well as high-resolution ultrasound used in open surgery. Surgeons use cryosurgery on cancerous, precancerous, and noncancerous conditions, both inside and outside the body. In fact, cryosurgery is applied to a wide range of conditions, including benign lesions, prostate cancer, skin growths, cysts, and so forth.

At the time of this writing, cryosurgery is considered an experimental therapy, and its long-term effectiveness remains largely unknown.

Candidates for cryosurgery should have the type of cancer that could be excised with surgery, were it not for the patients' age or medical conditions not related to the liver. The patients must not have any disease outside the liver. Ideally, the tumors should not be larger than five centimeters in diameter, and they must not be close to major blood vessels in the liver or the BILE DUCTS; otherwise, it is difficult to freeze the tumors completely safely. Although it is possible to freeze as many as eight small tumors, if there are four or more tumors present, it is quite likely that there are many other smaller tumors. Cryosurgery alone cannot successfully contain these tumors. In such cases, long-term disease control requires combining it with other therapeutic approaches, such as CHEMOTHERAPY.

Researchers are studying the effectiveness of cryosurgery in combination with other cancer treatments, such as hormone therapy, chemotherapy, radiation therapy, or surgery. As an example, a patient may be given radiation therapy or chemotherapy before cryosurgery is performed to remove the remaining tumors. It is believed that combining different modalities will produce a higher success rate in treating cancer and improve patient survival.

When the tumor is outside the body, liquid nitrogen can be applied directly to the growth with a cotton swab or spraying device. Treating liver tumors can be done as an open abdominal surgery, laparoscopically (using a tube with a light for viewing), or through the skin (percutaneously). General anesthesia is used for the procedure.

The tip of the cryoprobe—a hollow metal tube with ultracold liquid nitrogen or argon gas circulating through it—is placed directly into the tumor using ultrasound or magnetic resonance imaging (MRI) for guidance. The liquid inside the probe circulates at a temperature of −196°C. Cryoprobes are between three millimeters and three centimeters in diameter. The larger probes are used to treat larger tumors. Cryosurgery is generally performed for tumors that are no larger than five centimeters in diameter, but it is sometimes possible to treat tumors larger than six centimeters by placing multiple cryoprobes in different areas of the tumor. Some researchers are investigating to see whether tumors currently too large to freeze can be first reduced in size by chemotherapy injected into the vein, then frozen.

When the freezing probe is placed in the tumor, it creates an ice ball in its center that gradually expands outward to one centimeter beyond the tumor. This helps limit damage to the surrounding healthy tissues. Nevertheless, for this procedure to work, there must be enough margin of healthy tissue around the tumors. There will be some membrane damage.

Thawing of the frozen area results in further damage. After the frozen tissue thaws, it is naturally absorbed by the body. (Or in the case of external tumors, the frozen tissue dissolves and forms a scab.) Usually two cycles of freezing and thawing are done in each area to produce better results.

Risks and Complications

Although complications and side effects are generally not as severe as those for regular surgery or radiation therapy, they do occur. Some complications include those below:

- short-term elevation of LIVER ENZYMES
- mild fever
- cold body temperature
- fluid around the lungs
- blood-clotting problems (coagulopathy)
- high white blood cell count (leukocytosis)
- infection
- bleeding during the procedure
- delayed bleeding
- prolonged bleeding time (prothrombin time)
- damage to bile ducts
- bile leakage

Although not common, severe complication known as cryoshock syndrome—a potentially fatal multisystem failure—may occur. When that happens, the patient may experience persistent decrease in the number of blood platelets, renal (kidney) failure, and liver failure.

In rare cases, cryosurgery may interact badly with certain types of chemotherapy.

Outlook and Lifestyle Modification

Recovery time with cryosurgery tends to be shorter than with conventional surgery; the hospital stay is correspondingly shorter if there are no complications. Because the physician focuses on only a limited area, destruction of nearby healthy tissue is minimized. Patients also generally experience less pain and bleeding. If cryotherapy is done with a laparoscope—a small, tube-shaped, lighted instrument—through a small incision, the recovery time is even shorter. The procedure is also less expensive than conventional surgery.

Cryosurgery can be repeated if necessary, and given in combination with other, standard treatments.

Cryosurgery may be inadvisable in some situations, depending on the size, number, and location of the tumors. Although physicians can remove tumors that they can see (ultrasound or other imaging tests are used for viewing), microscopic cancer spread cannot be treated.

Further studies on cryosurgery are needed to determine its long-term effectiveness.

The incision wound should be cleaned several times each day for the first two weeks following surgery. Patients are advised to limit physical activity and should not do any heavy lifting for up to three months after surgery.

One-year survival rates for patients with primary liver cancer—HEPATOCELLULAR CARCINOMA (HCC)—are reported to range from 56 to 60 percent, and two-year survival rates are between 24 to 36 percent. Survival rates are somewhat higher for patients with liver cancer that has spread from the colon and rectum; survival rates are from 62 to 77 percent at one year and from 50 to 65 percent at two years.

depression Depression has often been called the common cold of mental illness. While anyone can suffer from depression, it can also be a symptom of a serious physical illness, such as chronic LIVER DISEASE. Moreover, people experience a great deal of stress when they are dealing with chronic illnesses such as HEPATITIS C, and chronic stress can play a major role in depression. Additionally, fatigue—one of the most common symptoms of liver disease—can often lead to depression.

When it comes to depression, individuals and their families often do not recognize the symptoms. To make matters worse, physicians are apt to overlook the emotional aspects of illness and minimize symptoms of depression. The management of often chronic health problems like liver diseases requires careful attention to the patient's mental health and quality of life.

Symptoms and Diagnostic Path

National Institutes of Health lists the following signs and symptoms of clinical depression. Answers of yes to three or more of the following questions may indicate depression. Anyone who has thoughts of suicide, or has expressed such thoughts, should consult a mental health professional as soon as possible.

- feel persistently sad

- feel that life is meaningless

- suffer from low energy

- no longer find pleasure in activities that were once enjoyable

- find it hard to fall asleep, or wake up in the middle of the night or early in the morning

- experience significant weight gain or loss

- feel helpless or hopeless

- feel more irritable than usual

- frequent bouts of crying

- suffer from chronic aches and pains that do not respond to medical treatment

- have thoughts of death or suicide

Health care professionals believe that alcoholism and drug addiction are often a mask for depression. In other words, alcoholics and drug addicts may be unconsciously drinking as a way to self-medicate. People who are not addicts may also drink or do drugs to escape from uncomfortable feelings. But alcohol and drug abuse is known to increase depression because it leads to the depletion of vital nutrients and key stabilizing chemicals in the body, thus creating a vicious circle. In addition, excessive consumption of alcohol and drugs can cause liver disease, which may in turn worsen any existing mood disorders.

Treatment Options and Outlook

Studies suggest that the best results are obtained with a combination of medication and psychotherapy, particularly cognitive-behavioral therapy that focuses on changing negative thought and behavior patterns.

Even in the absence of depression, counseling and psychotherapy may be beneficial in patients trying to cope with problems associated with serious or long-term illnesses. Various antidepressants (such as Prozac, Zoloft, Elavil, and Effexor) appear to be quite effective. Some patients try herbal remedies such as Saint-John's-Wort, which may be effective for mild depression. Another popular alternative is SAMe (S-adenosylmethionine), a natural substance derived from the amino acid methinonine.

Patients are advised to consult with their physician before taking antidepressants, nutritional supplements, or herbal remedies. Even substances that a normal liver can metabolize may worsen the condition of a LIVER already compromised by disease.

EXERCISE is almost always recommended in the treatment of depression, no matter what the root cause. Although vigorous exercise may not be recommended or even possible for some patients with liver disease, light exercise like walking can be quite beneficial.

Enough evidence has been collected to show that yoga and meditation reduce symptoms of anxiety and stress, and may in turn lift depression. Massage therapy is also beneficial in alleviating stress and, consequently, depression.

INTERFERON is often used to treat HEPATITIS B (HBV) and C (HCV). One of the unfortunate side effects of interferon is depression, especially in individuals who may have experienced bouts of depression prior to the treatment. Some patients find that they have to reduce the dosage or stop the treatment altogether. For this reason, patients with a history of mood disorders or other psychiatric illnesses are best referred to a psychiatrist for evaluation before beginning interferon treatment. Patients already on antidepressants for depression before being diagnosed for hepatitis B or C may find that their dosage for antidepressants needs to be adjusted.

Interferon can cause depression even in patients without a pre-treatment history of depression. Therefore, patients must be closely monitored. The interferon dosage may need to be reduced, or even stopped altogether. Depending on individual circumstances, the physician may prescribe antidepressants to continue with interferon therapy.

des-gamma-carboxyprothrombin (DCP)

Des-gamma-carboxyprothrombin (DCP) is currently being researched as an alternative tumor marker for LIVER CANCER—HEPATOCELLULAR CARCINOMA (HCC). Currently, the most widely used biochemical blood test for liver cancer is ALPHA-FETOPROTEIN (AFP). The problem with AFP is that it is not highly sensitive. Its sensitivity for liver cancer may be as low as 60 percent in many cases. Researchers J. A. Marrero et al. suggest that the poor performance of currently available tests for cancer accounts in part for the lack of improvement in survival rates of liver cancer patients in the last 20 years.

Researchers are hoping that DCP might be a more sensitive marker for liver tumor. Basically, DCP is an abnormal form of an important blood-clotting factor called prothrombin, which the liver secretes to stop bleeding.

To determine the accuracy of DCP, researchers conducted a study on 207 American patients. In their report published in the May 2003 issue of the journal *Hepatology,* they concluded that DCP was more sensitive and specific than AFP for differentiating HCC from nonmalignant chronic liver disease.

DCP appears to be complementary to AFP. DCP is often positive in some patients with liver cancer whose AFP level tests normal; in other cases, AFP shows positive where DCP is normal. Once the accuracy of DCP as a blood test has been confirmed, the combination of both AFP and DCP should help doctors detect tumor cells earlier.

Marrero, J. A., et al. "Des-gamma carboxyprothrombin can differentiate hepatocellular carcinoma from nonmalignant chronic liver disease in American patients. *Hepatology* 37, no. 5 (May 2003): 1,114–1,121.

Ando, Eiji, et al. "Diagnostic clues for recurrent hepatocellular carcinoma: Comparison of tumour markers and imaging studies." *European Journal of Gastroenterology & Hepatology* 15, no. 6 (June 2003): 641–648.

diabetes and liver disease

Connections between diabetes and LIVER DISEASE have long been noted, but the causes of those links are not always clear. Some drugs used to treat diabetes can damage the liver, and HEMOCHROMATOSIS—a disorder in which the body absorbs and stores too much iron—can affect not only the liver but the pancreas as well, which may lead eventually to diabetes. In addition, drugs used to treat liver conditions can raise blood sugar levels, prompting treatment.

One factor complicating the relationship is that liver disease associated with diabetes is insidious. There are rarely definitive symptoms, and the condition often goes undetected until it leads to a much more serious condition such as cancer.

A study published in the February 2004 issue of *Gastroenterology,* however, may have established a direct link between diabetes and liver disease. According to the study—the largest of its kind—males who have diabetes are at a significantly increased risk of developing chronic nonalcoholic liver disease and LIVER CANCER.

The study, conducted by researchers from the Department of Veterans Affairs (VA) and the National Institutes of Health (NIH), followed the hospitalization records of VA patients nationwide. The study population included all patients hospitalized between October 1985 and October 1990 with a diagnosis of diabetes. To reduce the chance of misleading or erroneous statistics, the researchers eliminated all patients who had been diagnosed with liver disease at any time before their hospitalization for diabetes, and all patients who were diagnosed with liver disease within one year after. The remaining patients—173,643 with diabetes, and 650,620 without—formed the study cohort, a statistical term that indicates a group being used for a comparative analysis. Most of the cohort—98 percent—were men, and patients with diabetes were older than patients without diabetes (62 vs. 54 years).

The study followed each member of the cohort through the year 2000, looking for the occurrence of chronic nonalcoholic liver disease (CNLD) and primary liver cancer, HEPATOCELLULAR CARCINOMA (HCC). In the case of CNLD, the study found that over a span of 1,289,716 person-years with diabetes, 2,339 patients developed CNLD, for an incidence rate of 18.13 per 10,000 person-years. *Person-years* is a term that researchers often use to describe a length of time of an experience (for a study) that subjects were observed. It is the sum total of the length of time that each person was exposed or observed. In terms of person-years, therefore, 100 people observed over a one-year period of time is the equivalent of 50 people observed for a two-year period of time.

In this study, when it came to more than 5,905,490 person-years without diabetes, 5,460 patients developed CNLD, for an incidence rate of 9.55 per 10,000 person-years. In other words, patients with diabetes were about twice as likely to develop chronic liver disease—including cirrhosis—than patients without diabetes.

The results for HCC were similar, if somewhat more dramatic. The HCC analysis showed that out of more than 1,324,444 person-years with diabetes, 317 patients developed HCC, an incidence rate of 2.39 per 10,000 person-years. For patients without diabetes, 515 developed HCC over a span of 5,925,098 person-years, for an incidence rate of 0.87 per 10,000 person years. Thus, diabetes patients were nearly three times as likely to develop liver cancer.

In both cases, the results were independent of other factors. Demographics, alcoholic liver disease, and viral hepatitis had no effect on the results.

Like most statistical studies, the VA study has its caveats. All the patients were veterans, and most were men. Consequently, the results cannot be generalized for nonveterans or women. In addition, the study was unable to address causes and could not uncover the mechanisms by which the liver disease developed. All those areas must be addressed by further studies before the links between diabetes and liver disease can be well established. In the meantime, the VA study strongly underscores the wisdom of monitoring diabetes patients for complications involving the liver.

El-serag, Hashem B., Thomas Tran, and James E. Everhart. "Diabetes increases the risk of chronic liver disease and hepatocellular carcinoma." *Gastroenterology* 126, no. 2 (2004): 460–468.

diabetic patients   See DIABETES AND LIVER DISEASE.

dietary concerns   See LIFESTYLE AND CHRONIC HEPATITIS C.

donating organs   Donation of one's entire body or transplantable organs after death, or of one or more organs while living, is a primary process by which medical schools obtain cadavers for research and teaching, and transplant centers receive new organs for transplant patients.

For many diseases involving the LIVER, lungs, kidneys, and heart, organ transplantation is the most reasonable treatment; for other such diseases, transplantation is the only treatment. Most organs for transplantation must be obtained from people who have recently died and have donated their organs for that purpose. Some organs, however, can be donated by a living person. The liver is one of those organs.

Donation after Death

Individuals can donate their organs or their entire bodies—or both—after death. Most people indicate their wishes on the backs of their driver's licenses. It is a good idea for a donor also to carry a donor card and to register with his or her state's donor registry, if there is one.

When considering whether to make a donation after death, it is essential to discuss the decision with family members. Even when donors indicate their wishes plainly, the next of kin may be required to give consent when death occurs.

A whole body donation—commonly called donating (one's) body to science—consists of giving one's cadaver to a medical school to be used as a teaching tool or for research purposes. A body donated in that way may be used for years after death. Whole body donation may exclude the possibility of organ donation, except for the eyes. If both types of donation are made, organ and tissue donations for transplantation take precedence over whole body donation.

There is no absolute age limit on the possibility of organ or tissue donation. There are a few medical conditions—such as human immunodeficiency virus (HIV, responsible for AIDS), actively spreading cancer, or current severe infections—that rule out organ donation. When death occurs, an assessment will be made of what organs might be recovered. Similarly, in the case of whole body donation, there are some situations in which the body may not be accepted, including contagious medical conditions, serious trauma to the body at the time of death, advanced decomposition, or autopsy.

Many sources on the Internet describe whole body and organ donation programs.

Living Donation

Living donation is possible because of characteristics of the human body or of the organ to be donated. A kidney can be obtained from a living donor, for example, because a human body normally has two, but can operate quite well with just one. A living liver donation is possible because of the uniqueness of the liver itself: It is the only solid organ able to regenerate missing tissue. In a LIVER TRANSPLANTATION involving a living donor, the patient's diseased liver is removed and replaced with part of the donor's healthy one. In about two months, the donor's liver regenerates the portion that was removed, and the portion that was transplanted into the patient regenerates its missing portion as well.

Living donor liver transplants have several advantages over harvesting livers from cadavers. Cadaveric livers are in short supply, to begin with. And even though the liver continues to function in people who have been declared brain dead, the length of time it remains in the body can compromise its quality, increasing the chance—however slightly—of unpredictable complications after transplantation. With living donors, the transplant team can be assured of receiving a liver that is in excellent condition. On the other hand, living donor transplants are not risk-free for the donor, and any decision to become a living donor requires careful consideration.

To form a good match between a donor and a recipient, the two must be the same blood type and should be fairly close in body size, with the donor being the larger. Generally, living donors are closely related to the patient. While a close genetic relationship is not strictly necessary, genetic similarity often enhances the chances for a successful transplant. In addition to those considerations, transplant teams look for donors who are over 18 and in good physical and mental health, and who have no hope or promise of financial gain from the donation.

The process for evaluating a donor typically consists of the following steps:

1. The donor is asked to complete a questionnaire, which includes attaching a copy of blood typing.
2. If the completed questionnaire indicates that the donor is suitable, and the blood type is compatible with the patient's, the donor is evalu-

ated by a liver specialist. That evaluation will include appropriate blood tests and urine tests.

3. If the donor is still considered suitable, the donor will be asked to take a CT (computed tomography) scan so a liver volumetric evaluation can be made.

4. The donor is interviewed by a social worker or a psychiatrist, or both, to help determine the donor's social and psychological readiness to donate.

5. The transplant team discusses the potential donation, and a final decision is made.

Living donation generally must be arranged with individual transplantation centers, and each has its own protocol and procedures. Individuals wishing to donate their liver to their loved one may obtain additional information from the transplant center or hospital where the operation is to be performed.

To obtain donor cards, contact:

Health Resources and Services Administration (HRSA)
U.S. Department of Health and Human Services (HHS)
(888) 275-4772
http://www.organdonor.gov

For information about whole body donation, contact:

Anatomical Board of the State of Florida
http://www.med.ufl/edu/anatbd

For information about organ donation, contact:

First Gov (government's organ donation site)
http://www.organdonor.org

United Network for Organ Sharing (UNOS)
http://www.unos.org

For other sources regarding donor programs, contact:

American Liver Foundation
(800) 464-4837 or (888) 443-7222 (24-hour helpline)

National Kidney Foundation's National Donor Council
(800) 622-9010 or (212) 889-2210

drug-induced hepatitis Drug-induced hepatitis, also known as toxic hepatitis, is caused by medications taken by mouth or by injection. Many different medications, as well as vitamins, herbal remedies, or food supplements, can be potentially toxic to the liver. Different drugs injure the liver in different ways, and present different clinical pictures.

It has been estimated that drug-induced hepatitis is responsible for up to 25 percent of cases of fulminant liver failure in the United States, and it accounts for 10 percent of hepatitis cases. In adults over 50 years old, the number rises to as much as 40 percent of cases.

Symptoms and Diagnostic Path

A person with drug-induced hepatitis experiences symptoms that are often very similar to acute viral hepatitis. Depending on the medication and the individual, negative effects of the offending medication may occur on the first day of its use or after several months. Usually the onset is quite sudden. The usual symptoms are loss of appetite, nausea, and vomiting, often with chills and fever. Symptoms may range from mild to severe, with more toxic patients experiencing more severe symptoms. In very mild cases, the only recognizable effect may be slightly elevated liver enzymes; in severe cases, there may be delirium, convulsions, and coma leading to LIVER FAILURE.

Common symptoms of drug-induced hepatitis include those below:

- abdominal pain
- anorexia (loss of appetite)
- clay-colored stools
- dark urine
- diarrhea
- enlarged and tender liver
- fatigue
- fever
- flu-like symptoms

- headache
- JAUNDICE (yellowing of the skin and eyes)
- joint pain
- nausea
- rash or itchy red hives
- sore muscles
- vomiting

Certain medications can at times cause injury to susceptible individuals with a personal or family history of liver disease, or who drink alcohol regularly or heavily. Unless otherwise directed by their physician, such individuals should avoid taking any known hepatotoxic medications. The physician will either determine that the benefit of the medication outweighs its risks or else work with the patient to discover other, equally effective treatment options or medications that are safer for the individual. When administering medications that are potentially toxic to the liver, the physician will want to monitor carefully the patient's health status. Any medication can affect liver function, and some individuals manifest sensitivity to drugs that are in general well tolerated.

When a patient presents with an acute liver disorder of unknown cause, it is critical for the doctor to take a careful history of all prescription and over-the-counter drugs and amounts consumed. This also includes vitamins, food supplements, and herbal preparations.

Blood tests may show elevated blood aminotransferase, alkaline phosphatase, and GGTP activities. A physical examination may reveal an enlarged liver and tenderness in the right upper quadrant of the abdomen.

Once the causative agent is identified and the exposure stopped, progress may be monitored with serial blood tests.

Treatment Options and Outlook

The offending drug should be immediately stopped. Generally, within days or weeks, the symptoms will gradually subside. There are no specific treatments for drug-induced hepatitis, other than supporting the patient until liver function recovers. Fluid and electrolyte balance is restored and main-

MEDICATIONS THAT CAN POTENTIALLY INDUCE HEPATITIS

allopurinol	gout
amiodarone	cardiac depressant
carbamazepine	trigeminal neuralgia and epilepsy
chropromazine	antipsychotic
cimetidine (Tagamet)	ulcers
ciprofloxin	antibiotic
clindamycin	antibiotic
coumadin	blood thinner
diazepam (Valium)	tranquilizer
erythromycin	broad spectrum antibiotic
halothane	inhalational anesthetic
HMG CoA reductase inhibitors (Statins)	lowers serum cholesterol
hydralazine	antihypertensive
ibuprofen (Motrin)	analgesic
isoniazid	tuberculosis
methotrexate	anticancer
methyldoa	antihypertensive
metronidazole (Flagyl)	antibiotic
naproxen (Anaprox)	analgesic
oral contraceptives	birth control
phenytoin	anticonvulsant
salicylates (aspirin)	analgesic
6-mercaptopurine	acute leukemia
tamoxifen	breast cancer
valproic acid	anticonvulsant

tained, and blood replaced, as needed. Intensive care is essential if there is liver failure, and LIVER TRANSPLANTATION may become necessary.

In the case of acetaminophen overdose (found in analgesics like Tylenol), N-acetylcysteine acts as an antidote. It is effective within 10 hours of the overdose, but probably ineffective after more than 24 hours.

Prognosis depends on the drug and the particular circumstances of the individual. If the toxin is identified early and removed, there may be little or no damage to the liver, and recovery should be rapid. But if there has been a longer period of exposure, the liver may be compromised and recovery more prolonged. There may be scarring though the liver heals. In rare cases, severe liver failure and death may follow.

Contact the doctor immediately if symptoms do not subside after stopping the medication, or if new symptoms develop.

Risk Factors and Preventive Measures

Never take more than the prescribed dosage of medication, whether prescription or over-the-counter. Significantly, some medications cause liver damage at doses not much higher than the therapeutic range. For instance, millions of people take Tylenol without experiencing any negative effects. But the active ingredient, acetaminophen, is associated with liver inflammation, and there have been cases of severe liver injury, even liver failure and death, after an individual has taken a slightly higher than recommended dosage.

If any signs or symptoms develop after taking a new medication, the doctor should be contacted immediately. The patient should keep a log of all medications (as well as vitamins and herbs) he or she is taking, being careful to note the date, time, and dosage, and any physical changes or symptoms. This makes it easier to track down offending substances. Showing the log to the doctor can greatly expedite matters.

drugs and liver disease Many chemical compounds, including certain medications and herbal preparations, are toxic to the LIVER. They can cause both acute and chronic inflammation of the liver, as well as other liver disorders, including CIRRHOSIS, tumors, and FATTY LIVER. The spectrum of symptoms can range from mildly abnormal liver-function tests to LIVER FAILURE leading to death. In the United States, drugs have outstripped viral hepatitis as the most common cause of hospitalization for acute liver failure, accounting for up to 25 percent of cases.

Substances known to be harmful to the liver are called hepatotoxins. Some medications contain ingredients that become hepatotoxic when taken in higher-than-recommended amounts. These are called dose-dependent drugs. The liver acts as a filtering agent, breaking down most toxins into harmless substances. But the reverse can happen sometimes. A harmless chemical can be broken down into by-products that are toxic to the liver. Damage to the liver can occur when these chemicals accumulate in the body because the patient takes a higher-than-recommended dosage of the medication, or takes it over a long period of time. The greater the overdose, the more likely the drug will cause liver injury.

How Painkillers Can Become Toxic

One class of drugs that is dose-dependent and therefore must be handled with caution is painkillers. Tylenol's active ingredient is acetaminophen, which is intrinsically toxic to the liver.

Acetaminophen is in fact the most common cause of drug-induced liver disease in the United States. It is also the most common over-the-counter drug associated with severe, acute liver failure. A number of cases have been reported in the United States of patients who have died as a result of taking too much Tylenol, which is used to reduce pain and fever. The journal *Annals of Internal Medicine* reported in December 2002 that more than 20 percent of cases of acute liver failure were caused by acetaminophen overdose in a study of 308 patients. In one case described in the June 2003 issue of the journal *Consultant,* a six-year-old girl lost her liver and had to receive a transplant as a result of taking a total of six grams of Tylenol in two days.

When the liver breaks down acetaminophen, a small percentage becomes a highly toxic compound N-acetyl-para-benzoquinoneimine. Normally, the liver is able to neutralize the poison. But if too much is ingested, it overwhelms the liver and causes massive liver cell death. There is a relatively narrow band between a safe and a dangerous dosage. Moreover, the potentially toxic dosage is lower for children and for people who regularly drink alcohol (acetaminophen should never be combined with alcohol), or are extremely malnourished or have been fasting.

Acetaminophen is an active ingredient in more than 200 other medications, including cough medicines like Nyquil and some cold remedies. Anyone taking over-the-counter medications should read all labels carefully so as not to double up by mistake. Add the amount of acetaminophen if taking several different preparations containing the chemical. Some cold and cough medicines contain acetaminophen; do not double up by mistake.

Taken properly, in small doses not exceeding four grams a day, popular painkillers like Tylenol are safe, and millions of people worldwide take them without experiencing any ill effects. But note that acetaminophens are dose-dependent drugs, and can turn dangerous if more than the recommended amount is taken.

Other widespread drugs are the aspirin (acetylsalicylic acid) and nonsteroidal anti-inflammatory drugs (NSAIDs) used to relieve pain and inflammation. Although overall the incidence is quite low, these analgesics also have the potential to cause liver disease, and nearly all of them have been associated with mild to severe liver injuries in some people. Women over the age of 40 seem to be particularly susceptible to the hepatotoxicity of NSAIDs and are best advised to avoid them. People with any type of liver disease should check with their doctors before taking any medications, including over-the-counter painkillers.

Medications and Their Risks

No drugs are without side effects, and they all have the potential to affect the liver adversely. Thus, taking medication is always a balancing act between gaining the therapeutic benefits of the drug and incurring the risk of side effects or potentially adverse consequences. The physician will help the patient weigh risks against benefits. For instance, for patients prone to epileptic seizures, or who have active tuberculosis, the physician may determine that the risk of not receiving treatment may be far greater than the risk of developing a liver disease. On the other hand, it may be inadvisable for patients who already have a liver disease to take any drugs that could further harm the liver. In such cases the physician may explore different medications or other possible treatment options.

Idiosyncratic Reactions to Drugs

Even medication not normally regarded as hepatotoxic, and taken in therapeutic amounts deemed safe, may trigger an adverse reaction. This hypersensitivity to a drug, much like an allergic reaction, is completely unrelated to the quantity of the drug ingested. Clinicians refer to such cases as idiosyncratic drug reactions. They are by their very nature unexpected, and the resulting damage to the liver is unpredictable. They can occur at any time during the course of treatment, though they usually develop after a few weeks. Idiosyncratic drug reactions can be mild or severe, and account for anywhere between 15 to 20 percent of acute liver failure. The patient often has fatigue, fever, and rashes.

When the causative drug is stopped, symptoms should gradually subside, but sometimes they may persist for as long as a year.

Symptoms of Drug Overdose

The same general symptoms appear for the specific liver disease, regardless of what may have caused it. That means that often the etiology—the cause of the illness—is not immediately apparent. A careful review of all prescription and over-the-counter remedies, as well as vitamins and food supplements, should be taken when there is unexplained damage of the liver. This is particularly true for patients over the age of 60 who are taking medications. The possibility of drug-induced liver injury should not be ruled out for any patient on medication. Prescription medication is the major cause of liver injury in adults older than 60 years of age, followed by blood transfusion.

In the case of acetaminophen overdose, the patient may initially experience loss of appetite, nausea, or a general feeling of malaise, much like the flu. Blood tests may show extremely high aminotransferase activities that rapidly return to normal. Although symptoms may disappear after the first day, it does not mean that the patient has healed. The symptoms may simply have gone underground, reappearing some 48 hours later in the form of jaundice, dark urine, and possibly coma. These are the signs of liver failure.

What to Do in the Event of an Overdose

In case of an accidental overdose, contact the poison center immediately. With acetaminophen overdose, N-Acetylcysteine administered intravenously (IV NAC) is an effective antidote. The antidote needs to be given fast, however, as it is effective only within 12 to 24 hours after the overdose. It is most likely too late if symptoms of liver damage have already appeared.

Anyone who has started taking a course of medication should go to the doctor immediately at the first suggestion of liver problem. Often fatigue, nausea, and vomiting or other unusual symptoms appear. Even if the dosage is not excessive, there may be an idiosyncratic reaction. As well, chronic use can sometimes lead to an accumulation of toxins, so symptoms should not be ignored.

Risk Factors That Increase Susceptibility to Drug-Induced Liver Disease

The following is a list of personal factors that can increase one's risk of sustaining drug-induced liver disease:

age	adults, particularly over 60, are more prone to liver injury than children. (However, children should never take an adult-size dosage of any medication.)
gender	female
genes	impaired ability to break drugs down into safe by-products, genetically inherited
health condition	obesity; poorly functioning kidneys; HIV infection; autoimmune disorders like rheumatoid arthritis; liver impairment or disease
nutritional status	severe malnourishment

Practices that make the liver more prone to injury from medications:

dosage	the higher the dose of any medication, the greater the chances for liver toxicity
duration	the longer a medication is used, the greater the chance of damaging the liver
alcohol	alcohol combined with drug ingestion, or regular consumption of excessive amounts of alcohol
cigarettes	cigarette smoking
drug interactions	taking multiple drugs known to be toxic to the liver
nutritional status	fasting (particularly vulnerable to acetaminophen)

Drugs Associated with Liver Damage

Literally thousands of medications affect the liver, so it is not possible to provide a comprehensive list of those that may be toxic to the liver. Patients using the following types of medications should have periodic checkups to ensure that their liver is not suffering from abnormalities.

TYPES OF DRUGS AND THEIR TOXIC EFFECTS ON THE LIVER		
Type of Drug	**Name of Drug**	**Possible Liver Damage**
anabolic steroids		rare form of liver tumor
analgesic	naproxen (Anaprox)	acute hepatitis, cholestasis
	ibuprofen (Motrin)	acute hepatitis
	acetaminophen (Tylenol)	acute hepatitis
anesthetics	halothane	mild hepatitis or serious liver damage, especially in repeated applications
	methoxyflurane	
	enflurane	disruption of liver function, similar to Halothane
antibiotics	erythromycin estolate	cholestasis
anticancer	tamoxifen	acute hepatitis
anticonvulsants	phenytoin (Dilantin)	acute hepatitis
hepatitis	valproic acid (Depekote)	acute fatty infiltration of liver
antihypertensive	alpha-methyldopa (Aldomet)	acute hepactocyte (livercell) necrosis

TYPES OF DRUGS AND THEIR TOXIC EFFECTS ON THE LIVER		
Type of Drug	**Name of Drug**	**Possible Liver Damage**
anti-inflammatory agents	corticosteroids (prednisone)	fatty liver
antituberculosis agents	isoniazid	hepatitis
antipsychotic drugs	chlorpromazine (Thorazine)	hepatitis, cholestasis
blood thinner	coumadin	hepatitis, cholestasis
cardiovascular drugs		hepatitis
cholesterol-lowering drugs	lovastatin (Mevacor)	hepatitis
	pravastatin (Pravachol)	
	simvastatin (Zocor)	
	fluvastatin (Lescol)	
	atorvastatin (Liptor)	
	cerivastatin (Baychol)	
immuno-suppressant	cyclosporine A	cholestasis
oral contraceptives	birth control	liver tumor, cholestasis
psoriasis	methotrexate	fatty liver, fibrosis, cirrhosis
rheumatic disease	methotrexate	fatty liver, fibrosis, cirrhosis
treats ulcers	cimetidine (Tagamet) omeprazole	Hepatitis, cholestasis

Other Toxins

Many other substances can be hepatotoxic, or toxic to the liver. These include recreational drugs, such as cocaine and Ecstasy. Cigarette smoking may also render the liver less effective at detoxifying dangerous substances.

Amanita phalloides mushroom can cause acute liver failure. People exposed to industrial cleaning solvents that contain trichloroethylene may also suffer liver damage.

Liver cancer and cirrhosis can be caused by the chronic ingestion of aflatoxin, a contaminant of a variety of nuts, particularly peanuts. Although this cause of liver disease is virtually unheard of in the United States, it is fairly common in other parts of the world.

Pyrrolizidine poisoning is also extremely rare in the United States. Pyrrolizidine is more often seen in Jamaica, where medicinal bush teas are prepared from poisonous plants.

Lee, W. "Acute liver failure." *New England Journal of Medicine* 329 (1993): 1,862–1,872.

Ostapowicz, G., R. J. Fontana, F. V. Schiedt, et al. "The US acute liver failure study group. Results of a prospective study of acute liver failure at 17 tertiary care centers in the United States." *Annals of Internal Medicine* 137 (2002): 947–954.

Rusyniak, D., W. Dribben, B. Furbee, and M. Kirk. "Survival after massive ingestion of acetaminophen presenting as coma and metabolic acidosis." *Journal of Toxicology: Clinical Toxicology* 38, no. 5 (August 2000): 569.

Sadovsky, M.D., Richard, R. M. Jasmer, et al. "Short-course rifampin and pyrazinamide compared with isoniazid for latent tuberculosis infection: A multicenter clinical trial, short-course." *Annals of Internal Medicine* 137 (October 15, 2002): 640–647.

embolization Embolization is a blockage of an artery that prevents blood flow to tissue supplied by the artery. Embolisms may form spontaneously, such as when blood clots are transported from the site of an injury to another part of the body, and these embolisms may cause serious medical problems, such as strokes.

Sometimes it is desirable, however, to place an embolism at a selected site within the body. This is done during a minimally invasive procedure in which a material is injected into a selected position in an artery to block blood flow past that position. Embolization is sometimes used to treat inoperable LIVER CANCERS, with the goal of starving the tumor of blood and nutrients by blocking the blood supply to the tumor. In these cases, it is usually combined with one or more CHEMOTHERAPY drugs, although it is also possible to perform embolization without the drugs. The combined treatment is called CHEMOEMBOLIZATION.

employment issues See ADVOCACY; FINANCING HEALTH CARE in APPENDIX I.

endoscopic retrograde cholangiopancreatography (ERCP) Endoscopic retrograde cholangiopancreatography is a test procedure that allows a physician to view a patient's BILE DUCTS in an X-ray. The procedure uses an endoscope—an instrument consisting of a long, hollow, lighted tube—to inject dye into the bile ducts, making them visible in an X-ray.

ERCP is used to diagnose and treat conditions of the bile ducts, including gallstones and cancer. It is particularly good for diagnosing PRIMARY SCLEROSING CHOLANGITIS (PSC), a chronic liver disease that damages the bile ducts, both those inside and those outside the liver.

ERCP involves passing an endoscope down the throat, through the stomach, and into the duodenum. Consequently, patients must be given both an anesthetic, to numb the back of the throat, and a sedative, to help them relax. Preparation for the procedure includes refraining from both food and drink for the immediately preceding six to eight hours, as well as following any special instructions from the doctor.

The test is usually given in an X-ray room. The patient lies on his or her left side and swallows the endoscope. The physician then guides the scope through the esophagus and stomach and into the duodenum, until it reaches the spot where the biliary tree enters. Then the patient is turned to lie face down, and the physician passes a narrow plastic tube through the scope. The tube is used to inject a dye into the bile ducts, and the X-ray technologist immediately begins taking pictures. If the X-rays reveal a problem, the physician can insert instruments into the scope to remove an obstruction or perform a biopsy.

Like any other invasive procedure, ERCP can have complications. Complications are rare but may conceivably include pancreatitis (inflammation of the pancreas), infection, bleeding, and perforation of the duodenum. Some patients have tenderness or a lump where the sedative was injected, but that usually goes away in a few days or weeks.

The procedure may take anywhere from 30 minutes to two hours. Patients typically suffer some discomfort, but the pain medicine and sedative should minimize the effect. After the procedure, the patient must stay at the physician's office for one to two hours until the sedative wears off and the doctor has made certain there are no signs of complications. If any kind of treatment is done during ERCP, such as removing a gallstone, the patient may be hospitalized overnight.

exercise Patients diagnosed with chronic LIVER DISEASE, or who are considered to be at risk for development of liver disease, can often ease their symptoms—perhaps slow or even halt the progress of the condition—by exercising regularly.

Regular exercise not only strengthens the body, it strengthens the emotional state as well. A well-conditioned body will help the patient battle depression, boost self-confidence, fight fatigue, and improve energy levels. For patients with joint pain, water exercise will help avoid stress on joints.

For certain liver conditions, the results can border on the dramatic. An article in the March 2004 issue of *Gut*, for example, announced the results of a 15-month study on the effect of weight loss and exercise on patients with nonalcoholic fatty liver disease (see FATTY LIVER). At the end of the 15 months, 21 of the 31 study participants showed both decreased levels of ALT, a liver enzyme, and decreased levels of insulin. High levels of ALT are associated with liver disease. Ten patients in the study showed increased ALT levels at the end of the study, but those 10 did not maintain the prescribed two-and-one-half hours of aerobic exercise each week.

Exercise and Cancer Patients

While the beneficial effects of exercise have become common knowledge, not many people, including physicians, are aware that exercise can benefit cancer patients, most probably because the effect of exercise on disease states is not an area that most researchers traditionally paid much attention to. But recent research has highlighted the beneficial effect of exercise on patients with cancer. In addition to lifting depression and in general helping the emotional state of patients who are bat-

tling cancer, exercise has been shown to improve immune system function and benefit patients both during and after treatment for cancer. Compared with cancer patients who did not exercise, those who regularly exercised were discovered to have the following effects:

- better function in certain immune cells
- better endurance
- less decline in physical performance
- greater muscle strength

More research is needed to find out whether exercise can reduce the risk of cancer recurrence.

Exercise can take many forms. Walking, yoga, and tai chi are generally good choices, but some cancer patients and patients with advanced liver disease may find certain forms of exercise difficult. A physical therapist should be able to design an exercise plan to accommodate the patient's limitations, while still conferring the advantages of exercise. Similarly, patients who have undergone LIVER TRANSPLANTATION may consult with their physical therapist for an exercise regime suitable for their condition.

For patients without special needs, the most important factors to consider include choosing exercise suited to them that they will enjoy. A variety of exercises is important as well, to help avoid boredom. As always, patients wishing to start an exercise regimen should consult their doctor.

Batty, David, and Inger Thune. "Exercise benefits cancer patients." *Cancer* 94 (2002): 539–551.

Hickman, I. J., J. R. Jonsson, J. B. Prins, S. Ash, D. M. Purdie, A. D. Clouston, and E. E. Powell. "Modest weight loss and physical activity in overweight patients with chronic liver disease results in sustained improvements in alanine aminotransferase, fasting insulin, and quality of life." *Gut* 53 (2004): 413–419.

failing liver   See LIVER FAILURE; FULMINANT HEPATITIS.

fatigue   See CIRRHOSIS; HEPATITIS; HEPATITIS C; HEPATITIS C TREATMENT; INTERFERON; INTRAHEPATIC CHOLESTASIS OF PREGNANCY; POST-TRANSPLANTATION CARE.

fatty liver (steatosis)   Fatty liver disease, as the name implies, is a condition in which too much fat accumulates in the LIVER. Large droplets (macrovesicular) of fat or tiny droplets (microvesicular) are deposited in the cells of the liver. Steatosis is the medical term for fatty liver. In severe cases, the liver may become comprised mostly of fat, compared with a normal liver, which has less than 5 percent fat. Fatty liver disease is categorized into two types: alcoholic- and nonalcoholic-related. Fatty liver caused by excessive drinking is called alcoholic fatty liver. If the steatosis is caused by something other than alcohol consumption, it is referred to as nonalcoholic fatty liver disease (NAFLD).

A recent estimate is that some 9 million individuals in the United States suffer from nonalcoholic fatty liver disease. Exact numbers are hard to know because many people may have fatty liver without being aware of it.

NAFLD can range from benign to severe inflammation with fibrosis or cirrhosis. When fatty liver exists concurrently with inflammation and injury of the liver, and the cause is non-alcohol-related, the condition is called nonalcoholic steatohepatitis (NASH). The term NASH was first coined by researchers at the Mayo clinic in 1980. The same condition caused by excessive drinking is referred to as alcoholic steatohepatitis (ASH). Distinguishing NASH from ASH is not easy because the results of LIVER BIOPSIES from people with NASH are frequently identical to those from people who have injured their liver through heavy alcohol consumption, yet people with NASH do not have a history of excessive alcohol use. Also, it is not clear just how much alcohol one needs to consume to induce fatty liver with inflammation. The amount varies considerably with the individual.

Risk Factors

A strong link appears to exist between "simple" fatty liver (NAFLD) and insulin resistance, which is recognized as a precursor to Type 2 diabetes. Studies indicate that nearly everyone with NAFLD has insulin resistance, even if not obese. Patients with Type 2 diabetes are also at increased risk for developing NASH (fatty liver with inflammation). The other greatest risk factor for NASH is obesity, particularly for individuals with excessive fat around their midsections. But only a minority of obese people go on to develop NASH. Other individual environmental and genetic factors play important roles in the progression to NASH.

Risk factors for fatty liver and NASH include elevated levels of fats in the blood (hypderlipidemia), rapid weight loss, starvation, prolonged intravenous feeding, use of steroids or estrogen, and altered GI anatomy such as weight reduction surgery (gastroplasty, jejunal bypass surgery), and surgical removal of the small intestine. Other causes for NASH are Reye's syndrome, fatty liver of pregnancy, rare inherited metabolic diseases, and Jamaican vomiting sickness (caused by a toxin from the unripened fruit of the ackee tree).

Certain medical procedures and medications also increase the risk for fatty liver and NASH:

- amiodarone (a heart medicine)
- tamoxifen (medication for breast cancer)
- methotrexate (a type of chemotherapy)

Symptoms and Diagnostic Path

Generally, there are no clear signs or symptoms, or they are nonspecific, such as fatigue and weakness. Occasionally, a person might complain of discomfort in the area of the liver.

No single tests can accurately diagnose NASH or NAFLD. Elevated ALT and AST (aminotransferase) activities in blood tests should alert the physician to possible problems with alcohol use. The blood tests are not definitive, however, and should be considered along with the patient's history and screening tests.

Fat accumulated in the liver can be detected by ultrasonography, computerized tomography (CT), or magnetic resonance imaging (MRI). But fat deposits can at times resemble cirrhosis or a tumor. Furthermore, none of the imaging studies can distinguish between a fatty liver alone and NASH, or determine the extent of fat deposits or severity of the disease.

Only liver biopsy can reliably diagnose fatty liver (NAFLD) and fatty liver with inflammation (NASH). A biopsy therefore remains the gold standard for diagnosis. Unlike other tests, a biopsy can provide information about the amount of fat accumulation and inflammation of the tissues. The distinction needs to be made between NAFLD and NASH because it is critical in patient management and prognosis. NAFLD is considered benign, whereas NASH can progress into CIRRHOSIS and lead to end-stage liver disease.

Once more research has been done, a substitute for a biopsy may be available to patients. The use of calibrated CT (tomography) may provide similar information about the architecture of the liver and the progression of the disease.

Treatment Options and Outlook

The basic approach to treating NAFLD and NASH is through weight loss (where appropriate) and physical activity. Studies consistently show the beneficial effect of a restricted diet and exercise in obese patients who have fatty liver with or without inflammation. Weight loss must be slow, not more than 1 kg a week. More rapid weight loss or "fad" diets, especially starvation techniques, can worsen or even cause fatty liver and NASH. All patients should strictly limit or avoid alcohol.

Diabetic patients can strive to control better their blood sugar for better overall health, though it generally will not improve liver abnormalities.

If medications or toxins were responsible for NAFLD and NASH, simply discontinuing the offending substances will generally reverse the condition. Cirrhosis, however, if already present, is not reversible.

Patients often show nutritional deficiencies, and these should be addressed.

Patients who develop complications of cirrhosis may be candidates for LIVER TRANSPLANTATION. Transplant patients should be careful to maintain a normal weight after the transplantation because there is a tendency, particularly among those prone to NASH, to gain weight after surgery.

Fatty liver is a relatively harmless condition that rarely progresses to NASH. There is no increase in mortality, and patients do not experience any liver-related complications. But it would be better to eliminate the condition, as the possibility of an increased susceptibility to liver diseases has not been completely ruled out.

NASH has an entirely different prognosis than just fatty liver. Follow-up studies show that up to 25 percent of patients may develop significant fibrosis and cirrhosis. Cirrhosis leads to permanent scarring and potential liver failure. Patients who have fatty normal and normal aminotransferase levels (AST and ALT) can also have inflammatory activity and signs of fibrosis.

Future Research

Insulin-sensitizing agents hold promise for future treatments. Individuals with insulin resistance have an impaired ability to utilize the insulin produced by their pancreas. Insulin resistance is regarded as the key player in the development of NASH. In pilot trials, the use of insulin-sensitizing agents in both diabetic and nondiabetic patients appeared beneficial.

Antioxidants also show promise as an alternative approach for treating patients with severe

NASH. Data from several trials also suggested that vitamins C and E could be of benefit.

Agrawal, S., and H. L. Bonkovsky. "Management of nonalcoholic steatohepatitis: An analytic review." Abstract. *Journal of Clinical Gastroenterology* 35 (2002): 253–261.

Ataseven, H., M. H. Yildrim, M. Ylniz, et al. "Correlation between calibrated computerized tomographic findings and histopathologic grade/stage in non-alcoholic steatohepatitis." *Journal of Hepatology* 38, suppl. 2 (2003): A3842.

Brunt, E. M. "Nonalcoholic steatohepatitis: Definition and pathology." *Seminar on Liver Disease* 21 (2001): 3–16.

Bugianesi, E., E. Leone, N. Vanni, et al. "Expanding the natural history of nonalcoholic steatohepatitis: From cryptogenic cirrhosis to hepatocellular carinoma." *Gastroenterology* 123 (2002): 134–140.

Cabakan, B., S. Ozgulle, I. Hatemi, et al. "Biochemical, radiological, and histological correlates in patients with non-alcoholic fatty liver disease with or without ALT elevation." *Journal of Hepatology* 38, suppl. 2 (2003): A3764.

Ipekci, S. H., M. Basaranoglu, and A. Sonsuz. "The fluctuation of serum levels of aminotransferase in patients with nonalcoholic steatohepatitis." *Journal of Clinical Gastroenterology* 36 (2003): 371.

Ludwig, J., T. R. Viggiano, D. B. McGill, and B. J. Oh. "Nonalcoholic steatohepatitis: Mayo Clinic experiences with a hitherto unnamed disease." Abstract. *Mayo Clinical Procedure* 55 (1980): 434–438.

McCullough, A. J. "Update on nonalcoholic fatty liver disease." *Journal of Clinical Gastroenterology* 34 (2002): 255–262.

Merat, S., R. Malekzadeh, M. R. Sohrabi, et al. "Probucol in the treatment of non-alcoholic steatohepatitis: A double-blind randomized controlled study." Abstract. *Journal of Hepatology* 38 (2003): 414–418.

Sasaki, N., T. Ueno, A. Morita, S. Yoshiok, E. Nagata, and M. Sata. "Therapeutic effects of restricted diet and exercise is of benefit to patients with non-alcoholic steatohepatitis (NASH)." *Journal of Hepatology* 38, suppl. 2 (2003): A4235.

Tahan, V., F. Eren, D. Yavuz, et al. "Rosiglitazone attenuates liver inflammation in a rat model of non-alcoholic steatohepatitis." *Journal of Hepatology* 38, suppl. A (2003): A4277.

Ueno, T. "Therapeutic effects of restricted diet and exercise in obese patients with fatty liver." Abstract. *Journal of Hepatology* 27 (1997): 103–107.

Yakaryilmaz, F., S. Gultier, S. Ozenirler, and G. Akyol. "Vitamin E treatment for patients with non-alcoholic steatohepatitis: Results of a pilot study." *Journal of Hepatology* 38, suppl. 2 (2003): A4216.

fibrosis   Fibrosis refers to the formation of scar tissue anywhere in the body. Body processes form such tissue as a reaction to a foreign agent, such as dust, or as an attempt to repair an injury. In the LIVER, the damage that starts what is called the fibrotic reaction can result from any of a number of causes, including excessive alcohol consumption, viral hepatitis, drugs that are toxic to the liver, and genetic or immunologic LIVER DISEASE.

This type of liver scarring tends to develop first in the area where damage to cells is greatest. In viral hepatitis, for example, fibrosis usually develops first in the inlet area of the sinusoid, the area where blood being channeled to the hepatic vein originates. The signal indicator of ALD is fibrosis at the opposite end of the sinusoid, in the outflow region; it suggests that the cellular injury of ALD is due to an impairment of oxygen delivery in the blood cells farthest from the oxygen-rich blood of the artery.

Fibrosis typically requires months or years of alcohol ingestion to develop. Cellular injury does not occur after a single binge, even of several days. Sustained injury is also required for liver fibrosis associated with viral hepatitis and genetic liver disease. It is not known for certain why sustained injury is necessary before fibrosis develops, but it may be that the production of scar tissue during chronic injury may eventually exceed the liver's capacity to break it down with specialized enzymes.

Only 10 to 15 percent of heavy drinkers develop fibrosis, but the risk increases with the overall duration of heavy drinking and the average daily intake of alcohol. Other factors that affect the development of fibrosis include gender—females are more susceptible than males—and the specific type of immune response—injuries involving some types of cells in the immune response seem to engender fibrosis more often than other types. In addition, several studies have shown that the development of fibrosis clearly accelerates in HEPATITIS B and HEPATITIS C patients who also drink to excess. The most likely cause is the cumulative effect of both types of injury, but a direct interaction between alcohol and the hepatitis virus cannot be ruled out.

There is overwhelming evidence that the proximate cause of liver fibrosis is a process known as stellate cell activation. Stellate—or star-shaped—cells are distributed throughout a normal liver, and are the primary storehouse of vitamin A. In the activation process, stellate cells lose their vitamin A and begin to multiply, producing large amounts of scar tissue and restricting the blood flow through the liver by constricting the sinusoid. The result is the disruption of the normal functioning of liver cells.

Some evidence suggests that fibrosis is reversible. The evidence is clearer in the case of autoimmune diseases of the liver (diseases that stimulate an inappropriate immune reaction), but it has also been observed in successful INTERFERON treatment of hepatitis B and hepatitis C. While the routine reversal of fibrosis is not yet a reality, research continues, and many researchers are hopeful that studies of stellate cell activation can eventually yield something approaching a cure.

The most effective treatment of alcoholic fibrosis is, of course, the cessation of drinking. Abstinence from alcohol can, in many patients, almost completely reverse the development of fibrosis. By contrast, continued alcohol use by patients who already have fibrosis virtually guarantees a worsening of the condition, often leading to CIRRHOSIS and end-stage liver disease.

Other treatment options focus primarily on inhibiting stellate cell activation, while much research focuses on preserving healthy cell matrix.

Inhibition of stellate cell activation has resulted in treatment with antioxidants, primarily vitamin E, to reduce the generation of free radicals, which can injure cells and set off the activation process.

Preserving healthy cell matrix is the subject of current research. Any effective treatment must prevent the degradation of healthy tissue while maintaining the rate of breakdown of scar tissue. Because the enzymes that degrade healthy matrix are different from those that degrade scar matrix, it may be possible in principle to develop inhibitors that selectively block the enzymes that disrupt the normal matrix, while leaving undisturbed the enzymes required for scar breakdown. To that end, it is necessary to identify specific enzymes and their cellular sources, an effort that is ongoing.

Arthur, M. J. "Pathogenesis, experimental manipulation and treatment of liver fibrosis." *Experimental Nephrology* 3, no. 2 (1995): 90–95.

Brechot, C., B. Nalpas, and M. A. Feiltelson. "Interactions between alcohol and hepatitis viruses in the liver." *Clinics in Laboratory Medicine* 16, no. 2 (1996): 273–287.

Day, C. P. "Is necroinflammation a prerequisite for fibrogenesis?" *Hepato-Gastroenterology* 43, no. 7 (1996): 104–120.

Evans, R. W. "Liver transplants and the decline in deaths from liver disease." *American Journal of Public Health* 87, no. 5 (1997): 868–869.

Friedman, S. L. "The cellular basis of hepatic fibrosis: Mechanisms and treatment strategies." *New England Journal of Medicine* 328, no. 25 (1993): 1,828–1,835.

Friedman, S. L. "Hepatic stellate cells." *Progress in Liver Diseases* 14 (1996): 101–130.

Lieber, C. S. "Pathogenesis and treatment of liver fibrosis in alcoholics: 1996 update." *Digestive Diseases* 15 (1997): 42–66.

Lieber, C. S., S. J. Robins, J. Li, L. M. Decarli, K. M. Mak, J. M. Fasulo, and M. A. Leo. "Phosphatidylcholine protects against fibrosis and cirrhosis in the baboon." *Gastroenterology* 106, no. 1 (1994): 152–159.

fulminant hepatic failure   See LIVER FAILURE; FULMINANT HEPATITIS.

fulminant hepatitis   Fulminant hepatitis is a severe form of LIVER FAILURE in which injury to the liver rapidly progresses to massive liver cell deaths (hepatic necrosis). Also known as acute fulminant hepatitis, it can result in liver failure and death.

Hepatitis is broadly divided into two types, acute and chronic. Acute hepatitis lasts for less than six months, while chronic hepatitis is defined as inflammation that lingers for six months or longer. In most cases of acute hepatitis, the illness resolves within six months, and the patient completely recovers. If the illness does not resolve, it turns into chronic hepatitis, a condition that could last a lifetime. In rare cases, however, acute hepatitis develops into fulminant hepatitis, which is potentially fatal. If proper treatment is not given, mortality is more than 70 percent. If support management—including LIVER TRANSPLANTATION when indicated—is not given within eight weeks of the onset of the disease, it can develop into fulminant liver failure, including hepatic necrosis, ENCEPHALOPATHY (mental confusion), and COAGULOPATHY (blood-clotting disorder).

Fulminant hepatitis is associated with the failure of the liver to regenerate. Many factors are involved in the processes that lead to such profound hepatic damage, including the age and susceptibility of the host and the extent of the injury to the liver. The proximate cause is either viral hepatitis or toxic hepatitis (DRUG-INDUCED HEPATITIS).

Fulminant hepatitis is most often caused by HEPATITIS A virus (HAV) or HEPATITIS B virus (HBV). However, HAV infection rarely causes fulminant hepatic failure unless the patient has an underlying liver disease. More usually, fulminant hepatitis is associated with SUPERINFECTION with HAV or HBV and HEPATITIS C.

Many researchers believe that the hepatitis C virus (HCV) can cause fulminant hepatitis by itself, and that when it does, the prognosis is not good. Not everyone agrees, however, that hepatitis C can be a cause. Among patients with fulminant hepatitis not caused by hepatitis A or B, roughly half show antibodies against HCV (anti-HCV) or HCV RNA in their blood. In Western countries, however, the figure is only 2 percent, including patients with hepatitis A, B, C, and D, as well as other infectious diseases, such as bacterial and parasitic infection, and rickettsial infection. (Genus of the family rickettsiaceae, when transmitted by lice or ticks, can cause a number of serious diseases like Rocky Mountain spotted fever and typhus.)

Other causes of fulminant hepatitis include ischemia (a low oxygen state or inadequate blood flow) or shock, BUDD-CHIARI SYNDROME (a condition of obstruction to the veins in the liver), nonalcoholic fatty liver, acute FATTY LIVER of pregnancy, and an acute form of WILSON'S DISEASE (copper metabolism disorder).

Symptoms and Diagnostic Path

The major symptoms of fulminant hepatitis are as follows:

- abdominal pain in the upper-right quadrant
- acute kidney failure
- acute pancreatitis (inflammation of the pancreas)
- anorexia (weight loss)
- ascites (abdominal swelling)
- bleeding
- cardiopulmonary (heart and lungs) failure
- coagulopathy (defect in blood-clotting mechanism)
- coma
- delirium
- encephalopathy (mental confusion and impairment)
- hypoglycemia (low blood sugar)
- JAUNDICE (yellowing of the skin and eyes)
- vomiting

In about 1 percent of cases, hepatitis B may progress to fulminant hepatitis B. Patients infected with various strains of hepatitis B or a mutation called precore mutant, who are experiencing coinfection (being infected by more than one infection at the same time) or superinfection (a second infection superimposed on an earlier one) with other viral hepatitis agents, or who are immunologically compromised, are more likely to progress to early CIRRHOSIS or severe chronic hepatitis, and may be more likely to experience fulminant liver failure. Their response to INTERFERON therapy may be variable.

It is uncommon for adults to survive fulminant hepatitis B, although when they do recover, they do so completely without any permanent liver damage and no chronic infection.

In general, the prognosis for children is better than for adults.

In managing the condition, the physician monitors blood glucose levels, corrects hypoglycemia, and prevents gastrointestinal bleeding.

Children and acute liver failure   Acute liver failure in childhood is rare but usually fatal. It may develop as a result of metabolic liver disease or an infection. The cause varies with the age of the child. Infection or metabolic liver disease is common in newborns; in older children, viral hepatitis and drug-induced liver failure are more likely.

Clinical presentation depends on the age and the cause. In neonates, jaundice and coagulopathy may be obvious, but there may be subclinical encephalopathy (mental confusion). Infants may be irritable, and their day and night sleep patterns may be reversed. Vomiting and poor feeding may be a sign of encephalopathy in metabolic liver disease. Older children may show aggressive behavior.

The development of effective medical therapy for certain metabolic disorders and the success of liver transplantation have improved the prognosis, but cerebral damage must be reversible.

Acute liver failure in newborns   Newborns may develop acute liver failure as a result of blood poisoning (septicemia). The causes of hepatitis in newborns include hepatitis B, adenovirus (virus with 40 different varieties, some of which cause the common cold), echovirus (a virus found in the gastrointestinal tract), and Coxsackie virus (causes a variety of diseases, including hand, foot, and mouth disease). Hepatitis A is rare in newborns.

Older children may suffer liver failure as a result of viral hepatitis A to G, acetaminophen (such as Tylenol) poisoning, autoimmune disease, or metabolic disorders such as Wilson's disease (disorder of copper metabolism).

Causes of fulminant hepatitis in newborns and children include those below:

- neonatal HEMOCHROMATOSIS, a defect of iron metabolism. Though rare, it is the most common cause of acute liver failure in infancy. In this condition, the infant accumulates excess iron in the liver, pancreas, heart, and brain. Within hours or weeks of birth, an affected infant develops jaundice, hypoglycemia, and severe coagulopathy. The infant must be given supportive management of liver failure and an antioxidant cocktail. Treatment is more effective if it is begun within 24 to 48 hours after birth. If the child does not respond to the treatment, then liver transplantation is recommended.

- tyrosinemia type 1, a defect in the metabolism of tyrosine, leading to the development of toxic metabolites (by-products of metabolism). Acute liver failure can commonly develop in infants between one and six months of age. The infant develops jaundice, hypoglycemia, coagulopathy, encephalopathy, and occasionally ASCITES (abdominal swelling).

- mitochondrial disorders, a group of rare disorders causing acute liver failure and diseases of multiple organs. The disorders are inherited, sometimes through the maternal DNA, but other modes are possible as well. An infant affected by a mitochondrial disorder develops jaundice, coagulopathy, and certain neurological features that are sometimes difficult to distinguish from those caused by hepatic encephalopathy. There is no treatment, and liver transplantation is ineffective due to multi-organ failure.

- familial erythrophagocytic syndrome, a rare disease that may be inherited or induced by a virus. Typically, an affected infant suffers jaundice, an enlarged liver, relapsing fever, skin rash, and multi-organ failure. Treatment is usually of a supportive nature. Liver transplantation is ineffective, but bone marrow transplantation may be possible.

Viral hepatitis is responsible for some 80 percent of liver failure in children of all age groups, and is the most common cause of fulminant hepatitis. Acute hepatitis A leads to liver failure more often than hepatitis B, but overall has a better prognosis.

Hepatitis B can cause fulminant hepatitis in infants. Hepatitis B is transmitted from mother to infant during pregnancy, with an overall transmission rate of 70 percent. The majority of infected infants become asymptomatic carriers. However, if the pre-core mutant virus is transmitted from mother to child, there is an increased incidence of fulminant hepatitis B, and the infant may develop it within the first 12 weeks of life. Fulminant hepatitis B may be prevented by vaccinating all infants whose mothers are carriers of hepatitis B.

Autoimmune hepatitis, particularly autoimmune hepatitis type 2, may present with liver failure. Wilson's disease is the most common metabolic cause of fulminant hepatic failure in the older child.

Treatment Options and Outlook

The management of acute liver failure includes providing support for the liver, assessing the prognosis for liver transplantation, and preventing complications while waiting for a donor liver, or for the liver to regenerate.

Many complications are associated with acute liver failure. These include a toxic condition resulting from the spread of bacteria (sepsis), gastrointestinal bleeding, brain swelling (cerebral edema), and kidney and heart failure. Gastrointestinal bleeding is frequent and may be prevented. The role of broad-spectrum antibiotics in the prevention of infection is controversial. N-acetyl-cysteine, which is particularly useful in acetaminophen poisoning, is reported to be successful in the management of acute liver failure.

Managing cerebral edema is critical for survival. Convulsions must be treated immediately. Whether to monitor intracranial pressure (pressure within the cranium) is controversial.

It is difficult to provide support for the liver. Artificial liver support appears to be useful as a "bridge to transplantation," but it is not clear that long-term outcome and survival are affected.

In the case of children with acute liver failure, patients with acetaminophen poisoning or hepatitis A have the best prognosis for spontaneous recovery compared with infants or children with metabolic liver disease. Prognostic factors for survival are less well established in children than in adults, but children with metabolic liver disease or severe coagulopathy are less likely to recover.

In newborns and infants, it is not so easy to demonstrate irreversible cerebral damage because the cerebral sutures will not have fused, and the classical signs of cerebral edema may not be present. The prognosis appears to depend on age and

the cause of hepatitis. The prognosis for adults is generally unfavorable if the patient is of advanced age, has respiratory failure or marked prothrombin time (time it takes for blood to clot), or the hepatitis was caused by exposure to halothane (anesthetic) or hepatitis C. If the patient goes into a coma, chance of mortality is 80 percent.

Patients with fulminant hepatitis must be considered for liver transplantation as early as possible to expedite the search for a donor. Recent advances in liver transplantation have eliminated the necessity to exclude children from surgery because of their age and size, but a shortage of matched organs for transplantation means that most children will receive a reduced or SPLIT-LIVER TRANSPLANTATION.

Auxiliary liver transplantation, in which part of the recipient liver is left within the patient's body to regenerate, remains a controversial treatment for fulminant hepatic failure. The advantage is that the graft may be removed if the original liver regenerates. Auxiliary liver transplantation, however, is not suitable for treatment of acute liver failure resulting from metabolic liver disease, as these livers are unlikely to recover. The recipient liver may have cirrhosis, and there is a risk of malignant tumor of the liver (hepatoma), which generally precludes transplantation.

Some centers perform living-related donation for acute liver failure. In a living-related donation, a portion of a liver from a living person, usually the patient's next of kin, is removed and transplanted into the patient. The drawback is that the case of acute liver failure, for which transplantation must be performed immediately, gives families and potential donors little time for preparation and counseling.

The survival rate of post-transplantation for acute liver failure has improved. Most recipients can expect a 70 percent five-year survival rate.

Omata, M., T. Ehata, et al. "Mutations in the precore region of hepatitis B virus DNA in patients with fulminant and severe hepatitis." *New England Journal of Medicine* 324, no. 24 (June 13, 1991): 1,699–1,704.

Vento, Sandro, M.D., et al. "Hepatitis A virus superinfection in patients with chronic hepatitis C." *New England Journal of Medicine* 338 (June 11, 1998): 1,771–1,773.

gallbladder The gallbladder is a pear-shaped, muscular sac about the size of a golf ball, attached to the lower surface of the LIVER. BILE flows from the liver to the gallbladder through a series of ducts. It leaves the liver through the left and right hepatic ducts. These ducts join to form the common hepatic duct. The cystic duct carries bile between the gallbladder and the common hepatic duct, and these two ducts join to form the common bile duct. The common BILE DUCT empties into the duodenum, or upper part of the small intestine, a few inches below the stomach, at a ring-shaped muscle called the sphincter of Oddi.

Bile is a combination of salts, electrolytes, pigments, cholesterol, other fatty substances, and waste products from the liver. It emulsifies fatty substances in the intestines, forming small fat globules that can be further digested in the intestines. It also helps digest and eliminate certain waste products, including pigments from destroyed red blood cells and excess cholesterol, and it helps digest and absorb fats and fat-soluble vitamins.

The gallbladder stores bile produced in the liver and performs a backup function for the stream of bile that is released continuously from the liver. The sphincter of Oddi is a control valve for bile flow into the intestines. Between meals, about half of the bile produced in the liver is diverted through the cystic duct into the gallbladder for storage, and the rest of the bile flows into the intestines. In the gallbladder, bile is concentrated, with up to 90 percent of its water absorbed into the bloodstream. When food enters the small intestine, nerves are triggered and hormones are released, causing the sphincter of Oddi to relax and release additional concentrated bile that has been stored in the gallbladder.

It may be removed surgically when it is diseased or damaged, if it is absolutely necessary to do so. One can live without a gallbladder.

The most common gallbladder diseases are cholecystitis, or inflammation of the gallbladder, and cholelithiasis, or gallbladder stones. Both of these diseases are more common in pregnant women, in people who are overweight, and in people who are over 40 years old. Symptoms of gallbladder problems include abdominal pain and a bloated feeling after eating high-fat foods. If bile flow is obstructed, it may also cause jaundice, a yellowish coloring of the skin and the whites of the eyes, and infection. Less common gallbladder diseases include tumors that block the bile ducts.

Gallstones usually consist of concentrated bile and cholesterol mixed with minerals and pigments. They usually do not cause symptoms unless they leave the gallbladder and enter the bile duct. If they get lodged in the bile duct, however, they can cause severe pain and interfere with the flow of bile.

Inflammation of the gallbladder without the presence of gallstones may be caused by an allergy. Many doctors are poorly informed about this allergic reaction and, as a result, order unnecessary gallbladder surgeries.

Some gallbladder problems can be treated with medications or herbs. Dandelion, nettle, turmeric (the yellow coloring found in mustard and curry powder), milk thistle, peppermint oil, quercetin, eucalyptus, celandine, yellow dock, wahoo, radish root, gentian, and artichoke have all been used as treatments for gallbladder problems. Most of these herbs increase bile flow. Pharmaceuticals made from some of these herbs and preparations combining several of the herbs have been shown to improve bile flow significantly in clinical studies.

Gallstones can be a serious condition, however, and a qualified health care professional should manage their treatment. Herbs may help move the stones along by increasing bile flow, but the increased bile flow may also move stones into the cystic duct, where they can get lodged. If a stone is already blocking the flow, the increased flow may cause additional problems. This is especially true if the patient uses a "liver flush" or "liver cleanse." This common home remedy or preventive measure for gallstones uses a combination of olive oil and lemon or grapefruit juice. People report passing numerous large stones with these treatments, but the "stones" are actually formed in the intestines from a chemical reaction among the oil, juice, and minerals.

Severe cases of gallbladder disease are treated by surgical removal of the gallbladder.

Gallstones may be caused at least partially by a diet that includes too much refined food and too little fiber. With such a diet, the bile secreted by the gallbladder is less acid than normal, and it does not dissolve cholesterol properly. The cholesterol accumulates in the gallbladder and forms stones. Gallstones are less common in vegetarians, probably because they eat large amounts of fiber.

gallstones See GALLBLADDER.

genotype See HEPATITIS C.

Gilbert's syndrome (GS) Gilbert's syndrome (GS) is an inherited disorder that interferes with the LIVER's ability to process BILIRUBIN, a greenish yellow bile pigment.

However, GS is not a disease per se, but a variation—within the normal range—in which individuals have benign elevations of bilirubin in their blood, especially during periods of stress and illnesses from viruses. Nevertheless, the diagnosis of GS is important. GS is not the only liver disorder that can cause JAUNDICE, and diagnosing GS eliminates other, more harmful, illnesses, such as hepatitis, as the problem.

Bilirubin is usually present in the bloodstream in small amounts. It is a product of the breakdown of hemoglobin, the red pigment in red blood cells. Bilirubin is carried to the liver, where it undergoes a series of chemical changes and eventually passes out of the body. When red blood cells break down excessively, or when something interferes with the liver's ability to process bilirubin, it builds up in the blood. Excessive buildup can cause the characteristic yellowish discoloration of the skin and eyes called jaundice.

GS affects about 5 percent of the population, and is an inherited condition in about half of its sufferers. It affects men much more often than women, and in most cases first appears in early adulthood.

GS has few symptoms and is frequently detected by chance through routine blood tests. Sufferers are often not even aware of a problem, although some may develop mild jaundice or complain of gastrointestinal problems, fatigue, or weakness.

A diagnosis can be made by a combination of clinical history, physical exam, blood tests, and urinalysis. A costly search for structural liver disease is unnecessary.

GS does not require any treatment. The liver remains unaffected by the condition, and people with GS lead normal, healthy lives, and have normal life spans.

grieving A patient diagnosed with chronic LIVER DISEASE often develops a sense of grief. It is a normal reaction. Patients with chronic disease must deal with the loss of the individual they thought they were and the lives they had envisioned for themselves, and adjust to their new reality. Grieving helps that adjustment to occur.

In the case of chronic liver disease, the process may be complicated by the effects of the disease itself. Fatigue, low energy levels, and loss of concentration may render patients more emotionally vulnerable and make them susceptible to depressive periods. Feelings of grief may recur with each new symptom or activity of the disease.

There is no correct or incorrect way to grieve, but for many patients the key is to talk about what is happening to them. Patients often keep journals or diaries, talk with friends, or join a support group on the Internet or in a clinical setting.

At the same time, it is important to watch for signs of DEPRESSION. Patients experiencing continuing loss of sleep, substantial changes in eating habits, or feelings of hopelessness should speak with their doctor. Serious emotional problems may require additional help from a professional counselor or mental health clinic.

helpful and harmful herbs Herbs are plants or plant parts believed to contain therapeutic properties. Herbs have played a long and revered role in the history of humankind, and their use is deeply rooted in many cultures. Indeed, the majority of the world's population still depends on herbal medicine for their primary medical care. In China today, it is used in conjunction with allopathic medicine to treat all types of ailments, including LIVER DISEASES, such as HEPATITIS and CIRRHOSIS. In Japan as well, *kampo*—traditional Japanese medicine derived from China—is an accepted practice, and medical doctors may prescribe *kampo* along with conventional Western medication. In the United States, where Native Americans have long used a wide variety of indigenous plants, there is a resurgence of interest in herbs. A 2002 survey by the *American Journal of Gastro-enterology* revealed that when patients with liver disease sought treatment outside of mainstream medicine, they were most likely to use herbs.

Precaution in Using Herbs

Most people have the misconception that herbs are natural and therefore completely safe, but concerns have been raised about the safety of certain herbal remedies. Just as with any medication, herbs are not to be used indiscriminately; they can be quite potent, and must be handled with respect. In fact, some herbs are naturally toxic to the LIVER. These include chaparral, also known as creosote bush or greasewood, and sold as a tea, tablet, or capsule. The Food and Drug Administration (FDA) reports that chaparral is associated with acute hepatitis, a rapid progression of liver disease. Germander, often used to treat obesity (it is usually mixed with other herbs), has also been associated with acute hepatitis. Other adverse effects on the liver include obstruc-tion of blood flow, such as may occur through the ingestion of comfrey, a long-leafed plant.

If injury to the liver is serious, it may lead to acute liver failure requiring LIVER TRANSPLANTATION.

The use of herbal medicine is not regulated. Unlike pharmaceutical drugs, herbs do not require approval by government regulatory agencies, and have not been subjected to the same type of rigorous studies that approved drugs undergo. The effectiveness of herbs in treating liver disease is mostly anecdotal; there have been few standardized double-blind, placebo-controlled studies. This is not to imply that the healing properties of herbs should be dismissed outright, but that more research is required before any definitive conclusions can be drawn. Meanwhile, individuals—particularly those already suffering from a liver disease—must take extra precautions when dealing with herbs. They should be administered only by qualified practitioners and be taken in recommended dosages. Patients are also advised to inform their physicians of any herbal remedies they are taking so as to exclude ones that are potentially harmful to the liver, or may interact adversely with their prescription medication.

Harmful Herbs

The following is a partial list of herbs that have been associated with toxic liver reactions:

- asafetida
- buckthorn
- chaparral
- comfrey (symphytum species)
- germander
- gordolobo yerba

- ho-shu-wu
- hops
- jin bu huan
- lobelia
- ma huang (ephedra)
- mistletoe
- nutmeg
- pau d'arco
- pennyroyal
- poke root
- ragwort
- sarsparilla
- sassafras
- senna fruit extracts
- skullcap
- sweet clover
- tansy
- valerian root
- woodruff

Helpful Herbs

Some herbs are believed to exert beneficial effects on liver function. These include, but are not limited to, the following:

- xiao-chai-hu-tang (also known as Sho-saiko-to in Japan) An herbal medicine used in China to treat chronic hepatitis. Research in Japan and China suggests that this herb may be useful in treating chronic hepatitis and preventing it from progressing to cirrhosis.

- milk thistle (*Silybum marianum*) The active extract of milk thistle, called silymarin, is believed to have medicinal qualities and antioxidant properties. Milk thistle is one of the most favorite herbs in the treatment of liver dysfunction, and is often recommended for "strengthening" or "protecting" the liver. The herb has been used to treat a wide range of liver diseases, including hepatitis, cirrhosis, and fatty liver. To date, there is insufficient evidence to show that milk thistle is effective in treating viral hepatitis, though animal studies seem to suggest that the herb may protect liver cells against toxic insult and have antifibrotic activity. Studies on humans are contradictory, with a few indicating significant improvement in LIVER ENZYMES, but others showing no improvement in histology (microscopic examination of liver tissue) or biochemical markers of liver function, and no reduction in mortality.

- licorice root (*Glycyrrhiza glabra*) Licorice root is the dried root of the licorice plant, which has as its primary active component a substance called glycyrrhizin. Licorice root has been used in China since the second and third century B.C. Some studies suggest that licorice root may improve liver function, reduce long-term complications of cirrhosis and chronic hepatitis C, and help prevent the development of LIVER CANCER. However, these benefits have not been conclusively demonstrated.

  On the down side, licorice taken for a week or longer can have serious adverse effects, such as high blood pressure. It can also cause water retention and worsen ascites—fluid buildup in the abdomen—a common symptom of chronic liver disease. Licorice may also contain iron, and is best avoided by people with iron overload disease.

- schisandra (*Schisandra chinensis* and *Schisandra sphenanthera*) is used in traditional Chinese and Japanese medicine. Most of the studies, performed on animals, appear to suggest that schisandra may protect the liver, improve some liver enzymes, and have an antioxidant effect.

- ginseng Asian ginseng (*Panax ginseng*) and American ginseng (*Panax quinquefolius*). Asian forms of ginseng include Chinese, Japanese, and Korean ginseng. It has been used for thousands of years in Asia to boost the immune system and increase stamina. Whether ginseng is useful in the treatment of viral hepatitis or other liver disease is not known, but it may improve overall health.

  Prolonged use of ginseng, especially combined with caffeine, may be associated with hypertension. Diabetic patients using insulin must be careful, as ginseng can lower blood sugar. Some studies have also shown ginseng to increase bleeding risk. It is therefore probably best to avoid using ginseng with NSAIDs (nonsteroidal anti-inflammatory drugs), such as aspirin and ibuprofen.

As yet, there is insufficient evidence that herbs can reduce the amount of virus in the blood of a patient with viral hepatitis, such as hepatitis C, though some herbs, like the milk thistle, may help lower the level of liver enzymes.

Overall, an analysis of studies published on herbal medicine show results that are intriguing and promising, but the majority of the studies are poorly designed and therefore interpretation of the results is difficult. Additionally, very few studies have tested whether herbs can prolong the life of the patient or show clearly measurable clinical improvements. Clearly, more research, especially in the form of controlled clinical trials, is needed before firm conclusions can be drawn in regard to their curative properties for liver disease. However, patients with chronic liver disease who are prescribed herbs by health care providers often report increased energy and an improvement in their overall sense of well-being. It is recommended that patients seek out clinics and hospitals that offer integrative medicine, which combines conventional allopathic medicine with herbal or other complementary and alternative treatments. At the very least, for the sake of safety, patients must inform their physicians of any herbal medicine—as well as vitamins and dietary supplements—that they are taking. This is especially true for patients with chronic liver disease, as the burden of metabolizing food and drugs falls on the liver.

Agency for Healthcare Research and Quality, Rockville, MD. Available online. URL: http://www.ahrq.gov/clinic/epcsums/milktsum.htm Accessed on January 3, 2005.

Lawrence, V., B. Jacobs, et al. "Milk thistle: Effects on liver disease and cirrhosis and clinical adverse effects." Summary, Evidence Report/Technology Assessment, no. 21 (September 2000).

Strader, Doris B., et al. "Use of complementary and alternative medicine in patients with liver disease." *American Journal of Gastroenterology* 97, no. 9 (September 2002): 2,391.

hemochromatosis   Hemochromatosis is a genetic disorder that causes a severe overload of iron in the body. The excess iron collects mainly in the LIVER, but also in the heart, joints, pancreas, and pituitary gland. It may collect in other organs as well.

If undiagnosed, excess iron can cause CIRRHOSIS, LIVER CANCER, enlarged heart, arrhythmia, arthritis, or other problems, eventually leading to death. The problem can be controlled, however, and a person who is diagnosed early can have a normal life expectancy.

An average American ingests about 10 to 20 milligrams of iron a day. The body, however, loses only about 10 percent of that through its normal mechanisms. Consequently, the amount of iron in the body is largely determined by how much the body actually absorbs.

The body can normally sense iron levels. If it senses that there is not enough iron, it absorbs more; if it senses too much, it absorbs less. Iron that has been absorbed but cannot be eliminated is stored in the organs, primarily the liver. When iron accumulates unchecked over a period of years—the condition called iron overload—it damages the organs where it has been stored.

Iron overload can be caused by nonhereditary factors, such as repeated blood transfusions (usually more than 50) or excessive use of dietary iron supplements. In the United States, however, the most common cause is hemochromatosis, a genetic defect in which the body absorbs more iron than it needs and loses its ability to sense iron levels.

Hereditary hemochromatosis (HHC) is associated with mutations in a gene called HFE. The mutations are called C282Y and H63D.

To be at risk, one must inherit two copies of the C282Y mutation, one from each parent. An individual who inherits only one copy of the mutation is a carrier. Carriers are normally not at a substantially increased risk for developing iron overload, but their offspring may be. Someone who inherits one copy of C282Y and one copy of H63D has a slightly increased risk.

The mutation is associated primarily with people of northern European descent, especially those of Irish, Scottish, Celtic, or British heritage. The defect is sometimes seen in other groups, however.

Men and women are affected equally, but men usually display overt symptoms earlier in life than women. That is probably because women lose significant amounts of iron through menstruation.

Symptoms and Diagnostic Path

The problem with hemochromatosis is that there are often no early symptoms. About 10 percent of men and 25 percent of women show no early signs at all. Before 1960, patients often were not diagnosed until the disease was well advanced and they showed the classic symptoms: so-called bronze diabetes, in which the skin develops a dark pigmentation; arthritis; LIVER DISEASE; and cardiac failure. Even today, with the increasing importance of laboratory testing, most diagnoses are accidental, made while testing for other conditions.

The most common early symptoms are weakness and fatigue. Some patients have reported decreased appetite and weight loss. Since the liver is the body's main storehouse of iron, it may be damaged early in the course of the disease, causing abdominal pain or nonspecific pain in the upper-right quadrant, where the liver is located.

Damage to other organs and glands usually occurs in later stages. Such damage may be manifested as a reduced interest in sex, impotence in men, or loss of menstruation in women. Iron deposits in the joints can cause joint pain and arthritis. People with HHC can also be prone to bone loss (osteoporosis).

Hemochromatosis was originally called bronze diabetes because in the latter stages of the disease, which was when most doctors first saw it, the patient develops both a grayish-bronze skin tone and symptoms of diabetes, including increased urination and increased thirst.

Advanced hemochromatosis may also cause heart arrhythmia, an enlarged heart, an enlarged liver, shrunken testicles, or swollen joints. Signs of cirrhosis or liver failure may be evident.

People with HHC may also have an increased risk of bacterial and viral infections, such as chronic hepatitis.

Because the early symptoms of hemochromatosis are either absent or highly nonspecific, early diagnosis is essential. The Iron Overload Diseases Association recommends that all Americans over the age of 18 be routinely screened for iron overload.

Elevated iron levels are detected by routine blood tests that look for three important values: the level of iron, the level of ferritin, and the transferrin saturation level. Ferritin is the form in which iron is stored; transferrin is a protein made by the liver that transfers iron through the body. The transferrin saturation level is the amount of transferrin that is saturated with iron.

If the ferritin and transferrin saturation levels are both elevated, it is a strong indication that a person has hemochromatosis, even if the iron levels are normal.

People with HHC often show elevated liver-function tests (LFTs) as well, but LFTs by themselves are not good indicators. In the early stages of the disease, LFTs are usually normal.

The presence of both the C282Y and the H63D gene mutations can be detected through a simple blood test. A tissue collection kit is also available that allows a patient to collect a sample merely by swabbing the inside of the mouth with a brush. The results of either test, of course, must be evaluated by a physician.

The gene for hemochromatosis is quite common. A family might be carriers over several generations without ever developing the disease. Consequently, whenever a person is diagnosed with HHC, his or her family members, especially siblings, should also be tested. The screening usually starts with blood tests. If any of those tests are abnormal, they can be followed by genetic tests.

A LIVER BIOPSY to determine iron levels is the best way to make a definitive diagnosis. A biopsy may not always be necessary, however. A young person who has been identified as a candidate through family member screening, for example, has probably not yet developed significant liver scarring, and may not need a biopsy. In those situations and similar ones, a diagnosis might be made using the usual blood tests.

Once a person has been diagnosed with hemochromatosis, a liver biopsy becomes an important tool. It will reveal both the amount of iron stored in the liver and the degree of liver damage already done, information that will help determine both prognosis and treatment.

Treatment Options and Outlook

Treating hemochromatosis involves removing excess iron from the body. That can be done with phlebotomies or by a process called chelation therapy. Some dietary restrictions are also in order.

A phlebotomy removes blood from the body through a catheter in the arm—a blood donation. The blood donated may be able to be reused, depending on factors determined by the Federal Drug Administration.

A person diagnosed with HHC will probably require phlebotomies for the rest of his or her life, though the frequency will vary. Normal maintenance usually involves a phlebotomy once every three months or so.

At the beginning of treatment, however, the usual regimen is the removal of one unit of blood each week. In some cases—if a liver biopsy reveals excessive scarring, for example—twice weekly or even more frequent donations may be needed to prevent cirrhosis.

How long that phase of treatment lasts depends on how much iron must be removed. Each unit of blood removed contains about 250 milligrams of iron. That means that it will take about 100 phlebotomies to remove 25 grams of iron—about two years of weekly treatments.

Each phlebotomy is followed by a blood test to determine ferritin and transferrin saturation levels. When those levels are acceptable—a ferritin level below 50 micrograms per liter and a transferrin saturation of less than 50 percent—the frequency of phlebotomies is reduced to a maintenance level.

Will phlebotomies relieve symptoms? They might, depending on the symptom. Most patients report improvement in the classic symptoms—fatigue, bronze skin coloration, abdominal pain, and liver enlargement. Elevated liver-function tests usually normalize. Heart conditions caused by hemochromatosis also usually improve, though are not cured. A progression toward cirrhosis may be halted, as long as cirrhosis was not present when the disease was first diagnosed. Diabetes

may become more manageable, though continued treatment will probably be required.

Arthritis associated with the disease usually does not improve, and may still develop even after the excess iron has been removed. Likewise, impotence usually does not resolve.

Chelation therapy involves the introduction of a chemical called deferoxamine into the body, either directly into a vein or just under the skin. The deferoxamine chemically binds with iron, which is then eliminated from the body in urine.

The problem with chelation therapy is that it removes much less iron from the body than phlebotomy—only about 10 to 20 milligrams per treatment. Chelation therapy is also much more expensive than phlebotomy, and may cause side effects such as diarrhea, increased heart rate, or disturbances in hearing or vision. For those reasons, chelation therapy is usually restricted to patients who cannot tolerate phlebotomy.

Other iron chelation agents can be taken orally. At this time, those agents are not recommended because they can be toxic.

Specialists insist that wholesale changes in the diet are unnecessary because hemochromatosis is effectively controlled with phlebotomy. Still, it would seem reasonable to make some changes, many of which are recommended by those same specialists. Among them are those below:

- Refrain from iron-rich foods such as red meat—especially liver. It is not necessary to avoid iron-rich vegetables; the iron in vegetables is not readily absorbed.

- Avoid vitamin C supplements. Vitamin C increases iron absorption.

- Patients should not take iron supplements. Anyone with the condition who takes a multivitamin supplement should make sure that it does not include iron.

- Avoid alcohol. Alcohol, aside from its well-known effect on the liver, can increase iron absorption.

Above all, patients should carefully read the labels on all substances that are to be ingested. Medicines, weight-loss products, and some herbs may contain excessive levels of iron and vitamin C. Even foods as seemingly innocuous as breakfast cereal may contain excessive levels of iron.

Hemochromatosis is potentially fatal. But early diagnosis and prompt treatment, which, are essential, will help a patient live a normal life span.

Early diagnosis cannot be overemphasized. A person with both hemochromatosis and cirrhosis is 200 times more likely to develop liver cancer than the general population, and an individual who has already developed cirrhosis when HHC is diagnosed has a significantly decreased life expectancy. If cirrhosis develops later, the HHC patient may develop complications, including liver cancer, even if iron levels have been successfully lowered. Complications of cirrhosis may make the patient a candidate for a liver transplant.

The heart can also be involved. A common cause of death in people with both hemochromatosis and cirrhosis is heart arrhythmia and heart failure. Heart involvement necessitates very aggressive treatment.

Chung, Raymond T., and Norton J. Greenberger. "Hereditary hemochromatosis—Early diagnosis can lead to cure." *Patient Care* 37, no. 8 (August 2003): 54.

hemophilia   See HEPATITIS B; HEPATITIS C.

hepatic artery infusion chemotherapy (HAI)
Hepatic artery infusion chemotherapy (HAI) is a type of CHEMOTHERAPY for patients with LIVER CANCER. Chemotherapy is a treatment with drugs that help to kill or suppress cancer cells, while minimizing damage to normal tissue. Systemic chemotherapy, the standard form of chemotherapy, delivers the drugs by injecting them into a vein or muscle. The drugs then circulate through the bloodstream, thus exposing most parts of the body to the chemotherapy. In the procedure known as HAI, instead of an injection, a pump and a catheter (a thin, flexible tube) dispense and infuse the hepatic (liver) artery with chemotherapy drugs. The intent is to increase treatment efficiency by

increasing the amount of chemotherapy drug delivered to the site of the tumor. When chemotherapy is administered locally, as with HAI, the tumors are directly targeted by the drugs, thus heightening their effect.

HAI is primarily used to treat patients with metastatic colorectal cancer (CRC). Colorectal cancer relates to cancer of the colon and rectum, which are part of the large intestine. This type of cancer often metastasizes (spreads) from its site of origin to distant places in the body, including the liver. In fact, the liver is the most common site of metastasis. Various studies have shown that patients with CRC benefit the most from HAI because the tumors that spread to the liver derive most of their blood supply—more than 80 percent—from the hepatic artery. HAI is therefore often used as an alternative for systemic chemotherapy in the treatment of metastatic colorectal cancer. Sometimes HAI is used in conjunction with systemic chemotherapy to increase the therapeutic potency. It may also be used after the removal of tumors (liver resection) that spread to the liver. A study reported in a 1999 issue of the *New England Journal of Medicine* showed that patients with metastatic colorectal cancer benefited from HAI. The authors of the report wrote, "Two years after undergoing resection of liver metastases from colorectal cancer, about 65 percent of patients are alive and 25 percent are free of detectable disease." The objective of their study was to find out whether giving patients a combination therapy of systemic chemotherapy and HAI could produce better results than systemic chemotherapy alone.

The study randomly assigned 156 patients who had, at the time, received resection of hepatic metastases from colorectal cancer, to receive six cycles of HAI and systemic chemotherapy, or six weeks of systemic therapy alone. The patients in the group for combination therapy received a hepatic arterial infusion of floxuridine (injection medication used to treat certain types of cancer) and dexamethasone (corticosteroid used to reduce swelling and inflammation) plus intravenous fluorouracil (chemotherapy drug), with or without leucovorin (faster-acting, more potent form of folic acid). Those in the second group, who received systemic chemotherapy alone, were administered fluorouracil intravenously, with or without leucovorin.

Two years after the cancer treatment, 86 percent in the combination therapy and 72 percent in the mono therapy group were still alive. The median survival was 72.2 months (about six years) for the patients given the combination therapy, and 59.3 months (a little under five years) for those receiving systemic chemotherapy alone. Moreover, 90 percent of the patients in the first group survived without any recurrence of the cancer in the liver, compared with 60 percent of the patients in the second group. Moderately severe side effects were similar in the two groups, except that the combined-therapy group experienced diarrhea more frequently.

Thus, according to this study, it is apparent that the combination of HAI (using the drug floxuridine) and systemic chemotherapy (injecting fluorouracil) can improve the outcome for patients with metastatic colorectal cancer.

Extensive studies are lacking, however, on patients who have primary liver cancer (tumors that started in the liver), or whose cancer metastasized from areas other than the colon or the rectum. Accordingly, HAI is infrequently administered to these patients.

Procedure

This procedure is done in an operating room as an open surgery, under general anesthesia, so the patient is asleep. A system of dispensing the cancer medication is fully implanted in the body. First, the surgeon has to open the abdomen and identify a branch of the hepatic artery that will be used to insert the catheter. After the catheter has been inserted, the pump is implanted under the skin (percutaneous) through a six-inch-long incision on the right side of the abdomen. The surgeon then attaches the catheter to the pump, which will be filled after surgery with chemotherapy medication.

During the course of the surgery, the surgeon will probably remove the GALLBLADDER. This is to prevent inflammation of the gallbladder that could result if the chemotherapy drug directed to the

liver travels to the gallbladder, which is connected to the liver by blood vessels.

This system permits the medication to be dispensed directly into the site of the tumor in the liver, over a period of time. The pump is periodically filled with the chemotherapy medication, usually about once a month, though the delivery schedule, as well as the medication used, varies according to the doctor.

The mechanism of the pump, in conjunction with the body temperature, will ensure that the drug is delivered steadily at a slow rate.

Various studies have shown that regional chemotherapy achieves higher concentrations of drugs at the site of the tumor, and is more effective in treating cancer, than systemic chemotherapy. Tumor growth is delayed, and patient survival rates are increased. The response rates for HAI are higher than with standard chemotherapy, as higher drug doses can be administered. At the same time, fewer side effects are experienced because the drugs are delivered directly into the artery of the liver. Not only can patients live longer, fewer side effects mean an improved quality of life. Even when the tumor continued to grow, with HAI, the uncomfortable physical symptoms of the disease tended to occur later.

Other advantages are that patients can participate in normal daily activities, and are fully mobile because the pump is implanted. The HAI system requires little or no home maintenance, and clinic visits are reduced.

Risks and Complications

Because the pump for delivering the medication must be implanted surgically, the complications of HAI are similar to those for most surgeries, such as reactions to anesthesia, wound infection, and incision breakdown. There may also be erosion of the skin over the pump. Sometimes, just as with regular chemotherapy, patients can have adverse reactions to the chemotherapeutic agent. These can include nausea and vomiting. Problems can also develop if too much or too little medication is delivered, due to improper handling or accidental damage to the pump. Because body temperature regulates the flow of the drug, if the patient develops a fever, more medication than prescribed could be pumped out.

Outlook and Lifestyle Modifications

As with any type of surgery, the patient should refrain from strenuous activity and lifting of heavy objects. Since the pump is implanted under the skin, patients should also avoid raising body temperature through hot tubs, steam baths, sauna, and heating pads. High altitudes can also affect the delivery of the drug. Full recovery can take up to three months.

At some hospitals, the catheter is placed in the hepatic artery with the laparoscopic method, which uses a laparoscope, a lighted tube. This technique substitutes small incisions for a large one needed to open the abdomen. It allows for faster recovery and less patient discomfort.

hepatitic coma, cholemia See HEPATIC ENCEPHALOPATHY.

hepatic encephalopathy (HE) Hepatic encephalopathy (HE) is a complication of LIVER disorders that causes brain and nervous system damage, resulting in mild to severe mental impairment. As a consequence of the abnormal brain function, the patient becomes mentally confused, with disorientation, difficulty in reasoning, erratic behavior, and changes in consciousness. If the encephalopathy is progressive, there is a gradual decrease in the level of consciousness, beginning with lethargy to sleepiness during the daytime and eventually reaching coma. Approximately 30 percent of end-stage liver disease patients go into a coma. When the onset of LIVER FAILURE is sudden, the prognosis is usually poor without a liver transplant.

HE occurs in both sudden-onset liver failure (fulminant hepatic failure) and in other conditions where blood circulation bypasses the liver or metabolism of toxic compounds is decreased within the liver because of poor functioning. Examples of these conditions include CIRRHOSIS, which causes permanent scarring of the liver, and HEPATITIS, which causes inflammation of the liver. In cirrhosis, abnormal architecture of the liver causes toxin-laden blood leaving the gut to bypass the liver. HE is seen in nearly 70 percent of patients with cirrhosis, and about 30 percent of cirrhosis patients die in hepatic coma.

The exact mechanism of HE is not known, but the condition probably results from a buildup of toxins that occurs when the diseased liver is unable to clear out these toxic products. Although the specific toxins responsible for this altered mental state have not been identified, several processes are thought to be involved with HE. First, metabolic toxins responsible for the mental confusion probably originate in the intestine, and the toxins may bypass the liver or be processed inadequately by a damaged liver. Second, excess ammonia in the blood may alter the blood's amino acid composition. Third, the blood-brain barrier normally keeps toxins out of the brain, but the blood-brain barrier in patients with encephalopathy is disturbed, allowing toxins to enter the brain. Fourth, liver production of compounds that maintain normal central nervous system function is reduced. Thus, the toxins carried in the blood exert either direct or indirect effect on the central nervous system. Some researchers believe that there may be multiple causes for this disorder, with a synergistic effect of toxic substances.

Ammonia neurotoxicity has the most support among researchers as a cause of HE. Ammonia is produced in the gastrointestinal tract, and, normally, the liver detoxifies ammonia. When the liver fails to clear ammonia from the blood, it may cause brain damage. However, studies have shown that the correlation between ammonia levels in blood and the severity of hepatic encephalopathy is inconsistent. Approximately 10 percent of patients with significant encephalopathy have normal ammonia levels, and many patients with cirrhosis have elevated levels of ammonia levels without evidence of encephalopathy. It is therefore unwise to rely on ammonia levels for diagnosis of HE. Nevertheless, whether this theory is totally or only partially correct, the most effective therapies for HE reduce ammonia in some way.

Symptoms and Diagnostic Path

In the early stages of HE, the changes are usually quite subtle. People suffering from HE often experience irritability, shortness of temper, mood swings, short-term memory loss, and changes in sleeping patterns. They may also be forgetful, confused, or disoriented, especially about time and place. In later stages, the confusion can become more severe, and the people so afflicted may even become violent. They may experience delirium (severe confusion with fluctuating levels of consciousness), changes in mood, decreased alertness, personality changes, and decreased ability to care for themselves. They may sleep for many hours and it may be difficult or impossible to arouse them. Encephalopathy accompanied by a significant loss of synthetic capability of the liver is a hallmark of severe acute liver failure (fulminant hepatic failure).

In addition to loss of cognitive function, the patients may lose certain simple motor skills, such as writing their own name or drawing a six-pointed star. This condition is called constructional apraxia. Another characteristic that doctors test for is liver flap, or flapping tremor. The patient is asked to hold his or her arms straight out with palms up and fingers spread apart, like a policeman stopping traffic. If the patient has encephalopathy, the hands may flap. Other conditions, such as drug toxicity, can also account for this involuntary movement. Another notable characteristic of HE is what is known as liver breath, or fetor hepaticus, where the patient's breath has a sweet, pungent, musty odor.

Physicians generally grade the symptoms of encephalopathy into the following five stages:

Grade 0—may appear normal, but tests show minimal changes in memory, concentration, intellectual function, and coordination

Grade 1—shows confusion and altered mood, with mood swings, irritability, decreased, and disordered sleep pattern

Grade 2—obvious personality changes with inappropriate behavior, some disorientation and drowsiness

Grade 3—markedly confused behavior, amnesia, stuporous but can be aroused; occasional fits of rage

Grade 4—coma

Some disorders, including effects related to alcohol consumption, mimic or mask symptoms of hepatic encephalopathy. These include intoxication, sedative overdose, alcohol withdrawal, and hypoglcyemica (low blood sugar).

Treatment Options and Outlook

Many patients may have other causes of encephalopathy in addition to HE, which makes it difficult to diagnose HE. Thus, generally accepted measures for the treatment of acute hepatic encephalopathy are to identify and immediately correct or eliminate any factors that could trigger encephalopathy or aggravate any existing encephalopathy. These factors include excessive use of diuretics; infection; constipation; bleeding in the gastrointestinal system; use of certain medications that act upon the central nervous system; electrolyte imbalances, such as low potassium level; kidney dysfunction; excessive alcohol consumption; stroke; hypoglycemia, or low blood sugar; organic brain damage; LIVER CANCER; and, rarely, excessive consumption of animal protein.

The standard therapy for treatment of HE is the administration of lactulose, an extremely sweet, synthetic sugar that is not absorbed from the gut. It is used to treat chronic constipation and disturbances of function in the central nervous system accompanying severe liver disease. Lactulose acts as a powerful laxative and also acidifies the stool, making it less favorable for ammonia and nitrogen-containing toxins. Usually, lactulolse is taken orally daily or twice daily. The doctor will probably advise the patient to take a sufficiently high dosage to have two to four loose stools per day. For comatose patients or anyone else unable to take the medication by mouth, lactulose may be administered as an enema.

Antibiotics that are not absorbed from the gut may also be prescribed. These antibiotics kill ammonia-producing bacteria in the intestines. Neomycin is one suitable antibiotic, although some studies question the effectiveness of this drug. Neomycin should be given only after beginning treatment with lactulose, and long-term treatment should be avoided because of possible adverse effects on organs or nerves involved in hearing or balance; it can also be poisonous to the kidneys. Other antibiotics that are sometimes given are metronidazole, paromomycin, oral vancomycin, and oral quinolones.

LIVER TRANSPLANTATION may be considered for patients with encephalopathy, particularly if the condition is caused by liver failure.

Since the early 1950s, standard treatment of hepatic encephalopathy has included restricting dietary protein. However, recent research appears to indicate that encephalopathy patients have an increased need for protein. Not only are high-protein diets well tolerated, they seem to help improve the mental state of patients. Moreover, patients with liver disorders tend to be malnourished to begin with, so further restriction of protein for a prolonged period may be detrimental. As a result of these considerations, the European Society for Parenteral and Enteral Nutrition (ESPEN) now recommends that traditional protein restriction should be abandoned in patients with hepatic encephalopathy. At the least, patients should not be on long-term protein restriction. Patients may turn to vegetarian sources of protein, because most experts believe that they are better than animal protein for anyone suffering from encephalopathy.

If the underlying liver disorder is corrected and treatment with lactulose is started in a timely fashion, encephalopathy can be reversed. When encephalopathy develops slowly with milder symptoms, patients can often recover completely. However, patients sometimes have a chronic form of encephalopathy, and, despite medical therapy, they continue to have symptoms. In contrast, acute hepatic encephalopathy associated with liver failure quickly progresses to profound coma. Once the patient reaches grade three or four, there is a high risk for swelling of the brain, which is very dangerous. There is a high mortality rate for patients with liver failure who receive only standard medical therapy. According to a report in the October 1992 issue of *Archives of Internal Medicine,* when a patient progresses to stage three or four encephalopathy, survival rates are poor, between 10 and 40 percent. But with liver transplantation, survival rates have increased to 60 to 80 percent. Therefore, effort should be made to identify patients for transplantation before they develop irreversible brain injury or other complications.

Basile, A. S., and E. A. Jones. "Ammonia and GABA-ergic neurotransmission: Interrelated factors in the pathogenesis of hepatic encephalopathy." *Hepatology* 25, no. 6 (1997): 1,303–1,305.

Nielsen, K., J. Kondrup, L. Martinsen, H. Dossing, B. Larsson, B. Stilling, et al. "Long-term oral refeeding of patients with cirrhosis of the liver." *British Journal of Nutrition* 74 (1995): 557–567.

Ong, J. P., et al. "Correlation between ammonia levels and the severity of hepatic encephalopathy." *American Journal of Medicine* 114 (February 15, 2003): 188–193.

Plauth, M., M. Merli, J. Kondrup, A. Weimann, P. Ferenci, M. J. Muller, and ESPEN Consensus Group. "ESPEN guidelines for nutrition in liver disease and transplantation." *Clinical Nutrition* 16 (1997): 43–55.

Riordan, Stephen M., and Roger Williams. "Treatment of hepatic encephalopathy." *New England Journal of Medicine* 337, no. 7 (August 14, 1997): 473(7).

Soulsby, Clare T., and Marsha Y. Morgan. "Dietary management of hepatic encephalopathy in cirrhotic patients: survey of current practice in United Kingdom." *British Medical Journal* 318, no. 7195 (May 22, 1999): 1,391.

Tarter, Ralph E., Switala, JoAnn, Plail, Joseph, Havrilla, Jeffrey, and David H. Van Thiel. "Severity of hepatic encephalopathy before liver transplantation is associated with quality of life after transplantation." *Archives of Internal Medicine* 152, no. 10 (October 1992): 2,097(5).

hepatitis   Hepatitis basically means inflammation of the LIVER. The word *hepatitis* simply means "inflammation [itis] of the liver [hepat]," and a diagnosis of hepatitis means nothing more than that the liver cells have become irritated or swollen; this condition results in an inflammation of the liver. It does not imply anything about the cause of the inflammation.

The five basic signs of inflammation include redness, warmth, swelling, tenderness, and loss of function. But while the inflammation of a joint is quite apparent, an individual may have hepatitis without being aware of it.

When most people think of hepatitis, they think of viral hepatitis, a LIVER DISEASE caused by various viruses. In addition to viruses, however, there are many other causes of hepatitis:

- autoimmunity (AUTOIMMUNE HEPATITIS)

- metabolic disorders, such as ALPHA 1-ANTITRYPSIN DEFICIENCY

- bacteria, fungi, or protozoa

- exposure to toxic agents (toadstool poisoning, for example)
- herbs, alcohol, or drugs (DRUG-INDUCED HEPATITIS)
- chemical poisons

Congenital defects, parasitic infections, metabolic disorders, and neoplasms may also result in hepatitis.

There are two main modes of transmission, blood-borne and fecal-oral routes. A blood-borne infection is spread by contact with contaminated blood; a fecal-oral route occurs when infection-laden stool from one person finds its way into the mouth of another. HEPATITIS A (HAV) and HEPATITIS E (HAE) are also known as fecal-borne hepatitis, for example, because of their mode of transmission.

Symptoms and Diagnostic Path

Because it performs so many functions, and because it plays a major role as a detoxifying agent, the liver is subject to a variety of environmental insults and toxins. It is one of the most frequently injured organs in the body.

Injury to the liver can cause a wide range of impairment to the liver's vital functions, yet in many instances of viral hepatitis, there are no symptoms. Many cases go undiagnosed because the symptoms suggest a flu-like illness, or they may be very mild or absent. And because the liver is so resilient, it gives little or no warning of its pathology until the damage is advanced. The liver generally continues to carry on its duties despite a significant amount of damage, but eventually the damage will lead to various types of dysfunction. When the liver suffers from inflammation, regardless of its specific cause, it leads to clinical manifestations that are often similar. Those classic symptoms include malaise, fatigue, mild fever, nausea, vomiting, anorexia (weight loss), vague abdominal pain (especially discomfort in the right upper quadrant above the liver), and sometimes diarrhea. There may also be muscle or joint aches and itching of the skin.

Hepatitis occurs in two general forms: acute and chronic.

Acute hepatitis Acute hepatitis is defined as hepatitis lasting fewer than six months. Acute hep-

atitis can be caused by bacterial, viral, and amebic infections, as well as by medicines and toxins. The condition usually comes on rapidly, with symptoms that may be severe, but it runs a short course. Autoimmune hepatitis, in which some liver cells (hepatocytes) are destroyed by the body's own immune system, can also occur as acute hepatitis. Hepatitis A, B, C, D, and E can all cause acute hepatitis.

In the early stages, the symptoms of acute hepatitis include the following:

- aching muscles and joints
- change in taste perception
- enlarged liver
- fatigue
- fever
- general malaise
- headache
- loss of appetite
- nausea
- skin rash

In later stages, symptoms include:

- dark urine
- jaundice (yellowing of the skin and whites of the eyes)
- light-colored stools

Acute hepatitis generally resolves on its own, but occasionally it can result in massive tissue destruction of the liver, leading to liver failure, or FULMINANT HEPATITIS.

Acute infectious viral hepatitis usually improves on its own. Fewer than one in 300 patients develops liver failure and, with it, the risk of death. Hepatitis caused by mononucleosis always improves on its own; acute hepatitis caused by medicines or alcohol usually improves once the patient stops taking the offending medicine or abstains from alcohol.

Chronic hepatitis Chronic hepatitis lasts longer than six months. A chronic condition usually comes on slowly and has a long course. The causes of chronic hepatitis are similar to that of acute hepatitis, but not all cases of viral hepatitis develop into chronic conditions. Contagious viral hepatitis such as hepatitis B, C, and D can cause chronic hepatitis. In addition, inborn metabolic disorders, such as WILSON'S DISEASE (a disorder of copper metabolism) and HEMOCHROMATOSIS (a disorder of iron metabolism) can lead to chronic hepatitis. Repeated exposure to toxins, such as alcohol and drugs, can also cause chronic hepatitis. Chronic inflammation, whatever the cause, may lead to advanced and irreversible scarring of the liver tissue known as CIRRHOSIS.

There may or may not be any symptoms. Many patients have no symptoms at first. When symptoms do develop, they include:

- abdominal pain
- aching muscles and joints
- enlarged liver
- fatigue
- increased need for sleep
- JAUNDICE (yellowing of skin and eyes)

Viral hepatitis Worldwide, viral hepatitis remains one of the leading causes of chronic liver disease, and is an area of active medical research. At least five distinct human hepatitis viruses have been identified, and they are responsible for the vast majority of cases of acute and chronic hepatitis. They have been named alphabetically in the order of their discovery: hepatitis A (HAV), B (HBV), C (HCV), D (HDV), and E (HEV). Two other possible hepatitis viruses, hepatitis F (HFV) and G (HGV), have been named, but they do not play a significant role in infection, and not all researchers agree that they even exist.

The primary target of a hepatitis virus is the hepatocyte, the major liver cell. It is there that the virus replicates, causing hepatocellular injury. Cell damage occurs either as a direct result of viral replication or as an immune-mediated response. (In an immune-mediated response, the body's attempts to eliminate the virus cause the inflammation of the liver and the problems associated with it.)

Many other viruses also affect the liver and cause inflammation, including infectious mononucleosis, yellow fever, herpes simplex, cytomegalovirus, Epstein-Barr, HIV (human immunodeficiency virus), and Ebola virus, which causes hemorrhagic fever. However, these viruses do not primarily target the hepatocyte. The vast majority of cases of viral hepatitis are caused by one of the hepatitis viruses (A, B, C, D, and E). Regardless of the cause, however, all instances of liver inflammation are classified as hepatitis. The patient may experience many of the same symptoms, though the duration and severity of the illnesses may differ.

The human hepatitis viruses are very different from one another. They cause different types of liver disease, and there are several possible ways to classify them. The common factor is that they are all viral in origin, meaning that the patient is infected by a virus.

Most people recover from hepatitis A and E. There may be mild flare-ups during the process of recovery, but a relapse does not necessarily preclude complete recovery. Hepatitis B, C, and D, on the other hand, can linger, becoming a chronic, possibly lifelong, infection. (An individual cannot become infected by hepatitis D unless he or she has already been infected by hepatitis B, or contracts hepatitis B and D at the same time.) Chronic hepatitis can lead to CIRRHOSIS and LIVER CANCER. Even those who are otherwise healthy may be able to infect others.

Hepatitis A Hepatitis A (HAV) is most commonly seen in children in developing countries, but its incidence has been increasing in the developed world. There are sometimes outbreaks of hepatitis A in restaurants or institutions where contaminated food has been served. People most often become infected by consuming contaminated food or water, by eating raw shellfish, or by using cooking utensils that have been contaminated. The incubation period is normally two to six weeks after exposure to the virus. Hepatitis A is an acute condition; it never turns chronic. Hepatitis A used to be called infectious hepatitis.

Hepatitis B HEPATITIS B (HBV) is a blood-borne disease, meaning that it is spread through exposure to an infected person's blood. It can also be transmitted through sexual contact. Hepatitis B can also be transmitted vertically, which means that it can be spread from an infected mother to her infant at birth. The incubation period is anywhere from four to 25 weeks.

About 10 percent of hepatitis B cases turn chronic; the rest are acute, and the patient recovers. When an individual is infected at birth or at a very young age, it is more likely to turn chronic.

Hepatitis C HEPATITIS C (HCV) used to be called non-A, non-B hepatitis before the virus was isolated. It is a blood-borne infection, primarily transmitted through direct blood contact. It is less commonly transmitted through sexual contact or vertical transmission from an infected mother to her child at birth. The incubation period is usually five to 10 weeks. The majority of hepatitis C cases are chronic; only about 25 percent of cases are considered acute. Symptoms may be nonexistent or may develop only later.

Hepatitis D HEPATITIS D (HDV) can infect only people who are already carriers of the hepatitis B virus. The incubation period is about two to eight weeks. It is found mainly in intravenous drug users, and can cause both acute and chronic conditions.

Hepatitis E HEPATITIS E (HEV) used to be known as enteric or epidemic non-A, non-B hepatitis. It is considered to be an acute condition.

Hepatitis F HEPATITIS F (HFV) may or may not exist. If the virus does exist, it appears to be transmitted by the oral-fecal route.

Hepatitis G HEPATITIS G (HGV) resembles hepatitis C but appears to be more benign. It is transmitted through blood and blood products.

Nonviral hepatitis There are two main types of nonviral hepatitis, alcoholic hepatitis and DRUG-INDUCED HEPATITIS (also known as toxic hepatitis). A third type, autoimmune hepatitis, is also nonviral but is uncommon.

Granulomatous hepatitis is sometimes mentioned as a nonviral hepatitis, but strictly speaking it is not a true hepatitis. In granulomatous hepatitis, white blood cells collect in the liver. The condition does not always cause liver inflammation, nor does it always cause fibrosis. Hepatic granulomas (a mass of granulated tissue usually associated with infections, particularly ulcerated infections) are found in about 3 to 10 percent of liver biopsies. Usually they indicate a systemic disorder rather than primary liver disease. There may be many causes, but the usual culprit is an infectious disease. The list of possible infections is long, and includes bacterial infections, such as tuberculosis and other mycobacterial infections; fungal infections, such as histoplasmosis and cryptococcosis; parasitic infections such as schistosomiasis—the most common worldwide—and toxoplasmosis; and, less commonly, viral infections, such as infectious mononucleosis. Other possible causes include Q fever, syphilis, and cat-scratch fever.

Autoimmune hepatitis In autoimmune hepatitis, liver inflammation is caused by the patient's own immune system. The condition is sometimes known as autoimmune chronic active hepatitis (CAH), idiopathic chronic active hepatitis, or lupoid hepatitis. Most patients with autoimmune hepatitis—about 70 percent—are women between the ages of 15 and 40.

Autoimmune hepatitis is a chronic and progressive condition, but the patient often shows symptoms of acute hepatitis, including jaundice, fever, and signs of severe liver dysfunction.

The reason for the immune system's attack is unknown, but researchers believe that genetic factors predispose some people to autoimmune hepatitis, as well as to other autoimmune conditions. Autoimmune hepatitis is often associated with the production of specific antibodies that can be detected by blood tests.

Autoimmune hepatitis is quite serious. The immediate result is liver inflammation. If untreated, it can result in long-term liver cell death, cirrhosis, and liver failure.

Alcoholic hepatitis Alcoholic hepatitis, a result of excessive alcohol intake, is the most common precursor of cirrhosis in the United States. Usually alcoholic hepatitis develops only after years, often decades, of alcohol abuse. That is not always the case, however. Some patients can develop hepatitis within a very short time of the onset of alcohol abuse, often within only a year.

Toxic hepatitis Toxic, or drug-induced, hepatitis is caused by inhaling or ingesting a toxic chemical. The symptoms are similar to viral hepatitis, but the damage to the liver tends to be more extensive.

Industrial chemicals toxic to the liver include carbon tetrachloride, vinyl chloride, and a variety of heavy metals. Toxic hepatitis can also be caused by poisonous mushrooms. The list of medications that can be toxic to the liver includes isoniazid (used to treat tuberculosis), methyldopa (a treatment for high blood pressure), acetaminophen (the pain reliever), oral contraceptives, and anabolic steroids.

Because of the similarity between viral hepatitis and toxic hepatitis, it is important for the physician and the patient to be wary. In any apparent case of viral hepatitis that does not conform to the usual demographic profile, or that does not respond to standard treatment, the possibility of toxic exposure should be investigated. The primary tools in that investigation include a history of exposure to hepatotoxic chemicals, medications, and other agents.

Neonatal hepatitis This uncommon form of hepatitis occurs only in newborns. NEONATAL HEPATITIS develops usually within two months of birth, and the cause can be difficult to determine. It may clear up within six months or cause permanent liver damage, depending on the cause and nature of the condition.

Signs and symptoms do not show the whole picture; the doctor therefore uses a variety of blood tests to determine the type of hepatitis the patient may be suffering from. The doctor may consider another possible diagnosis, such as syphilis, bacterial sepsis, leptospirosis (a type of bacterial infection), or schistosomiasis (a parasite infection).

Blood tests for detecting specific antigens and antibodies are necessary to demonstrate the agent responsible for viral hepatitis. Specific antigens test for viral proteins. The body's primary response to viral infection is to produce antibodies and T cells. At least three classes of antibodies are produced: immunoglobulin G (IgG), immunoglobulin M (IgM), and immunoglobulin A (IgA).

Viruses are very simple, and there is some debate as to whether they are truly life forms. Unlike most life forms, viruses do not have an independent metabolism and are unable to reproduce themselves. They must commandeer their host cells and can reproduce themselves only within their host cells by using the host's energy sources, chemical compounds, and protein synthesis machinery. In that sense, viruses may be likened to parasites.

One sign of virus is that it reproduces and randomly changes its genetic material. By doing so, a virus can evade the host's immune system.

Viruses are so tiny that they are measured in terms of nanometers. A nanometer is one billionth of a meter. The human red blood cell, one of the smallest cells in the body, is about thirty times the size of the largest virus. Viruses range in size from about 15 nanometers to 250 nanometers. Because viruses are so small, they cannot be seen under a regular microscope. They can be seen only with an electron microscope, an instrument that can produce enlarged images of tiny objects through a beam of electrons.

Viruses contain either ribonucleic acid (RNA) or deoxyribonucleic acid (DNA) as their genetic material. Animals and plants have only DNA as their genetic material. Most viruses have a core protein around which winds the viral RNA or DNA. Some viruses may be enveloped in a fatty (lipid) outer layer that contains specific viral proteins. Apart from the protein that is part of their structure, most viruses produce proteins to perform the biochemical functions necessary for them to reproduce.

Another characteristic of a virus is a property called cellular tropism. Tropism is an involuntary movement of an organism—or one of its parts—in response to an external stimulus. Tropism involves turning or curving toward or away from the stimulus. In the case of viruses, cellular tropism results in the virus preferentially infecting certain host cells. For example, the human immunodeficiency virus (HIV) has a preference for certain cells of the immune system. Viruses that cause hepatitis preferentially infect hepatocytes, the major cells of the liver, and are therefore referred to as primarily hepatotropic.

What makes viruses so lethal is their ability to mutate. Because they can reproduce rapidly, their mutation rates are high. That makes it difficult for the body to eliminate the virus from its system. Experts believe that mutation may be an important way that the hepatitis C virus escapes detection by the immune system. Mutation also makes it difficult to create vaccines or to design drugs, as the viruses can change the viral proteins that are normally the targets for drugs.

Another important characteristic of viruses that makes them lethal is a property called latency. Viruses may integrate their DNA, or a DNA copy of their RNA, into the DNA of the host cell. When they do so, the viruses propagate when the host cell divides. The viruses are not replicating, or are replicating only at a very low level, the viral particles that the host's immune system usually targets to kill. Consequently, the viruses remain in the body. These latent viruses can later be activated and begin to replicate again, making viral particles that are highly infectious. For instance, in hepatitis B, the virus can integrate into the host cell's DNA.

Furthermore, viruses commandeer the machinery of the cells they infect, using the host cell's energy and chemical compounds. That characteristic makes it extremely difficult to design drugs that can kill viruses. In the case of bacteria, antibiotics usually target the bacterial proteins that the bacteria uses to synthesize its proteins or for energy metabolism. But since a virus uses the host's protein synthesis machinery, drugs cannot be directed against the proteins to inhibit viral replication, because that would also kill the host cells.

All those characteristics can make viral causes of hepatitis difficult to detect and difficult to expel from the body. The long-term consequences of viral hepatitis may include CIRRHOSIS, which involves permanent damage to the liver structure and function, and LIVER CANCER.

Treatment Options and Outlook

The management of hepatitis primarily involves removing the patient from exposure to its cause, to the extent possible. Any drugs or substances known to be toxic, such as alcohol, should be immediately discontinued. Nonessential medication may be stopped; for other medications, the physician should determine a course of action on a case-by-case basis.

The patient may receive supportive care and rest as needed. General measures include a well-balanced diet. The doctor should evaluate any herbs or other substances the patient is taking, and weigh carefully the risk versus benefit of any medication or herbal product, especially if the patient has acute hepatitis.

Sedatives should not be given, especially if the patient shows signs of mental confusion or other altered mental status (encephalopathy). Sedatives can mask signs of fulminant hepatitis or even trigger it.

Dienstag, J. L. "Hepatitis non-A, non-B: C at last." *Gastroenterology* 9 (1990): 1,177–1,180.

Huppertz, H. I., et al. "Autoimmune hepatitis following hepatitis A virus infection." *Journal of Hepatology* 23, no. 2 (August 1995): 204–208.

Lee, William M., M.D. "Hepatitis B virus infection." *New England Journal of Medicine* 337, no. 24 (December 11, 1997): 1,733–1,745.

Radetsky, P. *The Invisible Invaders: Viruses and the Scientists Who Pursue Them.* Boston: Little, Brown, 1994.

hepatitis A   Hepatitis A is an inflammation of the liver caused by a virus known as the hepatitis A virus (HAV). While HAV is highly infectious, it is considered to be the most benign of the five major hepatitis viruses (A, B, C, D, and E). HAV causes an acute infection, generally mild and short-lived, though 15 percent of cases may be protracted, with some relapses over a six- to nine-month period. Most patients recover without complications. Unlike HEPATITIS B or C, hepatitis A does not cause a chronic liver disease, and there is no danger of developing cancer. Some people, however, can become gravely ill from contracting HAV. In about 1 percent of the cases, mostly in people over 50, the infection can lead to severe and acute liver failure and, in rare cases, death.

Hepatitis A is an exceptionally stable virus that replicates within liver cells. HAV was the first hepatitis virus to be identified, in 1973. Before that time, it was known by various names, including *infectious hepatitis, epidemic hepatitis,* and *epidemic jaundice,* but these terms are no longer used.

Hepatitis A is the most prevalent in underdeveloped countries, but it is also common in the United States, where HAV accounts for one-fourth of all viral hepatitis, with 25,000 to 30,000 cases of hepatitis A reported each year. These may be isolated cases of disease or epidemics. Roughly 22 to 26 percent of the infection source is household or sexual contact with a person infected with HAV.

All hepatitis A cases must be reported to the Centers for Disease Control and Prevention. But the infection is underreported because some people have no symptoms, while others mistake the infection for a bad case of the flu and never see a doctor.

When patients recover, they develop lifelong immunity to HAV. Developing resistance to one type of viral hepatitis, however, does not automatically confer immunity to other hepatitis viruses, such as hepatitis B and C. It is also possible for one person to be infected by several different hepatitis viruses.

Symptoms and Diagnostic Path

The patient may develop one or more symptoms: fatigue, abdominal discomfort, fever, loss of appetite, and sense of malaise (discomfort). Symptoms usually come on quickly. In some cases a person may notice darker urine and lighter stool a few days before the onset of jaundice. Smokers often report that they suddenly find cigarettes distasteful. Symptoms usually resolve within two months, though a few patients may be ill for up to six months.

The severity of the symptoms increases with age. Most infected children (75–95 percent) have no symptoms, while the majority of adults (75–95 percent) experience some symptoms. The infection is most serious in older patients and those with other health conditions, such as hepatitis B and C.

The incubation period—the interval between contracting the virus and the onset of illness—varies between 15 and 50 days. The average is about 30 days. Usually the more severe the infection, the shorter the incubation period.

The most infectious time is the middle of the incubation period and before the onset of symptoms, generally about two weeks preceding. The patient remains infectious a week or so following the development of symptoms.

HAV is transmitted primarily via the fecal-oral route. First, the virus is shed in the feces of the infected person. Then an unsuspecting person puts something in the mouth that has been contaminated by the infected stool. This happens quite frequently in third world countries, as HAV can remain virulent for a long period outside the host. Water and food can be easily contaminated in areas with poor sanitation or where personal hygiene is not strictly observed. Children in developing countries with inadequate sewage systems and poor sanitary conditions are almost universally infected, though few show clinical symptoms, and they then acquire lifelong immunity.

Periodic outbreaks of hepatitis A occur in developed countries as well, especially in restaurants and public institutions where large groups of people can become easily exposed to the virus. Foods often associated with HAV include lettuce, frozen strawberries, hamburger meats, raw oysters, and other shellfish. In 2003, hundreds of people were infected and three died after eating at a Mexican restaurant in Pittsburgh, Pennsylvania, believed to be the largest outbreak on record in the United States. Investigators suspect that raw or lightly cooked green onions imported from Mexico were contaminated with the virus. In other cases, the chef or other food handlers with hepatitis A unwittingly spread the virus through the food they served. It is generally difficult to trace the source because hepatitis A has a long incubation period.

Anyone living in the same household as an infected person or in communities with poor sanitary conditions are at risk for acquiring HAV.

Children are a major means of infection for both adults and other children, because people come into close physical contact with them, and because they often show no symptoms. Employees and children at day-care centers are thus particularly vulnerable to infection. It is estimated that in the United States, 14 to 40 percent of all cases of HAV infection are of children at day-care centers.

Institutions for the developmentally disabled have higher incidences of HAV infection because of crowded conditions and less than meticulous personal hygiene of the residents. The situation has improved, however, and fewer outbreaks have been reported.

Troops living under crowded conditions are also at high risk.

The use of intravenous drugs also increases the likelihood of infection. Other potentially risky behavior includes engaging in oral or anal sex. In rare cases there have been instances of HAV transmission through infected blood.

Nonhuman primates, such as apes and monkeys, can also transmit HAV to people who come in close contact with them.

A diagnosis cannot be based solely on symptoms and signs. Blood tests usually reveal elevated alanine transaminase (ALT) and asparate transaminase (AST). But that tells the doctor little other than that there may be a liver abnormality. The only way to make a definitive diagnosis is by checking for the presence of an antibody to HAV. Testing positive for IgM antibodies is an indication that the individual is currently infected with HAV. IgM is usually detected during the acute phase of the infection and for three to six months thereafter.

There is another HAV antibody called IgG. Testing positive for IgG shows that the patient has been exposed to or infected by HAV in the past. If the IgG is present but the IgM cannot be detected, the patient no longer has an active infection, is not infectious to others, and cannot become infected with HAV again.

No radiologic (imaging studies) or liver biopsy is necessary to diagnose hepatitis A.

Treatment Options and Outlook

For most people, getting plenty of rest and drinking lots of fluids is sufficient. Avoid alcohol or other drugs that can further damage the liver. Nothing can shorten the course of the illness. Antibiotics are not effective against viral diseases. The doctor may prescribe a short course of steroid treatment if there is any itching. If itching persists, the patient should be checked for the presence of other liver disorders.

Patients who become very ill may require hospitalization. In rare instances the patient may develop severe jaundice, mental confusion, stupor, and even coma. This is a sign of impending liver failure, and the patient should be hospitalized immediately into an intensive care unit. Prompt referral and preparation should also be made for a liver transplant.

The course and management of HAV is the same for pregnant women in developed countries, and they generally do quite well. In developing countries, however, the infection may prove fatal in pregnant women, possibly because of inadequate nutrition.

Risk Factors and Preventive Measures

Thanks to improvements in sanitation and sanitary systems throughout much of the world, the prevalence of HAV infections appears to be decreasing. Far fewer children are catching HAV, and the age at which infection is likely to occur is rising. Ironically, when infection is delayed and people contract hepatitis A as adolescents or adults, their symptoms are more severe. The likelihood of developing a serious liver disease is greater. Researchers warn that exposure to HAV at a later age could lead to more outbreaks and higher instances of death.

An individual can help keep hepatitis A from spreading in three ways. One is through good personal hygiene. Householders living with a hepatitis A–infected person should wash their hands after using the bathroom and changing diapers, and before eating and handling food. Restaurant staff should be particularly meticulous about hand washing. The same goes for workers at day care centers and institutions, who should observe commonsense measures about maintaining sanitary conditions.

When traveling to areas of high infection, drink only bottled water (make sure that ice cubes are made from purified water), peel fruits, and avoid raw foods and shellfish, that often live in contaminated water. A recent study suggests that microwaving foods may reduce the risk of HAV infection. But cooking vegetables in a microwave oven destroys most of the vitamin B, so it is not advisable as a long-term preventive strategy.

Despite the best precautions the possibility of infection remains. The other two preventive measures are vaccinations against hepatitis A and passive immunization with immune globulin.

Hepatitis A vaccine The FDA approved an inactivated hepatitis A vaccine in February 1995. This vaccine does not contain any live hepatitis viruses. It is regarded as safe and effective and provides long-term protection, probably about 15 to 20 years' worth. In the United States, the vaccine is licensed for use for adults and for children over the age of two. Children younger than that should not be vaccinated. If they are going to be at risk, they may receive immune globulin instead.

Two shots of hepatitis A vaccine are given spaced about six months apart. Should there be a delay in the second dose of vaccine for any reason, the person should try to obtain it as soon as possible. There is no need to repeat the first dose. There should be no problem if the second dose of vaccine is from a different manufacturer than the first one.

The vaccine gives protection four weeks after the initial dose. Anyone visiting high-risk areas on short notice (within fewer than four weeks) should also receive immune globulin at a different injection site. If long-term protection is needed, a second dose of hepatitis A vaccine should be given six months after the first.

Travelers who also need to be protected against hepatitis B virus (HBV), and who must depart on short notice, can receive an HAV-HBV combination vaccine on an accelerated schedule. This combination vaccine gives most people protection against both viruses within as few as two months after the initial dose. The vaccination consists of three doses. The second dose is given a month after the first dose, and the third dose, six months later. It also reduces the number of shots a person would otherwise need to complete the series. The combination is as effective as vaccines given separately.

In addition to immune globulin, other vaccines can be administered at the same time as the hepatitis A vaccine. But separate sites must be used for each injection. These include hepatitis B, diphtheria, cholera, rabies, Japanese encephalitis, yellow fever, and tetanus, to name a few.

There is no danger of adverse reactions if a person already immune to hepatitis A happens to be vaccinated. A person need not get tested for natural immunity unless the cost of the vaccine exceeds that of the test or there are other reasons to avoid vaccinations.

HAV vaccination is recommended for the following people:

- more likely to get hepatitis A
- more likely to get seriously ill if they do get hepatitis A
- have chronic liver disease
- international travelers
- sexually active gay men
- living with HAV-infected people

- sexual contact with HAV-infected people
- intravenous drug users
- workers at day-care centers

Regarding travelers, the U.S. Centers for Disease Control and Prevention (CDC) recommends HAV vaccine for people who will be visiting or living in Africa, Asia (except Japan), the Mediterranean basin, eastern Europe, the Middle East, Mexico, Central and South America, or the Caribbean.

Starting in 2000 in the United States, routine vaccination has been recommended for children born in states with twice the national average of HAV (20 cases of infection per 100,000). These states are Alaska, Arizona, California, Idaho, Nevada, New Mexico, Oklahoma, Oregon, South Dakota, Utah, and Washington. Vaccination is suggested in states that have infection rates 1.5 times the national average, namely, Arkansas, Colorado, Missouri, Montana, Texas, and Wyoming.

According to a report in *Liver Transplant* published in 2000, researchers at the Mayo Clinic found that some of the patients who receive liver transplants may lose their immunity to the hepatitis A virus after the transplantation. These findings "may have implications for future vaccine recommendation," M. Arslan and colleagues said in their report.

Immune globulin   Immune globulin is a preparation of antibodies (immune proteins) that can be given to provide short-term protection either before or after exposure to HAV.

Because HAV-infected people are at their most contagious before symptoms start, they often expose others, especially family members, to the disease without knowing it. Anyone who has had close personal contact with a person with hepatitis A, including household and sexual contacts, or infected persons in day-care centers and other institutions, or an infected food handler, are candidates for receiving immune globulin.

The following individuals may also consider getting immune globulin:

- anyone at risk of infection but who is allergic to hepatitis A vaccine, or otherwise chooses not to be vaccinated

- travelers who have to leave on short notice to a country where hepatitis A is endemic (it takes four weeks for the vaccination to take effect). A single dose of 0.02 mL/kg of immune globulin offers protection for up to three months. If the trip is expected to last longer than five months, travelers should receive an initial dose of 0.06 mL/kg. The injection should be repeated every four to six months

- anyone recently exposed to HAV but not vaccinated against the virus. The immune globulin should be given as soon as possible, but within two weeks after exposure to the virus for maximum protection. Doing so will prevent HAV infection more than 90 percent of the time

- children at risk under two years of age

Immune globulin can also be administered during pregnancy and breast feeding.

Associated disease Sometimes a person may suffer from an inflammation of the GALLBLADDER (cholecystitis) caused by the hepatitis A virus infecting certain cells of the gallbladder.

Approximately 10 percent of people who contract hepatitis A develop an illness called cholestatic hepatitis. This is characterized by a failure of bile flow accompanied by deep jaundice and severe itching.

HAV may also trigger a type of chronic AUTO-IMMUNE HEPATITIS in genetically susceptible individuals. This is a liver disease in which the body's antibodies attack components of its own liver cells. The liver fights back and becomes inflamed in the process.

There is also new evidence that a number of viral infections, including hepatitis A, are strongly associated with heart attacks and cardiovascular death.

Researchers are working to develop new, more convenient vaccines against HAV. There is an urgency to this search because currently available hepatitis A vaccines require multiple boosters and are not feasible in developing countries. This presents a problem because people in developing countries are losing their natural immunity to hepatitis A as sanitary conditions improve.

The World Health Organization has designated the creation of a better hepatitis A vaccine as part of its development program.

Arslan, M., J. B. Gross, J. R., J. J. Poterucha, R. H. Wiesner, and N. N. Zein. "Hepatitis A antibodies in liver transplant recipients: Evidence for loss of immunity post-transplantation." *Liver Transplant* 6, no. 2 (2000): 191–195.

Barzaga, B. N. "Hepatitis A shifting epidemiology in South-East Asia and China." *Vaccine* suppl. 1(2) (February 2000): S61–S64.

Centers for Disease Control and Prevention. "Foodborne transmission of hepatitis A." *Morbidity and Mortality Weekly Report* 52, no. 124 (June 20, 2003): 565(3).

Editorial Staff. "Hepatitis A breaks out in the west of Pennsylvania." *Contemporary Pediatrics* 20, no. 13 (December 2003).

Editorial Staff. "Hepatitis A picture is shifting globally." *Hepatitis Weekly*, March 13, 2000.

Mishu, Ban, Stephen C. Hadler, Valerie A. Boaz, Robert H. Hutcheson, John M. Horan, and William Schaffner. "Hepatitis A: Evidence that microwaving reduces risk?" *Journal of Infectious Diseases* 162, no. 3 (September 1990): 655(4).

Mourani, Samir, Stuart M. Dobbs, Robert M. Genta, Atul K. Tandon, and Boris Yoffe. "Hepatitis A virus-associated cholecystitis." *Annals of Internal Medicine* 120, no. 5 (March 1, 1994): 398(3).

Muhlestein, Joseph, M.D., et al. "Study links infections and cardiovascular death." *Antiviral Weekly* no. 1 (March 28, 2000): NA.

Nichols, Sonia. "Hepatitis A and B vaccine combo protects when accelerated schedule needed." *Vaccine Weekly*, February 13, 2002, p. 4.

Worcester, Sharon. "HAVgenes (Clinical Capsules)" *Internal Medicine News* 35, no. 18 (September 15, 2002): 16(1).

hepatitis B Hepatitis B is an inflammation of the LIVER caused by a virus called hepatitis B (HBV). Although hepatitis B was recognized as clinically distinct from hepatitis A in the 1930s, it was not until 1965 that the existence of the B virus was discovered accidentally by Dr. Baruch Blumberg and his collaborators. They found the protein of the hepatitis B virus in the blood of an Australian aborigine and called it the Australia ANTIGEN. (Antigens are chemicals that the body recognizes as a foreign substance and against which it sets off an immune response.) They did not realize then that it was a viral protein, but a few years later they proved that the antigen was associated with hepatitis.

Hepatitis B is a serious global health problem. Left untreated, chronic hepatitis B can lead to scarring of the liver, which can then progress to primary LIVER CANCER—cancer that originates in the liver. HBV is estimated to cause 60 to 80 percent of the world's primary liver cancer.

According to the Centers for Disease Control and Prevention, 1.25 million people in the United States are afflicted with chronic, or lifelong, hepatitis B, and every year some 5,000 people die from liver disease caused by hepatitis B. Approximately 350 million people worldwide have chronic hepatitis, and it is estimated that 250,000 die each year from hepatitis B–related LIVER DISEASE.

Different geographic areas of the world have different prevalence rates for HBV. HBV is highly endemic (always present) in Asia, the Pacific, and sub-Saharan Africa. Other regions with high rates of HBV infection include parts of eastern and central Europe, the Middle East, and the Indian subcontinent. In many of these countries, the majority of people acquire HBV as infants or children, whereas in northern European countries and North America, most people get the infection as an adult through the sharing of needles or having unprotected sex with an infected person.

The HBV is a small, spherical virus that primarily infects liver cells. The virus belongs to the family of Hepadnaviridae. Similar hepatitis viruses that belong to this same family can infect ducks, ground squirrels, and woodchucks. For this reason these animals have often been used for medical experiments related to hepatitis.

The HBV is an enveloped virus; it has a central, inner core surrounded by an outer shell. The outer shell, or envelope, is made up of a protein called hepatitis B surface antigen, or HBsAg. This outer surface of the hepatitis B virus triggers the body's immune response, and antibodies are produced to attack the virus. The hepatitis B blood tests can detect this surface antigen in the blood of infected individuals. A test result of HBsAg positive means that the person is infected with the hepatitis B virus.

The inner core is made up of a circular, partially double-stranded DNA and enzymes used in viral replication. These enzymes are called DNA polymerase. The core also contains a protein called the hepatitis B core antigen. It is given the designation HBcAg, shorthand for hepatitis B core antigen. HB refers to hepatitis B, c is core, and Ag, antigen. An antigen is a protein or carbohydrate that triggers an immune response in the body. It causes the production of antibodies to protect the body. Another protein contained in the core is hepatitis B e antigen (HBeAg). The hepatitis B e antigen is correlated with active replication of the virus, of how rapidly the virus is multiplying. The faster the virus multiplies, the more virus particles there are in the blood, and the more contagious the infected person. The B e antigen therefore serves as a marker for the virus's ability to spread the infection. When a person recovers from acute hepatitis B, the surface antigen disappears from the blood (HBsAg–). If the disease becomes chronic, the surface antigen remains in the blood (HBsAg+).

HBV is a blood-borne infection; its primary mode of transmission is through contaminated blood or blood products; sexual contact is also an important means of infection. The virus can be passed on through contact with the blood or body fluids, including the semen, vaginal discharge, saliva, breast milk, and menstrual blood of an infected person. HBV is also found in the urine, but only in low concentrations; there is none in the feces.

Because blood donations were not screened for HBV before 1975 (in developed countries), people who received a blood transfusion before then are at risk. But today, the risk of transmission is very low because all blood, organ, and tissue donations in developed countries are now routinely tested for HBV.

The nature of their occupation puts health care workers at risk, but patients can also be exposed to contamination through medical instruments and equipment. For instance, heart patients undergoing cardiac bypass surgery, transplant patients who receive organs, or women giving birth may all be more vulnerable to the disease. In the United States, the highest incidence of acute (short duration) hepatitis B is among young adults, and the most common means of transmission is through sexual intercourse.

Another common method of transmission among young people is through intravenous (using needles) drug use. Minute amounts of blood left on everyday objects can also result in inadvertent infection. Being quite stable, the virus remains on contaminated needles or surgical tools. So it is possible to acquire HBV by getting a tattoo, ear piercing, dental work, or acupuncture, if unsterile instruments are used. On the other hand, HBV cannot be spread by casual contact, such as hugging, kissing, shaking hands, and so forth. Accordingly, acquiring an HBV infection in an office environment is unlikely. Unlike hepatitis A, the virus is not spread through food or water, and sharing eating utensils or drinking glasses does not put one at risk for hepatitis B. Nor does eating food prepared by an infected person.

One of the most common means of hepatitis B (HBV) transmission is from mother to baby during childbirth. In many parts of the world, this is the most common method of infection. It is therefore recommended that all pregnant women be screened for hepatitis B. If an expectant mother has hepatitis B, arrangements can be made to have the proper medications ready in the delivery room for vaccinating the newborn. The vaccinations help the babies' bodies make antibodies to protect them. The majority of adults can eliminate HBV from their bodies, but the immune system of infants and children are still immature and cannot fight off the virus as effectively. This is why as many as nine out of 10 babies born to infected mothers end up being hepatitis B carriers for the rest of their lives. Moreover, people infected as infants or children do not respond as well to medication to suppress HBV, and are far less likely to have a remission of the illness. They are also more prone to developing advanced scarring and liver cancer.

As long as infants receive the proper vaccination, roughly 95 percent will be protected from hepatitis B. The baby should be given two shots within 12 hours of birth: the first dose of the hepatitis B vaccine, and one shot of the hepatitis B Immune Globulin (HBIG). The second dose of hepatitis B vaccine should be given when the infant is one to two months old, and the third dose at age six months, to ensure complete protection.

Occasionally, even when given the proper immunization, babies born to pregnant women with high levels of HBV DNA (the marker for hepatitis B) become infected. One study suggests that giving the expectant mothers short-term therapy with a daily dose of 150 mg of lamivudine (Epivir-HBV) in the last month of pregnancy can prevent infection to the newborn. This approach needs to be further evaluated.

In the past, infected mothers were discouraged from breast-feeding their babies because the virus can be found in breast milk. But only a small amount is present in breast milk. In fact, the benefits of breast-feeding outweigh the slight risk of infection—which can be further reduced by giving the vaccines. The Centers for Disease Control and Prevention (CDC) now recommend that women be encouraged to breast-feed their newborns to give them nutritional advantages unavailable from infant formulas. It is safe to start breast-feeding immediately if the baby has been given the proper shots. The mother should make sure that her nipple areas are not cracked or bleeding.

In countries where HBV is widespread or is persistently present in the population, such as in Southeast Asia and sub-Saharan Africa, infants commonly become infected at birth. The rate of infection is extremely high, nearly 100 percent. Moreover, about 95 percent of the babies will develop chronic HBV infection.

The U.S. Department of Health and Human Services recommends that the following people be vaccinated for hepatitis B because they have an increased risk for infection:

- individuals living in the same household with an infected person
- individuals having sex with more than one partner
- sex partners of people infected with the virus
- men who have sex with other men

- individuals who recently had a sexually trans-mitted disease, such as gonorrhea or syphilis
- illicit drug users who use needles and syringes
- individuals who get tattoos or body piercing
- travelers to countries where HBV is common (Asia, Africa, South America, the Pacific Islands, eastern Europe, and the Middle East)
- individuals emigrating from countries where hepatitis B is common (see above)
- families adopting children from countries where hepatitis B is common (see above)
- kidney dialysis patients
- individuals who use blood products for medical conditions, such as hemophilia
- individuals who received a transfusion of blood or blood products before 1975
- infants born to infected mothers
- health care workers and others whose job exposes them to human blood

Symptoms and Diagnostic Path

Like HEPATITIS C, hepatitis B is a silent disease. Almost 70 percent of infected people have no symptoms and feel quite healthy. When there are signs and symptoms, they are generally relatively mild and are often mistaken for a bad case of the flu. Because people are so often unaware that they are infected, they unknowingly pass the virus on to others; this is one reason that HBV has spread throughout the world.

The incubation period—the time between exposure to the virus and the first symptoms—of HBV is quite long. Symptoms occur from six weeks to six months after infection; they can range from mild to severe. People who become sicker generally have a better chance of recovering completely than those who have few or no symptoms. The infection often becomes chronic for people who appear not to be affected by the illness.

The following are some of the common symptoms of acute hepatitis:

- abdominal discomfort or pain around the liver area

- altered sense of taste and smell
- anorexia (loss of appetite)
- fatigue
- fever
- JAUNDICE (yellowing of skin and eyes)
- mild nausea
- muscle or joint pain
- vomiting

Doctors often refer to hepatitis that is accompanied by the yellowing of the skin as acute icteric (jaundiced) hepatitis.

Occasionally, before the actual onset of the symptoms of hepatitis, patients may develop ill effects that are seemingly unrelated to the infection. Called prodromal symptoms, they may resemble an allergic reaction or flu-like symptoms. Individuals may suffer from severe joint stiffness, swelling, and pain. These symptoms of arthritis usually appear suddenly and can be quite severe. Quite often, several joints are affected (polyarthritis), usually the hands and knees, but other large joints can be involved as well. In the majority of cases, the symptoms of arthritis spontaneously subside within a week or two with the onset of jaundice (yellowing of skin and eyes). It is essential to recognize that this arthritis is associated with hepatitis B, and will resolve itself with the hepatitis. This is important because regular treatments for arthritis such as steroids and other medications can aggravate the infection and cause the virus to replicate faster.

In rare cases (less than 1 percent of adults), acute hepatitis can follow a severe downward course, progressing to sudden-onset liver failure, called FULMINANT HEPATITIS. Signs and symptoms of LIVER FAILURE should not be ignored. The affected individual requires immediate hospitalization and emergency medical care. These include abdominal swelling from an accumulation of fluids (ASCITES), severe nausea and vomiting, COAGULOPATHY (bleeding disorder), and mental confusion or coma. Without prompt medical intervention and LIVER TRANSPLANTATION, about 80 percent of such patients die.

The course of chronic hepatitis B depends on many factors, including the patient's age at which the infection begins. The immune system of individuals infected at birth or as children—as is most commonly the case in some parts of Asia and Africa—does not react to the HBV, possibly because it does not recognize the virus as a foreign substance. This stage of the illness is sometimes known as the immune-tolerant phase, and can last for years. The affected individual does not have symptoms, and little or no damage is done to the liver. Ironically, the damage done to the liver when a person contracts hepatitis B is not directly caused by the virus but by the immune system's attack against the infected liver cells in its attempt to throw off the virus. Although there may be few symptoms in the immune-tolerant phase, tests will show measurable amounts of the hepatitis B surface antigen (HBsAg+), the hepatitis e antigen (HBeAg+), and HBV DNA.

People infected as adults, which is usually the case in more developed countries, never go through this phase. Instead, they go right to the next stage, in which the immune system works to eliminate the virus from the body. Those infected in childhood may enter this phase as late as the third or fourth decade of an infection. As a result of the injury to the infected liver cells by the immune system's aggressive attacks, tests measuring LIVER ENZYMES, such as the ALT and AST, become elevated. LIVER BIOPSY may also show significant inflammation and the formation of scar tissue. The severity of liver cell destruction depends on the duration and strength of the immune response.

After this, the viral infection enters a dormant, or quiescent, phase. During this time, the liver enzymes are normal or almost normal. There is an ongoing presence of HBV infection, and the individual generally remains positive for the B surface antigen. The HBV DNA level is low. The marker of viral reproduction, the B e antigen, will disappear; at the same time, the B e antibodies (anti-HBe) will appear. This quiescent phase can last many years, but the individual can revert to the more active phase.

Some people have detectable B surface antigens (HBsAg) in their blood, but have no signs or symptoms of hepatitis B. Lab tests reveal normal levels of the liver enzymes ALT and AST. If a liver biopsy

examining liver tissue is performed, about 25 percent of patients with no obvious symptoms may in fact have inflammation of the liver. The biopsy may even show advanced scarring of the liver. In about 75 percent of these patients, however, a biopsy may show no evidence of inflammation. Individuals with little clinical evidence of chronic hepatitis are called healthy carriers, and their chance of developing CIRRHOSIS and liver cancer is small, although somewhat higher than for those not chronically infected with HBV.

Healthy carriers can, however, transmit the disease to others, so they should exercise proper precaution. In very rare cases, and only in individuals who acquired HBV in adulthood, healthy carriers may spontaneously lose the surface antigen. This is typically associated with a cure.

It is also possible for a healthy carrier to experience a reactivation or "flare" when the virus becomes active again.

Acute hepatitis B An acute hepatitis B infection occurs when a person first gets infected with the virus. The illness from the infection lasts six months or less. During the acute stage, the infected individual can pass the virus to others. Most healthy adults, about 90 to 95 percent, are able to recover from HBV. They will develop protective antibodies against future infections of hepatitis B. (However, they can acquire other hepatitis infections.)

Individuals who have a stronger immune response are more likely to eliminate the virus and recover. This is why the person who has more severe symptoms and appears to be sicker usually recovers. A weaker immune response causes fewer symptoms but may fail to rid the body of the invading viruses. This explains why infants and children are much more likely to develop chronic HBV, but rarely show any symptoms.

On the other hand, a strong immune response can be a mixed blessing. While it can protect the body against invading viruses, it can also damage the liver. Ironically, in an HBV infection, it is the body's reaction to the virus, not the hepatitis B virus itself, that directly injures the liver.

Chronic hepatitis B By definition, if a person continues to be infected by HBV six months after its onset, the infection is no longer considered acute, but chronic. The person becomes a chronic carrier of hepatitis B. For unknown reasons, men are six times more likely than women to suffer from chronic hepatitis B. But the overall probability that an acute hepatitis B infection will turn chronic in adults is quite low, about 1 to 5 percent. As mentioned earlier, however, infants and children are much more susceptible. Because their immune systems are still immature, their bodies are less equipped to eliminate the virus. In infants, the likelihood of developing chronic hepatitis B is 90 to 95 percent; children have up to a 50 percent chance that the condition will become chronic.

Although HBV infection is relatively rare in developed countries, in other parts of the world, liver disease associated with chronic hepatitis B is one of the top-10 causes of death.

HBV-related cirrhosis of the liver Inflammation of the liver caused by the hepatitis B virus causes scarring of the liver. It is estimated that in 15 to 20 percent of patients, the scarring will become irreversible (cirrhosis) within five years. These patients will develop symptoms of cirrhosis such as fatigue, loss of muscle mass, and general weakness. A worsening of the patient's condition will lead to advanced cirrhosis and all its attendant complications. The condition is called decompensated cirrhosis. Complications can include swollen feet and ankles (edema), swollen abdomen (ascites), gastrointestinal bleeding, mental confusion (encephalopathy), and jaundice. In rare occasions, some patients can have breathing difficulties because of abnormal functioning of the lungs (hepatopulmonary syndrome) caused by cirrhosis. If the virus remains active, and scarring progresses to advanced cirrhosis, only 55 to 85 percent of patients survive for more than five years.

HBV and liver cancer Everyone who has chronic HBV is at higher risk for developing primary liver cancer—cancer that originates in the liver and not from another organ. But the patient with the advanced scarring of the liver that is the hallmark of cirirhosis runs an even higher risk of developing cancer. And if the virus is actively reproducing, rather than lying dormant, the individual is also more susceptible to liver cancer. Exactly how HBV can lead to cancer is not fully understood, but researchers believe that the HBV DNA somehow becomes incorporated into the DNA of the patient's liver cell.

The exact risk for developing cancer is not known; it is relatively rare in the United States. But in parts of the world where hepatitis B is widespread, liver cancer is the leading cause of cancer-related deaths.

Not everyone's chance of developing cirrhosis and cancer is equal. Aside, perhaps, from genetic susceptibility, individuals with compromised immune systems—patients whose immune systems are already weakened by receiving chemotherapy or taking immunosuppressive (anti-rejection) medications after transplantation—have a heightened risk. Others in this category are chronic carriers who were infected as infants or children. The physician may recommend that these patients be regularly tested for cancer. Screening is usually done by ultrasound and Alpha-FetoProtein (AFP), which tests for a liver tumor marker.

Some common symptoms of liver cancer include abdominal pain and swelling, weight loss, and fever. The physician may discover an enlarged liver, increased red blood cells (erythrocytosis), high blood calcium (hypercalcemia), and low blood sugar (hypoglycemia). Although there can be other causes for these symptoms, hepatitis carriers should be especially alert to any signs suggestive of cancer.

Even apparently healthy carriers of hepatitis B are advised to have regular medical checkups. Not only can the infection suddenly become active, but even when there is liver damage, there may be no symptoms, or symptoms that are so general and nonspecific that they are likely to be attributed to other causes.

Disorders of other organs In rare cases, chronic hepatitis B can also affect organs other than the liver, such as the kidneys. This is caused by the deposit within the body of something known as the HBV immune complex. This complex is formed as a result of the HBV antigen binding together with the HBG antibody. An antigen is a foreign substance that enters the body; and an antibody is produced by the white blood cells in response to the antigen. An inflammation is caused by the HBV immune complexes when they are deposited in the filtering elements of the kidney, causing a condition known as glomeronephritis.

Another type of kidney problem can occur when the immune complexes become deposited in the small arteries, causing inflammation of these blood vessels called polyarteritis nodosa. This can cause kidney problems leading to excess protein in the urine (proteinuria) and occasionally even to kidney failure. Because the arteries carry blood throughout the body, the inflammation can cause wide-ranging damage, including nerve damage, muscle weakness, deep skin ulcers, and fevers.

Treatment Options and Outlook

Chronic hepatitis B is regarded as an important public health problem in the United States and worldwide. It is estimated that one out of 20 people in the United States have contracted the hepatitis B; in other parts of the world, as many as one out of three are infected. Once a person has contracted chronic HBV—still a very common occurrence in parts of Asia and Africa—treatment with antiviral agents is the only known way to reduce diseases associated with HBV and to reduce mortality levels. Chronic hepatitis B can lead to progressive scarring of the liver and liver cancer.

No real cure for chronic hepatitis B exists at the present time, but most individuals with chronic hepatitis B who are actively infectious can begin antiviral therapy.

Even though complete eradication of the virus may not be possible, slowing down the virus slows the progression of liver disease and keeps liver damage to a minimum. When this is achieved, the patient is less likely to transmit the disease, has few or no symptoms associated with it, and has a much better long-term prognosis. Accordingly, the primary aim of therapy is to suppress the hepatitis virus to the lowest possible level. People with chronic hepatitis B usually have detectable levels of HBV DNA (as measured by an assay) and the B e antigen (HBeAg) in their blood. Detectable levels of B e antigen in the blood generally indicate that the virus is multiplying profusely. The goal is to "lose" the B e antigen so that the blood test shows negative for HBeAg.

After a course of therapy is completed, ALT activity, levels of B e antigen, and the surface antigen should be tested. ALT activities often decrease or normalize when inflammation subsides. When the blood test for the B e antigen is negative, but positive for the protective antibody against the Be antigen (anti-HBe+), the patient has recovered from the disease and has a low chance of infecting others. Patients may also lose the surface antigen (HBsAg–), but this happens in only a minority of cases.

The secondary goal of therapy is to avoid drug resistance—the drug may lose its effectiveness after prolonged therapy of a year or more because mutant strains resistant to the drug develop. The full suppression of viral replication and the avoidance of drug resistance are the two keys to successful treatment in HBV.

Patients most likely to respond to medication fit the following criteria:

- have chronic hepatitis B with positive B surface antigen (HBsAg+)
- actively replicating virus—tests positive for B e antigen (HBeAg+)
- have elevated aminotransferase levels (ALT and AST)
- have low levels of HBV DNA
- have not developed complications from cirrhosis, such as abdominal swelling, internal bleeding, and mental impairment
- have not been coinfected with hepatitis D (HDV)
- blood ALBUMIN levels are normal and stable
- have not been infected with HBV for more than three years

Although patients who do not meet these criteria may not respond as favorably to medication, they may still find therapy to be beneficial, depending on their individual circumstances. They can discuss their options with their physician, particularly since many new drugs are being tested and coming out on the market.

The general consensus is that patients who are HBeAg positive with normal levels of ALT or who have mild chronic hepatitis should not be treated. Treatment is usually indicated only for patients with moderate or severe disease.

Patients with extensive scarring of the liver with complications such as internal bleeding or abdominal swelling from fluid retention may not do as well with antiviral therapy. In fact, some people may become worse.

Patients with some scarring of the liver may benefit from INTERFERON; however, anyone with advanced scarring of the liver should avoid interferon. Most physicians prescribe one of the newer drugs for such patients.

At present, there are three FDA-approved treatments for hepatitis B in the United States:

- Intron A (Interferon [IFN] alfa-2b) by Schering-Plough. Introduced in the 1980s, it was the first treatment to be approved by the U.S. Food and Drug Administration (FDA) for chronic hepatitis B.

- Epivir-HBV (lamivudine; 3TC), an oral antiviral agent by GlaxoSmithKline. It was approved for treatment in 1998.

- Hepsera (adefovir-dipivoxil), an oral antiviral agent, similar to lamivudine. It was approved in 2002.

All three of the medications above can be used as initial therapy for chronic hepatitis B. Each drug has its own benefits and shortcomings. Issues that need to be addressed first are how effective and safe a drug is; other considerations include cost, convenience of administration, incidence of drug resistance, monitoring tests, and patient preference.

Pegasys (peginterferon alfa-2a), a newer version of interferon called pegylated interferon, has demonstrated superior results compared with conventional interferon, and is more convenient for patients to take. Manufactured by Roche Labs and Schering-Plough, it has not yet received FDA approval. Patients infected with the most difficult to treat mutant strain of hepatitis B virus (HBeAg negative) do better with Pegasys than lamivudine, according to results presented at the 54th American Association for the Study of Liver Disease Annual Meeting in 2003. And adding lamivudine to Pegasys did not improve efficacy.

The advantages of taking interferon are that there is a finite duration of treatment, the response is more durable, and drug-resistant mutants do not develop. Its disadvantages are its cost, side effects, and need to inject the medication.

After lamivudine (LVD) was introduced, it soon became the drug of choice, because, unlike interferon, it is taken orally and side effects are minimal. It is also more economical than interferon; it is the least expensive of the three drugs. But the disadvantages are that the benefits of treatment often do not last once the drug is discontinued; long-term therapy usually leads to the development of lamivudine-resistant mutations. Adefovir (ADV) is similar to lamivudine but less likely to lead to drug resistance; it is also effective against lamivudine-resistant HBV. One study showed drug resistance to be as high as 70 percent after five years of treatment with LVD. In contrast, after two years of treatment with ADV, drug resistance was 3 percent. Because drug resistance is less likely, experts often recommend it for long-term therapy. ADV also has few side effects, but there is the danger of potential kidney problems when taken for a long time. Its long-term safety has not yet been established. ADV costs more than LVD, but less than interferon.

Currently more than a dozen experimental drugs are being studied for the treatment of hepatitis B.

Patients with chronic hepatitis B must be monitored regularly by a liver specialist (hepatologist), whether or not they are currently undergoing medical therapy. If they are not taking medication, they need to be checked periodically for disease progression and to determine that complications such as permanent scarring of the liver or liver cancer have not set in. While patients are taking medication, they must be observed to see whether the therapy is working and to check for any side effects.

In deciding which drug to use as a first-line therapy for chronic HBV, the physician will take into account the characteristics of the disease, such as whether the patient has measurable amounts of B e antigen (HBeAg) in the blood, the severity of liver damage, and previous treatments.

In assessing how well the treatment is working, the more sensitive PCR assay may be useful for measuring blood HBV DNA levels so that even minute changes can be detected. This will help the physician in discovering whether a drug-resistant virus may be emerging, and in deciding whether to continue the treatment.

With three FDA-approved treatments in the United States, it is not always easy for physicians to understand what type of treatment they should offer their patients. Some issues they need to consider include the severity of the patient's liver disease and complications before initiating treatment. To address this problem, a panel of U.S. hepatologists (liver specialists) compiled recommendations for the treatment and management of the disease. Their results were published in the February 2004 issue of *Clinical Gastroenterology and Hepatology.*

According to these experts, "the new algorithm is based on new developments in the understanding of the virology of HBV, the availability of more sensitive molecular diagnostic testing, and an examination of the advantages and disadvantages of currently approved therapies. This algorithm is based on available evidence, but where data are lacking, the panel relied on clinical experience and consensus expert opinion."

First, the panel recommends that a baseline level of HBV DNA be established before treatment. Molecular assays can detect HBV DNA at levels as low as 100 to 1,000 copies (viral particles) per milliliter of blood. It is thus possible to monitor closely patients' responses to antiviral medication, and to discover early on whether drug resistance is developing.

The primary aim is the sustained suppression of HBV DNA to the lowest level possible. Generally, patients with hepatitis B e antigen (HBeAg+) and a level of HBV DNA equal to or greater than 10^5 copies (viral particles) per milliliter can be considered candidates for treatment if their ALT is also elevated. Interferon, LVD, or AVD can be used. (If the HBV DNA level is high, LVD or AVD is preferred.) If the patient has normal ALT, then none of the three drugs is likely to work well. Further evaluation through a biopsy can be considered; treatment can be initiated or not based on its findings. If treatment seems indicated, LVD or

ADV is preferred because either is more powerful at suppressing HBV and has fewer side effects than interferon.

For those patients who test negative for hepatitis B e antigen (HBeAg−), treatment is appropriate if they have HBV DNA levels equal to or greater than 10^4 per milliliter and their ALT is elevated. If the ALT is normal, then patients will probably not respond as well to any of the currently approved drugs. In that case, a biopsy might be performed, and if there is evidence of disease, treatment may be started. If the ALT is normal and the HBV DNA level is lower than 10^4 per milliliter, the patient should not be medicated but monitored every six to 12 months.

Compensated cirrhotic patients (they have advanced scarring of the liver but have not yet developed complications associated with it) are candidates for treatment if their HBV DNA is equal to or greater than 10^4. Whether the patients are HBeAg positive or HBeAg negative makes no difference in this case. Either LDV or ADV is a first-line option, but ADV is preferred for long-term treatments because of the lower risk of developing drug resistance. Compensated cirrhotic patients with HBV DNA levels lower than 10^4 can either be treated or monitored.

Decompensated cirrhotic patients (those with advanced scarring of the liver with complications associated with it) who have HBV DNA levels less than 10^3 or equal to or greater than 10^3 may be placed on waiting lists for liver transplantation. Meanwhile, they can be treated with either LDV or ADV. For long-term treatment, ADV is preferred.

In combination therapy, two different medications are taken simultaneously; sometimes one medication is taken by itself for a short period of time, then a second medication is later added to the regimen. A combination approach may also decrease or delay the incidence of drug resistance that occurs from viral mutation. Opinion is somewhat divided over how effective combination therapy may be in comparison with monotherapy (using only one drug) in suppressing viral replication. In theory, combination therapy should be more effective, and evidence seems to bear that out. Different medications act on different parts of the life cycle of the virus, so a combination of drugs should more effectively repress the reproduction of the hepatitis B virus.

Thus, most experts appear to be leaning toward combination therapy for future treatments of chronic hepatitis B. Many questions still remain to be answered, however, such as which medications to use and in what combination.

So far, pairing up lamivudine (LVD) with interferon (INF) is the most popular approach, but the benefit of conventional INF and LVD combination treatment over LVD monotherapy is not so clearcut. Several studies suggested that taking LVD and INF together was no more effective than just taking one or the other. However, several studies presented at the European Association for the Study of the Liver Consensus Meeting (EASL), held in April 2004, indicated that the combination of pegylated interferon (peginterferon alfa-2b)—the newer version of interferon—and LVD was associated with a significantly higher response than LVD or IFN monotherapy. These studies suggest that combination therapy causes significant reductions in the blood levels of both HBV DNA and one of the liver enzymes, ALT, which is used to follow progress in therapy.

Other combination therapies investigated included using LVD and AVD together, and LVD with famciclovir, a drug that has not yet been approved by the FDA.

More studies are now under way to explore the safety and efficacy of combination therapy.

Risk Factors and Preventive Measures

Hepatitis B is highly preventable. Individuals belonging to the risk group mentioned earlier should consider getting a hepatitis B vaccine. The HBV vaccine was approved by the U.S. Food and Drug Administration (FDA) in 1981. In the United States three shots are required to complete the vaccination for HBV.

Individuals who discover that they are infected with hepatitis B should have members of their household—or others they have been in intimate contact with—screened for viral markers by having a blood test performed. Vaccination is strongly urged for anyone who falls into the risk group.

Individuals who have not yet acquired immunity to HBV, or have not been vaccinated and inadvertently came into contact with contaminated blood, or had sex with an infected person, can still get protected if they get passive immunization within 30 days of exposure. This is called passive immunization, because it does not depend on the production of antibodies by the body.

Antibodies are produced by the white blood cells to fight off foreign substances. With passive immunization, a patient receives ready-made antibodies prepared by collecting the blood of individuals who have immunity to hepatitis B. These antibodies have been sterilized. The preparation, hepatitis B immune globulin (HBIG), is given by injection.

Wearing a latex condom when having intercourse may reduce the chance of catching or spreading the virus. Whether condoms can actually prevent transmission of hepatitis B is not known, but they prevent sexually transmitted disease, which can also make one more vulnerable to hepatitis B. It is unwise to share products that might have blood on them, such as razors and toothbrushes. Intravenous drug users have a higher rate of HBV infection (as well as other communicable diseases) than the rest of the population. Accordingly, drugs, needles, syringes, or other paraphernalia, including rinse cups, should never be shared. Users can seek help at addiction centers or from counselors specializing in addiction treatment.

Diagnosis Hepatitis B has been characterized as a "silent disease." People often learn that they have been infected by hepatitis B for the first time when they go to their doctor for a routine checkup.

The first thing the doctor does is conduct a physical examination, which may reveal that the liver and spleen are enlarged. If liver abnormalities are suspected, the patient is given a battery of tests including the COMPLETE BLOOD COUNT and complete blood chemistries. The tests for the aminotransferases ALT (alanine aminotransferase) and AST (aspartate aminotransferase) provide some measure of the extent of liver inflammation. With hepatitis B, ALT and AST are often elevated. In chronically infected patients, doctors have traditionally followed ALT the most closely. It can help determine the type of treatment that may be beneficial, and is used to evaluate how well the patient is responding to therapy. Other tests for BILIRUBIN, PROTHROMBIN TIME, and albumin level can show to some extent how well the liver is functioning.

The definitive test for hepatitis B, however, is made from the results of specific viral blood tests (serologies). These are not a part of routine tests; they are given if hepatitis is suspected.

The hepatitis B blood panel checks for the presence of hepatitis B surface antigen (HBsAg), hepatitis B e-Antigen (HBeAg) and hepatitis B e-Antibody (HBeAb). These protein products are made by the genes of the HBV. A discussion of the blood tests follows in the next section.

Because the blood test results can be complicated for the patient, it is suggested that the patient request a copy of the results from the doctor. The doctor can help interpret the results so that the patient knows whether he or she has a new infection or a chronic infection, or had a past infection and has already recovered from it.

Once hepatitis B has been determined, the doctor may also check for possible damage to the liver. He or she may order ultrasound and imaging, and possibly a liver biopsy. Although the imaging studies may not show any damage, this does not necessarily mean that the liver is not damaged. A biopsy is usually necessary to find out the extent of liver damage and is the only sure way to determine the presence of cirrhosis, or scarring. A biopsy may be helpful in cases of chronic infection, but is not necessary in acute infections where the patient is likely to recover relatively soon.

Other tests the doctor may order include ALPHA-FETOPROTEIN (AFP) to check for liver tumors, human immunodeficiency virus (HIV) to check for AIDS, and antinuclear antibody (ANA) to check for autoimmune hepatitis.

The doctor may also need to check for possible coinfection with hepatitis C (HCV) and HEPATITIS D (HDV), especially in the case of chronic hepatitis B where the patient appears to be getting worse. This knowledge is critical in planning the appropriate treatment for the patient.

For a new infection, blood tests may be repeated after six months to determine whether the infection has resolved itself or turned chronic.

In some cases people who believed they were healthy are alerted to a possible infection when they attempt to donate their blood and are informed that they may be infected with hepatitis B. To screen donor blood for hepatitis B infection, many blood banks use an antibody test that can show whether the donor has been exposed to the virus. But the test alone is not enough to tell whether the individual is actually infected. This is important because it can mean that the individual has been chronically infected with hepatitis B, is recovering from an infection, or has recovered from a past infection. It is also possible for the test to show a false positive. For a more definitive diagnosis, the individual should go to the doctor for more blood tests to be done.

Diagnosis is established primarily by finding the hepatitis B surface antigen (HBsAg) in the blood. The surface antigen, HBsAg, is the first marker of HBV infection to appear in the blood. It usually appears within four weeks after exposure to HBV. The presence of the surface antigen means that there is active HBV infection; if the surface antigen is absent, there is no active infection. HBsAg disappears after an acute infection when the body eliminates the virus. This usually occurs within four months after symptoms first appear. In chronic HBV infection, the surface antigen remains in the blood for more than six months.

When an individual has recovered from acute HBV, antibodies to the surface antigen (anti-HBs, or HBsAb) appear. The individual is also no longer contagious. These antibodies provide protection against future hepatitis B infection. Individuals who have been vaccinated against HBV will also produce anti-HBs.

The hepatitis B core antigen, HBcAg, is not readily detected in the blood of infected individuals, though it can be seen in liver cells. But when the virus is rapidly replicating in the liver, tests can detect a smaller version of this core antigen. This form is known as the B e antigen, or HBeAg. It is a much more serious and a more highly contagious version of hepatitis B. Patients with HBeAg in their blood are usually sicker, with more symptoms and a greater amount of inflammation in the liver. Their disease will also more likely progress to cirrhosis and liver cancer. Such patients are more infectious because of greater viral activity that puts more viral particles in the blood.

The body produces antibodies to the core antigen known as the hepatitis B core antibody (anti-HBc, or HBcAb). Measuring the blood for these antibodies is another component of the hepatitis B blood test. If the test shows positive for anti-HBc—these antibodies can be detected in the blood—it can mean that the person either is currently infected or had a past infection. (It could also be a false positive.) Anti-HBc is usually present in people chronically infected with hepatitis B.

Two types of anti-HBc antibodies are produced: IgM antibodies (IgM anti-HBc) and IgG antibodies (IgG anti-HBc). IgM antibodies are found in acute hepatitis B infections; IgG antibodies are found in chronic infections.

The IgM anti-HBc remains in the blood for up to six months after symptoms show. Only the IgM is used to diagnose acute HBV infection. The IgG antibodies are present in anyone who has ever been exposed to the virus. The IgG antibodies can remain in the blood after the infection is gone, often for a lifetime. But their presence in the blood does not mean that the individual has immunity to the hepatitis B virus. And vaccinations against HBV do not produce IgG antibodies. As mentioned above, individuals who have immunity to hepatitis B have antibodies to the surface antigen (anti-HBs). If only anti-HBs are found in the blood, it usually means that the individual has a vaccine-induced immunity.

Basically, if the surface antigen is no longer detectable in the blood (HBsAg–), and surface antibodies are present (anti-HBs+), then the patient has recovered from hepatitis B and is no longer contagious.

Measuring HBV DNA DNA is the genetic material for HBV. Checking the blood for the DNA of hepatitis B can reveal whether an individual has been infected. When HBV is reproducing actively, high levels of HBV DNA can be found in the blood. Low or undetectable levels of HBV DNA indicate that the HBV infection is in a dormant, or inac-

UNDERSTANDING HEPATITIS B BLOOD TESTS			
Tests	Results	Interpretation	Recommendation
HBsAg	negative	not immune—has not been infected but is still at risk for possible future infection. Need protection	Get the vaccine.
HBsAb (anti-HBs)	negative		
HBcAb	negative		
HBsAg	negative or positive	immune—surface antibodies present. You may have been already vaccinated, or you have recovered from a prior hepatitis B infection. You cannot infect others.	The vaccine is not needed.
HBsAb (anti-HBs)			
HBcAb (anti-HBc)			
HBsAg	positive	new infection or a chronic infection-positive surface antigen; hepatitis B virus is present. You can spread the virus to others.	Find a doctor knowledgeable about hepatitis B for further evaluation.
HBsAb (anti-HBs)	negative		
HBcAb (anti-HBc)	negative or positive		
HBsAg	negative	*unclear—Several different interpretations are possible. You may need to have these tests repeated. See below.	The vaccine may or may not be needed. Find a doctor knowledgeable about hepatitis B for further evaluation.
HBsAb (anti-HBs)	negative		
HBcAb (anti-HBs)*	negative		
*Positive Hepatitis B Core-Antibody Test Result (HBcAB+).			

Source: Hepatitis B Foundation, www.hepb.org.

tive, phase. HBV DNA is usually measured by the number of copies (particles) per milliliter of blood. When the infection is in an inactive phase, there are about a million viral particles per milliliter; in an active phase, there are several billion particles per milliliter.

Laboratory tests (assays) can measure the HBV DNA. The most sensitive assay is the polymerase chain reaction (PCR), which can detect levels as low as 50 to 100 copies of DNA per milliliter. When less sensitive measurements are needed, a different assay, the hybridization method, is used. It can detect HBV DNA only when there are enough viral particles for the infection to be active.

Diagnosing acute HBV In general, patients with acute infection test positive for the hepatitis surface antigen (HBsAg+), positive for the hepatitis core antibodies (IgM anti-HBc+), and possibly also for the hepatitis B e antigen (HBeAg+).

The B e antigen, as mentioned earlier, is a smaller form of the hepatitis core antigen. Its presence indicates that the individual is highly infectious. In addition to the antibodies to the surface antigen (anti-HBs), which grants immunity, and the core antigen (anti-HBc), the body can also produce antibodies specifically against the B e antigen. These are designated as anti-HBe, or HBeAb. The presence of these antibodies indicates that the virus is in a more inactive state, and the risk of transmission is much lower. It is not possible to detect both the e antigen (HBeAg) and the antibodies for it (anti-HBe) in the blood at the same time.

If an individual appears to be infected with HBV, but the test is negative for HBeAg, then differentiating it from the chronic, inactive "carrier state" becomes a little more difficult. There is also a possibility that the individual has been infected with a mutant strain of the virus, as discussed below. The patient should be monitored over a period of six to 12 months for ALT and HBV DNA levels.

Chronic mutant hepatitis B Some patients may test negative for the hepatitis B e antigen (HBeAg), but still be infected with hepatitis B, as shown by assays measuring HBV DNA, and perhaps by symptoms as well. In these cases, the patients may have been infected with a mutant strain of HBV, known as precore mutants. A mutation occurred to change the structure of the virus so that its core proteins are no longer able to produce the e antigen (HBeAg), even though the virus is rapidly replicating. (This is different from patients who test negative for the B e antigen because they have not been infected with the virus, or have already been successfully treated for it.) Therefore the diagnosis of hepatitis B cannot be made solely on the presence or absence of HBeAg in the blood. To find out whether the patient has been infected with this mutant version, the virus has to be isolated and examined for its DNA sequence.

The pre-core mutant form of the virus has always been more common in Asia and the Mediterranean region, but has been turning up with greater frequency in North America. When a person has been infected with this mutant strain, the disease follows a more aggressive course. It is highly infectious and more resistant to treatment, the rate of relapse is much higher than for the normal strain, and the prognosis is poorer. It is capable of causing severe liver damage; 60 percent of patients develop cirrhosis within six years. Since mutation of the virus can sometimes occur after a person has already been infected with the regular hepatitis B virus, some experts believe that it is better to begin therapy earlier in the course of HBV infection to prevent the mutant strain from becoming the prevalent one.

Diagnosing chronic HBV In chronic HBV infection, the hepatitis surface antigen (HBsAg) is detectable in the blood for more than six months. The testing for this surface antigen is the most critical component to establish or exclude chronic hepatitis B. As already mentioned, the IgG core antibody (IgG anti-HBc) will also be present in the blood. In the absence of the surface antigen, however, the detection of the IgG core antibody by itself does not mean that the individual has chronic hepatitis B. The surface antigen must be present also. If the patient does not test positive for the surface antigen, but still shows other signs and symptoms of hepatitis, then other causes of hepatitis must be found.

Usually, in chronic infection, the B e antigen (HBeAg) is no longer detectable in the blood because the virus is no longer replicating as actively as it did during acute infection. But in some cases of chronic infection, the virus continues to replicate rapidly and blood tests for B e antigen come out positive. Therefore, individuals who have been diagnosed with chronic hepatitis B should always be tested for the B e antigen.

Chronic carriers of hepatitis B can spontaneously convert from testing negative for the B e antigen (HBeAg−) to testing positive (HBeAg+). This is not a good sign; it indicates that the virus is actively reproducing, and is associated with a worsening of the disease. But the reverse can also happen; carriers can go from HBeAg positive to HBeAg negative. This is a desirable change, with a better long-term outlook. Although the individual may experience a flare, a temporary worsening of symptoms as the immune system attacks the virus, in the long run his or her condition will improve.

No special medical treatment exists for people with a mild or moderate case of hepatitis B. Most recover from acute cases of infection on their own within weeks or months. The speed of recovery depends on the individual, but it can take up to six months after the initial infection. For most people, getting enough rest and drinking plenty of fluids is enough. The doctor may ask to see the patient several times over the course of the infection.

On rare occasions, a patient may develop a sudden onset of acute liver failure, with symptoms of mental confusion, drowsiness, and stupor. In such an event, he or she must be hospitalized immediately, if possible at a facility that can perform liver transplants.

Fortunately, most patients do not suffer lasting ill effects from the infection. But they should return after six months to the clinic for more blood tests to make sure that the virus has disappeared. If the virus persists after six months, then the infection has entered the chronic stage. In that case, the doctor may recommend antiviral therapy.

A recovery from acute hepatitis B is confirmed when blood tests show that the person has lost the surface antigen (HBsAg–) and has developed protective surface antibodies (anti-HBs+). Blood tests measuring the liver function should also be completely normalized, and any symptoms that were present are resolved. The patient is now no longer contagious and cannot be infected by hepatitis B again. Yet this does not mean that he or she has immunity against other types of hepatitis, such as hepatitis A or C.

The recovered person can never give blood again, as the hepatitis B core antibody (anti-HBc) will always be present in the blood. The presence of anti-HBc reveals that the would-be donor has been infected in the past.

Patients with chronic hepatitis B are urged to visit their doctor regularly to check on their health status and screen for liver cancer. If advanced scarring of the liver (cirrhosis) has set in, they will be generally advised against receiving any treatments with interferon.

There is a possibility that chronic hepatitis B also carries the risk of bone loss, although the evidence is as yet inconclusive. Patients may benefit from bone mineral density tests.

Most doctors will advise anyone with liver disease to abstain from alcohol. Alcohol is generally toxic to the liver and causes ALCOHOLIC LIVER DISEASE, but it has an even more damaging effect on HBV-infected people. The hepatitis B virus may multiply more quickly, the disease process will be accelerated, and serious complications, such as scarring of the liver from cirrhosis, are more likely to occur. In turn, cirrhosis increases the odds for developing liver cancer.

Both cigarette smoking and marijuana smoking have also been discovered to be extremely injurious to the liver for anyone with hepatitis.

There is no special diet for people who have chronic hepatitis B. A weakened immune system can allow the virus to reproduce more rapidly, so patients should try to stay as healthy as possible by eating a well-balanced diet with plenty of vegetables. Raw shellfish should be avoided, because they can contain bacteria harmful to the liver.

Since coinfection can make the disease worse, anyone who has not had hepatitis A should be vaccinated for it.

For pamphlets about hepatitis B, call 1-888-4-HEP-CDC or visit the Web site at www.cdc.gov/hepatitis. Or write Centers for Disease Control and Prevention Division of Viral Hepatitis, Mailstop G37 Atlanta, GA 30333, or contact your state or local health department.

Chan, H. L. Y., and others. "A randominized trial of peginteferon alfa-2b nd lamivudine combination treatment versus lamivudine monotherapy in Chinese patients with HBeAg-positive chronic hepatitis B." Abstract 423. 39th annual meeting of the European Association for the Study of the Liver (EASL). April 14–18, 2004. Berlin, Germany.

Graham, W., and E. Cooksley, M.D. "The role of interferon therapy in hepatitis B." *Medscape General Medicine* 6(1) (March 8, 2004). Available online. URL: http://www.medscape.com/viewarticle/464685. Accessed on May 10, 2003.

"Hepatitis B and you." Department of Health and Human Services, Centers for Disease Control and Prevention, 2004.

Karatapanis, S., and others. "Interferon plus lamivudine versus lamivudine monotherapy in patients with chronic hepatitis B anti-HBe positive." Abstract 430. 39th EASL. April 14–18, 2004. Berlin, Germany.

Keeffe, E. B., and others. "Treatment algorithm for management of chronic hepatitis B virus infections in U.S." *Clinical Gastroenterology and Hepatology* 2 (2004): 87–106.

Keeffe, Emmet B., Douglas T. Dieterich, Steve-Huy Han, Ira M. Jacobson, Paul Martin, Eugene R. Schiff, Hillel Tobias, and Teresa L. Wright. "Management of chronic hepatitis B: A new treatment algorithm from a panel of US experts." *Clinical Gastroenterology and Hepatology* 2 (February 2004): 82–106.

"Lamivudine treatment during pregnancy to prevent perinatal transmission of hepatitis B virus infection." *Journal of Viral Hepatitis* 10, no. 4 (July 2003): 294–298.

Lavanchy D., and others. "Hepatitis B virus epidemiology, disease burden, treatment, and current and emerging prevention and control measures." *Journal of Viral Hepatitis* 11, no. 2 (March 2004): 97–107.

Papatheodoridis, G. V., and S. J. Hadziyannis. "Current management of chronic hepatitis B." *Alimentary Pharmacological Therapy* 19, no. 1 (2004): 25–37.

Perrillo, R., and others. "Continued safety and efficacy of adding adefovir dipivoxil (ADV) to ongoing lamivudine (LAM) therapy in compensated chronic hepatitis B (CHB) patients with YMDD variant HBV: 2-year results." Abstract 438. 39th EASL. April 14–18, 2004. Berlin, Germany.

Schiefke, Ingolf, Gudrun Borte, Manfred Wiese, Eva Schenker, and A. Fach. "Decreased bone mineral density in non-cirrhotic patients with chronic hepatitis B or C." *Journal of Viral Hepatitis* 11, no. 2 (2004): 97–107. 37th EASL.

van Zonneveld, M., and others. "Viral dynamics during Peg-interferon alone and in combination with lamivudine." Abstract 446. 39th EASL. April 14–18, 2004. Berlin, Germany.

hepatitis C Hepatitis C is a LIVER DISEASE caused by a virus known as hepatitis C virus (HCV), one of several viruses that can lead to hepatitis—inflammation of the LIVER. The virus attacks and kills the liver cells, which are replaced by scar tissue. The hepatitis C virus is found in the blood of an infected person, and the virus is passed on when another person comes into contact with the contaminated blood. While there may be no symptoms for years, the virus silently injures the liver, at times causing to liver cancer or liver failure. HCV, the most common chronic infection in the United States, is a growing global problem. The World Health Organization (WHO) estimates that hepatitis C infects some 8.9 million people in Europe. More than 170 million individuals, or 3 percent of the world population, are chronic carriers of HCV.

Hepatitis C is not a new disease. Doctors simply did not know about hepatitis C until 1989, when workers at the biotechnology company Chiron Corporation identified the hepatitis C virus using specialized genetic chemistry. Although they did not conclusively see the hepatitis C virus under an electron microscope, its existence was inferred through the cloning of its genetic material.

The discovery of hepatitis C virus was a long-awaited breakthrough. Researchers had long suspected the existence of an unknown infectious hepatitis virus. For instance, they noted that patients given blood transfusions would sometimes contract hepatitis even if the blood had tested negative for both HEPATITIS A and HEPATITIS B. For lack of a more specific term, they lumped together any hepatitis viruses that were not hepatitis A or B into a category known as non-A, non-B hepatitis (NANB). After its discovery, the new virus was named "hepatitis C." About 90 percent of all cases of non-A non-B hepatitis are caused by the hepatitis C virus. The first test for screening the HCV became commercially available in 1990. Two years later, an even more accurate screening of HCV was introduced.

The discovery of HCV revolutionized doctors' approach to treating patients with hepatitis C. Patients could finally be given a diagnosis and offered treatments that have been growing more effective over the years as researchers refine their understanding of the virus.

Of all the viral hepatitis varieties (A, B, C, D, and E) that can infect a person, hepatitis C turns chronic the most easily. Only about 15 to 20 percent of individuals who become infected will be able to shake off the virus after the initial infection. Chronically infected people now number million in the United States—about 1.3 percent of the population. By contrast, 1 million suffer from a chronic case of hepatitis B. One reason that HCV is so effective at becoming chronic is that, compared with other viruses, the hepatitis C virus has an extraordinary ability to avoid destruction by the body's immune defense system due in part to its propensity to mutate frequently. Thus, any antibodies the body manufactures are soon rendered impotent by the ever-changing virus.

Another difficult characteristic of hepatitis C is that most individuals do not even know they have been infected because they do not feel ill; HCV can infect people for long periods without causing any obvious symptoms. The Centers for Disease Control and Prevention (CDC) estimate that only 5 percent of infected individuals become aware that they are harboring the hepatitis C virus in their bodies. These infected individuals can unwittingly become a source of transmission to others. Moreover, they themselves are at risk for chronic liver disease or other HCV-related disorders. Although it can take decades, the inflammation of the liver can eventually lead to scarring and other liver damage. The early stage of scarring is called FIBROSIS. About 20 percent of patients with fibrosis will develop CIRRHOSIS, or advanced scarring leading to a structural distortion of the liver. Patients with cirrhosis are more likely to develop liver failure or the complications of cirrhosis, including HEPATOCELLULAR CARCINOMA, or liver cancer. Complications from chronic hepatitis and cirrhosis caused by HCV are the most common indications for LIVER TRANSPLANTATION in the United States and western Europe.

Former U.S. surgeon general Dr. C. Everett Koop characterized HCV "as a graver threat to public health than AIDS," responsible for more than one-third of all liver transplants, and infecting three times more people than does AIDS. Indeed, a study presented at the 54th annual meeting of the American Association for the study of liver diseases in October 2003 in Boston revealed that in the United States, hepatitis C virus is four times more common than human immunodeficiency virus (HIV), which causes AIDS. Moreover, while many HIV-infected individuals have been diagnosed and treated, HCV infection often remains undiagnosed and untreated.

The CDC estimates that 8,000 to 10,000 Americans die each year from complications of hepatitis C—and this figure is expected to triple by 2020. Slightly different conclusions, however, are reached by the above-mentioned study presented at the American Association for the Study of Liver Diseases (AASLD). Extrapolating from current trends, the study estimates that in the United States, HCV-related deaths will peak at 14,000 to 19,000 by the year 2030. In contrast, deaths from HIV will drop to between 4,200 and 6,700.

The increase in deaths from hepatitis C will result mostly from old infections reaching clinical stages. The medical bill for treating HCV-related disease is expected to exceed $13 billion for the years 2010 through 2019.

There is a bright side to this picture, however. The number of new cases of hepatitis C has diminished strikingly in the last decade or so. In the United States, hepatitis C has declined from a peak in the 1980s, with some 200,000 people infected annually, to about 28,000 in 1999. Although the reasons for this dramatic drop are not completely clear, the drop can be credited in part to a greater awareness of HIV infection (AIDS) and a change in the practice of injection drug users. Another reason is the availability of sensitive blood tests that can screen individuals at high risk for having HCV as well as detect any viruses in the blood supply to safeguard patients. This screening of blood and blood products has substantially reduced the incidence of patients becoming infected after receiving blood transfusions.

On the other hand, it is expected that during the next 10 to 20 years, the number of deaths caused by HCV-related chronic liver disease will triple. This is because individuals infected by HCV 10 to 20 years ago are reaching ages at which complications from chronic liver disease typically occur. Also, estimates of the number of people infected by HCV are considered to be extremely low because not all groups of people are adequately tested. For instance, infection rates are believed to be quite high among the homeless, who are generally not included in estimates of disease prevalence.

The number of cases of HCV infections in a population group varies with geographic location. The prevalence of HCV is much higher in countries such as Africa and Southeast Asia than in North America and Europe. In Scandinavia, the incidence of HCV is less than 0.5 percent of the population, while it is over 20 percent in Egypt.

In terms of age group, people between 30 and 49 years have the highest prevalence rates of HCV infection. Among ethnic groups, the rates are substantially higher among African Americans than Caucasians, and males of all ethnicity have a higher infection rate than females.

Various factors can also affect the prevalence of HCV infection among any population group. For example, the highest prevalence of infection is found among people who have repeated direct exposures to blood through the skin (percutaneous), most notably injection drug users, and hemophilia patients who were treated with clotting factor concentrates produced before 1987. In the United Kingdom, almost all patients with hemophilia who received pooled clotting factor concentrates before 1987 became infected with hepatitis C virus. Some of these patients suffer from end-stage liver disease and are being considered for liver transplantation.

HCV is basically spread through the blood. Now that blood and blood products are routinely screened for HCV, by far the most common mode of transmission is through intravenous drug abuse. Since 1990 all potential donors are screened for hepatitis C, and even more sensitive screening techniques were introduced in 1992. These screening tests for blood have reduced the risk of contracting HCV from a single unit of blood to less than one in 100,000. Another potential source of infection, sexual contact, appears to be low, particularly in the context of a monogamous relationship. People with multiple sex partners are at greater risk, however, and should use barrier protection (condoms).

The hepatitis C virus is a single-stranded RNA (ribonucleic acid) virus. Thus it has the RNA as its genetic material. The virus contains a single RNA molecule in its center surrounded by a fatty envelope that contains two viral proteins.

HCV is a member of the Flaviviridae, a large family of viruses with many members, including those that cause yellow fever and dengue. The virus mostly reproduces within hepatocytes—major liver cells—though they have been demonstrated to multiply outside the liver as well.

Compared with other viruses, there is a relatively low concentration of the hepatitis C virus in the blood. For example, an individual with an active hepatitis B infection has several hundred million to billions of virus particles per milliliter of blood, while the average number of hepatitis C viral particles ranges from hundreds of thousands to several million. This is one of the reasons it took scientists so long to identify HCV.

The members of the family of hepatitis C virus are classified into genetically distinct groups that have arisen during the evolution of the virus. Each member, called a genotype, is related genetically to the others, but they are not identical. They may differ in their genetic makeup from each other by as much as 35 percent. Scientists recognize at least six major genotypes, which they identify by number—genotype 1, 2, 3, and so on. Some scientists also believe that genotypes 7 through 11 exist, mostly in parts of Asia. Furthermore, each genotype has one or two subtypes. More than 50 different subtypes are designated by a lower-case letter. Genotype 1, for example, is subdivided into genotype 1a and 1b. These subtypes differ genetically from each other by about 15 percent. Certain subtypes are predominant in different areas of the world and among different groups of people. In the United States, roughly 75 to 80 percent of the infected population has genotype 1a or 1b, with 1a predominating slightly more than 1b, according to some estimates.

An individual can become infected with one or more different genotypes. Unfortunately, becoming infected with one genotype of hepatitis C does not provide immunity against getting infected again with different—or even the same—genotypes of the virus. This is why there is no IMMUNE GLOBULIN or vaccination available to protect a person from infection either pre- or post-exposure to the virus.

The genes that make up the hepatitis C virus can vary slightly from one virus to another, as a result of mutation in the viral RNA. The mutations occur while the virus is replicating. These different genetic variations of HCV are known as hepatitis C mutants, or quasispecies. "Quasi" means similar, or resembling.

An individual can be infected with an entire conglomerate of various quasispecies of hepatitis C. Generally, this virus population consists of one dominant group of virus and numerous other mutants that are all similar in structure, but slightly different from one another. Scientists believe that these frequent mutations are the reason that hepatitis C so often progresses into a chronic disease. Constantly changing its genetic sequences may allow the hepatitis C virus to trick and slip past the body's surveillance system. Additionally, it allows the HCV to mutate into a stronger quasispecies that can withstand attack by the host immune system. Variations of the same genotype within the same patient may originate from the same infecting virus that mutated over a period of time. The patient may also have become exposed to different genotypes of HCV at different times. This can occur, for instance, in a person who habitually injects drugs. He or she can become reinfected numerous times.

As the quasispecies become more diverse, the patient may become resistant to INTERFERON, the main drug used for hepatitis C treatment. Therefore, the emergence of quasispecies in an individual is usually associated with more aggressive disease and poor response to treatment.

No commercial laboratories are currently available to determine the quasispecies; tests for identifying quasispecies are restricted to research purposes.

Symptoms and Diagnostic Path

Patients may have no symptoms, at least no noticeable ones, until they have progressed to advanced cirrhosis and reached the end stages of liver disease. This process can take decades. This is the main reason that so many people who have hepatitis C do not realize they have contracted it. Typically, only after they have a physical examination for their health insurance or try to donate blood do they discover that they are infected. They are often incredulous at the news, finding it difficult to believe that they have a disease, as they may feel perfectly healthy, or reasonably so, certainly not carriers of a potentially dangerous disease.

The fact is that fully 80 percent of patients with an acute HCV infection have no discernible symptoms, and of those who do, the symptoms tend to be of a general nature. The first symptoms, if any, that most people experience are similar to the flu. Patients may have a low-grade fever; their joints and muscles may ache; and they may feel tired, nauseated, and lose their appetite. Unlike the flu, if hepatitis C becomes chronic, the symptoms never completely go away, ebbing and flowing over the years. Fatigue is also one of the most common early symptoms, but it can occur years after the initial infection, and is easily attributable to any number of other causes. Other symptoms are also nonspecific, such as abdominal pain, and not readily recognized as caused by hepatitis C. A few patients may have symptoms from organs outside the liver that have been affected by the infection, usually as a result of the body's attempt to eradicate the virus. All too often, signs and symptoms of hepatitis C are dismissed as stress or a minor, short-lived infection. Even if HCV-infected individuals do go to the clinic, doctors who are not familiar with hepatitis C may miss the symptoms of the disease.

In the later stages, usually after the development of cirrhosis, patients may notice a yellow tint to the skin and eyes (jaundice), abdominal swelling as a result of accumulation of fluid (ASCITES), and liver failure fulminant hepatic failure).

The following are some of the most common symptoms of hepatitis C:

- abdominal bloating
- abdominal pains and discomfort
- cognitive problems such as brain fog (encephalopathy)
- itchiness all over the body
- JAUNDICE
- loss of appetite
- loss of libido
- mild depression
- mild to extreme fatigue
- nausea and vomiting

Other symptoms that have been associated with hepatitis include these:

- arthritis
- blood circulation problems
- blood sugar problems
- chest pains
- dark urine
- diarrhea
- dizziness
- facial puffiness
- fluid retention
- headaches, frequent or continuous
- irritable bowel syndrome
- mental fatigue
- mood swings
- sore throat

Acute hepatitis C An acute case of hepatitis C is, by definition, an infection that lasts six months or less. Because there are usually no outwardly obvious symptoms and no clinically apparent disease, acute infection with HCV usually goes undiagnosed; it is generally not easy to identify patients with acute hepatitis C. Symptoms of HCV infection, if there are any, are usually similar to those that occur from any acute hepatitis, regardless of the cause. Some 20 to 30 percent might develop jaundice, while 10 to 20 percent may have more nonspecific symptoms. But the "silent" nature of the disease makes it difficult for patients to recall ever having an acute episode of jaundice or other warning signs of liver disease. Some people may have had nonspecific symptoms at the time of the infection—a general feeling of malaise, for example—but did not associate them with liver disease.

Acute hepatitis occurs most often among people aged 20 to 39 years, though anyone can become infected by HCV. The CDC reports that overall, Hispanic Americans have higher incidences of acute HCV than the general population, while African Americans and Caucasians have similar incidences of acute HCV. In contrast, chronic infection of HCV is more common among African Americans than whites.

In the United States, acute HCV infections account for about one-fifth of all cases of acute hepatitis today. There are an estimated 30,000 new acute HCV infections each year, but only about 25 percent are diagnosed properly.

The number of acute HCV cases has been continuously declining. Although it is not entirely clear why this is so, better screening tests for HCV have undoubtedly contributed to the decline. Another factor could be that intravenous drug users have become more careful about sharing drug paraphernalia because of the publicity regarding HIV (AIDS) infection through contaminated needles. This, in turn, has led to a drop in hepatitis C infections because HCV shares transmission routes similar to HIV.

Chronic HCV Chronic hepatitis C is a long-lasting infection of more than six months. About 80 percent of people who suffer from a bout of acute hepatitis C infection become chronically infected. In the case of hepatitis C, they usually are saddled with the infection for the rest of their lives. The virus will stay and replicate in the liver.

Individuals who have had hepatitis C for years may not experience any obvious symptoms, even if the disease has progressed to cirrhosis, or massive scarring of the liver. Therefore, the absence of symptoms is not a good barometer of the severity or the duration of the disease. Indeed, during the first 20 years after infection, with only occasional exceptions, the disease causes few problems. Infected individuals can feel perfectly healthy, and they do not appear to be sick. But HCV can progress slowly and silently, inflaming and damaging the liver. Individuals with chronic hepatitis C are at risk for cirrhosis, liver failure, and/or cancer.

That is not to say that the disease leads necessarily to a dire outcome. In the majority of cases, patients will not end up with debilitating disease or suffer an early death. People are just as likely to die *with* chronic HCV than they are *from* it. Only one out of every 400 to 500 patients dies from liver failure caused by HCV. Disease progression can vary dramatically between individuals. Some may be quite healthy, suffer from minimal liver disease, and never develop complications, while others may end up with cirrhosis and end-stage (advanced) liver disease. In the United States, cirrhosis caused by chronic hepatitis C is the most common reason for liver transplantation. Once a person has cirrhosis, he or she is at increased risk of developing hepatocellular carcinoma (primary liver cancer). Estimated rates of hepatocellular carcinoma occurring after cirrhosis range from 1 to 4 percent a year, but there seems to be considerable geographic variation. It is not possible at the present time to predict which patients will develop complications of advanced liver disease.

Diagnosis Individuals who believe they may have been exposed to hepatitis C, however long ago, would do well to be tested for the disease. Hepatitis C may be suspected in individuals who belong to the at-risk population for HCV and have abnormal laboratory tests suggestive of liver disorders. Some individuals who otherwise appear healthy seek out a doctor after being rejected for health insurance coverage or a blood donation because they tested positive for HCV antibody tests. The diagnosis of hepatitis C is through medical history, blood testing, and, in most cases, a liver biopsy. The doctor will take the following steps:

1. obtain a complete medical history of the individual. Questions will be asked to identify possible risk factors for hepatitis C.
2. give the patient a physical examination, which will include feeling and tapping around the area of the liver to determine whether there are any changes in the size and location of the liver. A shrunken, enlarged, or hardened liver could indicate a liver disease.
3. order a battery of blood tests

The blood tests consist of the following:

a. a liver-panel or LIVER-FUNCTION TESTS to obtain a profile of the liver
b. HCV antibody tests to detect antibodies against the virus (anti-HCV)
c. tests to detect directly the presence or absence of the virus (HCV RNA)

The liver-panel test may show abnormalities if HCV is present; in the majority of cases of chronic hepatitis C, the liver enzymes ALT and AST are elevated. Most characteristically, the ALT is higher than normal. But even normal levels of ALT and AST do not rule out the possibility of HCV. Only a diagnostic test for HCV can confirm whether a patient is infected.

Once a diagnosis of hepatitis C has been made, the doctor may decide to gather the following information before deciding on a course of treatment:

1. identification of the genotype, or genetic strain, of the virus
2. determination of the amount of the virus circulating in the bloodstream
3. assessment of the degree of inflammation of the liver, and the existence of cirrhosis, or advanced scarring of the liver, through a liver biopsy
4. presence of HEPATOCELLULAR CARCINOMA (primary liver cancer), if cirrhosis is present and there are suspicions of cancer

The hepatitis C antibody test is the first diagnostic test the doctor will order, as it is inexpensive and easy to administer. This blood test determines the presence of antibodies to hepatitis C virus in the body (anti-HCV, or HCV Ab). The test does not look for the virus in the blood, but for antibodies produced against certain protein substances called an ANTIGEN that provoke an immune response in the body. In about 70 percent of people, antibodies against HCV can be found when symptoms begin and, within three months after the start of symptoms, in about 90 percent of people. However, many people either have no symptoms or attribute the symptoms to some other cause because they are not specific to hepatitis C.

The presence of antibodies to one or more of the hepatitis antigens indicates exposure to HCV. But the antibody tests cannot distinguish between a new (acute) or long-term (chronic) infection, and an infection that has been cleared from the body. In all these cases, the antibodies remain in the bloodstream. Antibodies against the hepatitis C virus do not confer immunity; their presence only indicates that the individual has been exposed to the virus.

If an individual tests positive for an antibody test, it can mean one of four things:

1. The patient is currently infected with HCV.
2. The patient was infected in the past and has already cleared the virus. This is the case for only 10 to 15 percent of people, as hepatitis C so easily becomes chronic.
3. The test gave a false-positive. Although the test looks positive, it should really have been negative, as the patient is not infected with HCV. This scenario is more common in patients who have a low risk for hepatitis C, and who happen to get tested as part of a routine screening, such as blood donation. It is important therefore, to confirm the result with a supplemental test.
4. The person being tested is a newborn infant whose mother is HCV-infected. Antibodies from the mother could have been passed on, giving a positive reading. In such a case, the antibodies generally clear in three months, unless the infant has become chronically infected as well.

A negative test result can mean one of two things:

1. The person is not infected with hepatitis C.
2. The test gave a false-negative. Although the test looks negative, in fact, the person is infected with hepatitis C. This can occur in patients who have recently become infected and not yet developed antibody levels high enough for the test to measure. Or it may be that the individual lacks the immune response that produces antibodies that the test can measure. Such may be the case with patients whose immune systems are compromised for various reasons. They may have active HIV infection (the virus that causes AIDS), may need to be on renal (kidney) dialysis, or are undergoing CHEMOTHERAPY— anticancer drugs. If it appears that the test is a false negative, the doctor may order a hepatitis C viral RNA test that can directly detect the hepatitis C virus.

When a positive result is obtained, particularly in individuals with a low risk of HCV, the doctor will recommend one or more of the following tests:

1. either RIBA (detects antibodies), or a hepatitis C viral RNA test (directly detects the virus), to confirm the finding
2. a hepatitis C viral RNA test, which will clarify the following:
   a. whether the patient is currently infected, or was infected in the past, and has cleared the virus
   b. the amount of hepatitis C viral particles that may be circulating in the bloodstream

Two antibody tests are currently approved by the FDA for the diagnosis of HCV:

- ELISA test (enzyme-linked immunosorbent assay)

- RIBA test (recombinant immunoblot assay)

ELISA I became available in 1989 shortly after hepatitis C was discovered, but it was somewhat unreliable, at times showing a positive antibody for the virus when the individual did not have hepatitis C (false-positive result), or conversely, testing negative for the antibody when the individual in fact did have hepatitis C (false-negative result). The enzyme immunosorbent assays measure specific antibodies to small pieces of HCV proteins called antigens. ELISA I can detect anti-HCV about 16 weeks after exposure to HCV.

In 1993, ELISA I was supplanted by a more sensitive test called ELISA II. The more sensitive a test, the more cases it can detect. While ELISA I detects anti-HCV against one of the hepatitis C antigens, ELISA II can detect the antibody against four of the hepatitis C antigens in the blood. The test can be used approximately nine to 10 weeks after exposure to HCV. In 1996, ELISA III, an even more sensitive test, became available. ELISA III can detect the antibody against five of the hepatitis C antigens after about six to eight weeks after exposure to HCV. However, all tests have a small margin of error, and false readings are possible. When the test is positive, a diagnosis of HCV can be made with greater than 95 percent accuracy in cases where the patient has elevated LIVER ENZYMES (ALT and AST), and possibly also risk factors for HCV.

Both ELISA II and ELISA III are inexpensive and easy to administer, and are the first diagnostic test that the doctor will order.

RIBA (recombinant immunoblot assay) is best used as a supplemental test. It is more accurate than ELISA, as it detects the individual antigens against which the HCV antibodies are reacting. It was developed to help with the false-positive readings that can sometimes occur with ELISA. Certain patients may be retested with RIBA if ELISA results come back as positive for antibodies against HCV. These patients are low-risk for hepatitis C, have no symptoms, and also may have normal results for their liver-function tests. RIBA 2.0 has been commercially available since 1993. Recently, an even more accurate test, RIBA 3.0, was introduced. Test results come back as positive, negative, or indeterminate. An indeterminate result much be carefully evaluated by a specialist.

Because the RIBA test costs more than ELISA, it is usually used only to confirm the diagnosis, after a positive antibody test. Some hepatologists (liver specialists) may skip the RIBA test altogether and order a molecular test for the detection of the hepatitis C virus (HCV RNA) to verify infection.

For those unable, for whatever reason, to see a doctor to be tested, an over-the-counter (nonprescription) home test is now available to diagnose hepatitis C. Called the Hepatitis C Check, it has been approved by the Food and Drug Administration (FDA), and allows the user to collect a sample of blood at home and mail it to the appropriate laboratory for hepatitis C antibody testing. The home test kit contains everything necessary to take the test. Only a small sample of blood that can be readily obtained by pricking the fingertip is needed. The patient should be able to obtain the test result by calling the number provided in the kit after about 10 business days.

Because of the possibility of a false-positive or false-negative result, the individual may wish to confirm the diagnosis. Particularly if one falls into the high-risk group, one should be aware that there is a chance of a false test result.

If antibodies to HCV virus are found, the next step is to look for the actual presence of viruses in the blood. Several types of assays (tests) can identify the ribonucleic acids (RNA—the genetic material of HCV) in the blood and body tissues. Unlike antibodies to HCV antigens, which can remain even after the infection has been resolved, the presence of viral RNA indicates that the infection is current, and that the virus is actively replicating, that is, it is reproducing and infecting new cells.

These tests are known as qualitative HCV RNA assays. They are sometimes also referred to as molecular tests because they examine the virus at the molecular level. They tend to be more sensitive and more definitive than antibody tests, but are also more expensive, so they are usually used only after a positive diagnosis has been made with the antibody tests. They can detect HCV in the blood approximately three days to two weeks after exposure to the virus, while HCV antibody tests must wait six to eight weeks after exposure for a person to develop antibodies.

The tests determine the presence of HCV RNA in the blood, and are used to confirm chronic infection with HCV. If viral RNA is detected, a positive result is reported; if viral RNA is not detected, a negative result is reported.

Currently there are three systems for measuring HCV RNA:

1. the hepatitis C virus RNA polymerase chain reaction test (HCV RNA RT-PCR), or PCR assay for short
2. branched-chain DNA (bDNA)
3. transcription-mediated amplification (TMA)

The PCR assay and branched-chain DNA tests have been available since 1995. TMA is a more recent addition. All three tests can show whether the virus is present, and the actual amount of virus circulating in the bloodstream, known as the viral load of HCV in the blood. Information about the viral load allows the doctor to monitor how well a patient is responding to antiviral treatment. A person testing positive indicates current active infection, which also means that the patient is infectious to others.

PCR tests use a technique known as reverse transcription-polymerase chain reaction (RT-PCR). It amplifies several million times a small section of the nucleic acid associated with the virus using polymerase chain reaction (PCR), which brings it to measurable levels in the blood. PCR tests are very sensitive and can measure viral particles as few as 50 international units (IU) per milliliter (mL) of blood, though the detectable range can vary between laboratories. PCR assays can also be useful for identifying patients who may have received a false negative in the antibiotic test. But the PCR is not infallible. It may be more sensitive to certain genotypes of the virus than others. Moreover, PCR assays may vary among laboratories, and because the viral levels in the blood can sometimes fluctuate, the results may vary at different times.

Branched-chain DNA assay is used as a quick way to assess how much virus a person has, and it is also less expensive than the PCR assay. It is easier to apply to a large number of samples, but it is less sensitive than PCR, measuring only viral loads greater than 500 IU/mL. Testing negative for this does not mean there is no virus in the blood; it is possible for a person to test negative with the b-DNA, but positive with the PCR.

TMA, the latest addition, is even more sensitive than the PCR, measuring viral loads as few as five to 10 IU/mL. It is also easier and cheaper to use. This test uses targeted amplification techniques (TMA) to detect HCV RNA.

With any of the tests, a single negative result does not prove that a person is not infected, as there is a chance that the virus is present but was not found by the tests. A follow-up HCV RNA test may need to be performed. A single positive test, on the other hand, is enough to indicate that the person is infected with HCV, as these tests are more than 98 percent accurate for positive results.

Once the presence of the hepatitis C virus has been determined, physicians often recommend another test called quantitative HCV assays, usually either the quantitative PCR (qPCR) or branched DNA signal amplification assay (bDNA). They provide information about the amount of virus in a milliliter of blood, but they do not represent the actual number of viral particles. The results used to be expressed in various ways, using several different measurements, but to make comparisons easier, standardization has been introduced. Viral titers are now reported in international units per

milliliter, while previously they were often measured in numbers of copies. But some laboratories continue to express result in copies, or some other system of measurement.

It appears that patients with relatively high viral load are more likely to progress to cirrhosis, although various studies give somewhat contradictory results. This discrepancy is attributable to the fact that viral concentrations typically fluctuate within an individual and do not correlate with the degree of elevation of the liver enzymes (ALT and AST). Put another way, the viral load does not correspond to the severity of liver injury or fibrosis (scarring). A higher concentration of viral RNA does not automatically indicate that the patient has more liver inflammation and damage than one with a lower viral concentration. Therefore, the viral load is not a reliable predictor of the natural course or outcome of the infection; it cannot determine who will or will not develop cirrhosis, or who may develop disease outside the liver. Although the viral load generally does not correlate with the severity of liver disease, higher viral loads do appear to be associated with a higher risk of transmission, particularly from mothers to infants during pregnancy and birth.

The primary purpose of determining the viral load is to help the physician monitor the patient's response to therapy. Measuring the viral load before, during, and after treatment is useful because it allows the physician to do the following:

1. predict, to a certain extent, how well the treatment might work. In general, the lower the viral load, the more likely the patient will respond to therapy.
2. observe whether the viral load is increasing or decreasing during treatment. A decrease shows that the treatment is working. The goal of treatment is to reduce the viral load to an undetectable level. If there is an insufficient drop in viral load after 12 weeks of therapy, it is unlikely that the patient will be able to eradicate HCV from the body.
3. monitor for a relapse after treatment has been stopped. Sometimes, the virus may become detectable again after being reduced

to an undetectable level when treatment was completed.

In interpreting viral load test results, the HCV viral load is considered low if fewer than 800,000 IU/mL or less than 2 million copies. HCV viral load is considered high if more than 800,000 IU/mL or 2 million copies. Numbers in between are considered intermediate.

A person's viral load is said to be undetectable if no HCV RNA is found. This may mean that the individual has no HCV (has never contracted the infection, or has successfully eradicated it from the body), or that the blood still contains a very low viral load, even though it cannot be measured by the test used. Moreover, test results may vary depending on how a blood sample is handled and stored, and from laboratory to laboratory. When monitoring treatment response, experts recommend using the same laboratory each time so that the results are more comparable.

When the viral load changes from one test to the next, the change may be expressed in terms of logs. If there is a tenfold increase or decrease, there is said to be a 1-log change. According to this system, a change from 1,000,000 IU/mL to 10,000 IU/mL is a 2-log decrease.

The next step after a diagnosis of HCV is to determine the genotype, or genetic strain, of the virus. In the past, genotyping was conducted for clinical research only, but it is now available to physicians through commercial laboratories, and many liver specialists are running the test as a matter of routine. Once the genotype is tested, it need not be tested again, as it does not change.

Identifying the patient's genotype can be useful in several ways:

1. in defining the epidemiology of HCV
2. in making recommendations regarding treatment

Infection with different genotypes may have different clinical consequences. Therefore, knowing the genotypes can provide a rough guideline on how well a patient might respond to therapy and how long the treatment should last. Although genotyping cannot accurately predict success or failure of therapy for any individual person, the following observations have been made through research:

1. Genotypes 1a and 1b, the most common in the United States, are relatively resistant to antiviral therapy.
2. Patients with genotypes 1 and 2 appear to have a greater likelihood of developing cirrhosis, advanced scarring of the liver.
3. Genotypes 2 and 3 are associated with a better prognosis, and are more likely to respond to interferon therapy.
4. A six-month course of combination interferon and ribavirin treatment may be adequate in the case of genotypes 2 and 3, instead of the conventional 12-month course for genotype 1.

A LIVER BIOPSY is a procedure that allows the physician to assess the condition of the liver. It is a minor surgical procedure where a tiny sample of the liver is extracted with a needle and placed under the microscope for examination. Many liver specialists believe that a liver biopsy should be part of the work-up for patients with chronic hepatitis, because it allows the pathologist to determine precisely how much inflammation and scarring is in the liver. Currently, a biopsy is the only definitive way to assess the amount of damage that has been done to the liver as a consequence of the viruses. This is of particular significance in the case of hepatitis C, because patients may have considerable underlying liver disease without having any symptoms or abnormal physical or laboratory findings.

A biopsy is generally recommended before initiating treatment for hepatitis C infection, a position endorsed by the National Institutes of Health (NIH) Consensus Development Conference Panel in 1997. In 2002, another NIH consensus conference reiterated the earlier recommendation regarding the liver biopsy, noting that liver enzymes (ALT and AST) show little value in predicting fibrosis (scarring). In this regard, the biopsy "provides a unique source of information on fibrosis and assessment of histology. . . . Extracellular matrix tests can predict severe stages of fibrosis but cannot consistently classify intermediate stages of fibrosis. Moreover, only liver biopsy provides information on possible contribution of iron, steatosis [fatty liver], and concurrent alcoholic liver disease to the progression of chronic hepatitis toward cirrhosis."

Exceptions may be made, however, for patients with genotypes two or three. As NIH has observed, because 80 percent of such patients respond favorably to current antiviral therapy, a liver biopsy may not be strictly necessary before commencing treatment, as the pathology result from the biopsy will not likely change the prescription for treatment.

A standardized evaluation of liver histology (tissue examined under a microscope) is useful in HCV infection. Accordingly, biopsy results show the nature and severity of liver injury through a grading system that indicates the extent of structural damage the liver has sustained. The staging considers the amount of inflammation and fibrosis in the liver, graded on a scale of zero to four. Zero indicates no fibrosis, meaning that no damage has been done to the liver yet. One shows mild fibrosis, and four means that cirrhosis—advanced scarring and structural distortion—is now present. In the case of HCV, fibrosis is more predictive of progression to irreversible liver disease than inflammation. This information is useful to the physician in deciding whether the patient should be treated for hepatitis C. The guideline provided by NIH calls for treatment for any patients who have a fibrosis of grade one or more.

Finding out how much fibrosis is present can also help in the prognosis. The disease will probably progress slowly in patients with mild or no fibrosis; patients with severe fibrosis have more advanced disease and a greater chance that the scarring will develop into cirrhosis. Finally, patients with cirrhosis have a high risk of complications, especially of developing hepatocellular carcinoma, or primary liver cancer. The presence of cirrhosis is particularly relevant when a decision has to be made regarding treatment.

In recent years, some researchers and clinicians have questioned the utility of performing a liver biopsy in routine cases of HCV infection, and much discussion has revolved around this issue. Some contend that clinical and laboratory findings alone provide sufficient information to make a decision for or against antiviral therapy. A liver biopsy is certainly not needed to

establish the diagnosis of HCV infection—blood tests are sufficient—and indeed, a biopsy will not alter the diagnosis. On the other hand, it has been pointed out that clinical and laboratory tests are not particularly good at predicting the extent of liver damage caused by HCV infection. For example, elevations of ALT (alanine aminotransferase, a liver enzyme) generally indicate that liver cells are being destroyed. However, in patients chronically infected with HCV, there is a poor correlation between symptoms or levels of ALT and any damage to the liver tissue or to the architecture of the liver. Patients with completely normal levels of the liver enzymes (ALT and AST) may be found to have significant fibrosis or cirrhosis on biopsy. Laboratory findings such as the ratio of the liver enzymes (AST/ALT ratio) and platelet counts cannot often accurately predict the amount of liver injury. A liver biopsy is required to provide useful information about the degree of fibrosis in HCV-infected patients, information that is often critical for making decisions in the management of HCV infection, as well as in monitoring the effectiveness of the various treatments.

Determining the stage of the liver disease through a biopsy can help predict how long it may take a patient to progress from one grade (between zero to four) to the next. A patient whose biopsy shows grade-one liver injury (mild fibrosis) can take about 12 years on average to progress to cirrhosis. On the other hand, a patient at grade three will take only about 18 months on average to develop cirrhosis. In other words, the higher the grade, the faster the disease progresses. That means that a person with a milder liver injury may have time to wait before embarking on an antiviral treatment—a luxury that a person at stage three may not have. Thus, a biopsy can help the physician decide on the best course of action for a particular patient. A patient with only mild liver disease who is infected by genotype 1a or 1b of the hepatitis C virus may defer treatment, because these genotypes tend to be resistant to treatment, and the patient can afford to wait. If a treatment is begun and the patient reacts adversely to it, treatment can be safely stopped. But the physician will probably decide to offer treatment to a patient who has moderate or severe liver disease even if he or she has genotype 1a or 1b, particularly because it is impossible to know in advance definitively whether an individual will respond to therapy, and there is little time to waste.

In approximately 20 to 30 percent of HCV-infected patients, a biopsy shows that cirrhosis has developed. If cirrhosis is discovered, further examinations are usually necessary to rule out bleeding varices (veins) in the esophagus (the digestive tube from the mouth to the stomach) and liver cancer.

Various analyses have confirmed that a biopsy is critical for the proper staging of liver disease.

One study offered data supporting the need for a liver biopsy for the following reasons:

1. to establish the stage of liver disease
2. to make a general prognosis
3. to establish the appropriate treatment and management for HCV

Researchers at the Cleveland Clinic reviewed the records of 126 patients with HCV who underwent liver biopsy at the clinic between January 31, 1990, and February 1, 1997. The results of this analysis suggest that in the majority of patients, less invasive assessments were not as accurate as a biopsy at detecting the level of disease activity or in establishing the stage of liver disease, including the presence or absence of fibrosis or inflammation. The results also showed no major complications from the biopsies; the most frequent problem was mild pain in the area of the biopsy site. From this the researchers concluded that it was safe for patients with hepatitis C to undergo liver biopsies.

Although the liver biopsy is extremely useful in the assessment of liver disease in chronic hepatitis C, it still suffers from some major weaknesses:

1. Minor variations in the amount of fibrosis are often missed because of the noncontinuous scoring (finer gradations of liver injury may be missed).
2. False-negative results may be found in 10 to 30 percent of cases. This is possible if the size of the biopsy specimen was too small. Because the amount of liver tissue obtained by needle

biopsy is very small—expressed in number of cells, it is no more than 1/30,000 of the liver volume—it can be representative of the state of the liver only if the inflammation and fibrosis are uniformly distributed. But some studies indicate that fibrosis may not be uniformly represented in each biopsy specimen. For cirrhosis, sometimes up to three specimens may be needed for an accurate evaluation. Specimen lengths need to be closer to 25 mm for greater accuracy. Use of too fine a needle can also impede the accurate staging of fibrosis and lead to diagnostic error.

3. The procedure is relatively expensive, costing somewhere from $1,500 to $2,000. Because antiviral therapy for HCV is also quite costly, a biopsy may overburden patient resources.
4. There is a risk of complications. Liver biopsy is invasive and at times may cause side effects. Approximately 20 to 50 percent will experience significant pain. There may be major bleeding in a few cases, as well as accidental perforation of the kidney, colon, or gallbladder. Death from biopsy is extremely rare, however.
5. Patient and physician aversion to the procedure must be considered. Patients may be extremely anxious about the procedure, and this may prompt physicians to prescribe antianxiety medication. The prospect of a biopsy may also discourage patients from undergoing an evaluation for subsequent treatment. Some physicians may also be averse to the biopsy because of the concern about complications and patient's fear of the procedure.
6. Biopsies usually require a gastroenterologist or a radiologist, who may not be the treating physician.
7. There may be a lack of specific findings. Any abnormalities in the liver due to HCV infection can also be seen in other viral and nonviral liver diseases, and this makes interpretation of results difficult at times. If, for example, a patient was formerly a heavy user of alcohol but has been abstinent for several months, then the presence of significant fibrosis that was caused primarily by heavy alcohol use may be erroneously attributed to HCV.

In an attempt to bypass many of the disadvantages of a liver biopsy, investigators have been trying to stage HCV on less invasive means, such as biochemical markers. They have suggested that liver fibrosis in patients with HCV infection may be satisfactorily staged through these alternative methods in many, if not most, HCV-infected patients.

Various markers based on blood tests assessing the severity of fibrosis or the inflammatory activity of liver disease have been recently proposed and are currently under clinical evaluation. The results of several marker determinants have been compared with the results of liver biopsy. The performance of these markers appears to be acceptable when discriminating between no fibrosis or mild fibrosis and cirrhosis, but seems to be less satisfactory in the intermediate states.

At present, liver biopsy remains an important tool in the baseline evaluation of the HCV-infected patient. The biopsy has always been considered a part of the standard of care for hepatitis C patients before undergoing treatment, though experts differ in their recommendations with respect to follow-up biopsies at various intervals to restage the liver.

The search for less invasive ways to evaluate the risk of liver disease progression has intensified. In the near future, no doubt, noninvasive markers will replace liver biopsy when their performance improves and they are able to provide more accurate information on the natural outcome of HCV-related liver disease.

The incubation period—the time between exposure and the onset of symptoms of HCV (whether recognized or not)—ranges from 15 days to five months, with the average between six to seven weeks. If the patient is able to clear the virus from the bloodstream, it usually happens within eight to 10 weeks. Although by definition, acute hepatitis does not last longer than six months, in some rare cases the hepatitis virus may not be cleared until nine months after the initial exposure.

If tests detect the virus (HCV RNA), but not anti-HCV antibodies, it is a strong indication of acute hepatitis, especially if antibodies appear later. An acute infection is unlikely if antibodies are present and HCV RNA is absent. It may mean that the infection is no longer current, and the patient has already cleared the HCV at some time in the past. Or it could be that something other than HCV infection is causing the liver disease. The patient should be retested a few weeks later, as sometimes the HCV RNA becomes detectable on subsequent testing. When both antibodies and HCV RNA are detected, it is difficult to tell whether the patient is suffering from acute hepatitis C or having a "flare-up"—an acute exacerbation—of chronic hepatitis C. Another possibility is that the patient is a sufferer of chronic hepatitis C and is having a bout of acute hepatitis of another cause, either viral (infection with hepatitis C does not confer immunity to any other viral hepatitis) or otherwise.

When testing for HCV, antibodies to the hepatitis C virus can usually be detected within 15 weeks of the initial infection in 80 percent of patients. After five months, it can be detected in 90 percent of patients, and after six months, in 97 percent of patients.

If both antibodies and HCV RNA are detected, the individual almost certainly has chronic hepatitis C, particularly if he or she belongs to the high-risk population. If confirmation is needed, the individual can be tested again with either a PCR or TMA for the presence of HCV RNA.

Treatment Options and Outlook

It is preferable to be evaluated by a hepatologist (liver specialist) for diagnosis and possible treatment, as there is a great deal of ongoing research in this area, and new developments are often underway. Not everyone needs or benefits from antiviral therapy. Treatment, when recommended, is aimed at eradicating the virus and stopping or slowing the progression of the disease before any complications develop. At this time, the treatment of chronic hepatitis C is based on a combination of pegylated INTERFERON (IFN) alfa and ribavirin. Generally, treatment is expected to last for one to three months, depending on the HCV genotype and other factors. The optimal treatment schedule for acute hepatitis C—the type of interferon, the dose, and the duration of therapy—has yet to be established.

Because of the extraordinarily high incidence of progression to chronic disease—only about 20 percent of people infected by HCV are able to shake it off—it is important to identify and treat the infection so that the virus may be eliminated at the acute stage. Some studies suggest that a short course of interferon achieved a significant reduction of the likelihood of progression to chronic liver disease in sufferers of acute hepatitis C. For instance, one study showed that 41 percent of patients treated with interferon cleared the HCV virus from their bodies, while only 4 percent of those without treatment did so. It follows that anyone accidentally exposed to hepatitis C should be tested and offered therapy if necessary, to prevent the infection from becoming chronic. It is best to wait at least a week, preferably two, before testing.

Although a few people with chronic hepatitis C do recover without treatment—the virus disappears from the blood and their liver enzymes are normalized—the vast majority will not. Patients most likely to clear the virus from their blood spontaneously without treatment have usually shown symptoms of HCV infection (rather than being asymptomatic), have a high peak bilirubin level, and are of the female gender.

Viral clearance tends to occur most frequently within the first 12 weeks after symptoms appear. Treatment is advisable if the virus has not been cleared within three months, particularly if the patients are asymptomatic—have no symptoms indicative of HCV—though tests clearly show they have been infected. At the end of therapy, patients must be tested with a sensitive HCV RNA technique. Therapy is considered to be successful if no HCV RNA is detected.

In general, any adult with chronic hepatitis C and evidence of active inflammation, under the age of 70, and without cirrhosis may be considered for treatment. Whether patients with very mild disease and little or no liver inflammation are candidates for antiviral therapy is best determined on an individual basis. Patients suffering from advanced cirrhosis may be evaluated for possible liver transplantation.

HCV infection can follow a benign course in some, but in others it can lead to serious liver disease. Chronic infection with hepatitis C is now recognized as one of the most common causes of cirrhosis. Scarring of the liver is mostly the result of the liver's attempting to protect itself from chronic long-term inflammation caused by the virus. There is a great variation in the rate at which cirrhosis develops. Some people may never develop cirrhosis; others may get it within five years of becoming infected with HCV, while still others may take 50 or even 60 years to develop cirrhosis. On average, cirrhosis develops over a 20- to 30-year period, and at least 20 percent of chronically HCV infected patients can expect to get cirrhosis. Once scarring progresses to cirrhosis, the person has a 25 percent increased risk for hepatocellular carcinoma, primary liver cancer. This heightened risk applies to cirrhosis from all causes, not just HCV, and people who are infected with hepatitis C but who do not have cirrhosis have no greater risk for liver cancer than those without the infection.

The likelihood of complications developing seems related to environmental influences not yet fully understood. For example, environmental pollution and cigarette smoking possibly accelerate disease progression. Other factors may include the viral load (amount of virus in the body) and the genotype. Superinfection, or coinfection with other diseases, such as hepatitis B and HIV (AIDS) reportedly increases the severity of chronic hepatitis C and the risk of liver cancer. Research has shown that liver scarring progresses faster in the setting of HIV infection.

The course of acute hepatitis C is variable, with fluctuations in the levels of ALT (alanine aminotransferase, a liver enzyme). The ALT levels should eventually normalize, suggesting full recovery. If the ALT levels appear to normalize, only to rise again, it indicates that the infection has progressed to chronic disease. In most cases of acute infection, the patient should recover without significant adverse effects. In very rare cases, patients suffer from fulminant hepatitis C, a severe form of acute hepatitis C characterized by the sudden onset of liver failure. It is often accompanied by jaundice (yellowing of the skin and eyes) and encephalopathy (mental disorientation and confusion). In about 85 percent of cases, the patients will die unless given an immediate liver transplant.

The course of chronic HCV is variable and generally cannot be predicted in a specific case. Doctors cannot accurately predict who will do well and who will develop cirrhosis or cancer.

At this time, there is one clearly known risk factor for progression to cirrhosis: alcohol abuse. Patients who have problems with alcohol should be referred for counseling. Meanwhile, additional research is needed to identify other factors that may play critical roles in determining the course of hepatitis C infection.

Future therapies   Today an improved understanding of the structure and replication cycle of the hepatitis C virus has opened up a new generation of drugs and prospects in the development of novel therapies.

Combination therapies of interferon (injected) and the nucleoside analog ribavirin (taken orally) are current treatment standards. The major drawback to these therapies is the relatively low response rate—effective in about 55 percent of patients. Moreover, the drug regimen is expensive and often not tolerated well because of its significant side effects and the therapy duration—usually either six or 12 months. And many patients cannot even qualify for therapy, such as those with advanced liver disease. Clearly, more effective non-toxic and inexpensive drugs are urgently needed.

In creating new drugs for hepatitis C, one of the biggest obstacles had been the inability to grow the virus in the test tube for study or for testing potential drugs. Animal research has also been impeded because only chimpanzees, which are expensive to use, can be infected with hepatitis C.

To circumvent these problems, scientists developed an artificial viral system called the replicon, which simulates the replication process of HCV. The replicon does not create complete new viruses, but it has some of the RNA from hepatitis C virus and uses the same enzymes (protease and polymerase) to reproduce itself. This allows researchers to try out new drugs to see whether they can successfully disrupt the replication of the replicon.

The above is just one example of how scientists have been mapping out various strategies to eliminate the virus or to minimize viral damage. Some of these approaches include those below:

- enhancing response to current interferon-based therapies

- developing newer nucleoside analogs
- inhibiting enzymes critical to the virus
- creating drugs to reduce the progression of fibrosis (scarring of liver tissue)

These new treatment approaches will be available to the general public once their safety and efficacy is established, a process that can take several years.

Immunotherapy   Drugs that can boost the body's immune system are being evaluated. Immune modifiers, or immunomodulators, can alter the body's immune response to help prevent damage to the liver caused by the hepatitis C virus. Some immune modifiers are to be taken in combination with interferon. Drugs that have been tested include thymosin-alpha-1 and histamine dihydrocholoride.

Investigators are also looking at specific types of T cells (immune factors) that appear to play an important role in individuals who are able to resolve spontaneously hepatitis C, in other words, to clear the virus from their bodies. They are working on DNA vaccines that can stimulate cytotoxic T cell activity.

Protease inhibitors   New drug therapies are designed to target viral enzymes—proteins used in catalysis of chemical reactions. All the HCV enzymes are essential for HCV replication, so they are good targets for potential drug discoveries. Accordingly, the primary focus of many researchers is to stop these viral enzymes from functioning. Target enzymes include protease, helicase, and polymerase.

The hepatitis C protease enzyme snips large viral protein units into smaller segments during replication. A family of drugs being developed called protease inhibitors can interfere with this packing of viral genes into new viruses. Since protease inhibitors designed against human immunodeficiency virus, (HIV causes AIDS) have been quite successful, the same methodology is being used for new drug development studies for HCV. Protease inhibitors against HIV will not work against hepatitis C because the inhibitors must be tailored to a specific virus. Protease inhibitors may work especially well for the hard-to-treat population with genotype 1.

Helicase inhibitors Once the hepatitis virus enters the host cell, helicase enzymes unwind the viral RNA as the virus copies itself. Helicase inhibitors stop the double-stranded RNA from unwinding, thus disrupting the replication process.

Polymerase inhibitors Polymerase enzymes catalyze the synthesis of nucleic acids. They are the third type of enzymes critical to HCV replication. Polymerase inhibitors such as NM283 block the replication of HCV polymerase. The inhibitors seem to work well with difficult-to-treat HCV genotype 1. Early data suggest that a combination of NM283 and interferon may work synergistically.

IRES inhibitors Drugs are being developed that can block other steps in HCV reproduction. The internal ribosome initiation site (IRES) is found in every hepatitis C virus genotype, and an essential part of the viral replication process. Scientists are working to create an IRES inhibitor that would prevent the expression of viral proteins by blocking production of the virus.

Ribozymes Ribozyme is a small catalytic RNA molecule that can cut targeted genetic material of the hepatitis C virus, interrupting the life cycle of the virus. Researchers are studying one kind of ribozyme called hammerhead ribozyme. These ribozymes have been shown to inhibit viral replication by more than 95 percent if used alone, and more than 99 percent with the addition of interferon.

Inosine monophosphate dehydrogenase inhibitors One new drug is an oral inhibitor of an enzyme called inosine monophosphate dehydrogenase (IMPDH). It has anti-inflammatory and antiviral activities similar to the immunomodulator thymosin-alpha-1, as well as to ribavirin, the oral antiviral medication currently used in combination with interferon. Ribavirin is also an inhibitor of IMPDH, which is essential for the production of a compound that forms the building blocks of DNA and RNA. Thus, inhibiting IMPDH may block viral replication. In the initial findings of a study assessing this drug—VX-497—presented at the 55th annual meeting of the American Society for the Study of Liver Diseases (AASLD), significant reductions in serum alanine transaminase (ALT) values were achieved. It is much more potent than ribavirin.

Amantadine Amantadine is an oral antiviral medication that fell out of favor after a brief period of enthusiasm in hepatitis C therapy in the late 1990s. In recent years it has attracted renewed interest. Some investigators are studying the effect of adding amantadine to the interferon/ribavirin mix. Randomized controlled studies provide conflicting results, and its efficacy is still a matter of controversy.

Antisense neucleotides Antisense nucleotides is a type of gene therapy for viral hepatitis. Antisense drugs genetically interfere with the viral gene's synthesis of proteins that cause disease. The antisense DNA (a human-made copy matched to a viral gene) attaches itself to viral RNA, preventing the production of necessary proteins, thus interfering with its workings.

Drugs to prevent cell injury Since the most serious complications of hepatitis C result from cirrhosis, investigators have been researching drugs that can affect the liver's response to injury. There may be nonspecific cytoprotective agents that might block cell injury caused by the virus infection. Antifibrotic drugs can slow and prevent fibrosis. Recent studies suggest that it may be possible to reverse fibrosis—perhaps even early cirrhosis—to some extent.

Therapeutic vaccine Therapeutic vaccine is not for the prevention of hepatitis C, but to treat patients already infected with the disease. Several such vaccines currently being developed are said to stop, or even reverse, liver damage in patients with hepatitis C.

Stem cell therapy Research has shown that liver stem cells reside in the bone marrow of the body. Stem cells are undifferentiated cells that can be directed to form many different tissues of the body. An example of undifferentiated cells are those in early embryos. In theory, these bone marrow stem cells can be isolated and grown into liver cells that can be used to regrow damaged liver. Research is still in its early stages, however, and it may be decades before this type of therapy has practical application.

Risk Factors and Preventive Measures

Hepatitis C is a blood-borne disease. Currently the primary route of infection is through blood contact, perinatally—from infected mothers to newborns—and less frequently, through sexual contact.

Individuals who have one or more risk factors for hepatitis C are advised to get tested for hepatitis C. Treatments are available today that may help keep the infection from progressing into a serious liver disease. The following are considered risk factors for contracting hepatitis C:

- received blood transfusions before 1992
- received organ transplants before 1992
- had surgery, including oral surgery, before 1992
- treated for clotting problems with blood products made before 1987
- currently has, or had, occupational exposure to blood, blood products, or needles (for example, health care and public safety workers)
- born to an HCV-infected mother
- had long-term kidney dialysis treatments
- received a tattoo or body piercing
- diagnosed as HIV-positive
- injected illegal drugs, even once
- inhaled cocaine
- served in the military
- been in prison
- member of immediate family diagnosed with hepatitis B or C
- had multiple sex partners
- changed sex partners frequently
- had sex with an infected partner
- had unprotected sex with anyone fitting the above description

In addition to the above, people who received acupuncture treatments with nondisposable needles may be at risk.

The highest prevalence of HCV infection is found among those with large or repeated through-the-skin (percutaneous) exposures to blood, such as intravenous drug users and recipients of blood transfusions from HCV-positive donors. Those who received frequent but smaller percutaneous expo-

sures, such as long-term hemodialysis patients, have a moderate prevalence of infection. A lower prevalence is found among those with small, sporadic exposures, such as health care workers or people exposed through high-risk sexual practices.

The American Liver Foundation encourages anyone who may have hepatitis C to be tested. Anyone with one or more of the above-mentioned risk factors may have become infected with HCV.

Chronic hepatitis C is sometimes referred to as "the silent epidemic." More people are expected to develop serious complications as a result of infection with the hepatitis C virus. And yet, hepatitis C is a largely preventable disease. In addition to ongoing research to discover more effective drugs against hepatitis C, greater emphasis needs to be placed on educating the public so that proper precautions may be taken to stop spreading the hepatitis C virus and keep the disease from turning into a public health crisis. The goal should be to prevent people from acquiring the infection in the first place.

It is imperative that all health care and public safety workers be educated regarding the risk of hepatitis and other infections, and the means to prevent them. Moreover, trained health care professionals should educate patients about hepatitis C and make sure they understand, and are capable of, following appropriate infection-control procedures. They should make home visits to make sure the procedures are being followed properly.

There are no recommendations to restrict professional activities of health care workers with HCV infection. They should, of course, follow the precautions outlined below, being especially careful to wash hands, use protective barriers, dispose of instruments properly, and ensure that patients and others will not come into contact with blood or body fluids that contain blood.

Hepatitis C patients can refrain from inadvertently transmitting the infection to friends, family, and others by observing the following guidelines:

- Do not share personal items that may be contaminated by blood. These include razors, nail clippers, and toothbrushes. At the same time, people should be aware that sharing food, water, or eating utensils does not spread HCV.

- Carefully dispose of any blood-soaked items to make sure that no one else will come into contact with them.
- Cover all open wounds, sores, and cuts, particularly if playing contact sports.
- Stop using and injecting drugs.
- Do not share needles, syringes, water, or drug preparation equipment with anyone. Even a drop of blood so tiny that it cannot be seen by the naked eye may contain thousands of hepatitis C viruses. If the equipment has been used, first clean it with bleach and water.
- Notify immediately those with whom one has shared intravenous drug equipment and urge them to be checked for hepatitis C infection.
- Seek out a needle-exchange program or use only disposable needles and syringes that are non-reusable if one cannot stop injection drug use. Safely dispose of syringes after one use.
- Seek help at a drug rehabilitation center if one cannot stop abusing drugs.
- Avoid donating blood or plasma, sperm, tissues, or organs, as HCV can be readily transmitted to the recipient.
- Practice safer sex. Use barrier contraception each and every time when having sex, particularly in a nonmonogamous relationship. In people with multiple sex partners and those with a history of sexually transmitted disease, there is an estimated 15 percent risk of transmitting HCV. Because the chance of spreading HCV to a partner in a monogamous relationship is low (about 5 percent), condoms are not absolutely necessary but may be used for extra precaution. Oral sex appears to be safe. HCV is not spread by hugging or kissing.
- Advise intimate partner(s) of infection.
- Avoid anal sex and sex during menstruation since HCV is transmitted primarily by blood.
- Inform all medical and dental health care professionals about HCV so that they may take proper precautions when treating.
- Practice good hygiene. Meticulously wash hands after using the bathroom or before and after changing diapers.

Expectant women must realize that there is no treatment or vaccine that can prevent infected mothers from transmitting HCV to their infants during childbirth. However, the risk is relatively low, approximately 5 to 6 percent. If the mother is also infected by human immunodeficiency virus, (HIV the AIDS virus), the risk increases to an average of 14 to 17 percent. Studies evaluating the possibility of transmitting HCV from breast feeding show an average infection rate of 4 percent in both breast-fed and bottle-fed infants. Thus, breast feeding does not appear to pose a higher risk of infection for the infant.

Patients should be aware that infection with the hepatitis C virus does not prevent becoming infected with other viral hepatitis. Studies suggest that becoming infected with both hepatitis C and hepatitis B leads to a much more serious case of hepatitis. Moreover, HCV patients who come down with an acute case of hepatitis A can suffer from fulminant hepatic failure. To avoid worsening of the disease, consider getting vaccinated against hepatitis A and/or hepatitis B. The hepatitis B vaccine grants double immunity against both hepatitis B and hepatitis D, since hepatitis D cannot exist without the presence of hepatitis B.

Afdahl, N., and others. "Final phase I/II trial results for NM283, a new polymerase inhibitor for hepatitis C: antiviral efficacy and tolerance in patients with HCV-1 infection, including previous interferon failures." Abstract LB-03. 55th annual meeting of the American Society for the Study of Liver Diseases (ASSLD). October 29–November 2004. Boston. Available online. URL: http://www.hivandhepatitis.com/2004icr/aasld/docs/hcv/1101_a.html. Downloaded on February 1, 2005.

Asselah, Tarik, and Patrick Marcellin. "HCV protease inhibitors-BILN 2061: A major step toward new therapeutic strategies in hepatitis C." *Journal of Hepatology* 41, no. 1 (July 2004): 178–181.

Centers for Disease Control and Prevention. "Recommendations for prevention and control of hepatitis C virus infection and HCV related chronic disease." *Morbidity and Mortality Weekly Report* 47, no. RR-19 (October 16, 1998): n.p.

Comador, Lorraine, M.D., Frank Anderson, M.D., Marc Ghany, M.D., Robert Pevillo, M.D., Jenny E. Heathcote, M.D., Chris Sherlock, M.D., Ian Zitron, David Hendricks, and Stuart C. Gordon, M.D. "Transcription-mediated amplification is more sensitive than conventional PCR-based assays for detecting residual serum HCV RNA at end of treatment." *American Journal of Gastroenterology,* 96, no. 10 (October 2001): 2,968–2,972.

Dagan, S., and others. "In-vitro and in-vivo evaluation of HCV polymerase inhibitors as potential drug candidates for treatment of chronic hepatitis C infection." Abstract 53. 39th annual meeting of the European Association of the Study of the Liver (EASL). April 14–18, 2004. Berlin, Germany. Available online. URL: http://www.hivandhepatitis.com/2004icr/39easl/documents/0421/042104_hcv_b.html. Downloaded on February 1, 2005.

Deuffic-Burban, S., and others. "Comparing the public health burden of chronic hepatitis C and HIV infection in United States." Abstract 552. 54th AASLD. October 24–28, 2003. Boston.

Dev, Anouk, M.D., Keyur Patel, M.D., and John G. McHutchison, M.D. "Future treatment of hepatitis C: What's around the corner." *Infections in Medicine* 21, no. 1 (2004): 28–36.

Ferenci, P., and others. "Randomized, controlled, double-blind placebo-controlled study of peginterferon Alfa-2A (40KD) (Pegasys®) plus ribavirin (Copegus® and amantadine (AMA) or placebo in patients with chronic hepatitis C genotype 1 infection." Abstract 534. 55th AASLD. October 29–November 2004. Boston. Available online. URL: http://www.hivandhepatitis.com/2004icr/aasld/docs/hcv/110804_e.html. Downloaded on February 1, 2005.

Gerlach, Tilman J., Reinhart Zachoval, Norbert Gruener, Maria-Christina Jung, Klinikum Grosshadern, Axel Ulsenheimer, Winfried Schraut, Albrecht Schirren, Martin Waechtler, and Markus Backmund. "Acute hepatitis C: Natural course and response to antiviral treatment." Abstract 676. Conference Reports for NATAP AASLD. November 9–13, 2001. Dallas.

Ishak, K., A. Baptista, L. Bianchi, F. Callea, J. DeGroote, F. Gudat, H. Denk, et al. "Histologic grading and staging of chronic hepatitis." *Journal of Hepatology* 22, issue 6 (1995): 696–699.

Kaul, V., F. K. Friedenberg, L. E. Braitman, U. Anis, N. Zaeri, J. Fazili, et al. "Development and validation of a model to diagnose cirrhosis in patients with hepati-

tis C." *American Journal of Gastroenterology* 97 (2002): 2,625.

Lin, K., and others. "VX-950: A tight-binding HCV protease inhibitor with a superior sustained inhibitory response in HCV replicon cells." Abstract 137 (oral). 54th AASLD. October 24–28, 2003. Boston. Available online URL: http://www.hivandhepatitis.com/2003icr/03_asssld/docs/1029/102903_e.html. Downloaded on February 1, 2005.

National Center for Infectious Diseases. Viral Hepatitis Resource Center. Reviewed October 2003. URL: http://www.cedc.gov/ncidod/diseases/hepatitis. Downloaded in January 2004.

"Recommendations for prevention and control of hepatitis C virus (HCV) infection and HCV-related chronic disease." Centers for Disease Control and Prevention 47, no. RR-19 (October 16, 1998): 1–39.

Torre, F., R. Gisuto, A. Grasso, et al. "Optimal hepatitis C regimen would include interferon plus amantadine and ribavirin." *Journal of Medical Virology* 64 (2001): 490–496.

Saadeh, S., G. Cammell, W. D. Carey, and others. "The role of liver biopsy in chronic hepatitis C." *Hepatology* 33, no. 1 (December 2003): 196–200.

hepatitis C and children Hepatitis C (HCV) is regarded as a major global public health problem. The incidence of HCV in children is not clearly known, but it is estimated that some 240,000 children in the United States have been infected or exposed to the virus. Of these, 60,000 to 100,000 are chronically infected with HCV—they have been infected for six months or longer.

Many experts believe that HCV in children is an underestimated problem and that the number of children with HCV is increasing. It is not easy to determine because diagnosing the disease can be complicated in infants. In some infants, the virus may be in the body for only a short duration, which would seem to indicate that it is not a genuine infection. Others may have an acute infection that spontaneously resolves itself. Moreover, most chronically infected children have few or no symptoms. Their alanine aminotransferase (ALT) levels are often normal or only mildly abnormal.

The main route of HCV infection is through infected blood. Many people, including children, were infected through blood transfusions before 1991, before blood and blood products were screened carefully for HCV. Today, the major source of infection in children is the mother. A mother infected with HCV can pass the virus on to the baby during pregnancy. This process is known as vertical transmission. If the infection occurs around the time of birth, the process is called perinatal transmission.

Exactly how the virus is transmitted from the mother to the child remains to be clarified, but experts agree that the risk of infection is quite low. Estimates by various studies range from 3 to 6 percent. Japan, which has a more severe form of hepatitis C than does the United States, has a transmission rate of 6 percent among newborns. The risk, however, is much higher if the mother has a higher concentration of virus in her blood, and especially if the mother is also HIV-positive (human immunodeficiency virus that causes AIDS). Infants infected with HIV—and vertical transmission of HIV occurs much more frequently than it does for hepatitis C—are also more likely than those who are not to contract hepatitis C. In addition, such infants are also more likely to suffer from significant LIVER DISEASE.

In terms of overall risk of vertical transmission, researchers in Spain who conducted a meta-analysis of nine studies involving 1,010 infants showed that it was almost four times higher in infants born to mothers who are coinfected with hepatitis C and HIV than to infants born to mothers who had only hepatitis C.

Symptoms and Diagnostic Path

Test results for HCV in the first month of life are not particularly reliable because of the low sensitivity of the tests. Initially, about two-thirds of children show negative results even if they have been infected by HCV, but after one month a negative RNA test result is usually accurate. Some children can be negative at three months and later test positive. Doctors usually recommend that blood tests wait until after 12 to 15 months, because the mother's antibodies could temporarily accumulate in the infant's blood and skew the results.

Infants, whether infected or not, have been observed to have various anti-HCV patterns due to passively acquired maternal antibodies that may persist for months. These passively acquired antibodies are usually gone by 12 months. Because antibodies to HCV are transferred from the mother to the fetus in the womb and remain detectable for several months—sometimes for more than a year—after delivery, a recommended approach is to test infants for HCV RNA rather than to the antibodies.

In infants, HCV RNA can be detected as early as one to two months, and then persist or be cleared spontaneously. Spontaneous clearance occurs more frequently in infants and children than in adults, though the exact frequency is not known.

When interpreting test results, it should be borne in mind that the sensitivity of tests varies between laboratories.

Not enough studies have been done on children to know whether the course of HCV infection is the same as in adults. A review of infected children shows that in 60 to 80 percent of them, the HIV infection turns into chronic hepatitis C. On the other hand, the infection appears to be relatively mild in children. For the most part, infants do not exhibit symptoms of hepatitis C. When liver tissue is examined under the microscope, there are rarely any signs of advanced scarring of the liver (CIRRHOSIS) or liver cancer (HEPATOCELLULAR CARCINOMA)—at least, not during childhood and adolescence.

The course of the disease is associated with different genotypes. For instance, children infected with hepatitis C genotype 2 tend to have a biochemically mild disease, while genotype three appears to be associated with a spontaneous clearing of the virus in early childhood. Children with both types 2 and 3 respond to interferon (IFN) treatment for a sustained period of time. But more children with different HCV genotypes must be tested before statistically significant results can be obtained.

ALT levels are usually only slightly or moderately elevated in children, though they can be highly variable in children one year or younger, and are not good predictors of eventual outcome. At present, the long-term prognosis for children is not known because of the lack of long-term studies in which the children are followed up for 20 to 30 years.

Research suggests that the mode in which HCV was transmitted may also influence the course of the disease. A large-scale study that examined 231 Japanese children who received a contaminated blood transfusion before 1992, when blood was not screened for HCV, discovered that most had only minor liver damage regardless of how long they had had the infection. In this study, 60 to 80 percent of the children who tested positive for HCV eventually developed chronic hepatitis C. Generally speaking, when children contract hepatitis C before or shortly after birth, the infection becomes chronic. However, differences were not detected in the grade of inflammation or the stage of fibrosis of the liver, irrespective of the duration of the illness.

Treatment Options and Outlook

Although most studies show that children usually have a mild case of hepatitis C, some children can become very ill. And doctors caution that because there is a risk of developing cirrhosis and hepatocellular carcinoma in adulthood, the infection should not be ignored; therapy may help prevent some of these complications. At the same time, because children are more likely to convert spontaneously from HCV RNA positive to negative than adults, they should not be rushed into treatment. Some doctors recommend that children not be treated for HCV for the first two years of life. If children do clear the infection, they usually do so by 18 months of age; but for some children, the process can happen later. A waiting period gives the children the chance to clear the infection on their own. This is preferable to receiving medical treatment because interferon (IFN), the primary drug used to treat hepatitis C, is neurologically toxic to children. A liver biopsy may be considered to evaluate whether the child should be given treatment. Unfortunately, there is no reliable method of predicting which children would require treatment.

Therapy for treating children with hepatitis C was approved U.S. Food and Drug Administration (FDA) in 2004. Now a combination therapy of Intron a (INTERFERON) and Rebetol (ribavirin) is available for children three years and older who have one of the symptoms of liver disorder, and who have not previously been treated with alpha interferon. Rebetol can be taken orally.

Ribavirin is used with alpha interferon to stop hepatitis C virus from multiplying. Studies show that ribavirin can make alpha interferon work better, but it cannot fight hepatitis C on its own.

According to the drug manufacturer, Schering-Plough Corporation, Rebetol can be dosed according to the patient's body weight, and Intron A according to the patient's size measured in body surface. In the case of pediatric patients, the drug company recommends 48 weeks of therapy for those infected with genotype 1 virus, and 28 weeks for genotypes 2 and 3. The drugs should be discontinued if the patient does not respond after 28 weeks of treatment.

Schering-Plough reported that in a clinical study of previously untreated children, the combination therapy achieved a sustained virologic response (SVR) in 46 percent of patients. A sustained virologic response is when the virus cannot be seen in the blood for six months or more after completing hepatitis C therapy. In patients infected with genotype 1, 36 percent achieved SVR, and 81 percent of those with genotypes 2 or 3.

Rebetol should always be given in conjunction with Intron A, as it is not effective as monotherapy against hepatitis C.

All drugs should be administered with care because of the possibility of side effects and adverse reactions. In the case of Rebetol (ribavirin), it is associated with hemolytic anemia, a type of anemia caused from the reduced survival time of red blood cells. For such patients, taking Rebetol can worsen cardiac conditions.

It was discovered that when pregnant animals were exposed to ribavirin, the embryo was sometimes injured and suffered abnormal development or death, and the developing fetus would often manifest defects or other anomalies. The drug had what is known as embryocidal and teratogenic effects.

For the above reasons, pregnant women and male partners of pregnant women should not take Rebetol. Both female patients and the female partners of male patients who are taking Rebetol must take extreme precaution to avoid pregnancy during therapy and for six months after completion of treatment, because of the long half-life of Rebetol.

Alpha interferons, which include Intron A and Peg-Intron, are known at times to aggravate certain conditions, such as autoimmune and infectious diseases. Ischemic diseases—a low-oxygen state of local tissue due to an inadequate or obstructed blood flow—can also be negatively affected. Therefore, patients must be monitored closely and given clinical and laboratory evaluations. If patients show worsening signs and symptoms, the treatment should be terminated immediately. In the majority of cases, the adverse reactions should stop when the drugs are discontinued.

Risk Factors and Preventive Measures

Prevention remains the best method of disease management for adults and children alike. Since most children today acquire HCV at birth from their mothers who are HCV-infected, logically the primary target for prevention strategies should be perinatal transmission. However, aside from taking commonsense precautions against infecting others, once a mother has become infected with HCV, there are no reliable means to prevent transmission to her child. Fortunately, cross-sectional studies suggest that the risk is quite low. More information may be available in the future for prospective mothers on the best method of delivery for preventing infections.

Bortolotti, F., et al. "An epidemiological survey of hepatitis C virus infection in Italian children in the decade 1990–1999." *Journal of Pediatric Gastroenterology and Nutrition* 32, no. 5 (May 2001): 562–566.

———. "HCV genotypes and pediatric HCV infection." Abstract 464. 39th annual meeting of the European Association for the Study of the Liver. April 14–18, 2004, Berlin, Germany.

———. "Hepatitis C virus infection and related liver disease in children of mothers with antibodies to the virus." *Journal of Pediatrics* 130, issue 6 (1997): 990–993.

Conte, Dario, M.D., et al. "Prevalence and clinical course of chronic Hepatitis C Virus (HCV) infection and rate of HCV vertical transmission in a cohort of 15,250 pregnant women." *Hepatology* 31, no. 3 (March 2000): 751–755.

Gibb, D. M., R. L. Goodall, D. T. Dunn, M. Healy, P. Neave, M. Cafferkey, and K. Butler. "Mother-to-child transmission of hepatitis C virus: Evidence for preventable peripartum transmission." *Lancet* 356, 9233 (September 9, 2000): 904.

Hoshiyama, Atsuo, Akihiko Kimura, Takuji Fujisawa, Masayoshi Kage, and Hirohisa Kato. "Clinical and histologic features of chronic hepatitis C virus infection after blood transfusion in Japanese children." *Pediatrics* 105, no. 1 (January 2000): 62.

Kirchner, Jeffrey T. "Prognosis of children with vertically acquired HCV (hepatitis C virus). *American Family Physician* 61, no. 11 (June 1, 2000): 3394.

Kubetin, Sally Koch. "Hold off on treating the very young for HCV. (Most will clear infection by 18 months)." *Pediatric News* 35, no. 11 (November 2001): 16(1).

Moon, Mary Ann. "Could elective cesareans help prevent perinatal hepatitis C? (Panel calls for research)." *Family Practice News* 32, no. 18 (September 15, 2002): 25(1).

Papaevangelou V., H. Pollack, R. Brodie, B. Hanna, K. Krasinski, and W. Borkowsky. "Mother-to-infant transmission of hepatitis C in children born to mothers coinfected with HIV and HCV." *AIDS Weekly* (October 2, 1995): 21(1).

Pembrey, Lucy, Marie-Louise Newell, and Catherine Peckham. "Is there a case for hepatitis C infection screening in the antenatal period? (Review)." *Journal of Medical Screening* 10, no. 4 (Winter 2003): 161(8).

Poiraud S., et al. "Mother to child transmission of hepatitis C virus: a case-control study of risk factors." Digestive Disease Week, May 20–23, 2001. Available online. URL: http://www.natapiorg/2001/ddw/ndx_ddw.htm. Downloaded in March 2003.

Ruiz-Chercoles, E., J. T. Ramos, J. Ruiz-Contreras, C. Alvarez, M. J., Domingo, A. Fuertes, and V. Rodriguez-Cerrato. "Vertical transmission of hepatitis C in children born to HIV infected mothers." *Blood Weekly* (October 5, 1998): pNA. An abstract submitted by the authors to the 12th World AIDS Conference. June 28–July 3, 1998. Geneva, Switzerland.

Sadovsky, Richard. "Vertical transmission of hepatitis C virus infection." *American Family Physician* 57, no. 1 (January 1, 1998): 126(1).

Schering-Plough. "FDA approves Rebetol (ribavirin) oral solution for treatment of children with chronic hepatitis C." Schering-Plough Corporation press release, January 20, 2004.

Staff. "Long-term course of hepatitis C viral infections in children." Abstract. *Infectious Disease Alert* 19, no. 6 (December 15, 1999): 46.

Zein, NN. "Vertical transmission of hepatitis C: To screen or not to screen." *Journal of Pediatrics* 130, issue 6 (June 1997): 859–861.

hepatitis C and drug use   The number of cases of hepatitis C (HCV) among intravenous, or injection, drug users has declined dramatically since 1989, but the use of injection drugs is still the primary way that HCV is transmitted. Of people in drug treatment programs, 30 to 90 percent carry HCV antibodies, and it is not uncommon for as many as 85 percent of the patients in any given drug program to carry the virus.

Intranasal and crack cocaine use are also reported to be risk factors, but some researchers believe the apparent connection can be attributed to unreported injection drug use. Injection drug use is typically not surveyed among those users, and according to the Centers for Disease Control (CDC), intranasal cocaine use is usually combined with injection drugs. Thus, the final answer on the risk among intranasal users awaits the collection of more specific data.

There is no evidence that drug use by itself is a risk factor. The transmission mechanism involved is the sharing of syringes, either directly or through contaminated preparation equipment. Another potential method is the transfer of a drug from one syringe to another, called front loading. If intranasal drug use is confirmed as a risk factor, the likely culprit would be a similar situation, such as sharing contaminated straws. A contributory factor is that injection drug use is often accompanied by the drinking of ethanol, which increases the incidence of fibrosis.

Risk of exposure to HCV is greatest during the first period of drug use. People who have used injection drugs more than five years have a 60 percent chance of having been exposed to HCV. It is estimated that as many as 90 percent of five-year users may be infected with HCV.

Injection drug users are often exposed to other infectious diseases as well. Users infected with HCV are often infected with multiple strains or have simultaneous infections—called coinfections—with other viruses such as HEPATITIS B. Coinfection with HCV and HIV (human immunodeficiency virus) have been found to occur in 5 to 30 percent of injection drug users, depending on the prevalence of HIV in the geographical area under study. Among young drug users, however, the HCV infection rate is four times as high as the HIV infection rate. The more rapid acquisition of HCV is likely due to a high rate of HCV infection, and results in a higher rate of exposure.

Maternal injection drug use also endangers the developing fetus, according to an Italian study reported in the March 1, 2002, issue of the Journal of Infectious Diseases. The study identified 1,372 consecutive, unselected mothers who tested positive for HCV antibodies and their infants in 24 medical centers. Ninety-eight of the children were infected with HCV. Only injection drug use was significantly associated with HCV transmission. Age, birth weight, breast feeding, and method of delivery appeared to be unrelated to transmission rates. The presence of HIV antibodies also appeared to have no effect, but the study noted that the presence of those antibodies and a history of injection drug use appeared to be strictly related, a finding that could account for previous reports suggesting that the presence of HIV antibodies increases the risk of transmitting HCV to the fetus.

In the treatment of HCV, screening for substance use disorders is routine, and often includes screening for both drinking of alcoholic beverages and alcohol abuse and dependence.

The Alcohol Use Disorders Identification Test (AUDIT) is a well-established screening test for both nondependent heavy drinking and alcohol abuse and dependence. It is brief (10 items), self-administered, and easy to score. The AUDIT-C, composed of the first three items of the AUDIT, appears to accomplish much the same thing in a shorter format. Most other screening tests identify only those patients with possible abuse or dependence problems, and often miss nondependent heavy drinking. To be thorough, such screens must include questions about the quantity and frequency of drinking.

Screening tests for other drugs often restrict themselves to general questions about drug use, but are more effective if they include questions that specifically address each class of drugs. Any drug used more than five times in a lifetime is usually deemed to deserve further exploration. Screening may also include urine toxicology tests. Many screening procedures do not test for synthetic narcotic drugs, such as methadone. If a drug screen is positive but the patient denies drug use, the laboratory may be asked for a confirmatory test using gas chromatography or mass spectroscopy.

When a patient screens positive for a substance use disorder, further evaluation is needed to determine whether the problem is substance abuse or dependence. Evaluations may be done in the hepatitis clinic, or the patient may be referred to an addiction treatment specialist. For patients addicted to narcotics, the most effective treatment is generally considered to be opioid agonist therapy (OAT), a treatment method often equated in the public's mind with methadone maintenance programs. OAT combines the use of an "opioid agonist agent"—methadone is not the only choice, and not always the best one—with a comprehensive program of medical, counseling, and rehabilitation services. By administering an agent to help reduce withdrawal symptoms, OAT is able to achieve a much higher success rate than simple detoxification, even when the detoxification program is extensive and combined with enhanced psychosocial services.

If treatment for substance abuse is needed, it is best if medical and addiction treatment personnel are able to work closely together to support completion of both treatments.

Current guidelines ask for complete abstinence from injection drug use for a minimum of six months before the initiation of interferon treatment for HCV, but available evidence suggests that recent or even ongoing injection drug use has no effect on the success or failure of the treatment. In a 2001 study, for example, 50 individuals undergoing detoxification treatment for injected drug use

were recruited for hepatitis C treatment as well. Of the 50 patients, 18 showed excellent response to interferon treatment, and 39 missed no appointments. Of the 40 patients who eventually relapsed to using injected drugs, 20 continued to demonstrate excellent virologic response to the virus. Similarly, in a 2002 study—a five-year follow-up of 27 Norwegians who were successfully treated for HCV while injecting drugs—only one case of reinfection was found, even though a third of the patients had resumed or maintained their use of injection drugs. From that evidence, excluding current OAT patients who are former heroin addicts from interferon treatment seems counterproductive. Withdrawing from OAT programs to receive interferon treatments is often counterproductive as well, since the typical consequence of withdrawal is relapse.

One item often missing from HCV treatment regimens is psychiatry. Patients undergoing antiviral treatments experience a high rate of depression and other neuropsychiatric symptoms, and those with preexisting psychiatric symptoms often worsen during antiviral treatment. Thoughts of suicide often occur to HCV patients, especially if the disease does not seem to be responding to the treatment. As many as 30 percent of patients undergoing interferon treatments may entertain ideas of suicide, and although no data are available relating specifically to injection drug users, it seems logical to speculate that struggling to eradicate a drug habit would almost certainly aggravate that tendency. The psychiatric implications of antiviral treatment in general, as well as HCV treatment specifically, need further exploration so that patients at risk for psychiatric symptoms can be more easily identified and appropriately treated. One 2003 study identified the Beck Depression Inventory (BDI), given at two- to four-week intervals, as helpful in early identification of depression.

Antidepressants may be helpful, but there are no controlled trials available indicating which drugs might be the safest and the most effective. Case reports and clinical experience, however, suggest that selective serotonin reuptake inhibitors (SSRIs) may be helpful. SSRIs are antidepressant drugs that prevent a neurotransmitter called serotonin from being reabsorbed into cells in the brain. (A neurotransmitter is a type of molecule that carries signals between brain cells.) The SSRIs citalopram (Celexa) and sertraline (Zoloft) show promise, because they have few interactions with other drugs and tend to be well tolerated.

Raising Public Awareness

Although the incidence of HCV is declining among injection drug users, there is some evidence that public information campaigns, designed to educate drug users about the dangers of exposure to HCV, are ineffective, and some believe that new prevention strategies are needed. In the absence of new strategies, however, it is important that the old ones be used to maximum effect. The general public, and HCV patients in particular, have a continuing need to be reminded of the methods of preventing HCV infections, including safe sexual practices such as using condoms and avoiding the sharing of personal items such as razors. Drug users must continue to receive similar warnings about the dangers of sharing needles and other paraphernalia, including cookers, cotton filters, and nasal tubes. And pregnant women must be warned about the dangers to themselves and their fetuses from past or present drug use.

Willenbring, M. L. "Treating co-occurring substance use disorders and hepatitis C." *Psychiatric Times* 21, no. 2. Available online. URL: http://www.psychiatrictimes. com/p040253.html. Downloaded on November 8, 2005.

hepatitis carrier   See HEPATITIS.

hepatitis C methods of transmission   Basically, hepatitis C (HCV) is spread through blood-to-blood contact. If infected blood gains entry into the bloodstream of a person, that person can contract hepatitis C. The blood must either directly enter the bloodstream through injection or other means or somehow get through the protective covering of the skin.

There are many known risk factors for contracting hepatitis C, but some people do not know how they were infected, or fail to report the means of transmission. Estimates of unknown sources of hepatitis C vary considerably, ranging from 10 to 40 percent.

In many cases, individuals may deny knowing how they became infected because they fear being stigmatized by reporting past intravenous drug use. Others honestly do not know or remember how they might have been exposed to contaminated blood. With hepatitis C, there is rarely a severe initial attack of the infection that the patient can remember. For those who have no known risk factors, yet have contracted the disease, it is assumed that they were unwittingly infected through medical procedures. Other possibilities are as yet unidentified means of transmission.

Intravenous drug use   Now that blood and blood products are routinely screened for HCV, by far the most common mode of transmission is through intravenous drug use—through injecting illegal drugs. Intravenous drug use remains responsible for a substantial proportion of HCV infections. Currently, it accounts for 60 percent of HCV transmission in the United States, despite the fact that hepatitis C cases are reported to be declining in incidence among intravenous drug users.

Among people attending drug treatment programs, the prevalence of HCV infection ranges from 30 to 90 percent, with the average falling somewhere from 65 to 85 percent. For all injection drug users, the prevalence is estimated to be 85 percent—even 100 percent by some accounts. The magnitude of the problem can be seen when this figure is compared with 30 percent of injection drug users becoming infected with HIV, the virus that causes AIDS. The source of infection for drug abuses is contaminated needles and other drug paraphernalia. Viruses are extremely small, and a speck of blood that is so small as to be undetectable to the human eye can still contain numerous hepatitis C viral particles. Even if the drug paraphernalia appears to be clean, it may still contain infectious viruses.

Accordingly, active, recurrent users of injection drugs are at very high risk for contracting hepatitis C. Engaging in this activity even once in the remote past is enough to infect a person. Doctors often encounter professional middle-aged men or women from an upper socioeconomic class who have used intravenous drugs "only once" or "a few times" in college in the sixties or seventies when their peers were experimenting with drugs. Even though they are completely drug-free today and lead a clean, healthy lifestyle, when they try to donate blood or get life insurance, they are rejected because they are discovered to be HCV-positive. The news stuns them because as far as they are concerned, they are at low risk for hepatitis C infection. What they fail to realize is that once is enough for the virus to take root in their bodies.

The good news is that some doctors believe that individuals who are not habitual drug users may have a better prognosis because they are more likely to have lower amounts of the virus in their blood. In general, the greater the amount of blood involved in the infection, the greater the amount of virus in the blood. Long-term drug abusers tend to have a greater viral load—more viral particles in their blood—as well as multiple strains of the virus, which makes treatment more difficult.

Intranasal drug use   One study suggested that regular users of cocaine had high risk factors for hepatitis C. This is because cocaine is generally "snorted" through a straw, a rolled-up bill, or other similar instruments, and small blood vessels in the nose may break open and bleed. Chronic cocaine use can also lead to a rupture in the cartilage that separates the two nostrils, leading to bleeding as well as exposing the person to contaminated blood that may be present, allowing blood-to-blood transmission of the virus. Even a tiny droplet of blood can contain enough hepatitis C virus to cause infection. Therefore, when the straw or other instruments are shared, the virus can be passed from person to person.

This means of transmission has not been conclusively demonstrated, as it is not yet entirely clear whether individuals who use intranasal cocaine failed to report that they are also injecting illegal drugs, or have done so in the past. Nonetheless, it is possible that intranasal drug use can transmit the hepatitis C virus.

Blood and blood products   In the past, before donated blood was screened for HCV, blood transfusions accounted for a substantial proportion of hepatitis C infections—as much as one-third of patients in the United States in the 1960s. Hepatitis C had not even been identified before 1989, and was called Non-A Non-B hepatitis. In 1986, blood banks in the United States finally began screening blood donors for hepatitis by measuring the LIVER ENZYME ALT and hepatitis B core antibody (HBcAb). If the unit of blood had elevated ALT or the HBV core antibody was positive, the blood was excluded from the blood supply. Although not specific for hepatitis C, the screening tests vastly reduced the risk of acquiring hepatitis C, dropping to about 5 percent of patients receiving transfusions. But because these tests did not directly screen for hepatitis C, blood transfusion recipients were still at risk for infection. The Centers for Disease Control and Prevention (CDC) estimates the number of people in the United States infected through blood or blood products to be almost 300,000. Almost 1 percent of donors appear to be infected with HCV.

It was not until 1992 that a more accurate screening test for the actual hepatitis C virus became available. The risk is now only about one in 100,000 units of blood transfused. Eventually, the risk may drop to zero, as blood banks begin to use even more accurate molecular techniques to detect the hepatitis C virus.

Potentially infectious blood and blood products include packed red blood cells (PRBC), blood platelets, fresh frozen plasma (the fluid part of the blood), and IMMUNE GLOBULIN (IG)—proteins from the blood of people immune to a particular disease, used as a form of vaccine.

In the early 1990s, contaminated batches of an intravenous immune globulin product called Gammagard and Polygam caused hundreds of people across the United States, mostly children, to become infected. Fortunately, all current lots of immune globulin are considered free of hepatitis C virus.

Clotting factor concentrates, which were prepared from plasma pooled from a large number of donors, also used to pose a high risk not only for HCV infection, but also for hepatitis B and HIV. Finally, effective procedures were introduced that could inactivate viruses, including HCV. In 1985, measures were taken to inactivate viruses for Factor VIII and in 1987, for Factor IX. Hemophiliacs treated with blood products before they were inactivated for possible viruses have prevalence rates of HCV infection as high as 90 percent. People with hemophilia can bleed excessively because they lack certain clotting factors in their blood that help stop the bleeding. They must receive clotting factors to treat their bleeding disorder. Fortunately, the risk of transmitting hepatitis C today is zero because synthesized or genetically engineered clotting products are used.

Products derived from plasma, used for intramuscular administration, have generally not been associated with transmission of HCV infection in the United States. Plasma derivatives include ALBUMIN (proteins found in blood plasma) and immune globulin (IG). In the United States, there was one outbreak of HCV infection from immune globulin given intravenously during 1993–94. The IG had not been virally inactivated. Since then, all IG products sold commercially in the United States must either be inactivated for viruses or test negative for HCV RNA (ribonucleic acid), and there have been no further incidents of HCV outbreak from these sources.

Patients used also to be at risk from organ grafts, such as liver or heart, for transplantation. As with blood transfusion, donors infected with HCV could transmit the virus to the person receiving the organ. This risk of infection has been virtually eliminated since all organ and tissue donors have been screened for HCV.

Today, there are hardly any incidents of transmission through contaminated blood or blood products, thanks to the routine use of effective screening tests for blood. Since 1994, the risk of contracting HCV from a single unit of blood has been less than one in 100,000. While the likelihood of contracting HCV from a blood transfusion is miniscule, a small risk still exists. The risk remains because when a person first becomes infected with HCV, the antibody for HCV (HCV Ab) is not detectable in the blood for a short time. Screening tests check for HCV antibodies. Should the person donate blood during this period, or window of time, the test will fail to detect HCV antibodies, but the virus will be circulating in the blood. This is why the risk of infection cannot be zero.

Blood bank look-back program   In 1997, the U.S. surgeon general recommended that all hospitals institute a "look-back" program to identify and notify people who had a blood transfusion prior to 1992 from a HCV-infected donor. Blood banks across the nation were to check their records to locate any donors who had tested positive for hepatitis C. They were then to trace the records of all blood recipients from these donors back 10 years to find all the patients who had received blood from him or her. Recipients of tainted blood had to be notified by letter that they should be tested. But it is often difficult to track down all recipients. Patients often move and change doctors, for example. Accordingly, it is strongly recommended that anyone who received a blood transfusion or blood products before 1992 should be tested for HCV.

A critical point to remember is that patients who received blood transfusions before 1992 are at risk now for hepatitis C infection because hepatitis is often a silent, slowly progressing illness. The estimate is that some 290,000 Americans contracted hepatitis C from transfusions before 1990. Middle-aged or elderly people who were blood recipients early in life, no matter how remote the event may have been, could be infected without being aware of it.

Occupational exposure   Needle-stick injury—accidental pricking with a needle—is a commonly recognized occupational hazard for health care workers. Other documented transmissions include blood spills or contaminated medical instruments, such as colonoscopes (a flexible tube for the visual inspection of colons). Because of the possibility of such accidents, anyone regularly exposed to blood is considered to be at higher risk than the general population for contracting hepatitis C. This includes people who work at health care facilities such as hospitals, clinics, doctors and dentists offices, and laboratories that handle blood specimens. Others, such as paramedics, police officers, and firefighters, may also come into contact with blood due to the nature of their work.

The risks of hepatitis C infection through occupational exposure are lower than for hepatitis B (HBV). For HBV, the probability is estimated to be from 15 to 30 percent, while it is just 2 percent for HCV, though some estimates go as high as 16 percent. (In contrast, the risk of contracting HIV after a single accidental exposure is 0.3 percent.) As in all cases, the larger the amount of infected blood that enters the bloodstream, the higher the likelihood of contracting the disease.

Studies suggest that health care workers who received needle-stick injuries from a patient testing positive for HCV RNA (the ribonucleic acid of HCV) are at greater risk than if they got the needle stick from RNA-negative patients.

Even with the higher chance of coming into contact with contaminated blood, however, the prevalence of HCV infection among health care workers is no greater than that of the general population.

Although not in the same category as health care workers, barbers can also face the threat of hepatitis C from shaving infected customers if they use nondisposable, nonsterilized blades. At the same time, they are also putting other customers at risk. No data are available in the United States, but a 1995 article in the *Lancet* reported that in Sicily, Italy, as many as 38 percent of barbers tested positive for HCV.

Medical procedures Unsafe medical practices can be a breeding ground of HCV as well as for other types of infection. In the past, even in developed countries, unsafe practices were common. Fortunately, with advancing medical knowledge, appropriate hygiene practices have been instituted in developed countries, and it is rare, although not impossible, for patients to be infected from medical procedures. The widespread use of disposable needles, for instance, precludes this type of infection. In certain parts of the world, however, especially poorer areas where needles may be reused for economic reasons and where medical equipment may not be properly sterilized, HCV infection can be a problem.

In the United States, there have been a few recorded cases of hepatitis C transmission from surgeons to patients, such as in open-heart surgery, but the risk is not considered significant.

At much greater risk are patients who suffer kidney failure. Treatment usually involves the use of hemodialysis, which directly involves the blood. The patient's blood is removed through an artery, cleaned by the hemodialysis unit, then pumped back into the body through a special arterial-venous shunt (AV). The AV shunt is created by a surgeon usually on the arm of a patient by connecting an artery directly to a vein and bypassing arteride and capillary vessels. In the United States, some 20 to 30 percent of hemodialysis patients are infected with HCV. The hepatitis C virus could have been readily transmitted if any of the equipment used during the hemodialysis procedure was not adequately sterilized—a minute amount of blood can infect a patient. Another factor for the high prevalence rate of HCV in hemodialysis patients is the frequent blood transfusions they may have received before 1992. Fortunately, greater knowledge and precautions taken means that fewer patients are becoming chronically infected with HCV.

If an individual has no risk factors for hepatitis C, then unhygienic medical practices may be suspected. The possibility cannot be discounted even in advanced countries. For example, in Japan, a developed country, fewer than 10 years ago, it was common for dentists to treat patients without wearing latex gloves. Dentists were often observed treating patients without washing their hands or donning gloves even after performing oral surgery. Moreover, because it has been the customary practice of many Japanese dentists to treat multiple patients at one sitting, they would rotate from one patient to the next, increasing the likelihood of transmission.

Acupuncture treatments have also been implicated with transmission of hepatitis C in South Korea. Acupuncture is a common treatment in many parts of Asia, and has become increasingly popular in the United States and other Western countries as well. Most acupuncturists today, particularly those in developed countries, use disposable needles, but in the past, needles were often reused and were not adequately sterilized. Achieving safe acupuncture practice is a priority in places such as rural areas of South Korea with poor hygienic practices.

Tattooing and body piercing Practices that involve breaking the skin are potential sources of infection because a small amount of bleeding can occur. These include tattooing and body piercing. It is possible to transmit tainted blood from one customer to another through the reuse of needles, ink, or other equipment used during these practices if they have not been sterilized properly. The probability of contracting hepatitis B through this means is greater, but it is also possible to get hepatitis C. One factor that potentially increases the likelihood of infection is that groups at high risk for hepatitis C—such as the military, gang members, prostitutes, and prisoners—are more prone to getting body tattoos.

According to one study, tattooing has been overlooked as a widespread source of HCV infection. Dr. Robert Haley, chief of epidemiology at the University of Texas Southwestern Medical Center and coauthor of the study, concluded that people who had received a tattoo in a commercial tattoo parlor were nine times more likely to be infected with HCV than people who did not have a tattoo. Contrary to the assumptions of most researchers who accept that the greatest risk factor for hepatitis C is injection drug use, Haley believes that commercially acquired tattoos are responsible for more than twice as many infections as injection drug use.

The study also found evidence that the risk of HCV infection is further heightened for people with multiple tattoos or larger and more complex tattoos, as well as tattoos using white, red, yellow, or orange pigments instead of all black.

The study, which was reported at the Digestive Disease Week conference in May 2004 in New Orleans, investigated patients at an orthopedic spinal clinic because it gave the researchers access to a large number of people. The patients involved in the study were seeing a physician for reasons unrelated to blood-borne infection. The study found that 33 percent of patients who had acquired their tattoos in commercial tattoo parlors had HCV, as compared with only 3.5 percent for those with no tattoos.

The research involved 626 patients, among whom 18 percent, or 113, had tattoos. Fifty-two of the participants with tattoos had received them in commercial tattoo parlors. When tattooed participants who had received their tattoos at places other than commercial tattoo parlors are included, the number of infection drops to 22 percent—still significantly higher than for patients without a tattoo. The source of these patients' infections

could not be traced to past or present intravenous drug use, transfusions, or other known routes of exposure.

Up to 40 percent of hepatitis C infections are of unknown origin. The researchers who conducted this study suggest that tattooing could account for many cases in which the source of transmission is unknown.

In recent years, tattooing has been gaining popularity among the general public, especially among teenagers and young adults, as celebrities have imparted to tattoos a fashion and cosmetic appeal. Trend-setting actors and athletes have increasingly been receiving tattoos. The Canadian actress Pamela Anderson, who starred in the television series *Baywatch*, claimed that she contracted hepatitis C by sharing a tattoo needle with her ex-husband, the rocker Tommy Lee.

Another study conducted at the University of Texas Southwestern Medical Center with a cohort of 626 people further implicated tattoos in viral transmission. It appears that people with tattoos may be just as likely as intravenous drug users to be infected with hepatitis C. However, drug users were six times more likely to experience earlier symptoms of the infection, such as nausea, fatigue, and JAUNDICE. Perhaps infection in drug users is detected earlier because they have a massive infusion of HCV directly into the bloodstream, while tattoo needles introduce the virus into the bloodstream slowly and in smaller amounts, with the result that HCV symptoms may not appear until decades later.

Thus, anyone who wishes to receive tattoos or other body art should go to a reputable practitioner and make sure that the dye used is not shared among customers, and that the needle and anything else with which the body comes into contact has been sterilized to medically accepted standards. Consumers should also be aware that very few states have regulations for safe tattooing practices, and even among those that do, most are not enforced. Tattooing is not only a risk for hepatitis B and C, but also for syphilis, leprosy, and tuberculosis.

Sexual transmission Experts agree that sexual contact—whether oral, genital, or anal—is an inefficient means of HCV transmission, particularly when it occurs within the context of a monogamous relationship. It used to be thought that hepatitis C virus could not be detected in the saliva, semen, or urine of HCV-infected people, but researchers have now isolated HCV from bodily fluids, including vaginal secretions.

While low, the risk of infection from sexual contact is far from zero, as the potential of transmission through intimate contact exists if there are any breaks in the skin or in the lining of the mouth or vagina. Infection may occur if there are open herpes sores or rough sex, particularly anal intercourse. Moreover, because HCV has been detected in menstrual blood, HCV-infected women should avoid intercourse during menstruation and for several days afterward. Overall, it is easier for a man to infect a woman than vice versa. The risk for women is said to be three times that of their male partners.

Estimated infection rates for sexual contact for monogamous couples are not more than 2.5 percent over a prolonged period of time. But research suggests that HCV is detected with greater than average frequency among people who have multiple sex partners, change partners frequently, or have sex with prostitutes. In the absence of other risks, about one out of 20 among this group become infected.

Doctors do not particularly recommend that couples in long-standing monogamous relationships use condoms for the prevention of HCV. However, people practicing promiscuous sex are advised to use a condom with every encounter.

One study published in 2004 evaluated the risk of sexual transmission of HCV among 895 partners of chronically infected individuals. This long-term prospective study followed the individuals under investigation over a 10-year period, corresponding to 8,060 person-years. The couples were all heterosexual and monogamous, did not engage in anal intercourse or sex during menstruation, and did not use condoms. They engaged in sexual intercourse an average of 1.8 times weekly. Based on the study, the authors concluded, "Our data indicate that the risk of sexual transmission of HCV with heterosexual monogamous couples is extremely low or even null. No general recommendations for condom use seem required for individuals in monogamous partnerships with HCV-infected partners."

New research suggests that partners of HCV-infected patients who are also infected with HIV (human immunodeficiency virus, which causes AIDS) are at greater risk of contracting hepatitis C. To begin with, HIV-positive patients are much more likely also to be infected with hepatitis C, but via a mechanism not yet clearly understood HIV seems to enhance the sexual transmission risk of hepatitis C. The risk rate for contracting hepatitis C through sexual contact with a partner coinfected with HIV may be as high as 19 percent. However, more studies are needed to support this estimate.

Kissing and HCV More than a dozen articles have now been published demonstrating the presence of HCV RNA in saliva. But, concentrations of the virus are much lower than in blood, and none of the studies has found evidence of viral transmission from saliva. Other infectious viruses, such as hepatitis A, hepatitis B, and HIV, can also be detected in human saliva, but none of them is transmitted through kissing.

Household contact Not only is the hepatitis C virus difficult to kill, it can exist and survive in amounts of blood that are virtually undetectable. Thus, people who share the household with an HCV-infected person may have a somewhat higher risk of contracting HCV than the general population. It is possible to spread HCV through sharing common household and personal care items, such as toothbrushes, nail clippers, razors, or any other sharp instruments. Such items should be placed or stored in such a way as to minimize accidental use or contact. In particular, care should be taken to keep children from touching or playing with them.

Despite all the warnings, however, there is no unequivocal evidence for transmission by shared household items. To garner evidence, researchers in Germany tested the saliva of HCV-infected people before and after brushing their teeth under controlled conditions. The result was that with sufficiently sensitive methods, HCV RNA could be detected in a large portion of toothbrushes used by HCV patients. Although the study did not determine whether the traces of the virus on the toothbrush could infect another individual, it showed that transmission by contaminated everyday household objects is possible, and it added strength to the commonly issued warnings about not sharing possibly infected personal items. The study coauthor, Dr. Claus Hellerbrand of the University of Regensburg, and his associates also suggested the possibility of health officials regulating barbershop razors and other publicly used items.

In a related observation, veterans in an American hospital have been reported to engage in communal sharing of electric shavers without disinfection. This practice should be discouraged, especially because the prevalence of HCV in veterans may be higher than in the general population (about 7 percent, according to one survey).

The rate of transmission from accidental household contact is believed to be quite low—approximately 4 percent—for the majority of people living with an HCV-infected household member. This estimate is based on data from countries other than the United States, as it is not known in the United States how often people acquire the disease from a household member. In fact, in the United States at least, there has not been any evidence of HCV transmission among nonsexual partners within the same household. Even the 4 percent prevalence rate of chronic HCV infection obtained in studies from other parts of the world may be too high for the United States. These studies were done in countries where family members may have a history of similar exposure in the past to contaminated medical equipment.

A recent investigation in the United States discovered that an HCV-infected mother had transmitted the disease to her child. This case is an exception, however, because the infection resulted from the mother preparing a home infusion therapy for her child, who is hemophilic. The mother accidentally stabbed herself with the needle used for the therapy, then used the contaminated needle to treat the child. This case clearly demonstrates a need for better education and understanding of the nature of HCV infection. Being better informed would have kept the mother from unnecessarily exposing her child to the disease. At the other end of the spectrum, it would help friends and family of chronically infected people from being overly cau-

tious, such as refraining from hugging, or shunning all physical contact. In fact, kissing, hugging, sneezing, coughing, cooking together, sharing drinking glasses or utensils, and sharing food does not transmit HCV. (Hepatitis A can be transmitted from sharing or eating food cooked by an infected person. Hepatitis A, however, is quite treatable and never becomes chronic.) It is also safe to use the same bathroom as an infected person, work in the same office, or swim in the same pool. Infected people can safely take care of children. Any contact without exposure to blood is safe. There is no need to avoid or isolate the infected person. As long as the precautions mentioned above are followed, friends and family of an infected person do not have an increased risk of getting HCV; no behavior changes are necessary or warranted.

Pregnancy and childbirth Doctors talk about the vertical transmission of HCV if the virus is transmitted to the fetus during pregnancy. If it is passed on from a mother to her infant around the time of birth, it is called perinatal transmission.

One of the major concerns of women infected with HCV is that they might transmit the virus to their babies. The potential certainly exists for the mother's blood to mingle with the baby's blood at the time of delivery, thus spreading the virus to the baby. But for the most part, women can put their minds at ease, as experts agree that the possibility of either vertical or perinatal transmission is relatively low, if the mother is otherwise healthy. Moreover, some studies suggest that transmission to the newborn occurs only in HCV-infected women who have high viral loads (the amount of HCV viral particles per milliliter of blood) of at least 1 million.

A much higher risk exists for transmitting human immunodeficiency virus (HIV, which causes AIDS) from the mother to the newborn than for hepatitis C. The CDC estimates the likelihood of a mother passing on the virus to her newborn to be between 5 and 6 percent, but this figure can vary somewhat depending on the population groups under study. For instance, recent studies on European women have estimated the prevalence rates to be as high as 13.3 percent. Some of the discrepancies in findings can be explained by various factors, such as the presence of different genotypes of the hepatitis C virus, the presence of additional infections in the mother, the different methodologies, and the different sensitivities of the blood tests used. Research indicates that women who have HCV antibodies in their blood have a transmission rate of 1.7 percent, while women whose blood tests show the presence of HCV RNA have a higher transmission rate—around 4.3 percent. The CDC gives a somewhat higher estimate, of around 4 percent, for infants born to mothers with HCV antibodies, and 6 percent for mothers with HCV RNA in their blood. The one factor consistently associated with viral transmission from mother to infant is the presence of HCV RNA in the mother at the time of labor.

Some reports have quoted transmission rates as high as 40 to 90 percent among pregnant women who are hepatitis C antibody positive and also inject illegal drugs, while others have found the rate to be much lower—about 9 percent—though still exceeding the rates of women who do not use intravenous drugs.

A report published in the *Journal of Pediatric Gastroenterology and Nutrition* in November 2001, found vertical transmission to be far riskier for children than blood transfusions. According to the epidemiological survey, vertical transmission caused 46 percent of pediatric HCV cases in the past decade, while blood transfusions were responsible for 34 percent. The reason for the surprisingly high vertical transmission rate is that women also infected with HIV were included in the study. One-third of the 279 women in the study had a history of intravenous drug abuse, and 17 percent were infected with HIV, in addition to drug abuse. Regardless of geographic location, coinfected women—those who have another infection in addition to HCV—have higher rates than the general population.

The estimated rate of transmission hovers around 19 percent in HCV antibody-positive women who are coinfected with HIV. The exact reason for the higher risk associated with HIV coinfection is unclear, but it may be because the HIV compromises the immune system. The hepatitis virus more readily replicates when the immune system is weakened.

In the United Kingdom, a recent study showed that the rate of vertical transmission among mothers also infected with HIV ranged from 12 to 13 percent. This particular study included 279 women infected with HCV. One-third of them had a history of drug use, and 17 percent who used drugs were also infected with HIV.

As a general rule, the higher the viral load—the amount of HCV particles per milliliter of blood—the more likely the infection will be passed on to the baby. However, some studies suggest otherwise, and not all researchers agree that the viral load is associated with transmission. On the other hand, according to CDC, there is a consistent association in women coinfected with HCV and HIV between virus titer and transmission of HCV. Titer refers to the concentration of a substance in a solution, in this case, the virus in the blood.

The CDC estimates that the average infection rate for infants born to women who test positive for hepatitis C antibody, and who are also HIV positive, is 14 percent. But if the woman is HIV positive, and also tests positive for HCV RNA in her blood, then the average infection rate is 17 percent.

Nevertheless, a study from Italy published by Dario Conte, M.D., in *Hepatology,* contradicts such research, suggesting that HIV coinfection raised the infant's risk of contracting hepatitis C. According to the results of this study, the mother's coinfection of HIV did not increase the rate of transmission of hepatitis C.

Another study from Italy has come to similar conclusions. After studying 1,372 mothers who tested positive for HCV and their infants, in 24 medical centers, the researchers, Dr. Massimo Resti of the University of Florence and his colleagues, wrote in the *Journal of Infectious Disease* that coinfection with HIV does not significantly increase the likelihood of hepatitis C transmission to the infant. Rather, injection drug use by the mother, not the HIV infection, heightens the risk for the newborn. That being the case, the researchers speculate that previous reports may have noted the correlation between HIV coinfection and higher transmission risk because people who inject drugs are more likely to be HIV-positive.

Because infection from blood transfusions has been virtually eliminated, experts predict that within a few years the most common mode of transmission of childhood hepatitis will be perinatally acquired hepatitis C. Although perinatal transmission should be the primary target for prevention strategies, no effective methods have yet been proposed. First, more research is needed to clarify the relationship between mode of delivery and HCV transmission. Not enough is known at present, partly due to the conflicting results obtained from studies that are too divergent in design. The limited data available until recently suggest that there is no difference in infection rates between infants delivered vaginally compared with cesarean-delivered infants. However, many of these studies were not set up adequately. For example, they do not differentiate elective from emergency cesarean, and at times they also fail to document maternal HIV status, two factors that could be crucial in HCV transmission. Some researchers suspect that infants delivered via elective cesarean might have a lower risk of infection than ones who are delivered vaginally with forceps, an advantage that may not exist with emergency cesareans. It is certainly feasible that there is an increased HCV vertical transmission risk during vaginal delivery with use of forceps, compared with elective cesarean section, which delivers the baby before membrane rupture, since it appears that most transmission occurs around the time of delivery.

A case-control study conducted in France offers some supporting evidence that cesarean delivery—the study did not distinguish between elective and emergency cesareans—may offer an advantage over vaginal delivery for HCV-infected mothers. Researchers included 161 mother-child pairs between the years 1992 and 2000 in their study to evaluate risk factors for HCV vertical transmission. These included amniocentesis, vaginal or cesarean-section delivery, use of forceps, episiotomy (a surgical procedure on the vulva to ease delivery), and maternal breast feeding or bottle feeding. The research discovered that the only significant factor associated with vertical transmission of HCV was vaginal delivery with forceps. Reporting at the Digestive Disease Week conference in May 2001 in Atlanta, Georgia, the researchers concluded, "Our study demonstrates an increased HCV vertical transmission risk during vaginal delivery with use of forceps compared with caesarean-section delivery."

More recently, an analysis of 227 infants reported in the *Archives of Disease in Childhood* revealed that of the 31 children delivered by elective cesarean section, none of them became HCV infected. The estimated transmission risk was 7.7 percent for vaginal and 5.9 percent for emergency cesarean-section delivery. The apparent finding of a protective effect of elective cesarean section should be regarded as tentative because the number of children delivered by elective cesarean section is small. Larger studies are needed for a definitive answer.

Another point to consider is that even if the mother tests positive for HCV antibodies, if she is negative for HCV RNA, transmission to the infant is extremely rare. Under these circumstances, therefore, it is inappropriate to recommend elective cesarean section if the only purpose is to lower the risk of infection.

As to HCV-infected patients who may desire in vitro fertilization, data are currently insufficient concerning the risks of transmission to make any recommendations.

Breast-feeding for HCV-infected women   Breast-feeding has not been implicated in any of the studies as a means of transmitting HCV. Studies evaluating the incidence of HCV in infants born to HCV-infected mothers have compared breast-fed versus bottle-fed infants. They showed that in each group of infants, approximately 4 percent contracted hepatitis C. Although hepatitis C virus may be detected in breast milk, the baby's digestive juices and enzymes are likely to destroy the virus. Therefore, an HCV-infected mother should be able to breast-feed her baby safely. If her nipples are cracked or bleeding, however, she should avoid breast-feeding.

Unknown sources   The potential risk factor for hepatitis C can be identified in approximately 90 percent of cases. That means that 10 percent of infected people are unable to identify their source of infection. They do not know, or cannot recall, how they acquired the infection. These patients are classified as having sporadic hepatitis C. In some cases, the individuals may be afraid of confessing to the use of illegal drugs, or they may have tried drugs just once a long time ago and do not see that as a possible route of transmission. Still others may have received blood transfusions or injections with nondisposable needles as a child that they do not know about or recall. Or they could have been exposed to an infected person's blood without knowing it. Other potential sources of infection that people often do not think about are tattooing, body piercing, and manicures. It is also possible that some ways of transmission have not yet been identified.

Generally, sporadic hepatitis C is associated with low socioeconomic status, perhaps because of high-risk exposures to various infectious diseases. Unfortunately, this nonspecific nature makes prevention more difficult. In all cases, information about hepatitis and strategies to stop preventing infectious diseases need to be widely disseminated.

Homeless people and HCV   The homeless population is at greater risk for hepatitis C, as well as for numerous other health problems. For the homeless, the primary cause of HCV infection is injection drug use and other substance abuse. They may also be more prone to sharing personal care items, such as toothbrushes and razors.

One study assessed differences among HCV-negative and HCV-positive homeless men in the Los Angeles area. About half of them were chronically infected with HCV. The investigators discovered that the following characteristics were significantly and positively associated with having HCV infection:

- history of substance use (including injection and noninjection drug use)
- recent injection drug use, including sharing drug paraphernalia
- sharing personal care items
- homelessness severity
- tattoos
- sexually transmitted diseases
- history of incarceration in jail or prison
- greater age

Lifetime alcohol problems were not associated with HCV, though drinking can often aggravate any liver injuries. Although it is not surprising that injecting illegal drugs and sharing equipment is associated with HCV infection, it was alarming that the behaviors were recent. Those who work among the homeless need to be aware that the latter are engaging in high-risk behavior that makes them and anyone working in close proximity to them more vulnerable to HCV infection.

The investigators recommended that a substance abuse treatment be implemented for the homeless population. In addition, needle exchange and clean equipment for drug use should be encouraged in areas where the homeless congregate.

HCV and prison inmates   As with the homeless population, prison inmates engage in high-risk behavior that exposes them to HCV infection. In fact, inmates may now be at greater danger for hepatitis C than HIV. For example, health officials say that in Massachusetts prisons and jails, as many as 40 percent of all women and 30 percent of all male prisoners have been infected with the virus.

Alter, Harvey J., C. Conry-Cantilena, J. Melpolder, D. Tan, M. Van Raden, D. Herion, D. Lau, J. H. and Hoofnagle. "Hepatitis C in asymptomatic blood donors." *Hepatology* 26, suppl. 1. (1997) 295–335.

Centers for Disease Control and Prevention. "Recommendations for prevention and control of hepatitis C virus infection and HCV related chronic disease." *Morbidity and Mortality Weekly Report* 47, no. RR-19 (October 16, 1998): n.p.

Conte, Dario, M.D., et al. "Prevalence and clinical course of chronic Hepatitis C virus (HCV) infection and rate of HCV vertical transmission in a cohort of 15,250 pregnant women." *Hepatology* 31, no. 3 (March 2000): 751–755.

Kelly, C. R., M.D. "Electric razors as a potential vector for viral hepatitis." *New England Journal of Medicine* 342, no. 10 (March 9, 2000): 744–745.

Lock, G., and others. "Hepatitis C—Transmission by toothbrushes; A myth or a real possibility?" Digestive Disease Week. April 19–22, 2002. San Francisco.

Oronzo, C., et al. "Vertical transmission of hepatitis C virus in a cohort of 2,447 HIV-seronegative pregnant women: A 24-month prospective study" *Journal of Pediatric and Gastroenterology & Nutrition* 33, no. 5 (November 2001): 570–575.

Medeiros-Filho, J., et al. "Evidence of intrafamilial transmission of hepatitis C virus: Analysis of relatives and spouses of hepatitis C virus patients." 52nd annual meeting of the American Association for the

Study of Liver Diseases (AASLD). November 9–13, 2001. Dallas.

Moon, Mary Ann. "Could elective cesareans help prevent perinatal hepatitis C? (Panel calls for research)." *Family Practice News* 32, no. 18 (September 15, 2002): p25(1).

Poiraud, S., et al. "Mother to child transmission of hepatitis C virus: A case-control study of risk factors." Digestive Disease Week. May 20–23, 2001.

Resti, Massimo, A. Meyer, et al. "Maternal injection drug use increases risk of vertical hepatitis C transmission." *Journal of Infectious Diseases* 185 (2002): 567–572.

Stein, J. A. and A. Nyamathi. "Correlates of hepatitis C virus infection in homeless men." *Drug and Alcohol Dependence* 75, no. 1 (July 15, 2004): 89–95.

"Tattooing is a major route of hepatitis C infection, says researcher." Digestive Disease Week. May 15–24, 2004. New Orleans.

Tumminelli, F., et al. "Shaving as potential source of hepatitis C virus infection." *Lancet* 345 (March 11, 1995): 658.

Vandelli, Carmen, et al. "Lack of evidence of sexual transmission of hepatitis C among monogamous couples: results of a 10-year prospective follow-up study." *American Journal of Gastroenterology* 99, no. 6 (May 2004): 855–859.

Zverev, S. Y., et al. "Necessity of prevention for vertical transmission of hepatitis C virus among coinfected both HIV and HCV women." Program and abstracts of the XIV International AIDS Conference. July 7–12, 2002. Barcelona, Spain.

hepatitis C treatment Hepatitis C (HCV) is a serious disease, but if treated properly, it can be a manageable disease, and people have been known to live with it for decades. Indeed, more people die of causes unrelated to the illness than from hepatitis C itself.

In about 80 percent of cases, hepatitis C turns chronic, lasting at least six months, but generally lingering for decades. Since the disease progresses relatively slowly, and there are few if any symptoms, patients can lead normal lives while making any lifestyle and other adjustments that may be required the better to manage the illness. One frustrating aspect of the disease is that doctors cannot always predict its clinical course. Some fortunate individuals with chronic hepatitis C live out a normal life span with relatively few health problems, while others suffer debilitating effects from the illness, and still others experience end-stage LIVER DISEASE, eventually dying from LIVER FAILURE.

One factor, however, can reliably predict disease progression, and that is the consumption of ethanol, or alcohol. Research has shown that alcohol is extremely injurious to the liver and plays a strong role in the progression of liver disease. For example, the National Institutes of Health (NIH) in Bethesda, Maryland, studied the impact of alcohol consumption on liver disease progression in 836 patients with hepatitis C. The study found that overall, the risk of developing cirrhosis increased by 31.1 times for hepatitis C–infected patients who drank heavily.

While small amounts of alcohol on an occasional basis may be tolerated, anyone in the habit of regular and excessive consumption of alcohol must stop immediately. The continued ingestion of alcohol or other substances toxic to the liver will accelerate disease progression. Individuals with substance dependency should be encouraged to seek help.

Once an individual has been diagnosed with hepatitis C, the next step is to assess whether treatment is needed. Any individual with chronic hepatitis C infection is a potential candidate for antiviral therapy. But that is not to say that therapy is indicated for every HCV patient. Many different factors—such as age, how long infected, HCV genotype, and extent of existing liver damage—should be taken into account in deciding whether a patient needs therapy or can benefit from it. Unless the patient was recently infected with HCV and has acute hepatitis, the decision to treat is rarely a matter of urgency. Before embarking on a course of therapy, the patient must be fully informed of the risks and benefits of treatment. It should also be remembered that not all patients respond to treatment in the same way; about half the patients will not benefit from therapy, and others may not be able to tolerate it because of side effects, or be otherwise disqualified from therapy.

The decision to begin a course of antiviral therapy must be made on a case-by-case basis by a qualified medical doctor, preferably a specialist in the field. While information in books and Web sites can help patients understand their illnesses better, it cannot be used to make a medical diagnosis on an individual case.

In 1997, a Consensus Development Conference Panel convened by the National Institutes of Health recommended treatment for hepatitis C patients at greatest risk of developing CIRRHOSIS, or advanced scarring of the liver, as shown through histological evidence (microscopic examination of liver tissue) of progressive disease. Panel recommendations are that all patients with fibrosis (scarring) or moderate to severe degrees of inflammation and necrosis (death of cells) on LIVER BIOPSY should be treated. Patients showing less severe disease on biopsy should be managed on an individual basis.

Suitable candidates fit the following profile:

- A blood test shows antibodies for HCV.
- A blood test detects HCV RNA (hepatitis C virus).
- There is persistent elevation of LIVER ENZYMES, especially ALT.
- A liver biopsy shows either fibrosis or moderate to severe degrees of inflammation and necrosis.

Patients are not to be selected on the basis of their mode of infection, whether or not there are symptoms, the HCV RNA genotypes, or the viral load (amount of virus in the blood). Patients with the following characteristics do not fit the criteria for an ideal candidate for therapy but may be considered for research trials, depending on individual circumstances:

- suffer from compensated cirrhosis (no sign of liver failure—such as JAUNDICE, abdominal swelling, mental confusion, and bleeding)
- only mild inflammation shown by liver biopsy
- under the age of 18
- over the age of 60

Patients under the age of 18 and over the age of 60 should be individually managed. The effect of treatment on older individuals is not well known,

and side effects are generally worse for older individuals. However, older individuals are sometimes successfully treated for HCV.

A substantial number of HIV-positive patients (human immunodeficiency virus for AIDS) are coinfected with hepatitis C. This group was regarded as difficult to treat and often steered away from HCV therapy, but the practice now is to offer coinfected patients treatment as long as there are no contraindications among their medications. In fact, as improved treatments for HIV-positive patients have made death from end-stage liver disease increasingly common, the view today is that HCV therapy may offer significant benefit to patients before their HIV infection becomes too advanced.

A case of acute hepatitis C—when the infection is recent—calls for quick action because studies have shown that treatment is the most effective in the early stages of the disease. Caught early enough—within one to four months of onset—therapy can keep the infection from progressing into a chronic condition in the majority of cases.

But doctors rarely see acute cases, and the optimal dosage or treatment schedule for hepatitis C has not been established. Data from studies conducted more than a decade ago using conventional interferon (as opposed to the longer-acting pegylated version) suggest that at least six months of therapy may be necessary. As with chronic hepatitis C, blood samples must be taken to assess the sustained or transient nature of the response to treatment.

Treatment is not always advisable due to health considerations. Some patients may wish to ask their doctors about participation in clinical trials.

Patients with the following characteristics are usually discouraged from treatment:

- suffer from major depression or other neuropsychiatric syndrome
- have low blood counts
- have received a solid organ
- pregnant
- have other medical conditions, such as thyroid gland disease, autoimmune disease, heart disease, diabetes, or uncontrolled hypertension

In the past, patients with alcohol or drug-use issues were usually disqualified from hepatitis C treatment. This is no longer the practice today. NIH released guidelines in August 2002 recommending that all HCV patients be considered for antiviral therapy if they are at risk for hepatitis C progression. Departing from its guidelines in 1997, NIH no longer recommends against treatment for HIV/HCV-coinfected people or those who have issues with alcohol or illicit drugs. An abstinence of six months from the patient's substance of choice (alcohol or drugs) is desirable but not an absolute requirement for therapy. Strict abstinence from alcohol or drugs is recommended during therapy, but patients with continuing addiction issues may be considered for treatment if they can be treated in collaboration with substance abuse specialists.

Patients with cirrhosis but without complications such as ASCITES (abdominal swelling), BLEEDING VARICES, or HEPATIC ENCEPHALOPATHY may be given antiviral therapy. However, most studies do not show that therapy improves survival in such patients.

Patients with decompensated cirrhosis (advanced liver scarring with complications) are not suitable candidates for therapy. If they do receive antiviral medication, it should be in a controlled setting where they can be monitored carefully, preferably at a facility capable of liver transplantation if a transplant becomes necessary.

The aim of HCV therapy is to lower the amount of virus in the bloodstream to an undetectable level, as measured by qualitative HCV RNA assays that directly look for the presence of the hepatitis virus RNA. To monitor the effectiveness of the therapy, the doctor takes blood samples before, during, and after treatment to see whether the virus has been eliminated or reduced. The ultimate goal of therapy is to clear the blood of the hepatitis C virus so that survival may be prolonged and the quality of life improved. Therapy should keep the disease from progressing to cirrhosis and cancer. Eliminating the virus improves liver function as measured by tests and observed by the microscopic appearance of the liver tissue. There should be a marked reduction in inflammation and less scarring.

The best outcome is a sustained virologic response, or a sustained response (SR). This means that the virus (HCV RNA) cannot be detected in the blood or liver for six months or more after completing the treatment. At this point, the treatment is considered a success.

Even if the virus has not been completely eliminated, therapy may help to achieve the following:

- decrease the viral load (the amount of hepatitis C virus in the blood)
- decrease the amount of liver damage
- lower the alanine aminotransferase (ALT) liver enzyme level
- improve overall well-being

Medications

INTERFERON (IFN) has been the mainstay of antiviral therapy against hepatitis. The body manufactures interferons, a family of naturally occurring proteins to fight viral infection. Special cells in the body secrete interferon in an attempt to interfere with viral reproduction and to protect other cells that have not yet been infected. Supplementing the naturally produced interferon with synthetically manufactured interferon has been shown to provide benefit. Drug companies manufacture several brands of interferon.

Conventional interferon is absorbed and cleared quickly by the body. A new, longer-acting form called pegylated interferon (or peginterferon) was recently approved by the Food and Drug Administration (FDA). Pegylated interferon was chemically altered by binding polyethylene glycol (PEG) molecules to the interferon in a process called pegylation. This new type of interferon stays in the body substantially longer and at a more constant level, increasing its effectiveness in fighting the virus. The longer life allows dosing to be reduced as well; pegylated interferon must be administered as a shot only once a week, instead of three times a week, as with standard interferon. Overall results are better and patient compliance higher. These advantages have turned the injection of pegylated interferon into the treatment standard. Side effects are comparable to standard interferon; however, a few patients may experience more adverse reactions. Currently two types of pegylated interferon are used: pegylated interferon alpha 2b (Peg-Intron

A) and pegylated interferon alpha 2a (Pegasys). So far, there appear to be no significant differences between the two pegylated interferons in effectiveness and safety.

A nucleoside analogue called ribavirin (Rebetol) is also used to treat hepatitis C. Nucleoside analogues are oral antiviral agents. They are artificially made molecules used to trick the virus into slowing down reproduction. These artificial molecules resemble the building blocks of the viral genetic material (hepatitis C RNA). Ribavirin does not work very well when taken alone, but when taken with interferon, it increases the effectiveness of the treatment.

Three treatments have been approved by the Food and Drug Administration (FDA) to treat hepatitis C:

- interferon alone (interferon monotherapy)

- combination therapy using conventional interferon combined with ribavirin

- combination therapy using pegylated interferon alfa 2a or 2b in conjunction with ribavirin (sometimes called peg-riba)

Pegylated interferon is mostly used when given as monotherapy, as conventional interferon alone is generally considered to be outdated.

The treatment of choice for hepatitis C today is a combination of pegylated intereferon alfa (PEG-IFN alfa), 2a or 2b, and ribavirin (RBV). This therapy is generally suitable for people who have never been treated with interferon before, those who have been treated with interferon but relapsed after initially responding to the treatment, and those who did not respond at all to interferon. Although combination therapy is associated with more side effects, it is preferable in most cases. Interferon monotherapy is reserved only for patients for whom ribavirin is contraindicated.

Ribavirin is taken by mouth as capsules or pills; interferon must be injected. Overall, combination therapy is much more effective than interferon monotherapy, and patients who did not benefit from interferon alone may consider combination therapy. But combination therapy is not suitable for all patients with hepatitis C. The side effects may be intolerable for some.

Recent studies show that some 55 percent of patients who take ribavirin and interferon together achieve a "sustained response"—the hepatitis C virus has been cleared from their blood after stopping treatment. In the early days of interferon therapy, with standard interferon alone, a sustained response rate was only around 8 percent after six months of treatment (with interferon-alpha only) and 15 percent after 48 weeks. By contrast, with pegylated interferon alpha-2a alone, approximately 30 to 40 percent of patients can achieve a sustained response after 24 to 48 weeks of treatment.

It is generally agreed that the response rate differs depending on the viral genotype. Genotypes 2 and 3 are more responsive to treatment than genotype 1—the most common type in the United States—and require a shorter course of treatment. Some studies have shown that higher doses of ribavirin given to patients with genotype 1 are associated with a higher sustained virological response.

Standard combination therapy lasts either 24 weeks or 48 weeks, but the treatment may be terminated early if there are adverse effects, or if the treatment does not seem to be working. Generally speaking, individuals with genotypes 2 or 3 may only need 24 weeks of therapy, while those with genotype 1, which is more resistant to treatment, usually do better with the longer treatment duration of 48 weeks. Some experts recommend that if HCV RNA levels have not decreased by two log10 units (for example, from 2 million IU to 20,000 IU or from 500,000 IU to 5,000 IU or less) in patients with genotype 1, treatment can be stopped early, as it is unlikely that they will have a sustained response.

Treatment time for a clinical trial for new medicines depends on the study design, and will be explained at the time of patient participation.

Response

Treatment means taking medication to rid the body of the hepatitis C virus. Doctors use the term "treatment naive" to refer to patients who have not yet taken any medication to treat their illness.

Broadly, there are four different responses to antiviral therapy: sustained response, relapse, breakthrough nonresponse, and complete nonresponse. A sustained virological response, or sustained response, is the optimal one. A sustained response means that the HCV DNA cannot be detected in the blood six months after treatment. These patients are sometimes called complete responders. Studies show that some 98 percent of patients who test negative for the virus six months after therapy will enjoy an indefinite remission. This means it is highly unlikely that there will be a reappearance of HCV RNA in the blood. Only a small minority (about 5 percent) of individuals experience a relapse—reappearance of the virus—one year after therapy. Studies show that 10 years after treatment, people who have eliminated the virus from their blood continue to show normal levels of liver enzymes. Therefore, remission from hepatitis C may be comparable to a cure. However, because treatment for hepatitis C has not been available for very long, the remission cannot be declared a cure until more long-term research has been conducted.

Patients who do not completely clear the virus from their blood fall into a category of nonresponse to therapy, which is further divided into the following:

- relapse. The treatment works initially, but the virus is detected in the blood again, shortly after the medication is stopped (usually within a year). Patients who initially respond to treatment are called relapsers, or transient responders.

- breakthrough nonresponse. The therapy seems to work during the early period of treatment, and the virus seems to disappear from the blood. However, even before medication is stopped, the virus reappears. These patients are known as breakthrough nonresponders, or breakthrough responders.

- complete nonresponse. There was no response at all to therapy. The treatment failed to clear the virus from the blood.

Even if the virus fails to be completely eliminated, patients who show some response to therapy may see some normalization of liver tests, and perhaps relief of symptoms. There may also be an amelioration of liver injury and scarring. But whatever

improvements there may be are not nearly as substantial as in the case of sustained responders, and a favorable outcome cannot be predicted as long as the HCV RNA remains detectable.

Therapy can last either 24 weeks or 48 weeks—and sometimes up to two years—but some patients may show a significantly positive response to therapy after just 12 weeks. The virus (HCV RNA) may become undetectable, or there may be a significant reduction of the amount of virus in the blood. This is called an early response to therapy, or early virological response (EVR). Generally speaking, the EVR is predictive of treatment success. If the patient responds to therapy after a few months, there is about a 70 percent chance that a full course of therapy will eliminate the virus. But if the treatment is not working by 12 weeks at least, the doctor may conclude it is unlikely that continuing the therapy for an entire year will do any good and suggest termination of treatment.

Patients unable to eliminate the virus after the end of treatment may want to try another drug immediately, take a break before beginning with another drug, or decide to wait until better treatments become available. The decision depends on various factors, such as the results of liver tests and the biopsy.

One experimental approach to nonresponders is the use of long-term or maintenance interferon. This approach is advisable only if the patient can tolerate pegylated interferon, and if the therapy has a clear effect on blood levels of the liver enzymes, or if the microscopic examination of liver tissue shows improvement even without clearance of HCV RNA.

A good number of relapsers and nonresponders who have tried only interferon monotherapy find that combination therapy with pegylated interferon and ribavirin benefits them. Current medical therapy for hepatitis C is far from ideal, as almost half the patients fail to respond to treatment. Researchers are still trying different drugs, but so far, the only treatment that has been clinically shown to be effective in reducing viral load is interferon therapy, with or without ribavirin.

Even patients who do not completely clear the virus from their blood may enjoy benefits from therapy. Disease progression may be slowed and complications of liver disease, such as cirrhosis, liver failure, and liver cancer, may be deterred or prevented.

Certain patient characteristics were identified as favorable predictors for a sustained response to interferon monotherapy:

- recent infection with HCV
- genotype 2 or 3
- low viral load (HCV RNA of less than 1 million copies/ml)
- little or no quasispecies variation
- absence of cirrhosis
- no excessive iron revealed by liver biopsy
- females
- age under 40 years

This does not mean that people who do not have the above characteristics will not respond to therapy. Response to alpha interferon can be determined after 12 weeks of therapy; patients who have failed to respond by then are unlikely to respond even if more of the same therapy is given. Furthermore, patients given combination therapy of interferon and ribivarin often go on to have a sustained response even if they failed to clear the virus at week 12. Therefore, it is recommended that patients on combination therapy continue for at least 24 weeks.

HCV genotypes may be a factor in individual differences in treatment responsiveness. Genotype 1, the most common type in the United States, is generally regarded as the most difficult to treat. Many studies suggest that sustained response rates for genotype 1 are roughly 40 percent, compared with response rates as high as 70 to 80 percent for genotypes 2 and 3. In a more recent study, researchers achieved response rates as high as 51 percent for patients with genotype 1 by using a combination of pegylated interferon (Pegasys) and ribavirin for 48 weeks.

Another factor apparently is the amount of fibrosis—scarring—of the liver. Individuals with higher grades of fibrosis are less likely to achieve early virologic response than those with less fibrosis.

Race may yet be another factor. For reasons that are as yet unclear, African Americans have been observed to show poor rates of response to hepatitis medication. Recent studies indicate that response rates for African Americans may improve if the ribavirin dosage is determined on the basis of the patient's body weight.

Other factors that may influence treatment responsiveness include the following:

- viral load (the amount of virus in the blood). A high viral load does not necessarily mean that the patient is sicker or has worse liver damage than someone with a lower viral load. Some experts believe that lower viral loads are linked with better treatment success, but others dispute this. Studies so far are inconclusive.

- viral diversity. There are many different viral strains of hepatitis C, and different strains can be found within the same individual. These viral strains are called quasispecies, and some studies suggest that the more diverse the population of quasispecies, the greater the likelihood of progression to advanced disease.

- iron. Iron levels may predict treatment response. It has been observed that people with chronic hepatitis C have higher iron levels in their blood, particularly men. Perhaps this is due to iron being released by dying cells. It may also be due to individuals carrying a gene for hereditary iron overload, called HEMACHROMATOSIS. Individuals with high iron levels in the blood or in the liver cells generally do not respond as well to treatment with interferon. This could be because iron promotes the replication of the virus. Some studies suggest that reducing iron storage may help reduce liver cell injury. This is done through drawing blood (phlebotomy) or through chelation therapy. Phlebotomy is used for people with an iron overload disease, such as hemocrhomatosis. The iron level in the body can be easily checked with a blood test or a liver biopsy. No definite conclusions have been drawn as to the efficacy of iron-reduction therapy as an adjunct to interferon therapy for people with chronic hepatitis C.

- gender. Women are somewhat more likely to respond to treatment than men. Moreover, hepatitis C is four times more likely to progress into liver cancer in men than in women.

- age. The illness seems to progress faster in people becoming infected when they are more advanced in years, after the age of 55. People who acquire the virus before the age of 40 stand a better chance of recovery.

- length of infection. The longer a patient has been infected with the virus, the more likely he or she will suffer from complications of the illness. Thus, there seems to be a definite correlation between the time from presentation of the illness to start of therapy: the shorter the duration, the more likely a sustained response.

- routes of transmission. The route of HCV transmission may influence the course of the disease. People who acquired the virus through a blood transfusion seem to have an increased chance of developing liver disease than those who acquired it through other means. Perhaps this is because large amounts of HCV viral particles can be transmitted via blood transfusion. Similarly, people who acquire their infection through repeated injection drug abuse tend to have a worse course of illness because they are more likely to have a larger viral load, and a greater variety of viral strains.

- other hepatitis viruses. People coinfected with hepatitis C and hepatitis B are more likely to have an aggressive course of disease. Those with chronic hepatitis B who also become infected with hepatitis A can sometimes suffer from FULMINANT HEPATITIS, which can lead to death. Likewise, people infected with both hepatitis C and HIV (the AIDS virus) are at an increased risk for developing liver disease.

- environmental factors. Environmental toxins and pollutants from work and other areas can potentially accelerate disease progression in people afflicted with chronic hepatitis C.

Finally, there is no definitive way of predicting how hepatitis C will develop in any one individual. No one really knows why one person can live for decades without problems, while others progress rapidly to end-stage liver disease. The only way to keep track of how the disease is progressing is to perform periodic liver biopsies.

Side Effects

Almost all patients experience side effects from antiviral therapy. Side effects may range from mild to severe, and differ greatly from person to person. The most frequently cited side effects of antiviral therapy are the following:

- flu-like symptoms (chills, headache, muscle aches, general malaise)
- hair loss (reversible)
- appetite and weight loss
- nausea and vomiting
- chest pain
- shortness of breath
- fatigue
- irritability
- anxiety
- depression

Most of these symptoms should fade away after the first few weeks of therapy, but a minority of patients may need to drop out of therapy due to adverse reactions.

Less common side effects include the following:

- anemia
- low white blood cell count (leucopenia)
- low platelet count (thrombocytopenia)
- hypothyroidism (decreased thyroid function)
- hyperthyroidism (excessive thyroid function)
- bacterial infection
- acute psychosis
- seizures
- autoimmune disease
- hearing loss and tinnitus (ringing of the ears)

Rare side effects include kidney problems or failure, and rashes. Interferon may also impair fertility.

Doctors can counteract some side effects by using, for example, various hormones to halt the drop in blood cell counts.

Ribavirin is associated with side effects that include the following:

- nausea
- cough
- itching
- insomnia
- shortness of breath
- anemia (caused by destruction of red blood cells, known as hemolysis)

Anemia is probably the most serious side effect related to ribavirin. Because of the possibility of anemia that can exacerbate coronary disease, it is recommended that complete blood counts (CBC) be obtained at the start of therapy, and again at weeks two and four, or at whatever intervals are indicated. Patients should be particularly vigilant with follow-up visits to the doctor during the initial period after commencing treatment, because anemia is most likely to occur during the first few weeks of therapy.

Sometimes anemia may be managed by administering epoetin alfa (Procrit) at 40,000 IU once a week. Patients who have an existing condition of anemia, or other health conditions such as heart disease or kidney disease, may not be able to take ribavirin, and they may benefit from interferon monotherapy.

One potentially serious side effect of ribavirin is possible birth defects. Although there have been no reports of human birth defects to date, animal studies show that ribavirin collects in the ovaries and testes, causing birth defects. Malformations can occur in the skull, palate, eyes, jaws, limbs, and gastrointestinal tract, and survival of fetuses and offspring was reduced. For this reason, women of childbearing age must test negative for pregnancy. Additionally, women and their male partners must use contraceptives both during treatment and for at least six months afterward to prevent pregnancy.

Interferons may be excreted in human milk. Mothers are advised either to stop nursing or to discontinue treatment. A pregnant woman should explore the best option for herself with her doctor.

Patients should report any side effects to their doctor who may have advice or medications to reduce the side effects, or make necessary adjustments in dosage. Patients should never stop or reduce medication on their own without consulting their doctor, as there may be serious consequences.

Most side effects disappear after several weeks, but they may persist in some cases, or become so intolerable that therapy must be discontinued. Patients who have severe reactions to ribavirin may opt out of combination therapy and try monotherapy with pegylated interferon instead. Here are some suggestions given by health care providers on managing side effects:

- Take a painkiller a half hour before the interferon injection to lessen side effects. (Check with the doctor first to make sure the pain medication and dosing is appropriate. Overdosing can lead to liver failure.)
- Inject interferon just before going to bed to sleep through the side effects.
- Identify anything that appears to cause or worsen symptoms. Triggers can be loud noises, bright lights, drinking caffeinated drinks, going for too long without eating, and so forth.
- Avoid exposure to chemicals as much as possible. These include hair dye and permanents.
- Avoid hair and skin products that have strong scents. Use simple, unscented lotions, shampoo, and other products.
- Drink at least eight glasses of water a day.
- Avoid beverages with alcohol, caffeine, or a lot of sugar.
- Avoid greasy foods, such as fast foods.

Liver transplantation The leading cause of LIVER TRANSPLANTATION in the United States today is advanced liver disease associated with chronic hepatitis C. A major drawback to liver transplantation for patients with hepatitis C is the almost universal recurrence of the HCV virus in the blood after surgery. This is more likely to occur if the patient has a high viral load at the time of transplantation. About 25 percent of transplant patients will suffer from significant hepatitis, and these patients will develop cirrhosis within five years of their transplant. Taking immunosuppressive medication to prevent rejection of the grafted organ also enhances viral reproduction. Patients sometimes consider re-transplantation after the failure of the transplanted liver caused by the recurrence of HCV infection.

However, hepatitis C patients have comparable five-year survival rates as other transplant patients.

Patients who do not receive therapy   Individuals with chronic hepatitis C who choose not to receive therapy for whatever reason should visit their doctors regularly—about twice a year—to have their disease monitored. They should have a physical exam, some blood tests, and perhaps imaging studies, with a liver biopsy conducted every five years to check the progression of hepatitis C. These are general guidelines only; individual circumstances may require more frequent checkups.

Bodenheimer, H. C., et al. "Tolerance and efficacy of oral ribavirin treatment of chronic hepatitis C: A multicenter trial." *Hepatology* 26 (1997): 473–477.

Davis, Gary, et al. "Interferon alfa-2b alone or in combination with ribavirin for the treatment of relapse of chronic hepatitis C." *New England Journal of Medicine* 339 (1998): 1,493–1,499.

Delwaide, J., et al. "Treatment of acute hepatitis C with interferon alpha-2b: Early initiation of treatment is the most effective predictive factor of sustained viral response." *Treatment of Acute Alimentary Pharmacology and Therapeutics* 20, no. 1 (July 1, 2004): 15–22.

Dev, A. T., and others. "Hepatic fibrosis influences early virological response rates in chronic hepatitis C (CHC)." Abstract 1159. *Internet Conference Report,* Digestive Disease Week. May 15–20, 2004. New Orleans. Available online. URL: http://www.hivandhepatitis.com/2004icr/ddw2004/docs/0607/060904_b.html. Downloaded on September 1, 2004.

Hadziyannis, S. J., et. al. "Peginterferon Alfa-2a (40KD) (Pegasys) in combination with ribavirin (RBV): Effi-

cacy and safety results from a phase III, randomized, double-blind, multicentre study examining effect of duration of treatment and RBV dose." Abstract 536. 37th annual meeting of the European Association for the Study of the Liver. April 18–21, 2002. Available online. URL: http://www.hivand hepatiits.com/hep_c/news/041902a.html. Downloaded on January 30, 2005.

Lee, William, et al. "Early hepatitis C. Virus-RNA response predict interferon treatment outcomes in chronic hepatitis C." *Hepatology* 28 (1998): 1,411–1,415.

Rowell, Diana, et al. "Should chronic viral hepatitis with persistently normal aminotransferase levels be treated?" *Viral Hepatitis Reviews* 3, no. 3 (1997): 189–199.

Seeff, Leonard B., et al. "Heavy alcohol use greatly increases cirrhosis risk in hepatitis C-infected patients." *Annals of Internals Medicine* 134 (2001): 120–124.

hepatitis D   Hepatitis D virus (HDV) is a "passenger virus" that needs the HEPATITIS B virus to live and to reproduce. It cannot cause infection on its own in the absence of coating material from the hepatitis B virus. Hepatitis D can either infect an individual who is already infected with hepatitis B (superinfection) or infect someone at the same time the individual becomes infected with hepatitis B (coinfection). HDV can cause both acute and chronic conditions, and coinfection with HDV tends to increase the severity of disease progression. However, it can lower the patient's risk of becoming a hepatitis B carrier, because HDV tends to repress the reproduction of the hepatitis B virus.

Patients with chronic hepatitis B who also become infected with HDV often also become chronically infected with the hepatitis D virus.

The hepatitis D virus was discovered in 1977 by Dr. Mario Rizzetto. HDV, also called delta hepatitis, is a small circular RNA virus belonging in the Deltaviridae family. It is estimated that 70,000 people in the United States are infected with HDV. HDV is endemic in areas such as the Middle East, the Mediterranean, and South America, but has a relatively low incidence in the United States.

Epidemics of hepatitis D usually occur in developing countries. When these outbreaks occur, the infection is extremely severe, and liver failure may occur rapidly. In such cases, mortality is close to 20 percent.

The transmission route of hepatitis D is similar to hepatitis B. HDV is spread mostly through contaminated blood, and can also occur during sexual contact or from an infected mother to her child during childbirth, but much less frequently than with hepatitis B.

The hepatitis D virus has also been found in the saliva, semen, and vaginal secretions of infected individuals. An individual infected with hepatitis D can spread both hepatitis B and hepatitis D to another person at the same time. Thus, a person who had previously been uninfected can contract both hepatitis B and hepatitis D from the same source.

High-risk groups include injection drug users, hemophiliacs, and homosexual men.

Symptoms and Diagnostic Path

The symptoms are practically indistinguishable from hepatitis B but are typically more severe, as hepatitis D tends to follow a particularly aggressive course. There may be mild jaundice, weakness, fatigue, appetite loss, nausea, vomiting, and abdominal pain.

People infected with both chronic hepatitis B and chronic hepatitis D have a much higher risk that their disease will progress into CIRRHOSIS, an extensive scarring of liver tissue. Perhaps as many as 80 percent will develop cirrhosis; moreover, they will do so at a much faster rate and a younger age than those with only HBV infection, and are more likely to develop complications. An estimated 75 percent of patients will experience complications of cirrhosis, compared with about 25 percent for patients infected with hepatitis B alone. These include conditions such as ASCITES (accumulation of fluid in the abdomen) and swollen, distended varices or BLEEDING VARICES.

In cases where hepatitis B is accompanied by hepatitis D, the patient may develop a sudden, severe liver failure.

Microscopic examination of liver tissue shows that coinfection or superinfection results in a more severe liver disease than hepatitis B alone.

It is not immediately obvious that a patient has been infected with hepatitis D, but superinfection with HDV may be suspected if there is a sudden worsening of liver disease, and symptoms such as JAUNDICE and abdominal pain. Examination may show an enlarged liver and spleen; LIVER ENZYMES alanine transaminase (ALT) and aspartate transaminase (AST) may be elevated. Infection with hepatitis D may also be suspected if a patient presents with a very severe acute hepatitis B, as coinfection generally causes a more severe acute disease. A coinfected patient also suffers a higher risk of developing a sudden, acute liver failure compared with those infected with hepatitis B virus alone. Diagnosis can be confirmed by blood tests for antibodies to the hepatitis D virus and HDV RNA.

Treatment Options and Outlook

Treatment for hepatitis D is the same as for hepatitis B. But studies to date show only a poor response to treatment with interferon-alpha, and therapy is currently unsatisfactory. Even when interferon is given for one year, most patients experience a significant relapse when therapy is stopped; the viral count goes up again, and they are unable to sustain the improvements shown during treatment.

Lamivudine, an oral nucleoside analogue that is quite successful at inhibiting hepatitis B, has been tried, but seems ineffectual at reducing either the viral load in hepatitis D or the disease activity. So far, no drug therapies have proven effective against hepatitis D, but research for new drugs is underway.

Patients who are not on drug therapy should be monitored with regular follow-up visits with the doctor, as well as periodic liver biopsies to check on the status of the liver.

LIVER TRANSPLANTATION may be attempted as a last resort if the patient is suffering from multiple complications or the disease progresses to liver failure. Because hepatitis D appears to inhibit replication of the hepatitis B virus, coinfection with both HBV and HDV may lower the risk of disease reinfection. Generally, when a hepatitis patient undergoes liver transplantation, the liver graft becomes reinfected.

Risk Factors and Preventive Measures

The best way to prevent hepatitis D is by preventing hepatitis B infection, since HDV cannot be contracted in the absence of hepatitis B. Individuals who are already infected with hepatitis B should lower their risk of transmission by reducing their exposure to blood and practicing safer sex by using barrier contraception. Patients already infected with hepatitis C are advised to consider vaccination against both hepatitis A and hepatitis B, as coinfection with multiple hepatitis viruses accelerates the disease progression and, in some cases, proves fatal.

An individual who contracted hepatitis B and recovered from it, or who has been vaccinated against hepatitis B, has also been conferred immunity to hepatitis D.

Fisher, Thomas, M.D. "Hepatitis D." Available online. URL: http://health.discovery.com/encyclopedias/246. html. Downloaded on January 5, 2005.

Weltman, M. D., A. Brotodihardjo, E. B. Crewe, G. C. Farrell, M. Bilous, J. M. Grierson, and C. Liddle. "Coinfection with hepatitis B and C or B, C and delta viruses results in severe chronic liver disease and responds poorly to interferon-alpha treatment." *Hepatology* 30, no. 2 (August 1999): 546–549.

hepatitis E　Hepatitis E (HEV) is a common cause of acute hepatitis that can sometimes lead to LIVER FAILURE, though it is usually a mild disease. Hepatitis E is similar to HEPATITIS A in its symptoms and clinical manifestations. Like hepatitis A, HEV causes only acute, short-lived LIVER DISEASE, and does not produce a chronic form of hepatitis.

The hepatitis E virus is an enteric virus; it is introduced into the body through the digestive system. It is spread mainly through contaminated water, though it can be spread through food as well. As with hepatitis A, poor sanitation is the most significant factor in the spread of the disease. But unlike hepatitis A, the transmission of hepatitis E through person-to-person contact is rare.

Hepatitis E is sometimes referred to as epidemic non-A, non-B hepatitis, because it is a major cause of epidemic hepatitis in many areas of Asia, Africa, and Mexico, where HEV is considered endemic. Formerly, hepatitis E was also called enterically transmitted non-A, non-B, and waterborne non-A, non-B hepatitis.

The hepatitis E virus was discovered in 1987. Two main geographic strains of the virus, Asian and Mexican, have been recognized.

The virus enters through the gastrointestinal tract, where it starts to divide, but it grows mostly in the liver. The nonenveloped, spherical virus has a single-stranded RNA approximately 32 to 34 nm in diameter. HEV has been classified in the Caliciviridae family. But as the HEV genome differs substantially from that of other viruses in the family, it will most likely be reclassified eventually into a separate family.

Worldwide, HEV is the most common cause (greater than 50 percent in HEV-endemic countries) of acute viral hepatitis. The virus is endemic in countries with poor sanitation where the drinking water is not purified and may be contaminated with human waste. Large epidemics of HEV involving thousands of people occur in developing countries. These epidemics often break out during or after periods of heavy rain, when drinking water becomes contaminated with feces. Outbreaks have been most commonly identified in southern and central Asia, northern Africa, and Central America. In the United States, the virus is generally considered to be imported. Reported cases of HEV in the United States are of people who recently traveled to HEV-endemic areas. Recent research suggests that HEV may be more prevalent in industrialized countries, however, than previously considered. Blood samples taken in recent years from residents of North America, the United Kingdom, and certain parts of Europe, such as Italy, Greece, and Spain, have been shown to harbor HEV strains that differ genetically from strains found in developing countries. More studies are needed before any conclusions can be drawn.

Symptoms and Diagnostic Path

Patients may develop sudden symptoms such as loss of appetite, nausea, vomiting, fever, feelings of malaise, and from fatigue 15 to 60 days after suspected exposure to the hepatitis E virus. The average incubation period is 40 days. There may also be discomfort or pain in the upper-right area of the abdomen where the liver is located. Symptoms may include jaundice, or yellowing of the skin and eyes, though jaundice tends to be rare among patients under 14 and over 50 years of age. Indeed, the disease itself is quite uncommon in the elderly and children, though children seem to be the reservoir for the virus during epidemics. The infection rate is highest in the age group between 15 and 40, particularly in young adults between the ages of 20 and 30.

Diagnosis is made through blood testing. Several diagnostic tests are available at the U.S. Centers for Disease Control and Prevention (CDC) in Atlanta, Georgia, or in research laboratories to detect IgM and IgG anti-HEV in the serum. During early recovery, the level of IgM antibodies declines rapidly, and can be used to diagnose acute hepatitis E, while IgG antibodies persist for some time after infection and may provide at least short-term immunity against the disease. Other tests for hepatitis E infection are available in the United States on a research basis, including polymerase chain reaction tests (PCR) to detect the hepatitis E viral RNA in the blood and stool during infection.

Treatment Options and Outlook

There is no specific treatment for hepatitis E. In most cases, the disease is mild, and the patient recovers without treatment. The doctor will most likely recommend rest and drinking a lot of fluids. Hospitalization may be necessary if the patient is too sick to eat or drink. Intensive care is necessary in the uncommon event of fulminant hepatic failure. In such an event, LIVER TRANSPLANTATION is the only treatment.

HEV is a self-limiting infection, resolving without treatment within two weeks or so. It is not usually fatal in the United States, but serious complications are possible, and about 1 to 2 percent of those infected can die of advanced liver failure. The hallmark of hepatitis E is its high fatality rate in pregnant women—an average of 20 percent and up to 30 percent. This is not the case for any other type of viral hepatitis. Rates for FULMINANT HEPATITIS and death are particularly high in the third trimester of pregnancy, as well as during labor. Terminating pregnancy does not appear to improve the survival rate of the patient.

Risk Factors and Preventive Measures

Prevention depends on avoiding contaminated food and, especially, water. Travelers to endemic regions should avoid drinking water from local water supplies, ice of unknown purity, uncooked fruits and vegetables, and shellfish. Pregnant women should take particular precautions because they are more vulnerable to fulminant hepatitis. No vaccines or post-exposure prophylactic immunoglobulins are available as yet, but recombinant vaccines are currently being prepared.

It is not clear whether having hepatitis E once guarantees against future HEV infection.

Clemente-Casares, Pilar, Sonia Pina, Maria Buti, Rosend Jardi, Margarita Martin, Silvia Bofill-Mas, and Rosina Girones. "Hepatitis E virus epidemiology in industrialized countries." *Emerging Infectious Diseases* 9, no. 4 (April 2003): 447–448.
Wu, J. C., C. M. Chen, T. Y. Chiang, I. J. Sheen, J. Y. Chen, W. H. Tsai, Y. H. Huang, and S. D. Lee. "Clinical and epidemiological implications of swine hepatitis E virus infection." *Journal of Medical Virology* 60, no. 2 (February 2000): 166–171.

hepatitis F It is not clear at the present time whether there is such a thing as a hepatitis F virus (HFV). Technically, it is a nonexistent virus, but a place has been reserved for it in the viral hepatitis nomenclature.

Scientists began suspecting the existence of a new hepatitis virus from observations of sporadic and post-transfusion viral cases that could not be attributed to hepatitis A, B, C, D, or E. The virus appeared to be transmitted through the intestines.

Investigators from various countries began looking for this mysterious virus. The first report came from India in 1983, followed by reports from England and France in 1987, and Italy in 1988. In 1992, investigators from Japan reported discovery of a new hepatitis virus that they called hepatitis F, but, their claim has not been substantiated. In 1993, other reports from Japan suggested that the hepatitis F virus may be a mutant form of hepatitis B. Then a handful of cases from France in 1994 described what was believed to be hepatitis F. Later that year, investigators reported that they injected the unknown virus into rhesus monkeys and recovered the viral particles in the stools of the monkeys. However, no one has been able to replicate the experimental transmission to primates.

If hepatitis F virus does exist, its origin, prevalence, effect on the liver, and clinical importance remain unknown.

Desmet, V. G. M., et al. "Classification of chronic hepatitis: diagnosis, grading and staging." *Hepatology* 19 (1994): 1,513–1,520.

hepatitis G A recently discovered strain of viral hepatitis, the hepatitis G virus (HGV) has been described as a "distant cousin" of HEPATITIS C, though studies suggest that hepatitis G is more common and milder than hepatitis C.

Hepatitis G is also called the GB virus C or HGBV-C. It is an RNA virus in the Flaviviridae family, and has been associated with both acute and chronic hepatitis, and tends to coexist with other kinds of hepatitis infections. But there is some controversy as to what extent the virus can cause hepatitis in humans. The infection appears to be "clinically silent" in that it does not worsen the clinical course of already existing liver disease. Several studies comparing patients who have HGV infection alone and people who are coinfected with hepatitis C and G show similar results on liver-panel tests and LIVER BIOPSIES. There is also little difference in patient response to medications for HEPATITIS, such as INTERFERON. Accordingly, HGV does not appear to be overtly infectious or to cause significant LIVER DISEASE.

The transmission of hepatitis G is believed to parallel that of hepatitis C, though the nature and frequency of infection remain unclear. HGV is spread through transfusions and exposure to blood and blood products; it is often transmitted with hepatitis C. Hepatitis G can also be transmitted from an infected mother to her infant during childbirth.

HGV, present in the U.S. volunteer blood donor population, is found in approximately 1.5 to 1.7 percent of blood donors, compared with 1 percent for hepatitis C. Due to the shared risk factors of infection—such as through transfusions or intravenous drug use—many HGV patients may have also become infected with hepatitis B or hepatitis C virus. Accordingly, many patients with hepatitis B or C may be at increased risk for contracting hepatitis G.

Although hepatitis G is recognized as a blood-borne pathogen, the overall rate of HGV infection in individuals who have had multiple transfusions is relatively low. This means that the risk factor for such individuals are also lower than previously assumed. Even with patients on hemodialysis—some of whom are HIV-infected and whose immune system is not functioning well—the rate of infection is not as high as might be expected. Recipients of blood products contaminated by HGV show little evidence of persistent infection. So why does the general population have a high rate of HGV infection? Investigators have yet to reconcile this paradox.

It is likely that HGV may be transmitted through sexual, as well as other, as yet undefined routes. Further studies must be made to understand why there is such a discrepancy in rates of transmission between hepatitis C and hepatitis G.

In 1995 and 1996, researchers reported discovery of several novel human RNA viruses that apparently could cause both acute and chronic hepatitis. These new viruses were similar to, but clearly distinct from, hepatitis C. Investigators at Abbott Labs in the United States identified three viruses that they termed GB-A, GB-B, and GB-C. "GB" is taken from the initials of a Chicago surgeon who contracted a previously unknown hepatitis virus—distinct from hepatitis A, B, C, D, and E—and who later died from the disease. Blood taken from the surgeon infected tamarin monkeys with hepatitis. GB-C is probably the same as hepatitis G. GB-A and GB-B are probably tamarin viruses. The precise role of HGV/GB-C in human disease is currently under investigation.

Hepatitis G is commonly found in the general population and is distributed globally, including Australia, Asia, Europe, and North America.

Symptoms and Diagnostic Path
What, if any, kind of infection HGV causes remains controversial. No symptoms may occur or they may be brief and mild.

The only test available today that is specific for hepatitis G is polymerase chain reaction (PCR) assay, which can show whether an individual is currently infected. But the test is relatively expensive, and in view of the fact that hepatitis G appears to be a benign disease, experts believe that in most cases the expense is not justified.

Treatment Options and Outlook

At present, there are no proven treatments for hepatitis G. Studies suggest that HGV RNA levels decrease during therapy with interferon-alpha. However, as with hepatitis C (when treated with interferon monotherapy), only a minority of patients had a sustained response. In other words, when treatment was stopped, HGV RNA was once again detectable in the blood of most patients.

Fortunately, unlike hepatitis C, hepatitis G is mild and transient, and usually does not become chronic. Even when chronic, the likelihood of hepatitis G infection progressing to CIRRHOSIS is probably quite low. On the other hand, a small study has implicated the hepatitis G virus in the development of FULMINANT HEPATITIS. The study, involving six Japanese patients, is too small to be definitive but at least suggests the possibility that hepatitis G may be the cause of fulminant hepatitis in Japan, and possibly in other parts of the world as well. To date, the role of HGV in fulminant hepatitis remains unresolved. More research is needed to understand better the risk factors for hepatitis G and its significance in causing disease in the liver or in other parts of the body. No clear guidelines can be formulated at the present time in the management of hepatitis G.

Alter, M. J., M. Gallagher, T. T. Morris, L. A. Moyer, E. L. Meeks, K. Krawczynski, J. P. Kim, and H. S. Margolis. "Acute non-A-E hepatitis in the United States and the role of hepatitis G virus infection." *New England Journal of Medicine* 346 (1997): 741–746.

Alter, H. J., Y. Nakatsuji, J. Melpolder, J. Wages, R. Wesley, W. K. Shih, and J. P. Kim. "The incidence of transfusion-associated hepatitis G virus infection and its relation to liver disease." *New England Journal of Medicine* 336 (1997): 747–754.

Goeser, T., S. Seipp, R. Wahl, H. M. Muller, W. Stremmel, and L. Theilmann. "Clinical presentation of GB-C virus infection in drug abusers with chronic hepatitis C." *Journal of Hepatology* 3 (March 26, 1997): 498–502.

hepatoblastoma   See LIVER DISEASE.

hepatocellular carcinoma (HCC)   Hepatocellular carcinoma (HCC) is a cancer of the hepatocytes, or liver cells. It is a primary cancer, originating in the LIVER rather than somewhere else in the body. It is a common cancer worldwide, but quite rare in the United States, northern Europe, Australia, and New Zealand. The highest incidences of HCC occur in eastern Asia (China, Hong Kong, Korea, Mongolia, and Japan), central Africa, and some areas of western Africa.

People living in these high-risk regions are five times more likely to get HCC than residents of developed countries. The main reasons are the prevalence of chronic HEPATITIS B and C, and exposure to food contaminants called aflatoxin. In all ethnic groups, men are at higher risk for HCC than women. The ratio is about 10 to one overall, though it varies depending on the ethnic groups and regions.

Although Japan has long since joined the ranks of industrial nations, it has a higher incidence of HCC than other developed countries, perhaps due to the comparatively higher numbers of people infected with viral hepatitis. Chronic hepatitis B (HBV) and HEPATITIS C (HCV) are associated with HCC. It is believed that many Japanese contracted HCV after World War II because of the use of common syringes to vaccinate against tuberculosis. This was in the days before the hepatitis C virus had been identified, and when the role of contaminated needles in spreading communicable diseases was not widely known.

In the United States, HCV is most commonly transmitted through intravenous (injection) drug use and sexual contact. Since the early 1980s more people in the United States have been diagnosed with hepatocellular carcinoma, an increase that is also mirrored in Japan. It is not clear what caused this jump, but researchers believe that it is related to a rise in hepatitis C virus infections that people acquired in the 1960s and 1970s. If that is the case, then HCC rates may continue to increase for many years. It generally takes 20 to 40 years of chronic hepatitis B or hepatitis C infections, or many years of excessive alcohol consumption before cancer develops. In the United States, the rise in the number of new cases of LIVER CANCER was seen in all ethnic groups and in most age groups over 40; however, the largest increases were in white men between the ages of 45 and 54, from 1995 to 1998.

The greatest risk in developing hepatocellular carcinoma is chronic infection with hepatitis B and hepatitis C. Certain parts of Africa and Asia have the highest risks for the primary liver cancer HCC mainly because of the prevalence of hepatitis B (HBV). In fact, HBV may increase the risk of developing hepatocellular carcinoma up to 200 times, and is probably the single most frequent cause of death from HCC. In some developing countries, as much as 60 to 90 percent of the population may have chronic hepatitis B, and the incidence of HCC is proportionately high.

Although severe scarring of the liver is present in almost all people with hepatitis B who develop HCC, cancerous tumors in the liver have been reported even in individuals without CIRRHOSIS.

Although it is an established fact that HBV and HCV are associated with the development of hepatocellular carcinoma, some researchers are now beginning to think that these hepatitis viruses may actually have been underestimated as risk factors for primary liver cancer. Most epidemiological studies used conventional radioimmunoassay that was not as sensitive as today's tests based upon the polymerase chain reaction (PCR). The older tests used only the detection of hepatitis B surface ANTIGEN (HBsAg) as the marker for chronic hepatitis B. But a recent European study discovered that, with more sensitive testing, nearly half of the patients with HCC who tested negative for the hepatitis B surface antigen in their blood were nevertheless found to have detectable HBV DNA in their livers. Similarly, among patients who had no evidence of antibodies to hepatitis C virus, 7 percent had detectable HCV RNA in their blood, and 26 percent had it in their livers. Thus, more cases of HCC may be related to hepatitis B or hepatitis C than were believed originally.

In one study in China published in 2002 in *Cancer Epidemiology Biomarkers and Prevention,* eight-year survival analysis showed an association between tobacco smoking and women with HCC, but the connection was not seen in men.

Researchers are also seeing evidence that when hepatitis B virus is actively reproducing, the infected person is at an increased risk of HCC. One study published in the 2002 issue of the *New England Journal of Medicine* showed that the presence of hepatitis B e antigen (HBeAg), a marker for active viral replication, is associated with an increased risk of HCC.

The risk factor for HCC also appears to be linked with the genotype of hepatitis B virus. Genotypes are slightly different strains of a virus. According to a study done in Japan, hepatitis B genotype B is seen mostly in people who are carriers of the infection but have no symptoms. By contrast, genotype C was associated with chronic liver disease. Among individuals infected with the hepatitis B virus genotype C, 60 percent had HCC, and 63 percent had cirrhosis. The likelihood of the asymptomatic carriers of genotype B developing HCC is comparatively low. More studies are needed to confirm these findings. They may prove to be a useful tool in identifying patients who have a heightened risk for developing HCC.

Yet another study from Japan showed that for some patients at least, the most predictive factor for the development of HCC was the viral load, the concentration of viruses in the blood. It appears that the higher the concentration, the higher the risk of HCC. Patients also had a higher risk that their disease would progress to cirrhosis. The severe liver scarring of cirrhosis is itself the leading cause of HCC.

Because of the risk of developing HCC, patients with chronic hepatitis B or hepatitis C may wish to be screened regularly for cancer.

Symptoms and Diagnostic Path

Early signs and symptoms, if any, are vague and nonspecific. They are usually not present until the later stages of the disease. The leading causes of HCC (viral hepatitis and cirrhosis) typically also lack warning signs that could alert the patient. This long period between the time the tumors start to grow and the first signs of illness is one reason for the high mortality. Fortunately in the United

States, patients with chronic liver disease like cirrhosis are usually under a doctor's care, and the tumor may be detected when it is still small and more likely to be operable. In developing countries, however, where HCC predominates, many people are not even aware that they have been infected by viral hepatitis, and so often do not discover the tumor until it is in the later stage when acute symptoms present themselves. Patients then suffer a rapid decline, as HCC can be quite aggressive. Acute symptoms include excruciating abdominal pain caused by the tumor stretching the membrane surrounding the liver. The pain sometimes extends into the back and shoulder. If the patient has cirrhosis, some complications from the extensive liver scarring may manifest, such as mental confusion (ENCEPHALOPATHY). More general symptoms are a high fever, fatigue, loss of appetite, weight loss, and swelling of the abdomen (ASCITES). The doctor may discover an enlarged, nodular, and rock hard liver, and some internal bleeding of the digestive tract. Jaundice—yellowing of the skin and eyes—may develop in some patients, and the urine may turn dark.

In addition to the above signs and symptoms, anyone who experiences the following should see the doctor:

- a hard lump in the area of the liver (just below the rib cage on the right side).

- pain around the right shoulder blade area

- frequent feeling of fullness after just a small meal

- a worsening in the condition of chronic hepatitis or cirrhosis

A very small number of people may experience a condition known as paraneoplastic syndromes. These are symptoms that manifest as a result of the secretion of hormones and other substances by the liver tumors. These are carried to other parts of the body through the bloodstream, affecting them. The two most common symptoms are low blood sugar (hypoglycemia) and high cholesterol levels (hypercholesterolemia). Less common symptoms include high calcium level (hypercalcemia),

elevated red blood cell count (polycythemia), and breast enlargement and other signs of feminization in men (gynecomastia).

Treatment Options and Outlook

Hepatocellular carcinoma is largely preventable. The most effective way is to avoid excessive alcohol consumption and take necessary precautions against contracting hepatitis B or hepatitis C, one of the major risk factors for development of HCC. People at high risk should be vaccinated against hepatitis B. HBV vaccination has been shown to be effective in decreasing infection rates and preventing progression into chronic HBV carrier status.

There are no comparable vaccines for hepatitis C viral infection, unfortunately. This is all the more reason that one should take precautions against using contaminated needles and syringes, and practicing safe sex.

Decreasing or abstaining from alcohol can prevent not only liver cancer but many other chronic LIVER DISEASES as well.

In developing countries, aside from reducing the incidence of viral hepatitis, measures need to be taken to reduce exposures to the carcinogen aflatoxins, mold spores often found in contaminated peanuts and grains.

For more information on cancer that begins in the liver, contact the National Cancer Institute.

El-Serag, H. B., J. A. Davila, N. J. Petersen, and K. A. McGlynn. "The continuing increase in the incidence of hepatocellular carcinoma in the United States: an update." *Annals of Internal Medicine*, no. 139 (November 18, 2003): 817–823.

Evans, Alison A., et al. "Eight-year follow-up of the 90,000-person Haimen City cohort: I. Hepatocellular carcinoma mortality, risk factors, and gender differences." *Cancer Epidemiology Biomarkers & Prevention* 11 (April 2002): 369–376.

Ishikawa, T., T. Ichida, S. Yamagiwa, et al. "High viral loads, serum alanine aminotransferase and gender are predictive factors for the development of hepatocellular carcinoma from viral compensated cirrhosis." *Journal of Gastroenterology and Hepatology Aims and Scopes* 16 (2001): 1,274–1,281.

Marrero, Jorge A., M.D. "Hepatocellular carcinoma." *Current Opinions in Gastroenterology* 19, no. 3 (2003): 243–249.

Sakugawa, H., H. Nakasone, T. Nayayoshi, et al. "Preponderance of hepatitis B virus genotype B contributes to a better prognosis of chronic HBV infection in Okinawa, Japan." *Journal of Medical Virology* 67 (2002): 484–489.

Tai, D. I., C. H. Chen, T. T. Chang, et al. "Eight-year nationwide survival analysis in relatives of patients with hepatocellular carcinoma: Role of viral infection. *Journal of Gastroenterology and Hepatology Aims and Scopes* 17 (2002): 682–689.

Yang, H. I., S. N. Lu, Y. F. Liaw, et al. "Hepatitis Be antigen and the risk of hepatocellular carcinoma." *New England Journal of Medicine.* 347 (2002): 168–174.

hepatomegaly The term *hepatomegaly* means enlargement of the LIVER. In most healthy adults, the liver lies in the upper abdominal cavity, the majority of it protected by the right side of the rib cage. The widest part of the liver occupies the right side of the upper abdomen. The triangle-shaped organ then extends across the abdomen, with the smallest corner lying just to the left of the midline of the body, above the stomach. Under normal circumstances, the liver cannot be felt beyond the lower edge of the ribs. With hepatomegaly, the liver may be felt more easily during a medical examination, as its larger size extends the lower border of the organ beyond its normal position in relation to the ribs.

As an organ that is required for sustaining life, the liver has many functions. It filters all of the blood circulating in the body, removing toxins and wastes. It helps the body get the energy to do its work by breaking down substances and storing energy. It makes bile, which is necessary for food digestion. The liver also plays a critical role in blood clotting. Hepatomegaly is not a disease in itself, but a symptom of another disorder that is negatively affecting the liver. Because of the critical role of the liver, new or worsening liver enlargement requires prompt medical evaluation.

Hepatomegaly can be caused by many conditions. It can be the direct result of a disorder of the liver, or an indirect result of another health problem that affects the liver. In fact, almost any liver problem can cause hepatomegaly. Common liver problems resulting in enlargement include hepatitis of any origin, CIRRHOSIS (scarring of the liver), liver cancer, benign tumors, cysts, an abscess (pus buildup caused by an infection), or an excess amount of fat in the liver (FATTY LIVER). Since a primary role of the liver is to filter blood, stress on the liver caused by toxins—such as chronic alcohol use, medication overdose, or poisoning—can lead to hepatomegaly. Blood disorders, such as sickle-cell anemia, hemochromatosis, or polycythemia, can also stress the liver and cause hepatomegaly.

Diseases elsewhere in the body can also cause liver enlargement. Diabetics—especially those on high doses of insulin or who have poor glycemic control—may have a higher risk of hepatomegaly. Cardiac problems such as congestive heart failure (CHF) and circulation problems may force blood to back up into the liver, causing enlargement of the organ. Likewise, a backup of bile—a fluid made by the liver to aid in digestion—can cause hepatomegaly. Bile may not flow properly if there is obstruction or cirrhosis of the bile ducts.

Many infections can cause hepatomegaly. Hepatitis is the most common, but other infections include Epstein-Barr virus (EBV), malaria, Reye's syndrome, and mononucleosis.

In diabetic patients, poor insulin compliance may lead to hepatomegaly and elevated LIVER ENZYMES. A swollen or enlarged liver is sometimes reported in adult and pediatric patients with type 1 diabetes.

A swollen spleen sometimes accompanies hepatomegaly. When both the liver and the spleen are enlarged, the resulting condition is called hepatosplenomegaly.

Symptoms and Diagnostic Path

The accompanying symptoms of hepatomegaly depend on the cause of the enlargement. Abdominal discomfort may or may not be present, and is often more pronounced with hepatomegaly caused by cancer or acute hepatitis. Dysfunction of the liver may cause symptoms such as jaundice (yellowing of the skin and eyes), vomiting, or a change in stool color.

A physician may initially diagnose hepatomegaly during a physical examination. Further tests are required to find the etiology and complications of the liver enlargement, such as a wide variety of blood tests, abdominal X-rays and scans, and an abdominal ultrasound. Treatment depends on the initial cause of the liver enlargement.

Yu, Y. Miles, and Campbell P. Howard. "Improper insulin compliance may lead to hepatomegaly and elevated hepatic enzymes in type 1 diabetic patients (Observations)." *Diabetes Care* 27, no. 2 (February 2004): 619.

hepatorenal syndrome (HRS) Hepatorenal syndrome (HRS) is acute kidney failure in patients with advanced LIVER DISEASE. HRS is the most serious complication of liver disease involving the kidneys, and may result in death if liver function is not improved, usually through LIVER TRANSPLANTATION. Kidney dialysis may be necessary as a temporary measure until the liver transplant can be performed.

There are two major filtering organs in the body: the liver and the kidneys. A damaged liver puts significant stress on the kidneys, and many kidney disorders are the result of underlying liver damage, especially CIRRHOSIS (irreversible scarring of the liver). In HRS, there is a drastic reduction in the flow of blood to the kidneys, but the reason for the flow reduction is not known. The structure of the kidneys remains unaffected, and they will often regain their normal functioning if the underlying liver disease is corrected.

HRS occurs in about 10 percent of patients hospitalized with liver failure, and in about 4 percent of patients with complications of cirrhosis, such as jaundice or ENCEPHALOPATHY (mental impairment and confusion). The incidence rate increases to 7 to 15 percent when the complications include ASCITES. All races and both genders are affected equally when chronic liver disease is involved. Age is generally not a factor, except that the scant amount of data available on children suggest that they may suffer a lower incidence of HRS, and that it may be less severe when it does occur.

Symptoms and Diagnostic Path

The main symptom of HRS is decreased urine production, which if untreated leads to uremia (retention of waste products in the bloodstream). Other symptoms may be present, especially symptoms of liver failure, and may include dark-colored urine, JAUNDICE, weight gain, abdominal swelling, nausea, vomiting, and changes in mental functioning.

HRS is diagnosed when other causes of kidney failure have been ruled out. A physical examination may reveal signs of liver failure in addition to the reduction in kidney function. There may be abnormal reflexes, indicating nervous system damage. Tapping on the abdomen (percussion) may yield a dull sound, and exploration by touch (palpation) may generate a visible fluid wave, both signs of ascites (fluid accumulation in the abdomen). Breast tissue may show an increase and the size of the testicles may show a decrease (gynecomastia).

Diagnostic tests may indicate both kidney failure and LIVER FAILURE as well. Signs of kidney failure may include those below:

- low urine output (fewer than 400 cc per day)
- low sodium concentration in the urine
- high specific gravity and osmolality (concentration of particles) of urine
- fluid retention in the abdomen (ascites) or extremities (edema)
- increased levels of both creatinine (a breakdown product from muscle tissue normally eliminated in urine) and blood urea nitrogen (BUN—a breakdown product of protein metabolism)

Liver failure may be indicated by the following:

- low levels of albumin (a type of protein) in the blood
- abnormal prothrombin time (PT—how long it takes blood to clot)
- high ammonia levels
- ascites

Treatment Options and Outlook

HRS itself may be treated in the same way as kidney failure from any other cause. All unnecessary drugs are stopped, especially diuretics and anti-inflammatory drugs such as ibuprofen. Dialysis may improve symptoms, and medications such as dopamine may be used to improve liver function temporarily. A Levine shunt (alternate pathway), placed between the peritoneum (abdominal cavity) and the jugular vein or the superior vena cava, the vein that drains the upper part of the body, may relieve some symptoms. Regardless of the treatment for kidney failure, however, additional treatment is required to improve liver function and to ensure that blood volume and heart function are adequate. A liver transplant may be necessary to restore normal kidney functioning.

The prognosis of HRS is poor. It depends partially on which of two types of HRS is involved, but the prognosis of neither is encouraging. Type I, usually a result of spontaneous bacterial peritonitis (SBP), carries a median survival expectancy of two to three weeks without treatment. Type II HRS proceeds more slowly, and occurs mainly in patients in whom liver function is relatively unimpaired. The median survival expectancy of patients with Type II HRS is three to six months.

hepatotoxin   See DRUG-INDUCED HEPATITIS; HELPFUL AND HARMFUL HERBS; HEPATITIS C AND DRUG USE; OCCUPATIONAL LIVER DISEASE.

hydatid cyst   Hydatid cyst, also known as hydatid disease or echinococcosis, is a parasitic infection caused by the larvae of a microscopic tapeworm. The term *hydatid* refers to the characteristic multicystic lesion—a large, roughly spherical, hollow cyst filled with fluid—that occurs after infection. There are four known species of tapeworms of the genus *Echinococcus*, three of which are medically important in humans: *Echinococcus granulosus, Echinococcus multilocularis,* and *Echinococcus vogeli.* Although human hydatid cysts are found worldwide, the disease is most closely associated with countries where dogs are used to herd sheep. There is no correlation between the rate of infection and race or sex.

The tapeworm life cycle usually alternates between herbivores, such as cattle and sheep, and carnivores, such as dogs, foxes, coyotes, and cats. The herbivore generally becomes infected by eating grass contaminated with tapeworm eggs. The eggs hatch in the small intestine, and larval tapeworms burrow through the intestinal wall and travel through the bloodstream to the LIVER or other organs. The cyst wall consists of an outer laminated layer that supports the cyst and a germ layer that forms brood capsules containing larval worms. The larval worm is called a protoscolex (protoscolices for multiple worms). The brood capsules may rupture, releasing protoscolices into the cyst fluid, or they may separate from the cyst wall and form free-floating daughter cysts that are identical in form to the parent cyst.

It takes about one to two years for cysts to produce infective protoscolices. Carnivores are infected by eating cyst-containing organs, either by direct predation or by scavenging a dead, cyst-bearing cadaver. The protoscolices attach to the intestinal walls of the host and form segmented worms, with both male and female reproductive organs in the last segment, called a proglottid. The worms are small; adult worms of the species *E. Granulosis* are only about three to six millimeters in length. Egg-laden proglottids detach from the ends of the worms and spill eggs into the host animal's intestine. The eggs then pass out in the host animal's feces.

A single cyst may contain from hundreds to tens of thousands of protoscolices, with a huge reproduction potential. Each protoscolex is capable of forming a new cyst if it moves to another location in the intermediate host or of growing into an adult worm when ingested by a dog or other definitive host. In addition, daughter cysts can move to new locations. Thus, if a hydatid cyst ruptures, the consequences for the intermediate host can be significant. Ruptures in humans can occur from trauma to the abdomen or from damage during surgery.

Human infection by the tapeworms usually happens accidentally, for instance, when a child transfers tapeworm eggs from feces to his or her mouth or when humans eat vegetables contaminated by egg-laden dog feces. The organs affected most often are the liver (63 percent of infections), lungs (25 percent), muscles (5 percent), bones (3 percent), kidneys (2 percent), brain (1 percent), and spleen (1 percent). In general, an infected human ends the life cycle of the tapeworms, and they are not normally passed on to a carnivore. However, human infection can cause serious symptoms and death in the human host.

E. granulosus causes cystic echinococcosis (CE), and this organism accounts for most human infections. *E. granulosus* is endemic and most common in the southern part of South America, Iceland, Australia, New Zealand, and southern parts of Africa. It is also endemic in the Mediterranean countries, the Middle East, and northern Alaska. Although it is not endemic in the United States and northern Europe, infected individuals are found as a result of changing immigration patterns and improved intercontinental transportation, and the incidence of the disease is rising in areas where it is not endemic.

In endemic areas, infection with *E. granulosus* ranges from one to 220 cases per 100,000 inhabitants. Two forms of *E. granulosus* are recognized, depending on the geographic location and the type of intermediate host. In the northern type, large deer serve as the intermediate hosts, and wolves, dogs, and coyotes serve as the definitive hosts. Transmission to humans occurs in areas where reindeer are domesticated. In the European type, which is more common, camels, pigs, sheep, cattle, goats, horses, and other animals may be intermediate hosts, and dogs, foxes, hyenas, and jackals can be the definitive hosts.

Most hydatid liver cysts caused by *E. granulosus* are located in the right lobe, and there usually are multiple cysts in an infected individual. Initially, the cysts can be as small as five millimeters in diameter, and there are no symptoms. However, the cysts can become quite large. Cysts as large as golf balls are fairly common, and cysts as large as basketballs have been observed.

Because the cysts grow slowly, symptoms may not develop until years later, depending on the size and location of the cysts. Hydatid cysts in organs other than the liver, such as the brain, are more serious. Cysts are rarely diagnosed during childhood or adolescence unless they occur in the brain. CE is most commonly diagnosed in adults between 30 and 40 years of age.

E. multilocularis causes the infection alveolar echinococcosis. Although rare, it is the most virulent form of *Echinococcus* infection. The adult stage of *E. multilocularis* occurs mainly in foxes and rarely in wolves, coyotes, lynxes, cats, and black bears. The intermediate hosts for *E multilocularis* are rodents. The parasites are usually diagnosed in adults, with an average age at diagnosis greater than 50 years. The mortality rate is 50 to 60 percent, reaching 100 percent in untreated or poorly treated infections. Sudden death has been reported in asymptomatic patients, based on autopsies. The incidence of the disease ranges from 0.03 to 1.2 cases per 100,000 people. The cysts are usually solitary masses, and they can involve large portions of the liver, causing narrowing of intrahepatic (within the liver) BILE DUCTS, the hepatic vein, and the portal vein.

Echinococcus vogeli is the rarest type of echinococcol infection and occurs mainly in the southern parts of South America, with normal transmission between the bush dog and the paca, a South American rodent.

Symptoms of hydatid cysts may arise when the cysts cause pressure on adjacent structures and organs, resulting in dysfunction of the organs. Hydatid liver cysts may cause biliary obstruction, as well as cirrhosis (advanced scarring of the liver), alone or together. The cysts may become infected or rupture, resulting in anaphylaxis or sepsis. Cysts can also rupture and spill their contents into the bile ducts, causing obstructive JAUNDICE. Trauma may cause a rupture into the free peritoneal space.

Symptoms and Diagnostic Path
Patients with hydatid liver cysts are often asymptomatic for years, and the first symptoms generally appear during adulthood, even if the patient was infected as a child. A few small cysts may go unnoticed, but a single large cyst may be fatal. Hydatid disease is far more serious when the cysts are found in organs other than the liver, particularly the brain.

The symptoms of hydatid liver cysts depend on the location, size, and parasite load of the cyst or cysts. Hydatid cysts can become quite large and cause pressure on the surrounding liver tissue and bile ducts. Most symptomatic cysts are larger than five centimeters in diameter.

Often, the first observed symptoms are the result of pressure from the cyst on surrounding tissues. Initial symptoms may include an enlarged liver, a dull ache over the right upper quadrant of the abdomen, and weight loss. Pressure effects may include nonspecific pain, cough, low-grade fever, and the sensation of abdominal fullness. As the cyst grows, the symptoms become more specific because the cyst compresses or obstructs specific organs. Large cysts can compress the main bile ducts and the vessels, causing abdominal pain, obstructive jaundice, atrophy of the liver lobe in which they are located, or portal hypertension. The symptoms of hydatid cysts can also mimic liver cancer or cirrhosis.

In alveolar echinococcosis (AE), when the cysts are caused by *E. multilocularis,* the symptoms can closely mimic those of cirrhosis or carcinoma (cancer). Symptoms of progressive liver dysfunction can ultimately lead to liver failure over a period lasting from weeks to years.

Secondary complications may occur if the cyst leaks or becomes infected. Minor leaks lead to increased pain and a mild allergic reaction characterized by flushing and hives. Major rupture leads to a full-blown anaphylactic reaction, which is fatal if not treated promptly.

The hydatid cyst may rupture spontaneously or from a traumatic impact to the abdomen, and ruptures are usually fatal. If a cyst ruptures into the bile ducts, the classic symptoms are biliary colic, jaundice, and hives, resembling symptoms of choledocholithiasis (the presence of gallstones within biliary tract) and cholangitis (inflammation of the bile duct). Daughter cysts may grow in the bile ducts and obstruct them, causing cholangitis.

Cysts can also rupture into the free peritoneal space. The protoscolices (larval worms) can then migrate to other organs, such as the lung, brain, or bone. After a cyst ruptures, the cyst membranes may be eliminated from the body through vomiting or in the stools.

Hydatid cysts can become infected either by primary infection or via a leak into the biliary tree.

The symptoms of an infected cyst range from mild fever to full-blown sepsis.

Often, the signs and symptoms of hydatid liver cysts are nonspecific, and the disease may be difficult to diagnose. However, proper diagnosis of hydatid liver cysts is important. In regions where the echinococcus worms are not endemic, a hospital's or a doctor's lack of experience can have catastrophic effects, particularly if a procedure is performed that results in spillage of cyst contents.

A physical examination of a patient with echinococcosis generally does not reveal specific findings characteristic of worm infestation of the liver. Rather, the physician will discover the effects of the cyst or cysts on the anatomy or the function of the affected organ or organs. There is the possibility that the patient will suffer from an acute allergic reaction if the cyst contents are leaking. Possible signs of hydatid cysts include these:

- jaundice (yellowing of the skin and eyes), which could be a sign of biliary obstruction

- spider angiomas (spidery web of veins), indicating portal hpertension secondary to either biliary cirrhosis or obstruction of the inferior vena cava

- itching

- fever, indicating a secondary infection or an allergic reaction

- hypotension (low blood pressure) accompanying an anaphylactic allergic reaction to the contents of a leaking cyst

- abdominal tenderness, which may be a sign of a secondary infection of the cyst, especially if accompanied by fever and chills

- enlarged liver or a palpable mass

- ascites (abdominal swelling), which is rare

- an enlarged spleen (splenomegaly), which may be the result of a cyst or cysts in the spleen or of portal hypertension

Because a physical examination of a patient with hydatid liver cysts may not reveal any specific indicators, a diagnosis depends, at least in part, on clinical suspicion. The suspicion may be based on the patient's history of living in or visiting an area where the disease-causing worms are endemic or where there is exposure to the parasite by ingesting foods or water that might be contaminated by feces of a definitive host animal.

Routine laboratory blood tests do not yield results specific for hydatid liver cysts. However, an elevated bilirubin or ALKALINE PHOSPHATASE level may be observed with an infected cyst. About 25 percent of infected people have elevated blood levels of eosinophils, a type of white blood cell, and about 30 percent have low levels of gamma globulin (immunoglobulin, type of antibodies).

Several specific diagnostic blood tests have been evaluated for their effectiveness in detecting echinococcosis. The indirect hemagglutination test and the enzyme-linked immunosorbent assay (ELISA) are the initial screening tests of choice, and they have a sensitivity of about 90 percent in hepatic echinococcosis. Other tests that are sensitive to antibodies to antigen 5 may be used to confirm a diagnosis. The Casoni test is an intradermal skin test that was used previously, but it has a sensitivity of only about 70 percent and can cause severe local allergic reactions.

Various radiologic tests are used in diagnosis, as well as to determine the presence of complications and plan treatment. Hydatid cysts can be identified by the presence of daughter cysts within a thick-walled main cavity.

- Standard X-ray films may reveal a thin rim of calcification that indicates the presence of an echinococcal cyst from an infestation with *E. granulosus* or *E. multilocucaris.*

- Ultrasound scans are an important diagnostic tool for hydatid cysts, but the accuracy depends on the skill of the operator. Debris and daughter cysts may be observed inside the cyst. Ultrasound evaluations may also be helpful for recognizing the presence of complications and for planning treatment.

- CT scans have an accuracy of about 98 percent and are sensitive enough to detect daughter cysts. In addition, CT scans can differentiate hydatid cysts from amebic and pyogenic (pus

producing) cysts in the liver. In infestations of *E. multilocularis,* CT scan findings are sometimes indistinguishable from those of hepatocellular carcinoma. CT scans may also reveal complications arising from hydatid cysts, and they may be helpful for planning treatment.

- MRI images reveal the cysts but do not provide advantages over the images available with a CT scan.

The CT or MRI scans are used to determine the number, size, and location of cysts. Such radiological imaging can also detect daughter cysts in the bile ducts.

A procedure called endoscopic retrograde cholangiopancreatography (ERC) may help diagnose a hydatid cyst that has ruptured into the liver.

Treatment Options and Outlook

The modern treatment of hydatid cyst of the liver includes a variety of approaches and types of procedures, including medical therapy, drainage of cysts through the skin (percutaneous), puncture, aspiration, injection, and reaspiration (PAIR) technique, and surgery. Both laparoscopic and open surgical techniques have been used successfully. In general, the treatment goals for a patient with symptomatic hydatid liver disease include elimination of the cyst or cysts and the prevention of a recurrence. Because hydatid liver disease is relatively uncommon outside endemic geographic areas, the treatment providers should be experienced in handling hydatid liver disease for the best chances of obtaining appropriate treatment. Thus, the medical staff should be experienced, and treatment should be obtained in a medical center with well-equipped wards for patient care, operating rooms, radiology facilities, and laboratory facilities. It should also be noted that cystic echinococcosis (CE) is managed differently from alveolar echinococcosis (AE).

Drug therapy may be effective in treating hydatid liver disease, particularly in younger adults. The primary drugs are antihelminthic (antiworm) benzimidazoles, albendazole, and mebendazole, used along with praziquantel, an isoquinoline derivative. The drugs may be used either as a primary treatment or to prevent recurrence after other forms of treatment. Drug treatment may be the only option in some cases, such as in patients with inoperable liver cysts and in patients with cysts in one or more additional organs. Drug therapy may not be recommended for patients in early pregnancy or who have bone marrow suppression, chronic liver disease, large cysts with the risk of rupture, or inactive or calcified cysts. An infectious disease specialist may be consulted for administration of drug therapy for hydatid cysts.

Albendazole (Albenza) decreases production of the energy-storing chemical adenosine triphospate (ATP) in the worms. The worms are immobilized and eventually die. The standard treatment regimen is oral administration twice a day for 28 days, followed by a 14-day period without the drug, and this cycle is repeated for three to six months. Recent studies in China indicate that continuous administration may also be effective.

Mebendazole (Vermox) causes worm death by blocking the uptake of nutrients from the patient's intestine. It is usually administered daily for three to six months. Mebendazole may disturb liver function, and patients should be monitored with periodic liver-function tests.

Praziquantel (Biltricide) is a trematodicide that increases the permeability of cell membranes in susceptible worms. As a result, there is a loss of intracellular calcium, accompanied by massive contractions and paralysis. Praziquantel also causes the worm's skin to disintegrate. It is administered with albendazole and mebendazole to enhance their effectiveness.

Patients taking albendazole, mebendazole, or praziquantel, alone or in combination, should be monitored regularly with CBC and liver enzyme tests to check whether the drugs are producing toxic effects. Imaging studies may be used to follow the morphologic status of the cyst or cysts.

In some cases, hydatid liver cysts can be drained and treated percutaneously (via a catheter inserted through the skin). After the cyst contents are drained, saline solution or alcohol may be injected into the cyst. One variation of percutaneous treatment is the puncture, aspiration, injection, and reaspiration (PAIR) technique, particularly for cysts caused by infestations of *E. granulosus* with relatively simple structures. In the PAIR technique, either ultrasound or CT images are used to insert a special cannula into the cyst and drain the contents. Next, an agent that kills the protoscolices is injected and allowed to remain in place for at least 15 minutes. The fluid is again drained from the cyst, and the procedure is repeated until the drained fluid is clear. Then saline solution is injected into the cyst. PAIR treatments are followed by treatment with benzimidazole drugs, such as albendazole and mebendazole, for one to three months.

A variety of scolicidal agents have been used to sterilize cyst cavities, including formalin, hydrogen peroxide, hypertonic saline, chlorhexidine, absolute alcohol, and cetrimide. Each of these agents has caused complications.

The PAIR technique is significantly less expensive than surgery and generally requires a shorter hospital stay. However, there is a risk of the cyst contents spilling outside the cyst, possibly accompanied by anaphylactic reactions, sclerosing cholangitis (inflammation of bile ducts), and development of passages between the cyst and the exterior of the liver.

Surgery to remove the germ membrane of the cyst is the traditional and generally recommended treatment for hydatid cysts, and it usually results in a complete cure of the patient. The rest of the cyst wall is usually left in place, because removal of the entire cyst wall or removal of a portion of the liver significantly increases risks to the patient. Surgery can be performed by the conventional or laparoscopic approach. The outcome depends on the surgeon's experience with both worm infestations and the surgical procedure used. Inexperienced surgeons have a higher rate of complications, including spillage of the cyst contents. The hospital where a patient is treated should be well equipped with the proper equipment and laboratory facilities, diagnostic and interventional radiology, pharmacy, and medical specialists. If these requirements are not met, the patient should ask to be transferred to another facility that meets them.

If possible, an antihelminthic drug, such as albendazole, is administered to the patient for several weeks before surgery to kill the protoscolices in the cyst or cysts. During surgery, special care should be taken not to spill the hydatid fluid. The tissue around the cyst is cut so that the hydatid cyst protrudes. Then the cyst is usually held with a sponge holder and the inner membrane is carefully removed, with the daughter cysts inside. The residual pericystic cavity can be partially excised, filled with saline, and closed with sutures. If there is any evidence of daughter cysts in the common bile duct, the bile duct is cleared and drained. It is essential to empty completely the primary cyst and remove all daughter cysts.

Other types of surgery may be used for CE patients with large liver cysts with multiple daughter cysts, superficially located single liver cysts that may rupture (traumatically or spontaneously), liver cysts with biliary tree communication or pressure effects on vital organs or structures, and infected cysts. Possible procedures include totally removing the cyst, removing a part of the liver that contains the cyst or cysts, or inserting a drainage tube for infected or communicating cysts. Regardless of the procedure used, it is very important to prevent spillage of the cyst contents to prevent seeding and formation of new cysts. If the cyst is opened or removed, the goals are to remove the parasites, sterilize the cyst cavity, and protect the surrounding tissues. The more extensive the surgery, the lower the risk of relapses and the greater the risk of complications.

Surgery is not recommended for patients who are very old, very young, pregnant, or have severe preexisting medical conditions; for patients with multiple cysts in multiple organs; or for cysts that are inaccessible, dead, calcified, or small.

For patients with alveolar echinococcosis (AE, caused by infestation with *E. multicularis*), surgery is usually the preferred treatment if imaging studies show that the portion of the liver containing the cyst can be removed. The only chance for cure is radical surgery with complete removal of the cyst. However, surgery may not be a suitable approach if the cyst is inoperable, very large,

or extends outside the liver and involves other organs. In some cases, part of the liver may be removed to decrease the parasite load, which increases the effectiveness of drug treatments. In other cases, surgery may be performed to improve organ function. Removal of the liver and transplantation may be considered. However, transplantation is an option only if there is no sign of infestation in other parts of the body, because the immunosuppressant drugs taken by transplant recipients can result in formation of new cysts if the organism is present.

Regardless of the type of infestation, postoperative care is similar to that for other surgical procedures that involve either or both the liver and the biliary tree. If the cyst was infected or if any signs of postoperative infection occur, antibiotics will be prescribed. Further, the patient will be given benzimidazoles, such as albendazole and mebendazole, to make sure that there are no remaining live protoscolices present. If the patient was infested with *E. granulosus* (CE), benzamidazoles are usually taken for about one month. If the *E. granulosus* patient had an incompletely resected cyst, spillage occurred during surgery, or metastatic lesions are present, or the patient had a complete resection for *E. multicularis* (AE), benzamidazoles are prescribed for a longer period, ranging from three months to two years postoperatively. An AE patient who had a partial resection or a liver transplant, or whose cyst was not operable will probably take benzimidazoles for three to 10 years.

Patients are usually monitored with follow-up ultrasound or CT scans. Also, patients on benzimidazoles are usually monitored with periodic CBC and liver enzyme tests to monitor for drug toxicity. In addition, they usually have periodic ELISA or indirect hemaglutination tests to screen for recurrence or aggravation of the disease.

Hydatid cyst patients may experience complications from either the parasite infestation directly or from treatments. Parasites may move to other locations and cause metastatic cysts. Even after treatment, an infestation may recur, either because the treatment did not remove or kill all the protoscolices present, or because the individual became reinfected by ingesting more eggs. Cysts can become infected, and their contents can spill if there is communication into the bile ducts or if the cyst ruptures. Spilled material can migrate to new locations and form new cysts. Also, the patient may experience an allergic reaction to the spilled cyst contents. Such reactions can be severe, including anaphylactic shock—a serious, often life-threatening allergic reaction. Five to 10 percent of hydatid cysts rupture spontaneously into the biliary tree, causing obstructive jaundice and cholangitis, inflammation of the bile duct. Infrequently, a rupture can cause acute pancreatitis, inflammation of the pancreas.

The antihelminthic drugs used to treat echinococcosis infestations may be toxic to the liver and other organs. Symptoms of toxicity include chemical sclerosing cholangitis, anemia, low platelet levels in the blood, and hair loss. The drugs are toxic to embryos and may cause birth defects.

Percutaneous drainage and PAIR treatments may have complications including hemorrhage, mechanical damage to other tissue, and infection. If the contents of the cyst spill, there may be an allergic reaction or anaphylactic shock, as well as persistence of daughter cysts that were not treated during the procedure. Sudden decompression of cysts can lead to biliary fistulas, or passages between the cyst and the biliary tree.

Complications of surgery include all the usual complications related to the surgical procedure and anesthesia, such as wound infection and chest infection. The residual cavity may become infected. Also biliary obstruction or biliary fistulas may occur. Biliary obstruction and biliary fistulas are treated by inserting a supporting tube into the bile duct.

The prognosis for patients infested with CE (*E. granulosus*) is generally good with complete surgical excision and no spillage of the cyst contents. Spillage occurs in 2 to 25 percent of cases, depending on the location of the cyst and the surgeon's expertise. A small percentage—0.5 to 4 percent—of patients die from surgery.

AE patients, infested with *E. multilocularis*, have a worse prognosis. Early detection and complete surgical removal of the cyst can cure patients.

When complete removal is not possible, long-term drug therapy has a 10-year survival rate between 10 and 90 percent.

Risk Factors and Preventive Measures

Human infection with *Echinococcus* results from ingesting food or water contaminated by the feces of an infected definitive host or by poor hygiene in areas where the *Echinococcus* worms are endemic. Thus, infestation can be prevented with the following steps:

- teaching the population at risk about proper hygiene and about the disease—its hosts, how it is transmitted, and how it can be prevented
- properly cleaning uncooked food and avoiding consumption of raw foods when possible
- ending the practice of feeding pet dogs the viscera of intermediate hosts, such as sheep
- controlling pet dogs to prevent them from eating material from sheep
- avoiding uncontrolled dogs
- periodically treating pet dogs for intestinal echinococcosis with praziquantel
- controlling the dog population
- regulating livestock butchering

Current Research

The December 15, 2003, issue of the *Journal of Infectious Diseases* reported on recent efforts to develop immunodiagnostic assays suitable for rapid, large-scale testing of people in areas where echinococciosis is endemic. Such tests could detect infections at an early stage, where they may be more treatable.

Dandan, Imad S., M.D., Assaad Soweid, M.D., and Firass Abiad, M.D. "Hydatid cysts." Emedicine.com. Available online. URL: http://www.emedicine.com/med/topic1046.htm. Downloaded on November 4, 2004.

Kacheriwala, S. M., K. D. Mehta, B. Pillai, and Y. Jain. "A rare presentation of primary hydatid cyst." *Indian Journal of Surgery* 66 (2004): 47–49.

Kumar, M. J., K. Toe, and R. D. Banerjee. "Hydatid cyst of liver (case report)." *Postgraduate Medical Journal* 79, no. 928 (February 2003): 113.

Li, Jun, Wen-Bao Zhang, Marianna Wilson, Akira Ito, and Donald P. McManus. "A novel recombinant antigen for immunodiagnosis of human cystic echinococcosis." *Journal of Infectious Diseases* 188, no. 12 (December 15, 2003): 1951.

Wagholikar, Gajana D., Sadiq S. Sikora, Ashok Kumar, Rajan Saxena, and Vinay K. Kapoor. "Internal drainage of liver hydatid-concerns and solutions." *Indian Journal of Surgery* 65, no. 5 (September–October 2003): pNA.

Wong, L. S., O. Braghirolli-Neto, Min Xu, J. A. C. Buckels, and D. F. Mirza. "Hydatid liver disease as a cause of recurrent pancreatitis." *Journal of the Royal College of Surgeons of Edinburgh* 44 (December 1999): 407–409.

immune globulin (IG)   Immune globulin (IG) is a sterilized solution that contains immunoglobulins, or antibodies, from pooled human blood plasma. (Plasma is the fluid in which blood cells are suspended.) The antibodies are substances that fight infections, and treatment with IG allows a patient to benefit from the antibodies formed by others against certain disease-causing agents. The protection is temporary and passive, unlike an immunization, where the patient's own body forms antibodies. Immune globulin formulations are produced from donors with high levels of antibodies against specific diseases, such as HEPATITIS A, HEPATITIS B, rabies, tetanus, and varicella (chicken pox). Immune globulins may also be called gamma globulins or immune serum globulins.

Unlike vaccines, which are usually administered to healthy people before any known exposure to diseases, IG is generally administered to people who have been exposed to certain infectious diseases or who are likely to be exposed. The IG products are highly effective, but they do not provide 100 percent protection. Thus, recipients of IG may be advised to take certain precautions to prevent the possible spread of the disease for which they are receiving treatment, such as avoiding donating blood for several months after the IG treatment.

IG preparations are carefully tested for evidence of viruses, such as hepatitis B, HEPATITIS C, and human immunodeficiency virus (HIV, which causes AIDS), that can be transmitted via blood. These preparations are sterilized, and there is no evidence that diseases such as AIDS have been transmitted via IG preparations. In the United States, IG is considered to be a safe and effective preventive measure against disease.

Immune globulin should not be administered to those who have had serious allergic reactions to thimerosol or other immune globulins, to people with blood-clotting disorders that would make an injection unsafe, or to people with IGA (immunoglobulin A) deficiency.

IG may interfere with the body's ability to develop good protection from vaccination for measles, mumps, rubella, or varicella. Thus, these vaccinations should not be administered for three months after an IG injection. Also, if IG is given within two weeks after an immunization, the immunization should be repeated after about three months.

IG is usually administered as an intramuscular injection. Side effects include localized pain, tenderness, itching, and swelling, which usually last less than one day. The protection lasts for several months. IG may be administered intravenously in patients with poorly functioning immune systems.

Immune Globulin for Hepatitis A

Immune globulin (IG) for preventing infection by hepatitis A is sold in the United States under the names Gamastan and Gammar. The protection is more than 85 percent effective in preventing hepatitis A if the injection is given within two weeks of exposure to the virus. The sooner the treatment is administered after exposure to the virus, the more likely it is to provide immunity. The immunity lasts for three to five months, and retreatment may be necessary if the threat of exposure still exists. IG is a safe and effective way to prevent infection with hepatitis A, even for women who are pregnant or breast feeding.

IG is administered by intramuscular injection to the following groups of people:

- household and sexual contacts of people who have been diagnosed with hepatitis A

- staff and residents of child care centers, hospitals, group residences, prisons, and food service settings where there is an outbreak of hepatitis A

- travelers visiting countries where sanitary conditions are questionable and hepatitis A is a known problem. Travelers who expect to stay in countries where hepatitis A is common might want to consider receiving hepatitis A vaccine, which provides longer-lasting benefits.

- people who need protection against infection with hepatitis A and are allergic to the vaccine

- children younger than two years who need to be protected against hepatitis A infection

Common side effects from IG injections for hepatitis A include soreness and swelling at the injection site and low-grade fever. Rarely, life-threatening allergic reactions can occur, and these are more likely if the IG is accidentally injected into an artery or vein.

In the United States, there are no reported cases of transmission of human immunodeficiency virus (HIV) or hepatitis B virus through IG. IG prepared in other countries may not be as safe.

Hepatitis B Immune Globulin

Hepatitis B immune globulin (HBIG, Nabi-HB) is prepared from the concentrated blood of donors who have a high level of hepatitis B antibodies. It is used to prevent infection by hepatitis B after exposure to the virus. The protection is short term, lasting three to six months. It is administered by an injection into the muscles of the arm, thigh, or buttocks.

HBIG is generally administered to the following groups of people:

- sexual partners of people diagnosed with hepatitis B

- people who may be exposed to hepatitis B through contact with blood, blood products, or human bites, including health care workers, employees in medical facilities, patients and staff

of live-in and day-care facilities, morticians and embalmers, police and fire department personnel, and military personnel

- household members of patients with acute hepatitis B

- babies less than 12 months of age whose caregiver tests positive for hepatitis B

- babies born to mothers who test positive for hepatitis B

- patients who have had liver transplants

HBIG should not be given to people who have a known hypersensitivity or allergy to HBIG or other gamma globulin products. Other medical problems, particularly bleeding, may affect the use of HBIG, because the intramuscular injection may cause additional bleeding. The effects of HBIG on fetuses and infants are not known.

Common side effects include pain and inflammation at the injection site, backaches, general discomfort, headaches, muscle aches or pain, and nausea. Less common side effects include abdominal or stomach cramping, burning, heat or redness at the injection site, chills, diarrhea, joint pain, lightheadedness, skin rash, and unusual fatigue or weakness. Although less frequent, severe hypersensitivity reactions may occur.

Other medicines and vaccines may interact with HBIG. Patients should inform their doctor if they have recently taken any vaccines made from a live virus, because HBIG may reduce the effectiveness of the vaccination.

Anderson, Kenneth R. *Mosby's Medical, Nursing, & Allied Health Dictionary*. 5th ed. St. Louis, Mo.: 1998.

immune status See IMMUNE SYSTEM; SUPERINFECTION AND COINFECTION.

immune system Over 200 years ago, Edward Jenner, a country doctor, observed that milkmaids generally did not become ill with smallpox. He took fluid from sores on cattle infected with cowpox, also called vaccinia, and injected the fluid into humans. The injected humans did not become sick with smallpox. Although Jenner probably did not fully understand why his method worked, he had discovered immunization, a way to work with the body's immune system to increase resistance to disease.

Since Jenner's discovery, the immune system has become much better understood. It works to fight many types of diseases, both infectious diseases and cancers. If it is not functioning properly, invading infectious cells can multiply, and one can become sick more easily. Also, cancer may develop.

Autoimmune diseases result when the immune system's ability to distinguish cells that are normally present from invading cells fails, and the immune system attacks the body's own cells. There are many autoimmune diseases, some causing minor annoyance and others being life-threatening. It is believed that autoimmune hepatitis (AIH), primary biliary cirrhosis (PBC), and primary sclerosing cholangitis (PSC) are autoimmune diseases in which the liver and associated tissues are attacked. Other autoimmune diseases include asthma, thyroid dysfunction, Sjögren's syndrome, lupus erythematosis, rheumatoid arrhtitis, and vitiligo. People who develop one autoimmune disease often are more likely to develop others.

The immune system uses two lines of defense to protect the body from foreign invaders, such as bacteria, viruses, and cancer cells, that are not normally present. First, the skin, mucous membranes, and lining of the respiratory tract provide a physical barrier to entry into the body. The barrier works in the same way for all invaders, and its response to an invasion does not depend on the type of invader. The second line of defense takes over when the first one fails and responds in a specific way to each type of invader. This part of the immune system recognizes invaders at a cellular level and then develops specific ways to fight them. Several organs play roles in the immune system: spleen, lymph nodes, tonsils, bone marrow, and white blood cells.

Immune system cells include lymphocytes (white blood cells), found in the blood and other parts of the body, in addition to other immune cells. There are several types of lymphocytes, each with a different function. Types of lymphocytes include B cells, T cells, natural killer cells, and monocytes.

Two kinds of protein are produced by immune system cells: antibodies and cytokines. Antibodies bind with ANTIGENS, with a specific antibody matching a specific antigen, similar to pieces of jigsaw puzzle or a key fitting into a lock. Cytokines communicate with other cells. Lymphokines, INTERFERONS, interleukins, and colony-stimulating factors are all types of cytokines.

- B lymphocytes, or B cells, mature into plasma cells that secrete antibodies called immunoglobulins, which are proteins that recognize and attach to foreign substances known as antigens. Each type of B cell makes one specific antibody, which recognizes one specific antigen.

- T lymphocytes, or T cells, attack infected, foreign, or cancerous cells directly. They produce proteins called lymphokines, which help regulate the immune response by signaling other immune system cells. One type of T lymphocyte, a cytotoxic (anticancer) T cell, releases a cytotoxic cytokine that can attack cancer cells directly.

- Natural killer cells (NK cells) attack any foreign invader, without first recognizing a specific antigen. They produce chemical substances that bind to and kill any foreign cells.

- Monocytes surround and digest microscopic organisms and particles, a process called phagocytosis. Monocytes can travel into tissue and become macrophages, or "big eaters."

Current research in immunology is focused on better understanding how immune system cells exchange messages and finding ways to make the messages more effective. Researchers are taking advantage of the characteristic of the immune system to develop BIOLOGICAL THERAPIES to treat cancer.

immunosuppressants Although an immune response protects people against viruses and bacteria of all kinds, there are situations in which the body mounts a response targeted at proteins or tissues that are not pathogenic (disease-causing.)

Immunosuppressants are powerful drugs that suppress the body's immune response. They are often prescribed to control inflammation, which may accompany some LIVER DISEASES, and they are a mainstay of treatment after organ transplantation.

When a person receives a donor organ to replace his or her failing LIVER, the presence of foreign tissue triggers a natural and automatic response in which the body's IMMUNE SYSTEM attacks the new organ and attempts to reject it from the body. This is what doctors mean when they talk about organ rejection. The rejection reaction can damage or even totally destroy the new liver. To stop the activity of the immune system and prevent damage to the new organ, transplant patients are given drugs from the group known as immunosuppressants. However, organ rejection can occur even with the drugs and was, in fact, the major cause of transplant failure up until 1983, when powerful new immunosuppressants became available. These new medications have improved the odds tremendously for the survival of the graft and therefore for the patient.

Many immunosuppressant drugs are available, and treatments almost always include a combination of drugs. Immediately after transplantation, medications are given in large doses to prevent acute rejection. Most incidences of rejection occur right after the surgery and during the first year afterward. But these doses are quite high for long-term use. Therefore, some of the drugs may be discontinued and/or the doses may be adjusted for long-term maintenance. Different medications are often used for maintenance than the ones prescribed immediately after the transplantation or given to treat rejection episodes.

Immunosuppressant drugs have many possible side effects, some of which can be serious. These effects can sometimes be controlled by changing doses or medications. Normally, the treatment regimen takes into account the patient's past medical history, level of side effects currently experienced, and type of transplant. But unless it is absolutely necessary to switch medications, it is not advisable, as doing so will result in added cost from an increased number of office visits because the transplant team must monitor the patient's progress and side effects.

Corticosteroids (steroids), such as prednisone, are synthetic hormones. They fight against inflammation and also stop the body's normal reaction to foreign tissue and infection. When organ transplants first became possible, patients were required to take corticosteroids for the rest of their lives. Now that other medications are available, the trend is to discontinue the corticosteroids as soon as possible because numerous and often debilitating side effects are associated with their long-term use. By discontinuing corticosteroids as soon as possible, the potential side effects are minimized. How soon patients can stop taking them after the transplant surgery is determined on a case by case basis at each transplant center. Factors that influence the decision include the underlying liver disease that led to the transplant. Patients with HEPATITIS B and C fare much better if the steroids are withdrawn earlier because they stimulate the replication of both hepatitis B and C viruses. On the other hand, patients who needed a transplant because they suffered from AUTOIMMUNE HEPATITIS (AIH) may be advised against discontinuing too early because of the possibility that AIH may recur in the new liver. In fact, immunosuppressants are sometimes given as treatment to patients with AIH.

Most centers stop requiring the patient to take corticosteroids anywhere from three months to one year after transplantation. This early discontinuation does not appear to affect adversely the survival rate of either the graft or the patient, and the occurrence of medication-induced side effects is significantly less. For instance, the incidence of high blood pressure, one of the side effects, is almost half in patients taken off the medication earlier, compared with those who continue the steroid therapy. Also, the chance of developing diabetes appears to be negligible if the medication is stopped about three months after the transplant.

The antirejection drug tacrolimus is often used with corticosteroids. Sometimes, a third immunsuppressive agent is used. It often was azathiprine, but today, mofetil has mostly replaced it. Mofetil may also be used as an alternative to cyclosporine or tacrolimus if the side effects to these drugs seem unbearable.

Cyclosporine (Sandimmune), one of the drugs introduced in the 1980s, targets anti–T-lymphocyte activity more specifically than does the earlier generation of immunosuppressive drugs. With the use of cyclosporine, there is less need to inhibit other host defenses, and there may be less suppression of bone marrow production. When bone marrow production is suppressed, there is a decrease in red and white blood cell levels.

Immunosuppressants	Some possible side effects
tacrolimus (prograf)	abdominal cramping diarrhea fatigue flushing hair loss itching insomnia high glucose (blood sugar) level some possibility of diabetes increased incidence of infections nausea night sweats rash seizures tremors
cyclosporine (sandimmune; Neoral)	heart disease high blood pressure (hypertension) increased facial and body hair increased risk of cancer kidney failure seizures tingling in hands and/or feet numbness
corticosteroids (predinose; Solu-medrol)	acne bruising diabetes eye problems (cataracts and glaucoma) facial or body hairiness facial puffiness high blood pressure fatty liver impaired wound healing
azathioprine (imuran)	hair loss mouth sores stomach upset
mycophenolate mofetol (Cellept)	bleeding bone marrow suppression (decreased white and red cell levels) digestive disturbances leg pain risk of infection skin rash weakness

Other medications Transplant patients must take many other types of medications, including antibiotics, antifungal medications, anti-ulcer medications, and diuretics. Depending on the patient's condition, additional drugs may be needed to treat various side effects of the medications.

infected blood See HEPATITIS; HEPATITIS C; HEPATITIS C METHODS OF TRANSMISSION.

infection See HEPATITIS; HEPATITIS B; HEPATITIS C METHODS OF TRANSMISSION.

inherited liver disease See BILIARY ATRESIA; BUDD-CHIARI SYNDROME; LIVER DISEASE; TRYOSINEMIA; WILSON'S DISEASE.

interferon Interferon is a naturally occurring protein whose name derives from its ability to "interfere" with the replication of viruses. When a virus infects a cell, the cell releases interferon into the bloodstream or the intercellular fluid. The interferon causes healthy cells to produce an enzyme that attempts to counter the infection by preventing the virus from replicating.

Interferon was identified in 1957. Human interferon was first produced for research purposes by extracting it from the body, but the extraction technique was costly. By 1980, interferon had been replicated through genetic engineering, and a synthetic product became widely available. In 1991, the Food and Drug Administration (FDA) approved the use of a synthetic alpha interferon in the treatment of HEPATITIS C.

Types of Interferon

There are three different types of interferon. Initially, the different types were thought to be produced in different places in the body, and were called leukocyte, fibroblast, and immune interferon, after the presumed production sites. When the presumption was proved wrong, their designations were changed to alpha, beta, and gamma, respectively.

Alpha and beta interferons are known as Type 1, and gamma interferon is known as Type 2. Alpha interferon is effective against both HEPATITIS B and hepatitis C, beta interferon, less so. Chronic hepatitis does not respond to gamma interferon.

Although there is only one form of beta interferon and one form of gamma interferon, there are many forms of alpha interferon. The forms are related, but differ slightly in their structure. Those structural differences are the basis of the distinctions among the three synthetic products currently approved by the FDA. The FDA is expected to approve more synthetic interferon products in the future because current data suggest that all forms of alpha interferon are similarly effective against hepatitis; the forms appear to differ mainly in the prevalence of their side effects.

In addition to hepatitis B and hepatitis C, alpha interferon is used to treat other disorders, notably genital warts; hairy cell leukemia, a blood disorder; and Kaposi's sarcoma, a skin cancer that occurs mainly in the elderly and in people with acquired immunodeficiency sydrome (AIDS).

Effectiveness of Interferon
Treatment of Viral Hepatitis

Interferon works by binding to another type of protein called a membrane receptor. The act of binding starts a chemical event that eventually results in certain cellular activities being enhanced. In particular, lymphocytes become better at killing target cells, and infected cells are better able to prevent the virus from replicating.

The treatment can stop inflammation of the liver, and sometimes rids the patient of the virus. It cannot reverse liver damage that has already been done, but studies suggest that interferon treatments may improve survival rates and reduce the risk of developing LIVER CANCER in patients who have already developed hepatitis-related CIRRHOSIS.

A study in Japan involving 2,889 patients with hepatitis C, reported in *Gastroenterology* (volume 123 [2002]), suggests that interferon treatments prevent liver-related deaths. That conclusion is supported by the results of another Japanese study reviewed at a conference of the American Association for the Study of Liver Diseases (AASLD) in Dallas, Texas, in 2001. This study reported that

interferon treatments reduced the risk of death from all causes by 62 percent, and from liver-related causes by 59 percent. The same study reported that patients treated with interferon had lower rates of liver cancer, and a better overall survival rate.

The effectiveness of interferon treatments, however, is known to be affected by the genotype of the virus. The genotype of a virus is a classification based on its genetic makeup. The hepatitis C virus, for example, has six different genotypes. The prevalence of the different genotypes varies widely from country to country, and can even vary between regions within a country. The most prevalent genotype in America, for example, is Type 1. About 75 percent of American hepatitis C patients are infected with the Type 1 virus. The most common genotype in Japan, however, is the Type 2 virus.

While all six genotypes respond to interferon treatment, each one responds differently. Those differing responses complicate research into hepatitis C treatment. Study results in one country or region may not be strictly comparable to results from similar studies elsewhere. Studies that compare response rates between patients with similar genotypes have yet to be conducted.

Overall, only about 25 percent of patients respond favorably to interferon treatments. Among the patients who do respond favorably, almost all suffer relapse when the treatment is discontinued. Experts now believe that suppressing a chronic viral infection requires prolonged therapy, retreatment of relapses, and maintenance regimens.

Effectiveness also depends on a number of other factors. Early detection and aggressive treatment for a period of 12 to 18 months increase the chances of a favorable response, for example. And interferon treatment seems most effective on patients who:

- have low levels of virus RNA (ribonucleic acid) in the blood before treatment (lower than 2 million/milliliter)

- have a genotype 3 infection

- have no cirrhosis

In general, a patient who will respond favorably to interferon treatment does so within the first two months of treatment. Failure to respond within the first four months indicates that the current round of treatment should be stopped because the virus will never respond to it.

Who Can Take Interferon

Interferon treatments are recommended for the following kinds of patients:

- those who have had hepatitis B for more than six months and are e-antigen positive, or patients who have either acute or chronic hepatitis C
- those whose levels of the aminotransferase liver enzymes ALT and AST are greater than one and a half times normal
- those who have had no more than two alcoholic beverages per week for the preceding six months.

A number of factors might influence the doctor's decision against interferon treatment. A woman who is pregnant or may become pregnant, for example, should not take interferon because little is known about its effect on the fetus. Similarly, nothing is known about its effect on sperm, and men should not try to conceive children while on interferon. A patient with advanced liver disease, such as severe cirrhosis, should not take it either, because it might worsen the disease. In addition, interferon is not recommended in the following situations:

- advanced age (over 60)
- heart, lung, or kidney disease
- organ transplantation and antirejection medication
- a history of depression
- autoimmune disease such as diabetes or psoriasis
- an accumulation of fluid in the abdomen (ASCITES)
- bleeding from dilated veins in the esophagus (variceal bleeding)
- mental impairment and confusion (ENCEPHALOPATHY)

Treatment with Interferon

Before treatment begins, a blood test is taken to determine three important numbers:

- the white blood cell (WBC) count. White blood cells, which fight infection, are measured in thousands per cubic millimeter of blood (K/mm³). A normal WBC count ranges from 3.4 to 9.6 K/mm³.
- the hematocrit value. This is the percentage of red blood cells in relation to total blood volume. A normal hematocrit ranges from 31.8 to 42.3 percent.
- the platelet count. Platelets help blood to form clots. A normal platelet count is in the range 162 to 380 K/mm³.

Treatment will not begin unless those counts are acceptably high. Interferon treatments affect the bone marrow, which is where blood is manufactured, and reduce the counts. If the counts are already low, the patient runs the risk of infection, bleeding, and anemia. The doctor should monitor those counts closely during treatment, especially during the first few weeks.

Interferon is administered by injection. It is usually given subcutaneously (beneath the skin), but the injection can be intramuscular (into a muscle). Interferon is ineffective when taken orally, so there is no pill form of the medication. Patients may be injected by a doctor or a nurse, or may be taught to inject themselves using the same type of needle diabetics use to self-inject insulin.

The recommended dosage differs for Hepatitis B (HVB) and Hepatitis C (HVC). For patients with HVB, the usual dosage is 5 million units of interferon per day, or 10 million units three times a week, for 16 weeks. For patients with HVC, the standard dosage is 3 million units three times a week for a minimum of six months.

Side Effects

Interferon treatments may have significant side effects. Even though interferon is a naturally occurring protein, the elevated levels associated with treatment can have profound effects on the body.

It is important to remember, however, that the side effects of any drug are highly variable from one individual to the next. Some people may feel very ill while undergoing treatment, while others may feel no effect at all. A few patients even feel better while undergoing treatment. Patients who do feel side effects may not feel them all the time. Only about 2 to 5 percent of patients feel side effects so severe that they abandon their treatment.

For most people taking interferon, side effects are worst during the first few weeks of treatment. Consequently, it is best to try to stick with the treatment for a month or two, to give the body time to adjust. Side effects of interferon are also often related to dosage: when side effects cannot be managed effectively, reducing the dosage may sometimes give some relief.

In general, patients with advanced liver disease or advanced scarring like cirrhosis are at the highest risk for significant side effects from interferon treatment. Those patients may feel fewer effects if they start out with a relatively low dosage.

The side effects of interferon treatments include the following:

- flu-like symptoms. This is the most commonly reported side effect, and may involve mild fever, headache, chills, muscle pain, and aching joints. The symptoms are usually worse at the beginning of treatment, and mitigate after a few injections. Staying well hydrated can often lessen the severity of such symptoms. Many patients can lessen the symptoms by taking acetaminophen—two regular-strength Tylenol tablets or their equivalent suffices just before the injection. Some patients find injecting themselves about an hour before bedtime and taking acetaminophen to be an effective strategy.

- fatigue. Symptoms of fatigue and malaise may develop after a few days of treatment, and may be accompanied by changes in cognition, or mental functioning. There is no treatment for such symptoms, but they are usually mild. About 10 to 15 percent of patients find the chronic effects so intolerable that they discontinue treatment.

- psychiatric symptoms. Interferon treatments may cause depression, or may worsen underlying depression. Treatments may also cause irritability, lack of initiative, apathy, confusion, impaired concentration, and other neuropsychiatric symp-

toms. They are not usually severe, and their frequency may be reduced by administering the interferon shortly before bedtime. Severe depression is a possibility, especially in patients with a history of depression.

- gastrointestinal symptoms. Weight loss may develop as a result of gastrointestinal side effects such as loss of appetite, changes in the sensation of taste, nausea, abdominal discomfort, diarrhea, and other effects. Such side effects are relatively common, having been reported by as many as 40 percent of patients.

- diabetes and thyroid disorders. Patients with diabetes mellitus or thyroid disorders may experience aggravation of their condition by interferon treatments. Diabetes sufferers should be especially careful about monitoring their blood sugar levels during treatment, and thyroid patients should get regular blood tests for thyroid function.

Additional side effects that have been reported include elevated triglyceride levels, rashes or itching, decreased libido, painful menstruation, and mild hair loss.

In some cases, interferon can also induce thyroid abnormalities. Usually people who are prone to autoimmune disorders are at the most risk. The treatments can induce either hypothyroidism—a slow-acting thyroid—or hyperthyroidism, a fast-acting thyroid. Many of the symptoms of those disorders are similar to side effects of the treatment itself, so it is important that patients undergoing interferon treatment discuss observed side effects with their physicians.

Interferon and Children
Interferon is not licensed for use in children under the age of 18. Some controlled trials have been conducted to examine interferon use in children. Most experts recommend against treating children under 10 not only because of side effects, but also because hepatitis is generally mild in children. Unless treatment is urgently needed, parents should consider waiting until the child is older. And newer treatments may become available in the years to come.

Interferon treatment for children with hepatitis B Hepatitis B (HBV) infection is less common in children than in adults, but several studies have suggested that the possibility of chronic infection is inversely proportional to age at the time of infection. Chronic hepatitis B infection is one of the major causes of cirrhosis in children, and it may also lead to HEPATOCELLULAR CARCINOMA (primary liver cancer) later in life.

The treatment goal for chronic HBV infection is generally to inhibit viral replication before irreversible liver damage and/or cancer develops. The hepatitis B e antigen (HBeAg) is associated with hepatitis B infection, and an individual who tests positive for hepatitis B e antigen is potentially infectious. The presence of the B e antigen is considered to be an indicator of viral replication, and eliminating HBeAg appears to stop the progression of liver damage. However, even if the B e antigen is absent, the patient may still be a carrier of HBV.

There is another antigen called the hepatitis B surface antigen (HBsAg). This is distinct from the B e antigen. The body produces antibodies to hepatitis B surface antigen as part of the normal immune response to infection. It is the presence of antibodies to the B surface ANTIGEN that are detected when a person tests positive for a hepatitis B blood test. Eliminating this B surface antigen appears to decrease the probability of developing hepatocellular carcinoma and increase the survival rate in adults.

Interferon (IFN) alpha has been approved for treatment of chronic HBV infection since the 1980s, and it is effective in treating chronic HBV in adults. Clinical evidence for its effectiveness includes clearance of the hepatitis B virus (HBV DNA) and the B antigen, as well as improvement in blood levels of alanine aminotransferase (ALT), a liver enzyme. IFN-alpha also seems to be an effective treatment for children with chronic hepatitis. Interferons are substances produced naturally within the body that help fight infections and tumors. Synthetic and recombinant interferons are also available.

Study results Several research studies have been conducted to determine whether IFN-alpha is a successful and well-tolerated treatment for children with HBV. In general, IFN-alpha treatments resulted in a loss of HBV DNA and the B e antigen in some, but not all, patients, with the results extending a year or more past the end of the treatments. Additional beneficial results were found in some children who lost B surface antigen and had improved levels of ALT. There is some evidence that higher doses of IFN-alpha bring better results.

Several factors seem to correlate with better responses to IFN-alpha treatments. The preferred candidates seem to be children who are more than two years old, have low to intermediate levels of HBV DNA and B e antigen, and have abnormal ALT values. There is some evidence that female children respond more favorably to treatment than males and also that younger children with lower levels of HBV DNA respond better. There is no evidence of correlation with ethnic origin. Although treatment can accelerate the clearance of the hepatitis B e antigen in some patients, it does not necessarily help to clear the B surface antigen.

One study noted that after five years, there was no difference between treated and untreated children in the proportion who sustained a clearance of the B e antigen. Thus, it appears that IFN-alpha may accelerate clearance but does not affect the longer-term results. IFN-alpha did improve the rate of B surface antigen loss in children with more extensive disease activity who responded early to treatments.

Another study investigated treatment with a large dose of IFN-alpha together with levamisole, an antiviral drug, for children with chronic hepatitis B. Some of the patients had severe side effects, and the results were no better than treatment with IFN-alpha alone.

Treatment with IFN-alpha is not usually advised for children with decompensated liver disease (advanced liver disease, such as abdominal fluid accumulation), cytopenia (reduction in the number of cells circulating in the blood), severe renal (kidney) or cardiac disorders, or autoimmune disease. Also, if the patient does not respond to the first course of treatment, re-treatment usually is not indicated.

Interferon treatment for children with hepatitis C Fewer children than adults are infected with hepatitis C (HCV), and infected children are less likely than adults to have symptoms from HCV infection. Prior to the institution of blood screening for HCV in 1992, some children became infected through blood and blood products. New infections in children still occur via perinatal transmission from the mother—the virus is passed on during childbirth. If chronically infected children do have symptoms, they are generally nonspecific, such as fatigue and/or abdominal pain. Children with HCV infection generally have normal or mildly abnormal liver enzyme levels.

Children with chronic hepatitis C virus infection are at risk for fibrosis (scarring) and cirrhosis (advanced scarring), similar to the risk faced by infected adults. HCV can progress to hepatocellular carcinoma (primary liver cancer) in adults, and probably also in infected children.

Interferon alpha has been used effectively to treat adults with chronic hepatitis C. However, sustained response six months after the end of treatment, with persistent viral clearance and normalization of the aminotransferase liver enzymes, is observed in only 15 to 20 percent of patients. There is little data for the use of IFN-alpha to treat HCV infection in children. In general, the response rates from different studies with different treatment protocols were between 0 and 56 percent.

Treatment with interferon alone Clinical studies of the effects of treatment of children with IFN-alpha have not been conducted on a large scale. In one study, 11 children received interferon (based on mega-units per square meter of body surface) three times per week for six months and followed for a total of 24 months, including the treatment period. At the end of the six-month treatment period, 36 percent had normal ALT levels, and at the end of 15 months, 90 percent had normal ALT levels. However, five of the children relapsed by the end of the two-year study. All the children had biopsies after treatment showing significant decreases in histological activity—after an examination of tissue under the microscope. The children who did not have HCV antibodies had different patterns of ALT levels than the children who did have HCV antibodies. Another study reported virological responses—how therapy affects the amount of virus circulating in the bloodstream—in only 8 percent of children tested. A study of IFN-alpha treatments for children with underlying malignant disease reported a range of 0 to 38 percent in complete sustained remissions.

The response rate of adults treated for hepatitis C with a combination of IFN-alpha and ribavirin is significantly better than in adults treated with just IFN-alpha. Ribavirin is an oral nucleoside analog, a class of drugs with a synthetic molecule that resembles a naturally occurring compound that shows activity against several RNA viruses and also can lower aminotransferase (a class of liver enzymes) activity levels in adults with chronic HCV infection.

Several studies have been conducted where children were treated with a combination of IFN-alpha and ribavirin. One study of 12 patients with chronic hepatitis C showed promising results, with half the children maintaining sustained virologic and biochemical remission after 12 months—the virus was cleared and signs and symptoms of the disease disappeared. The researchers concluded that the combination therapy was an effective and safe option for children and adolescents with chronic HCV after malignancy.

IFN-alpha, administered either by itself or in combination with antiviral drugs such as ribavirin, has been shown to be effective in treating children with chronic hepatitis C. But the rate of sustained response is low, and it may be better when a combination of drugs is administered. These results have not been confirmed by large-scale clinical trials.

The success of the treatment appears to depend on several factors:

- genotype of HCV; one study suggested better success in treating genotype 1b, and another indicated a better response rate for genotypes two and three

- absence of fibrosis on LIVER BIOPSY

- lower pretreatment HCV RNA titers

- underlying hematooncologic disease (cancer related to the blood)

- relatively short disease evolution

- mode of transmission

If, within the first two months of treatment, the transaminase levels return to normal and HCV RNA becomes undetectable, the response is considered to be good and continuation of treatment is recommended.

Treatment is not recommended for children younger than two years of age, because up to 12 percent of children infected perinatally (during childbirth) may spontaneously clear the virus during this period.

Information about IFN-alpha As with other drugs, it is important to make sure that the doctor knows about other medical problems, including these:

- previous unusual or allergic reactions to IFN-alpha
- bleeding problems, which may become worse during treatment with IFN-alpha
- chickenpox (including recent exposure) or herpes zoster (shingles), which create a risk of severe disease affecting other parts of the body
- history of convulsions (seizures) or other problems that affect the central nervous system
- diabetes mellitus
- heart disease
- kidney disease
- lung disease
- problems with overactive immune system
- thyroid disease
- other medications the child is taking, both over-the-counter and prescription

If a child is taking this medication daily, the dose should be given at approximately the same time each day. If a dose is missed, check with the doctor for further instructions. The doctor may also want the patient to drink enough water.

The most frequent side effects observed from IFN-alpha include flu-like symptoms, fever, headaches, musculoskeletal pain, loss of appetite, fatigue, dry skin and/or itching, persistent cough, tingling or numbness, unusual or depressive thoughts or behaviors, swelling of the hands or feet, and unusual weight gain. In children interferon can also result in growth retardation; therefore, extreme precaution needs to be exercised. The child's doctor should be contacted if these symptoms are persistent or bothersome.

The doctor should be called immediately if any of the following reactions occur: severe sore throat; severe nausea, vomiting, or diarrhea; difficulty breathing; severe weakness or fatigue; unusual bleeding or bruising; black tarry stools; blood in urine or stools; pinpoint red spots on the skin; confusion; seizures; or rash.

In addition to the symptoms listed above, the drug can cause lower hemoglobin levels, lowered leukocyte and platelet counts, and neutropenia (reduction in the number of white blood cells). In general, these effects are mild to moderate and last for a relatively short time. The child's growth rate may decrease during treatment, but usually the growth rate returns to normal after the treatment has ended. IFN-alpha may cause a temporary loss of some hair. After treatment has ended, normal hair growth should return.

The risk of bleeding or infection can be reduced by taking simple precautions, such as avoiding contact with people who have infections; taking care when brushing, flossing, and picking teeth; washing hands prior to touching the eyes or the inside of the nose; using care with sharp objects to avoid cuts; and avoiding contact sports or other situations where bruising or injury could occur.

American Association for the Study of Liver Diseases. "Effect of interferon therapy on the risk of hepatocellular carcinoma and mortality in patients with chronic hepatitis C: A large retrospective cohort study of 3296 patients." Conference for the National AIDS Treatment Advocacy Project (NATAP). 2001. Dallas.

Bortolotti, F., P. Jara, C. Barbera, G. V. Gregorio, A. Vegnente, L. Zancan, L. Hierro, C. Crivellaro, G. M. Vergani, R. Iorio, M. Pace, P. Con, and A. Gatta. "Long term effect of alpha interferon in children with chronic hepatitis B." *Gut* 46, no. 5 (May 2000): 715–718.

Dusheiko, Geoffrey. "Side effects of interferon alpha in viral hepatitis." NIH Consensus Development Conference on Management of Hepatitis C. 1997. Bethesda, Md. Available online. URL: http://www.hepnet.com/nih/dusheiko.html. Downloaded in January 2003.

Ertem, D., Y. Acar, Karaa E. Kotilo, E. Karaa, and E. Pehlivano. "High-dose interferon results in high HBsAg seroclearance in children with chronic hepatitis B infection." *Turkish Journal of Pediatrics* 45 (2003): 123–128.

Lackner, Herwig, M.D., Andrea Moser, M.D., Johann Deutsch, M.D., Harald H. Kessler, M.D., Martin Benesch, M.D., Reinhold Kerbl, M.D., Wolfgang Schwinger, M.D., Hans-Jurgen Dornbusch, M.D., Karl-Heinz Preisegger, M.D., and Christian Urban, M.D. "Interferon-a and ribavirin in treating children and young adults with chronic hepatitis C after malignancy." *Pediatrics* 6, no. 4 (2000). Available online. URL: http://www.pediatrics.org/cgi/content/full/106/4/e53. Downloaded on August 15, 2004.

Liberek A., and others. "Tolerance of interferon-alpha therapy in children with chronic hepatitis B." *Journal of Paediatrics and Child Health* 40, no. 5–6 (May 2004): 265–269.

Pensati, P., R. Iorio, S. Botta, et al. "Low virological response to interferon in children with chronic hepatitis C." *Journal of Hepatology* 31 (1999): 604–611.

Ruiz-Moreno, M., M. J. Rua, I. Castillo, M.D., García-Novo, M. Santos, S. Navas, and V. Carreño. "Treatment of children with chronic hepatitis C with recombinant interferon-alpha: a." *Journal of Paediatrics and Child Health* 40, no. 5–6 (May 2004): 265.

Shiratori, Y., et al. "Interferon therapy after tumor ablation improves prognosis in patients with hepatocellular carcinoma associated with hepatitis C virus." *Annals of Internal Medicine* (February 18, 2003): 299–306.

Tilg, H. "New insights into the mechanisms of interferon alfa: An immunoregulatory and anti-inflammatory cytokine." *Gastroenterology* 112 (1997): 1,017–1,021.

Yoshida, H. Y., M. Sata Arakawa, et al. "Interferon therapy prolongs life expectancy among chronic hepatitis C patients: National surveillance program in Japan." *Gastroenterology* 122 (2002): A T1375.

interferon treatment   See INTERFERON.

intrahepatic cholestasis of pregnancy   Intrahepatic cholestasis of pregnancy (ICP) refers to a specific LIVER condition in which the normal flow of BILE is impaired in a woman's body; this results in severe itching and, in 10 to 20 percent of cases, JAUNDICE.

Bile is the greenish yellow fluid secreted by the liver. The bile is transported through the biliary tree (passages to convey the bile) to the intestine. In the intestine, bile is important for absorbing fat-soluble vitamins and disposing of fat-soluble waste products. Normally, most of the bile acids are reabsorbed and travel back to the liver. However, in cholestasis, bile flow from the liver is decreased, and bile constituents accumulate in the blood. In addition, fat-soluble vitamins, such as vitamin K, are not absorbed. If the reduced bile flow occurs during pregnancy, the risks increase for maternal postpartum hemorrhage and fetal intracranial hemorrhage. ICP is also known as obstetric cholestasis (OC), cholestasis of pregnancy, or *pruritus gravidarum*.

In general, about one to two pregnancies per 1,000 are affected by ICP, but its incidence varies from country to country, with a clear racial and genetic predisposition. The incidence is about 0.01 percent in the United States, but it is higher in Scandinavia and South America and highest among the Araucanian Indians of Chile. ICP is rare in black patients. Increased risk factors include a family history of ICP involving mothers or sisters and a pregnancy with twins or more multiples. If a woman develops ICP during a pregnancy, her risk of developing it in later pregnancies is much greater, with some estimates as high as 90 percent.

ICP usually begins during the third trimester, although it has been observed as early as a few weeks into a pregnancy. Often the only symptom is itching, which is annoying but does not cause long-term health problems for the mother. But the condition can be fatal to the baby if it is not treated adequately. The fetal risk may be due to the transfer of bile acids across the placenta from the mother to the baby. The baby may need to be delivered early, at about 36 to 38 weeks' gestation. Usually, the itching disappears within a week or two after the baby is born. Obstetric cholestasis may be associated with cholesterol gallstones.

Many obstetricians consider itching to be a normal symptom of pregnancy, and they may not recognize ICP. The condition may be extremely stressful for the mother, and it should be taken seriously because it carries significant risks for the baby. In addition to possible hemorrhaging in both the mother and the child, ICP may lead to premature births in up to 60 percent of cases, to fetal distress in up to 33 percent of cases, and to intrauterine death in up to 2 percent of patients. Usually, acute lack of oxygen causes the fetal death.

ICP refers to a condition in which the mother's serum levels of primary bile acids, especially cholic acid, are preferentially raised. In addition, bile acid levels are also raised in the fetal serum, amniotic fluid, and the first stools of the newborn (meconium).

The causes of ICP and its actual incidence are not yet known, and current research is investigating possible roles of genetic, hormonal, and environmental factors.

There is a family history of the condition in 33 to 55 percent of ICP patients. Recent research has found mutated genes in some women who have had ICP. Furthermore, ICP in the mother is often associated with children who suffer from several rare cholestatic syndromes, such as progressive familial intrahepatic cholestasis (PFIC) type three and recurrent familial intrahepatic cholestasis. PFIC appears to be an autosomal recessive condition with abnormal bile production. In an autosomal condition, an abnormal gene is found in one of the "non-sex" chromosomes, i.e., in a chromosome that is not involved in sex determination. When the autosomal condition is recessive, the disease is not exhibited. The child must inherit the gene from both parents to have symptoms of the disease. The child is a carrier if he or she inherits the gene from only one parent.

The presence of certain estrogen and progesterone metabolites is associated with ICP. In other words, the end products of the metabolism of female sex hormones may play a role in ICP. One theory is that the liver cannot cope with the high female sex hormone levels that occur during pregnancy, particularly since the hormone levels and the ICP symptoms disappear soon after delivery. However, pregnant women with and without cholestasis have similar levels of circulating estrogen and progesterone, and it is believed that ICP results from either increased sensitivity to the normal hormone levels or to the action of a hormone metabolite.

There appear to be environmental factors in the development of ICP. The incidence of ICP is higher in winter than in summer, and some studies have linked the disease to low blood serum levels of selenium.

Symptoms and Diagnostic Path

The main symptom of ICP is itching, or pruritis, which classically begins during the second or third trimester of pregnancy and increases in severity until delivery or treatment. Usually, the itching begins with the palms and soles of the feet. It may spread to other parts of the body such as the face, back, and breasts, and it may become generalized. Often, it is worse at night and when blood flow increases, and in some cases, the itching becomes unbearable, interfering with sleep and making patients so uncomfortable that they scratch themselves until their skin bleeds. It may also interfere with daily activities and cause lack of appetite. It is believed that the itching is due to bile salts accumulating in the blood. Usually, the itching disappears completely within two weeks after delivery, but it may last longer.

Some itching during pregnancy is normal and is probably due to hormonal changes and the abdominal skin stretching as the baby grows. In contrast, ICP itching may be all over the body. If a woman believes she is itching more than normal, particularly if there is no accompanying rash, she should contact her doctor as soon as possible and request a serum bile acid test.

In addition to itching, other symptoms may be observed with obstetric cholestasis, varying in severity and type. The most common symptoms include the following:

- jaundice. A small percentage of ICP patients develop jaundice, with yellow appearance of the skin or eyes. If jaundice occurs, the patient should seek medical attention.

- dark urine and or pale, grayish stools. The increased levels of bile acids in the blood may alter the color of urine and/or stools. The dark urine may also result from dehydration.

- fatigue or exhaustion. Although fatigue is common during pregnancy, ICP may cause fatigue due to stress, loss of sleep, and some vitamins and minerals not being absorbed properly.

- premature labor. Although mothers with ICP are often encouraged to deliver early, this can be dangerous. The doctor may order a steroid injection to aid lung development in the baby.

- loss of appetite

- mild depression

Less common symptoms include pain in the upper-right quadrant of the abdomen, nausea, and severe depression

ICP usually is not associated with a rash, other than one caused by scratching. Moreover, ICP should not become worse after delivery, although it may take as long as a year for blood test results to return to pre-ICP levels. If the symptoms become worse after delivery, more testing should be done to rule out another liver disorder. Also, if the itching is accompanied by a rash, other possible causes should be investigated.

If a pregnant woman suffers from itching that is not just abdominal itching resulting from skin stretching, she should contact her doctor. Usually, the itching from ICP begins during the last 10 weeks of pregnancy, although it can start much earlier. It has been described as constant and sometimes intolerable. In such cases of itching that are not clearly from the stretching of the woman's abdominal skin, the doctor should consider ICP.

ICP is usually diagnosed on the basis of blood test results, particularly a bile acid test and liver-function tests. If the tests are negative, they should be repeated; sometimes the itching begins before the blood tests show abnormal results.

The most sensitive indicator of ICP is the serum bile acid (SBA) test. Elevated bile acid levels in the blood cause the intense itching of ICP, and usually the level of bile acids in the patient's blood increases before there are changes in liver-function tests. This test should be administered after a period of fasting, because some foods may increase bile production. The SBA test requires specialized equipment and is available only from a few laboratories worldwide. Thus, the results may not be available

immediately. Bile acid levels have been observed to triple in less than one week, so the doctor should consider the possibility of a delay in receiving the test results when planning treatment, particularly if the patient is 34 weeks or more into her pregnancy, has experienced itching for more than about two weeks, has a family history of ICP, or has previously experienced a stillbirth. Preferably, the bile acid tests are repeated at least weekly until delivery and also after delivery to rule out other liver problems.

Liver-function tests measure the blood levels of enzymes produced by the liver. A diagnosis of ICP should not be based solely on liver-function tests, however, because test results may be normal even when ICP is present. Indeed, the increased liver enzyme levels are the result of elevated serum bile acids. The tests are often repeated once or twice a week. The standard liver enzymes tested include the following:

- alanine aminotransferase (ALT). ALT is produced by liver cells. When liver cells are damaged, ALT leaks into the bloodstream, and ALT test levels increase. Although the ALT test is a sensitive indicator of liver cell damage, the ALT level may not correlate with the degree of cell damage.

- aspartate aminotransferase (AST). AST levels in the blood also increase when liver cells are damaged. However, the blood levels are affected by other conditions than liver disease. The ratio of ALT to AST is useful in evaluating abnormal liver enzymes.

- alkaline phosphatase (ALK). ALK levels are usually elevated in the blood during pregnancy, and they are usually not considered to be important in diagnosing ICP.

Routine liver-function tests show raised liver enzymes (ALT and AST) in 60 percent of ICP patients and a slight increase in bilirubin (another liver enzyme) serum concentrations in about 90 percent of ICP patients.

A diagnosis of ICP may be based on test results showing more than 12 to 14 micromoles (one millionth of a mole; a mole is a physical unit of quantity used for very large amounts of extremely small things, such as molecules) of bile acids per millimeter of blood. In addition, the ALT and AST levels may be two to four times as high as normal. A history of previous itching associated with the patient's menstrual cycle or use of oral contraceptives may help confirm a diagnosis of ICP.

Other tests may be ordered to help determine the appropriate treatment for ICP. PROTHROMBIN TIME, which measures the rate at which blood clots, should be checked at least weekly as the delivery date approaches and at delivery to detect malabsorption of vitamin K. A decreased ability for blood to clot can cause maternal hemorrhage as well as an intracranial hemorrhage in the infant, either before or after delivery.

An ultrasound test may be ordered to check for gallstones that could be blocking the bile ducts, with the itching resulting from the blockage of bile flow. This test uses high-frequency sound waves to image the baby and the mother's internal organs. Although gallstones are rare during pregnancy, women who develop ICP are at increased risk for developing gallstones.

Other tests may be ordered to examine fetal movements, fetal heart rate, and blood flow in the fetus and the mother.

Itching during pregnancy can have other causes than ICP, and it is important to consider them. ICP is a diagnosis of exclusion, and the condition is diagnosed by ruling out other causes of the itching and other symptoms. Other underlying liver diseases include viral infections, such as cytomegalovirus—a virus that is most frequently transmitted to a child before birth; Epstein Barr virus—a virus that can cause fatigue; and hepatitis—inflammation of the liver. Other causes include toxicity due to drug or alcohol use. Autoimmune liver disease may present with itching and similar blood test results. The presence of antismooth muscle antibodies indicates chronic active hepatitis, and the presence of antimitochondrial antibodies indicates primary biliary cirrhosis. Furthermore, allergies and a variety of skin conditions can cause itching.

If the itching does not disappear or becomes worse after delivery, an underlying liver disease other than ICP should be considered. Postpartum bile acid and liver-function tests are useful in determining when another disease is present.

In general, ICP in mothers and the drugs used to treat it do not have long-term effects on the babies they bear. But ICP patients are often deficient in vitamin K, and this deficiency increases the risk of premature labor, intracranial hemorrhage in the infant, and stillbirth.

In one study of 40 ICP patients, 32.5 percent were reported to have preterm labor. Other researchers have cited figures as high as 60 percent in ICP patients. Previous pregnancies with ICP and twin or triplet pregnancies appear to increase the risk of preterm labor.

The risk of stillbirth appears to increase after 36 weeks of pregnancy. One study reported intrapartal fetal distress in 22 to 33 percent of affected pregnancies and stillbirth in 1 to 2 percent. One possible cause of stillbirth may be that the elevated bile acid levels in ICP patients increases the incidence of meconium passage, which can result in sudden stillbirth. Also, meconium passage may be associated with constriction of blood vessels, which reduces umbilical blood flow. ICP patients often report meconium staining, a sign of poor prognosis for the fetus. If meconium staining occurs, the obstetrician should be contacted immediately. Another mechanism leading to stillbirth may be a decrease of heart muscle cell contraction caused by bile acid. However, medication and early delivery reduce the risk of stillbirth.

Treatment Options and Outlook

Treatment of ICP is oriented toward reducing abnormal bile acid levels and improving liver function. Elevated serum bile acids associated with ICP can be treated with ursodeoxycholic acid (URSO, ursodiol, UDCA, or Actigall). UDCA is a naturally occurring bile acid that improves liver function, reduces serum bile acid levels, and relieves itching. In addition to relieving the mother's symptoms, URSO also benefits the unborn baby by improving bile acid transport across the placenta, which reduces the risk of fetal distress and stillbirth. In one small study, fetal outcomes improved when the mothers took URSO.

URSO does not appear to have adverse effects on the mother or the fetus. It is classified by the U.S. Food and Drug Administration (FDA) in pregnancy category B, which means that it is not expected to harm an unborn baby. The most common side effect is occasional, mild diarrhea. Aluminum may interfere with the effects of URSO, and the patient should check with her doctor before taking antacids, such as Rolaids, Maalox, and Mylanta, while taking URSO. Also, the patient should make sure that her doctor is aware of her other medications.

In the past, cholesterol-lowering agents, such as cholestyramine (Questran or Cholestipol) were used to treat ICP. But it now appears that these drugs are less effective than URSO in lowering bile acid levels. Moreover, these drugs have potentially dangerous side effects, including inhibiting absorption of fat-soluble vitamins. One fat-soluble vitamin, vitamin K, is essential for blood clotting, and ICP patients are already at risk for vitamin K deficiency. This deficiency puts the mother and the baby at risk for hemorrhaging.

Bile plays an important role in absorbing vitamin K from food, and vitamin K is necessary for proper blood clotting. When a pregnant woman has ICP, both the mother and the baby are at increased risk of bleeding, both before and after delivery due to vitamin K deficiency. The bleeding may occur as hemorrhages, which can be life-threatening.

Thus, vitamin K therapy is often recommended for ICP patients. Oral, water-soluble vitamin K supplements are available for the mother. Breast milk does not contain much of this vitamin, so newborns are given vitamin K injections.

Soon after birth, the baby of a mother with ICP will be given a vitamin K injection to reduce the risk of bleeding.

If a woman is diagnosed with ICP, certain things may help to relieve the symptoms, particularly itching.

- diet. Although there is no medical evidence that indicates diet helps relieve itching, patients are advised to follow a well-balanced diet that includes lots of vegetables, fruit, and whole grain foods. It is possible to reduce stress on the liver by cutting back on dairy products and fried and fatty foods. Water helps flush toxins out of the body, so it is recommended to drink plenty of water.
- nutritional supplements. Milk thistle and dandelion root are believed to be safe to take during pregnancy, and they have been shown to provide benefits to the liver. SAMe (S-

adenosylmethionine) is a naturally occuring substance in the body involved in many biochemical reactions] has been shown to bring some benefits, but is not as effective as URSO. Black cohosh [(Actaea racemosn) herb used as a dietary supplement, often used to treat symptoms of menopause] is known to be beneficial to the liver, but it can contribute to premature labor, and it should be avoided before about 36 weeks' gestation.

- rest and stress reduction. Rest will not cure ICP, but relaxing and sleeping as much as possible may help, particularly when the itching raises stress levels and interferes with sleep.
- reduce skin irritation. It may be helpful to reduce skin irritation, such as by using moisturizers, using a humidifier to maintain adequate humidity, and wearing cool, loose cotton clothing. Lowering the ambient temperature reduces blood flow. Ice packs and cool baths may bring comfort. Mentholated skin lotions may be soothing. Treatments for "normal" itching, such as Aveeno baths and antihistamines, do not help with the itching of ICP. If the patient must scratch herself, a baby's hairbrush or other soft implement can reduce the chance of skin damage.

After a pregnant mother is diagnosed with ICP, she will probably have regular tests to monitor the baby's heartbeat (cardiotocography), as well as ultrasound scans and blood tests. The mother may be hospitalized to ensure adequate monitoring of the fetus. She may also have a series of prothrombin tests to monitor her blood-clotting ability.

Increased blood levels of bile acids are associated with a risk for premature labor. Because babies of mothers with ICP are usually delivered by 36 to 38 weeks to reduce the risk of stillbirth, there is a chance that the baby's lungs will not be fully developed at birth. Steroids, particularly oral dexamethasone, administered before 32 weeks' gestation help the fetal lungs to mature. The steroids may also reduce the mother's itching.

ICP patients should realize that proper treatment greatly reduces the risks of both fetal and maternal symptoms. Reducing the bile acids in the bloodstream and delivering the baby as soon as lung maturity will allow are both major aspects of treatment.

ICP does not seem to cause permanent liver damage, and the mother's symptoms and blood chemistry usually return to normal a week or two after giving birth. But the liver may be more sensitive to changes in hormone levels. Some women report itching during the menstrual cycle, either just prior to ovulation or just prior to menstruation. Usually this itching is mild. Oral contraceptive pills may cause a similar condition. Additionally, there is also a high probability that the mother will again develop ICP during a subsequent pregnancy. So far, there is no evidence that hormone replacement therapy for menopause causes ICP-like symptoms.

The mother may be asked to have a follow-up liver-panel test six to 12 weeks after delivery to confirm that the condition was obstetric cholestasis, rather than another liver disease. If the symptoms and blood chemistry do not return to normal, other reasons for poor liver function should be investigated.

ICP recurs in up to 90 percent of pregnancies in women who have previously had ICP. The itching may begin earlier and become more severe. If a woman has had OC, she should work with an obstetrician who is familiar with the condition during any subsequent pregnancies.

Brites, Dora. "Intrahepatic cholestasis of pregnancy: Changes in maternal-fetal bile acid balance and improvement by ursodeoxycholic acid." Concise Review. *Annals of Hepatology* 1, no. 1 (January–March 2002): 20–28.

"Focus on Intrahepatic Cholestasis of Pregnancy." *San Gabriel Valley Perinatal Newsletter* 1, no. 2. (April 1, 2003). Available online. URL: http://www.obfocus. com and http://www.perinatology.com. Downloaded on August 20, 2004.

Gendrot, C., Y. Bacq, M.-C. Brechot, J. Lansac, and C. Andres. "A second heterozygous MDR3 nonsense mutation associated with intrahepatic cholestasis of pregnancy. *Journal of Medical Genetics* 40 (2003): 32.

Lammert, Frank, Hanns-Ulrich Marschall, Anna Glantz, and Siegfried Matern. "Intrahepatic cholestasis of pregnancy: Molecular pathogenesis, diagnosis and management." *Journal of Hepatology* 33, no. 6 (2000): 1,012–1,021.

intravenous drug abuse   See HEPATITIS B; HEPATITIS C.

J–K

jaundice Jaundice is a condition in which the skin, the mucous membrane, and the whites of the eyes (sclerae) take on a yellowish cast. Jaundice is not a disease per se but is one of the symptoms of various diseases. The yellow pigment is caused by high levels of a substance called BILIRUBIN in the blood. Bilirubin is essentially a waste product that remains after old red blood cells are destroyed. When bilirubin builds up in the body, its yellow pigment becomes visible and results in jaundice.

Mild jaundice is best observed by examining the whites of the eyes in natural light. Jaundice usually becomes detectable when bilirubin levels in the blood reach 2 to 2.5 milligrams per deciliter.

Although jaundice can be a common symptom of LIVER DISEASE, other causes, such as malaria, may be responsible for the yellow pigmentation. Sometimes if an individual consumes too many carrots, the skin may take on a yellowish cast, due to the beta-carotene in carrots. But in this case, the whites of the eyes will not be affected, only the skin.

Conditions that cause jaundice include the following:

- overproduction of bilirubin. For example, in hemolytic anemia, in which red blood cells are destroyed at an abnormally rapid rate

- blockage of the BILE DUCTS, called CHOLESTASIS. A common cause of this is gallstones and cancer of the pancreas.

- inflammation of bile ducts, resulting in a disruption of bile flow and an accumulation of bilirubin. Diseases that may inflame the bile ducts include PRIMARY BILIARY CIRRHOSIS and PRIMARY SCLEROSING CHOLANGITIS.

- inflammation of the LIVER. Diseases that may inflame the liver include viral hepatitis, DRUG-INDUCED HEPATITIS, ALCOHOLIC LIVER DISEASE, and AUTOIMMUNE HEPATITIS. Alcohol and certain drugs, such as the painkiller Tylenol, may also cause inflammation.

- hereditary condition, including GILBERT'S SYNDROME, WILSON'S DISEASE, and ALPHA-1-ANTITRYPSIN DEFICIENCY

- NEONATAL JAUNDICE. Many neonates have some jaundice within the first few days or week after birth. This is generally normal, but it may be pathologic in certain cases.

- Less common disorder, including LIVER CANCER originating in other parts of the body.

Diagnosis is made through clinical and laboratory assessment, including imaging studies of the biliary tract using ultrasound, computed tomography (CT), and/or magnetic resonance imaging (MRI). The physician must determine whether the jaundice is caused by primary liver disease or by a systemic disorder that involves the liver.

Treatment of jaundice depends on its specific cause, with different underlying causes necessitating different treatments. For example, gallstones blocking the bile duct must be removed.

kernicterus See LIVER DISEASE.

199

lifestyle and chronic hepatitis C HEPATITIS C is often not diagnosed until decades after exposure to the virus because symptoms are either nonexistent or are so general that patients fail to realize that they are suffering from a chronic LIVER DISEASE. When they find out, they may be shocked and dismayed; there is usually a period of adjustment before they finally accept their condition. But even after they do so, patients may be more susceptible to periods of depression, especially if, as the disease progresses, they start to experience physical symptoms that may hamper them in their daily activities.

The good news is that many people with hepatitis C can live full, productive lives. With currently available antiviral therapy, about half of patients suffering from hepatitis C can enjoy an indefinite remission (see HEPATITIS C TREATMENT). Even those who cannot totally eliminate the virus from their bodies can experience some benefits from therapy. Because hepatitis C is one of the most researched areas in medicine, patients who are not helped by current therapy may soon be able to take advantage of new drugs or treatments.

By the time people become diagnosed with hepatitis C, most have had it for decades. The clinical course of patients with hepatitis C is difficult to predict. Some may never have serious liver problems, while others develop liver inflammation and FIBROSIS (scarring of liver tissue), and still others progress to serious liver disease including CIRRHOSIS (advanced, irreversible scarring), LIVER CANCER, and/or LIVER FAILURE.

Although doctors cannot accurately predict who will develop serious liver disease, they do know that taking good care of the liver and one's overall health plays an important role in how slowly or quickly hepatitis C progresses.

Catching the disease early, although not a guarantee, can mean a better chance of survival and leading a normal life. People with risk factors for hepatitis are advised to be screened for the disease even if they have no symptoms.

If the diagnosis is positive, consult a liver specialist for available treatment options. Unlike a general practitioner, a specialist in liver disease can give advice based on the most current research. In some people, the proper treatment can reduce the risk of liver damage and even reverse it.

The keys to managing any chronic liver disease, including chronic hepatitis C, are listed below:

1. obtaining proper medical care
2. making lifestyle changes
3. getting support from family, friends, and/or support group(s)

Obtaining proper medical care In interviews, hepatitis C patients often express doubt as to the medical competence of their physician. They sometimes mention that they were treated unkindly by their doctors; they felt they were not listened to, were misunderstood, or were somehow stigmatized by their illness, that they were negatively stereotyped as sexually promiscuous or drug addicts. The perception was that the doctor blamed them for their illness—in fact, a few patients were told point-blank that they were to blame because of their own lifestyle choice. Such complaints highlight the importance of seeking a specialist who is knowledgeable about hepatitis and does not harbor common misconceptions about the disease. Just as important, the doctor should be able to respond to patient's questions with empathy and sensitivity, not irritation, blame, or indifference. It is up to the doctor to explain hepatitis C in language that the layperson can understand, as well as teach the patients self-care skills so that they can better manage their illness. The patient has the right to obtain correct advice concerning treatment options, the expected clinical course of the illness, and whether he or she is a candidate for antiviral therapy.

When a patient is first diagnosed with hepatitis C, the doctor should address the following basic questions:

- Is the patient a good candidate for antiviral therapy?
- What new medications are on the horizon if not a candidate for therapy?
- What are the pros and cons of treatment?
- What is the likelihood of treatment success?
- What are the possible side effects of treatment?
- What is the patient's viral load?
- How often should the viral load be checked to monitor the disease?
- What is the genotype of the virus (a onetime test)?
- What are the results of LIVER-FUNCTION TESTS? How do the results compare with normal levels?
- How often should liver-function tests be performed?
- Is a LIVER BIOPSY necessary?
- How much scarring is there, and how might it affect treatment options if there is FIBROSIS or CIRRHOSIS?
- Is there immunity to hepatitis A and/or B?
- What is the advisability of VACCINES if not immune to hepatitis A and/or B?

Making Lifestyle Changes

It is important to care properly for the liver, as the health of the liver has a major bearing on the health of the entire body. Dietary changes are one of the first places to start. To begin with, avoid foods with saturated fats and hydrogenated oils. Eating fast foods is a good way to harm the liver. Foods such as french fries, potato chips, and doughnuts should be avoided. The following are important tips on caring for the liver:

- See a hepatologist (liver specialist) or a gastroenterologist (specialist in digestive disorders) at the scheduled time to monitor progress.

- Avoid excessive alcohol consumption. It is best to abstain from alcohol altogether. Although scientists do not yet fully understand the mechanisms of liver disease, one substance is a known toxin to the liver, and that is alcohol. Studies have shown that alcohol can lead to cirrhosis and liver cancer. People with hepatitis C who also drink have an especially accelerated course of the disease. It appears as if alcohol promotes the replication of the hepatitis C virus. Alcohol can also interfere with hepatitis antiviral medication. Even social drinkers who do not consume alcohol in excess may suffer because there is a wide variation in how alcohol affects individuals. In addition, people often believe that they are consuming less than they truly are.

- Stop smoking. Smoking's harmful effects on the lungs are well established, but most people are not aware that smoking can also be deleterious to the liver. For those already suffering from liver disease, smoking will likely make it even more difficult for the liver to repair itself. Some studies suggest that cigarette smoking may be a factor in promoting hepatitis C progression.

- Avoid toxins to the liver. Some people are exposed to toxins in their workplace that are potentially damaging to the liver. Individuals with liver disease should limit their exposure to these substances. Substances that can be toxic to the liver if exposed in high levels are auto exhaust, gasoline oil, pesticides, heavy metals, some chemicals in beauty parlors, air pollution, and certain prescription drugs, among others.

- Use aerosol sprays with caution because the liver filters everything that is breathed. When painting or cleaning with aerosol products, make sure the room is well ventilated or wear a mask. The same holds true for all other chemicals including bug sprays, paint sprays, and mildew sprays.

- Take care of what gets on the skin, as chemicals can pass through the skin and into the liver, destroying liver cells. Insecticides, for example, can be very harmful to the liver. When handling insecticides, or in an area that has been sprayed, cover the skin with gloves, long sleeves, a hat, and a mask.

- Use caution with medicines. Some medications, including prescriptions, over-the-counter medicines, and herbal remedies, can be toxic to the liver. And medications may interact in a harmful way. Therefore, always consult with a physician before taking any medicine. These include painkillers.

- Limit coffee consumption. Coffee may be sprayed with high levels of pesticides, and carcinogenic hydrocarbons may be produced during roasting.

- Avoid crash diets and/or binges. Learn to limit calories while eating a variety of healthy foods. Eat small, healthy meals. They are easier to digest.

- Eat a well-balanced diet with plenty of fresh fruits and vegetables, as well as whole grains, legumes, nuts, and seeds. To prevent bone loss, which can be a problem for people with hepatitis C, make sure there is plenty of calcium in the diet. Consider taking calcium supplementation as well. (Check with the physician first.)

- Exercise regularly. Appropriate EXERCISE is helpful for anyone; when recovering from a liver disease, check with the doctor to find out what exercises are beneficial. For people suffering from hepatitis C, weight-bearing exercise is particularly important because there seems to be a prevalence of bone loss in HCV.

- Avoid appetite suppressants and herbal medicines designed to lose weight, as they may damage the liver.

- Avoid taking vitamins, mineral supplements, or herbs without first checking with the health care provider. Special care must be taken with fat-soluble vitamins like vitamins A, D, and E. They are stored in the liver, and excesses of these vitamins can injure the organ. Avoid megavitamins unless taken under the guidance of a physician.

- Avoid any vitamins, supplements, and foods with added iron (including iron-fortified breads and cereals). People with hepatitis C sometimes also have iron storage disorders, in which they have excesses of iron in their bodies, and there is some evidence that too much iron can worsen hepatitis C.

- Avoid cooking with iron pots or other utensils that leach iron into the food.

- Restrict sodium, particularly if suffering from cirrhosis.

- Check with doctor to see how much protein to consume if one has cirrhosis. Too much or too little can be a problem.

- Drink plenty of water unless on a fluid-restriction diet. (Patients with cirrhosis may have to restrict their fluid intake.) Water should be plain—or with a twist of lemon for variety. Caffeinated drinks are dehydrating.

- Practice birth control diligently while on interferon and ribavirin combination therapy, as ribavirin can cause birth defects. This applies to both the patient and his or her partner. Consult with the physician before attempting to get pregnant.

- Avoid exposure to blood or blood products. Having hepatitis C does not make a person immune to being reinfected by hepatitis C or other viral hepatitis. Becoming infected with hepatitis C for the second time can mean that the viral load (the amount of viruses in the blood) will be higher, or there will be several different strains of the virus—both of which make the disease harder to treat. And being coinfected with another viral hepatitis or HIV (the virus that causes AIDS) may lead to accelerated disease progression.

- Get vaccinated against hepatitis A and hepatitis B if not already immune. The same recommendation applies to patients' family members.

Here are some suggestions for dealing with symptoms of hepatitis C, as well as the side effects of interferon:

Fatigue This is one of the common symptoms of hepatitis C, and a side effect of antiviral therapy. There is little that Western medicine can do to relieve fatigue, but alternative and complementary treatments such as herbal remedies may help alleviate it and increase energy. Exercise, taking naps, massages, and relaxation techniques such as deep breathing and meditation are also recommended. Those individuals who have never exercised should start slowly, doing only as much as they can handle. Regular physical activity helps with insomnia as well.

Nausea Sometimes nausea, if constant, may lead to weight loss. Identify the various triggers for nausea, such as smells, tastes, or eating greasy, fatty, spicy, or sugar-laden foods, and avoid them as much as possible. Ginger can be very helpful for combating nausea. Ginger can be taken in the form of capsules (purchased at the health food store), as tea, or cooked in foods.

Eating too much or going too long without eating can both cause nausea. Small, frequent meals are easier for the stomach to digest and keep the blood sugar under control.

Depression DEPRESSION is also one of the most common and debilitating side effects of interferon therapy. Treatment is available for depression and no one should hesitate to seek help. It helps to share the burdens of a chronic illness with family, friends, or a support group. Today, there is no reason for anyone—with or without physical illnesses—to suffer from prolonged depression.

Obtaining support Getting diagnosed with hepatitis C can be a frightening experience. Sharing the burden by discussing the diagnosis with family and close friends is a good approach to take. Since hepatitis C is a contagious disease, anyone likely to be at risk must be informed; however, this does not include casual acquaintances and coworkers in most cases. Hepatitis C is not spread by sneezing, coughing, casual hugging, or sharing eating utensils. As there is still some prejudice and misconceptions surrounding the illness, patients may wish to be selective in whom they confide. But whenever possible, it is important to obtain support from family.

Anticipating mood fluctuations and periods of depression will make it easier for the patient, as well as family members, to cope. GRIEVING is natural when one is first diagnosed with hepatitis C. Patients may experience mood swings that mirror fluctuations in the amount of hepatitis C

virus in their blood; there may be variations in viral load for unexplained reasons. Keeping a daily log of health conditions and changes in mood is an excellent device to monitor chronic illness. Instead of stuffing down emotions, it is better to express them in a healthy way, such as through journaling (writing down one's thoughts and feelings) or speaking to counselors or trusted friends and family members.

Maintaining a positive attitude can diminish the impact of stress. Learn through cognitive therapy how to change negative thinking, as well as unrealistic attitudes and expectations. Find an experienced counselor or therapist who uses cognitive therapy; or else find literature on the subject in libraries and bookstores.

Chronic illness is stressful for the entire family as well as the patient. Furthermore, family members are most likely to know little about hepatitis C and may not be as informed as they could. Patients are encouraged to have frank discussions with the people around them about the nature of the disease and the realities of living with it. Be aware that others may be fearful, or unwilling to offer support, and be prepared to educate them.

Being as informed as possible about hepatitis C makes it easier to obtain support from the right sources. Keep abreast of the latest developments in the treatment of hepatitis C; check out newsletters, magazines, books, and Web sites with information on the disease.

liver The liver is the largest organ in the human body. It plays a critical role in all aspects of metabolism, and consequently in overall health. It detoxifies poisons, manufactures proteins, and routinely performs more than 500 functions to regulate cell metabolism. It performs many other complex functions as well, so many, in fact, that it uses as much as 12 to 20 percent of the body's total energy.

Structure and Function

The liver is a wedge-shaped organ sheltered by the rib cage in the upper-right side of the body, below the lungs and above the kidneys. It weighs about four pounds in an adult male, making up about 2 to 3 percent of the total body weight. It is about the size of a football.

The liver is composed of two sections, or "lobes." The two lobes, referred to as the right lobe and the left lobe, are separated by a membrane called the falciform ligament. The right lobe is about six times as large as the left one.

The surface of a healthy liver is quite smooth, and its color is a rich reddish brown. It gets its color from the volume of blood it typically handles. About one-quarter of the blood in the body—more than a pint—passes through the liver every 60 seconds.

Blood enters the liver through two main "highways": the portal vein and the hepatic artery. Blood from the portal vein—about two-thirds of the liver's blood supply—is carried to the liver from the gut, and is rich in nutrients. Blood from the hepatic artery comes to the liver directly from the heart and lungs, and is rich in oxygen. The nutrient-rich blood from the portal vein and the oxygen-rich blood from the hepatic artery combine in the liver.

The portal vein is connected to the splenic vein, which drains the spleen. The spleen stores and sometimes manufactures blood cells. If there is an obstruction and the blood cannot flow properly, the blood backs up into the spleen.

The blood in the liver exits through the hepatic vein, enters the vena cava, the largest vein in the body, and returns to the right side of the heart.

The liver also has permeable capillaries called sinusoids.

The most numerous type of cell in the liver is a specialized cell called the hepatocyte. Hepatocytes perform the critical biochemical operations that largely define liver function. The action of the hepatocytes is tested the most often in the diagnosis of liver disease. Two main functions of the liver, for example, are the synthesis of a blood-clotting factor, necessary to clot the blood and stop bleeding, and the synthesis of ALBUMIN, the main protein in the blood and a key substance in regulating fluid balance in the blood vessels. Both those functions are performed by the hepatocytes, and the measurement of both products figures importantly in the diagnosis of liver disease.

The Liver and Toxins

The liver filters pollutants and toxic substances and converts them into waste that can be excreted through the urine or feces. It also processes drugs and medications and processes them into forms that the body can use.

Because of its filtering function, the liver is in the front line of assault by toxins. It is the first organ to receive drugs and toxins the body may have absorbed, and it plays a major role in metabolizing those drugs and purifying the blood. The liver is able to handle such toxins day in and day out because it is tough and resilient. It is one of the few organs that can regenerate damaged tissue. But it is not infallible.

The liver faces particularly dangerous assaults in a modern world in which pollution is increasing, drugs are proliferating, alcohol is widely available, and junk foods are the standard diet for many people. Liver disease may cause as many as 40,000 deaths each year in the United States. Even people who never suffer clinical manifestations of liver disease, such as JAUNDICE, fatty liver disease, or CIRRHOSIS, may well suffer from unhealthy liver conditions resulting from the continual assault by pollutants and stress.

Liver and Nutrition

The liver plays an important role in nutrition. It converts food into stored energy, and it secretes chemicals necessary for life and growth.

The liver stores carbohydrates as glycogen. The body taps into this stored glycogen as energy.

The liver continually secretes BILE, a greenish yellow fluid containing acids, salts, and other substances. The bile is carried by ducts from the liver to the GALLBLADDER, a tiny, saclike organ whose main function is to store and concentrate bile. Bile is released into the small intestine as needed, where it breaks down fat so it can be absorbed by the intestines. Bile is also essential in the absorption of fat-soluble vitamins such as vitamins A, D, E, and K. People with liver disease must sometimes follow low-fat diets because their diseased livers are unable to digest fat properly or completely.

The liver is the main regulator of protein metabolism. Proteins reach the liver in the form of amino acids. The liver converts certain amino acids into sugar, which is used by the muscles for energy.

Some proteins are converted into ammonia, a toxic by-product of metabolism. The liver converts that ammonia into urea, to be excreted in the urine by the kidneys. Too much ammonia can cause death. One of the complications of liver disease is HEPATIC ENCEPHALOPATHY, a state in which there is mental impairment and dysfunction, such as confusion, disorientation, impaired memory, and personality changes. This is believed to be primarily because of the buildup of ammonia in the body as the liver is no longer able to convert ammonia into urea.

The liver is also the main organ for breaking down hormones, such as estrogen, after they have served their purpose as messengers to certain cells. Among the hormones processed by the liver is insulin. If the insulin is not quickly broken down and removed from the system, it lowers the blood sugar. Lower blood sugar can result in hypoglycemia.

liver biopsy   A biopsy is a procedure in which a sample of a living tissue is taken from a patient for examination. Before the 1950s liver biopsies were rarely done, but the procedure has become quite commonplace since then. In a liver biopsy, a special needle removes a tiny piece of liver tissue. The tissue sample is then sent to a laboratory, where a pathologist examines it under a microscope to detect abnormalities that may be overlooked with other, less invasive tests. Biopsies are useful for diagnosing some LIVER DISEASES, such as CIRRHOSIS (advanced scarring of the liver), HEPATITIS (liver inflammation), and tumors.

Most liver diseases affect the entire organ, so a small tissue sample does not look much different from the rest of the liver. Consequently, sampling errors, where the selected tissue does not provide an accurate picture of the rest of the liver, are very rare.

Liver biopsy provides critical information that is not available with other, less invasive tests, such as computed tomography (CT) and magnetic resonance imaging (MRI). As the best method for establishing a definitive diagnosis, liver biopsy can also estimate the duration of the disease and determine the stage it has reached. It can also confirm or exclude the presence of coexisting liver disorders. For example, a biopsy can determine whether chronic hepatitis is due to alcohol, a viral infection, or a combination of both. Liver biopsy remains the gold standard in detecting liver disease.

A biopsy should be performed if cirrhosis is suspected, as it is the only way to confirm the condition, and it is also often required to confirm a diagnosis of LIVER CANCER. Doctors may also decide to perform a biopsy if blood tests show unexplained elevations of AMINOTRANSFERASE levels. In addition, it is the definitive test to confirm the diagnosis of specific diseases, including the following:

- HEMOCHROMATOSIS (iron overload)
- chronic viral hepatitis
- WILSON'S DISEASE (a rare hereditary disease)
- FATTY LIVER (liver with accumulations of fat)

Biopsies can also monitor the progress of treatments for diseases such as chronic hepatitis—the presence of viral infection for at least six months. They often help to make sure there are no other causes of liver disease and to provide information about the extent of inflammation. Another use for biopsies is to monitor the progress of liver inflammation, for instance, in patients with chronic hepatitis B. Although the optimal interval between biopsies is unknown, doctors typically wait five years before conducting another biopsy. However, some experts feel that three-year intervals may be more appropriate for patients with chronic hepatitis C, because the disease seems to accelerate in later stages.

Liver biopsies are not required in all cases of liver disease, and are more helpful in cases of chronic than acute liver disease. They should be avoided in patients for whom a biopsy would provide no additional insight into the treatment or prognosis, or if a biopsy would actually harm the patient, for instance, if the patient is not in a physical condition to tolerate an invasive procedure like a biopsy. Biopsies are also dangerous for people who have severe COAGULOPATHY (blood-clotting disorder). But if examining a liver sample is critical in the diagnosis or management of the liver disease, the doctor can use a method other than straight-needle technique to reduce the risk.

In certain situations, such as patients with HEP-ATITIS A, a biopsy is unnecessary because it will not change the recommended treatment protocol. For patients with drug-induced liver disease, the best tactic generally is to discontinue taking the medication and wait to see whether the problems resolve themselves. Should the problems persist, then a biopsy can be performed.

The doctor determines that a biopsy is needed after a thorough examination, including a physical checkup and blood tests, suggests that there may be abnormalities with the liver. As noted above, there should always be a medically sound reason for performing a biopsy. Although the procedure is quite safe, there are risks involved as with any invasive procedure.

Coagulation studies and platelet counts help make sure that the patient is not suffering from blood-clotting disorders or other types of illnesses that can make biopsy risky.

Procedure

One month before a biopsy, the patient will be asked to stop ingesting any alcohol. And 10 days before the procedure, the patient must stop taking any medications that may affect the test. These medications include blood thinners, aspirin, non-steroidal anti-inflammatory drugs (NSAIDs), ibuprofen, and others. (A small amount of Tylenol can be taken for pain relief.) In addition to prescription drugs, vitamins and supplements, particularly vitamin E and the herb gingko biloba, must also be avoided. Finally, at least eight hours before the biopsy, the patient must stop eating. But patients may drink water.

Although the procedure itself takes no more than 10 to 20 minutes from start to finish, the patient is usually asked to arrive at the clinic at least one hour before the procedure and to schedule a rest period of at least six hours afterward. An arrangement should be made with family or friend to accompany the patient home. The patient is requested to avoid physically strenuous activities for at least 48 hours afterward.

More than 90 percent of biopsies are performed with the percutaneous stick method. Percutaneous means through the skin. If desired, the patient may be sedated, either orally or by injection, but should remain conscious during the procedure. A local anesthesia is given to numb the area around the lower ribs on the right side of the body. The doctor percusses—or taps—the patient's abdomen around the liver to find a suitable spot for the biopsy. The place is then marked, and the skin in the area is cleaned with antiseptic solution. The doctor makes a small incision and then quickly inserts a special, thin needle into the liver. The needle goes in and out very quickly, usually in less than a second. The patient will be told to hold the breath and remain very still for five to 10 seconds while the needle goes into the liver, so the physician does not puncture or nick nearby organs, such as the lung or gallbladder. Some pressure and a dull pain may be felt.

The needle retrieves about 20 to 80 milligrams (mg) of wet liver tissue. In an adult, the liver normally weighs about 150,000 mg, and removal of this small sample has no effect on liver function. Because the liver is a large organ, an experienced doctor can usually find a suitable spot without difficulty. Many liver diseases affect the liver uniformly throughout, so most any part of the liver is a good sample. Sometimes the liver sample is too small for analysis, however, and the doctor has to reinsert the needle. This usually happens only when it is difficult to obtain a sample, for instance, if the patient is extremely obese or the liver has become rock hard from cirrhosis or has atrophied.

In some situations, a specific localized abnormality in the liver is targeted, and greater sampling precision is required, for example, if a sample has to be obtained from a liver tumor. To make sure that the liver sample is taken from an appropriate spot, imaging techniques such as CAT or MRI will be used for guidance. Other situations requiring more precise sampling include patients whose liver architecture is distorted by advanced cirrhosis and patients with a prior history of surgery in the right upper abdomen. Unless these special circumstances arise, imaging procedures are not needed for routine liver biopsies; they only add to the time and cost of the biopsy.

Transvenous liver biopsy Instead of a simple needle biopsy, the doctor may recommend transvenous biopsy for a patient who has severe abdominal swelling (ascites) and may be at increased risk for bleeding, or who has a PROTHROMBIN TIME (the time it takes for the blood to form a clot) that is prolonged by more than three seconds, or whose platelet count drops to less than 60,000. In transvenous biopsy, also called transjugular biopsy, a catheter (tubular medical device) is inserted into the jugular vein, in the neck, and directed to the hepatic vein, which drains the liver. A tiny biopsy needle is then inserted through the catheter and into the liver for the retrieval of a small biopsy specimen. These biopsies are usually performed by specialists called interventional radiologists.

Laparoscopic liver biopsy If a patient needs an abdominal surgery for reasons unrelated to the liver disorder, a biopsy may be done at the time. In such a case, a general anesthetic is given. The surgeon makes a small cut near the belly button and then inserts a thin, lighted tube, called a laparoscope, into the abdominal cavity. A biopsy needle is inserted through the lighted tube. The doctor guides the scope to view the liver directly. When liver cancer is suspected, or if the doctor finds any unusual growth on the liver, a tissue sample is taken from the suspicious growth and sent to the laboratory for analysis. Otherwise, the needle will retrieve some tissue from anywhere in the liver.

Risks and Complications

After the procedure, the patient's blood pressure, pulse, and breathing are monitored at the hospital. The patient is expected to lie on the right side or flat on the back for four to six hours in a hospital room to be observed for complications, including bleeding, which tend to occur during the first few hours after a biopsy.

There may be some pain in the side, or an aching sensation in the right shoulder, which is referred pain. Any discomfort should subside within an hour or two.

After going home, the patient is expected to lie still and avoid unnecessary physical exertion for a week. Aspirin-based products and ibuprofen should be avoided for a week or so, because they can increase the chance of bleeding. To relieve pain, the patient may take a small amount of acetaminophen (Tylenol).

Complications of biopsies are rare, occurring in fewer than 1 percent of cases, with excessive bleeding being the most common. Death from a biopsy is virtually unheard of.

In rare cases, a patient may have an allergic reaction to the drug used in the anesthesia. There is also a risk of infection at the site of the needle insertion. If a fever develops, or pain lingers for more than 24 hours after a biopsy procedure, or if there are any worsening of symptoms or changes in the patient's condition, such as unusual drainage from the biopsy area, the doctor should be contacted immediately.

Levin, Jules. "How often should you do a liver biopsy?" Conference reports for NATAP, American Association for the Study of Liver Diseases. November 9–13, 2001. Dallas. Available online. URL: http://www.natap.org/2001. Downloaded on November 3, 2003.

liver cancer (metastatic *liver cancer*) Malignant liver tumors are masses of abnormal cell growths that are cancerous and potentially fatal. They are what is commonly referred to as liver cancer.

The term *liver cancer* is a broad, nonspecific phrase that does not distinguish among the types of cancer in the liver. These distinctions change the types of treatment indicated and the outcome. Liver cancers can be broadly classified into two types, primary and metastatic, or secondary. Primary liver cancers originate in the liver itself; it is a disease in which malignant cells start to grow in the tissues of the liver. Metastatic liver cancers start somewhere else in the body, in another organ or area, and then spread to the liver.

Generally, primary liver cancer is categorized in two types. The first is HEPATOCELLULAR CARCINOMA (HCC), also called hepatoma or hepatocellular cancer. This cancer develops within the hepatocyte, a major type of liver cell. The other type of primary liver cancer is intrahepatic CHOLANGIOCARCINOMA, also called cholangiomas, or cholangiocarcinomas. The cancer arises from the bile duct cells within the liver rather than from the hepatocytes. The BILE DUCTS carry BILE into the intestines to help in digestion. There is some dispute as to whether these cancers actually come from "liver stem cells" that later grow to become either hepatocytes or bile ducts.

There is a rare subtype of HCC called fibrolamellar hepatoma. It occurs mainly in younger people, and is not associated with cirrhosis or any other liver disease. It has a better prognosis than other forms of HCC.

About 80 to 90 percent of primary liver cancer is hepatocellular carcinoma. It is still quite rare in the United States, representing about 4 percent of newly diagnosed cancers, but it is one of the most common malignant tumors in other parts of the world. The incidence of HCC has been increasing throughout the world, as well as in the United States, which is seeing a rapid increase especially among white men 45 to 54 years of age. An estimated 1 million cases are reported every year.

When tumors metastasize, they have spread beyond the primary, or original, site of the cancer and have established themselves at one or more different parts of the body. Cancer spreads through the lymph and vascular (blood vessel) systems. Cancer cells travel through the bloodstream, circulating throughout the body and lodging in other organs where they start to grow. Because blood comes into the liver for filtration from all areas of the body, the liver is readily accessible to cancer cells, and is a common site of metastasis. The rich blood supply also helps to nourish the cancer cells.

In the United States, metastatic cancer, also called secondary liver cancer, is 20 times more common than primary liver cancer, in which the cancer originates within the liver. Metastatic cancer is a leading cause of fatal liver disease, second only to cirrhosis, advanced scarring of the liver.

Cancer is most likely to spread from the colon, rectum, esophagus (the tube running from the mouth to the stomach), pancreas, lungs, breast, and skin. Since the liver is usually the first site to which cancer spreads, it is sometimes possible to catch the cancer earlier in this stage, before it has been deposited in multiple organs. Generally speaking, however, if the cancer has spread to the liver, it is probably already widespread within the lymphatic and circulatory systems, even if tests fail

to detect tumors elsewhere in the body. Patients should remember that the tests are not definitive—they cannot detect malignant tumors 100 percent of the time.

Symptoms and Diagnostic Path

There may be few or no symptoms, or there may be symptoms related to where the cancer began. For example, in the case of colon cancer, there may be altered bowel habits and rectal bleeding. Symptoms may also relate to liver injury, with general feelings of weakness, abdominal pain, and swelling. The individual may lose weight.

Almost half of all metastatic tumors in the liver originate from the colon and rectum. These are called metastatic colorectal carcinoma (CRC). CRC spreads most frequently to the lymph nodes; the liver is the second site, and the lungs, the third. CRC is the culprit in the majority of cases when an individual develops liver cancer that came from another site.

CRC is also the second most common cancer in developed countries such as the United States. The American Cancer Society estimates that every year, about 175,000 people develop colon and rectal cancer, and 35 percent of these patients die.

Liver resection (surgery) appears to be the only treatment currently available that can produce long-term survival in patients with CRC and offer a potential cure. Two years after undergoing surgery, about 65 percent of patients are alive and 25 percent no longer have any detectable disease.

Most patients with colorectal cancer are not good candidates for potentially curative surgery, however; they should be referred for novel treatment strategies and combinations of therapies. For the majority of patients with advanced colorectal cancer, the goal of surgery is not to cure but to improve survival and the quality of life.

Treatment Options and Outlook

By the time cancer has spread from the primary site to other locations in the body, it is in the highest stage of progression. Cancer that has advanced to this stage is the least responsive to treatment and has the worst prognosis. Without intervention, metastatic deposits in the liver most probably will grow in size and quantity, and start spreading to other sites as well. If the tumors are limited in number and size, and are contained within the liver, then aggressive surgical intervention may be possible. Before undergoing such treatment, however, patients should have a thorough diagnostic workup, especially with a PET scan.

The most common metastatic liver tumors that can at times be treated with surgery or other therapies directed at the liver include CRC and neuroendocrine neoplasms. Indeed, liver resection has become a fairly common treatment for localized colorectal liver metastases, as long as there is only a single tumor. Otherwise, patients with metastatic liver cancer are rarely treated with the surgical removal or destruction of the tumors in the liver, because treatment directed at the liver does not prolong the patient's life in these situations. Quite often, there are microscopic cancer cells within the lymph or circulatory system.

In recent years, however, the trend is to attempt surgical removal of tumors (liver resection) even for metastatic liver cancer. Reporting on the value of a more aggressive approach in the 2003 issue of the journal *Annals of Thoracic Surgery,* I. DiCarlo and colleagues wrote, "Recent improvements in hepatic surgery have made resection of metastases a safe procedure and it should certainly be considered whenever there is an isolated lesion."

Should patients have metastatic cancer cells that cannot be surgically removed (unresectable liver metastases), better options are systemic treatments that travel through the bloodstream and can reach cancer cells throughout the body. Systemic treatments include those below:

- *Biological therapy (immunotherapy)* Biological therapies fight cancer by using the body's immune system, either directly or indirectly. Interferon alpha (also used to treat viral hepatitis) and cytokines (produced by the immune system) are two examples, but there are numerous therapies for different types of cancer; many are still in the early stages of research.
- *Systemic chemotherapy* Chemotherapy fights cancer by using the body's bloodstream to deliver drugs. It is the most widely employed treatment for metastatic liver cancers that cannot be oper-

ated on. The drugs most often used for systemic chemotherapy are 5-fluorouracil (Adrucil, Efudex) or methotrexate (MTX, Mexate). A cure cannot be expected, but the aim is to prolong the patient's life. Whether the procedure will significantly lengthen the patient's survival time is still being debated, and may be best assessed on a case-by-case basis.

- *Hormone therapy (endocrine therapy)* Synthetic hormones or other drugs fight cancer by slowing or stopping the growth of certain cancers.

In addition to systemic treatments, metastatic tumors may also have to be treated locally if severe symptoms are present and are not resolved by other means. Some of these treatments may include the following:

- *Cryosurgery (cryosurgical ablation)*—freezing and removing the tumors with a probe containing extremely cold liquid
- *Radiofrequency ablation*—killing the tumors with extremely high temperature
- *Hepatic arterial chemotherapy*—administering chemotherapy locally through a pump that has been surgically implanted. This technique makes it possible to inject much larger concentrations of the cancer drug to be carried to the tumor than is possible when the drug has to be carried through the bloodstream. The drug most commonly used with the pump is floxuridine (FUDR). It is given for 14 days, followed by a 14-day period of rest. The cycle is repeated many times.

Some therapies may also be given in combination, depending on individual circumstances.

Generally speaking, patients with metastatic cancer are not good candidates for liver transplantation, because the cancer almost always comes back even after a new liver has been grafted. The more advanced the cancer, the greater the chances of recurring after the surgery. If the liver cancer fits the following criteria, transplantation is not recommended:

- There are more than three tumors.
- The tumors are larger than five centimeters.

- The tumors have grown into the portal vein that brings blood into the liver.
- The tumors have grown into the hepatic vein that carries blood out of the liver.
- The cancer has spread to the lymph nodes or other organs.

Neuroendocrine tumors usually arise in the lungs, the pancreas, or the intestine, and often spread to the liver. Sometimes it is not possible to identify the origin of these tumors, despite a thorough search. As a rule, neuroendocrine tumors grow quite slowly. But a troublesome aspect of such tumors is that they often produce hormones or other substances that cause considerable discomfort, such as stomach ulcers, low blood sugar, and diarrhea. In such cases, a liver transplant may be considered—but only after other treatments have been tried, such as surgical excision of the tumors, or chemoembolization treatments, in which the blood flow is blocked off from the tumors to starve them. Periodic chemoembolizations may give patients some symptom relief so that they can live a fairly normal life for quite some time. If the tumors continue to grow, or if the symptoms do not get any better, then a transplant might be an option.

One rare form of cancer is a blood vessel tumor that often begins in the bone marrow or the spleen and may spread to the liver. Called epithelioid hemangioendothelioma, the tumor grows very slowly. In such a case, the best treatment option might be to wait. But if the cancer progresses and causes severe symptoms, a liver transplant may be performed on the assumption that while the surgery will not cure the patient, it may prolong the patient's life.

Metastatic liver cancer is not an easy disease to treat. Patients with liver cancers that metastasized from cancer in the colon tend to live slightly longer than those whose cancers spread from cancers in the stomach or pancreas.

In the case of CRC, in a small minority of patients, the cancer spreads only to the liver and not to any other organs. (Thorough testing must be done to ensure that tumors are not present elsewhere.) If so, these patients may be fortunate enough to have the liver tumors completely removed, or if that is not possible, to obtain other treatments directed specifically at the tumors. (See LIVER CANCER, TREATMENT OF.) For CRC, the complete removal of the tumor from the liver by surgery (resection) most significantly prolongs survival. Their five-year survival rate after surgery is 25 to 40 percent. But generally, only about 5 percent of patients with CRC qualify for surgical removal of tumors; the majority of patients with CRC in the liver also have cancer in other organs as well. In such a case, simply treating the liver tumors does not improve survival.

When CRC spreads beyond the lymph nodes to the liver or any other site, the cancer has already advanced to stage IV, the last stage. By the time cancer has reached that stage, only about five out of 100 patients will live five or more years. (See CANCER STAGING.)

CRC comes back in some people but not in others; the reason is unknown. If surgery is undertaken to remove the tumors and CRC recurs in the liver, the majority of patients experience a recurrence within two years.

When CRC does recur, if it comes back after more than two years and spreads only to the liver but nowhere else, then the prognosis is better than in cases where the CRC comes back in the liver within the first year after the original surgery. One study reported in 2003 discovered that if patients with CRC are carefully selected for radical surgery, they could expect a 20 percent chance of long-term survival. If surgery is combined with new chemotherapy agents, the outlook should be even better.

DiCarlo, I., et al. "Liver metastases from lung cancer: Is surgical resection justified?" *Annals of Thoracic Surgery* 76, no. 1 (2003): 291–293.

Elias, D., J. F. Ouellet, N. Bellon, et al. "Extrahepatic disease does not contraindicate hepatectomy for colorectal liver metastases." *British Journal of Surgery* 90 (2003): 567–574.

liver cancer, treatment of An early diagnosis helps in treating liver cancer. The types of treatment depend on many factors, such as whether the liver cancer is primary or secondary. In primary liver cancer, the abnormal growth of cells began within the liver. In secondary, or metastatic, liver cancer, the cancerous cells started growing some-where in the body other than the liver.

To determine the most appropriate treatment, the doctor also has to know the stage of the disease. Cancer at an earlier stage is more easily treatable; when it has reached an advanced stage, the tumors grow larger and spread to other organs and areas in the body. If the metastatic cancer originated elsewhere in the body, then the site of the primary cancer must be located. Other factors to take into account are the patient's age, health status, whether the cancer recurred after treatment, the type of previous treatments (if any), and the presence of coexisting diseases, such as cirrhosis, scarring of the liver.

Broadly, there are four stages to adult primary liver cancer: localized resectable; localized unresectable; advanced; and recurrent. If the primary liver cancer is localized resectable, then the tumor (or tumors) is found in one place in the liver and can be resected (surgically removed). Certain patients may need LIVER TRANSPLANTATION. Localized unresectable refers to cancer found in only one place in the liver, but it cannot be completely removed in an operation. Advanced cancer precludes surgery because the tumors have either already spread throughout the liver, spread to other organs in the body, or spread to both the liver and beyond. There are no standard treatments, but the doctor may recommend chemotherapy and radiation therapy, as well as various new therapies, such as biological therapy.

Even after treatment, cancer often returns, either in the liver or in another part of the body. Treatment for these patients depends on a variety of factors, such as the kind of treatment they received before, the part of the body in which the cancer has recurred, and whether the liver has cirrhosis. Patients may wish to partake in a clinical trial for a new treatment.

Some treatments are standard (those currently used), and some are being tested in clinical trials. A treatment clinical trial is a research study that many hospitals perform to help develop new treatments or to improve current treatments. Patients may wish to take part in a clinical trial to take advantage of emerging therapies that are not otherwise available. New treatments discovered through clinical trials may become the standard treatment in the future.

Treatment generally involves LIVER RESECTION, cutting out the portion of the liver containing the tumor, or targeting the tumors for destruction with radiation, drugs, heat, cold, or alcohol. A third option is obtaining a healthy liver from a donor for transplantation. Each treatment has its risks and advantages, and not all patients are suitable candidates for them. Some of these treatments are still relatively new, and their long-term effectiveness has not been established. To achieve the best results, physicians today often apply treatments in many varying combinations; patients should discuss the best treatment strategy for their condition with their health care providers.

Basically, standard cancer treatment falls into four categories:

1. liver resection. Surgery to remove the portion of the liver containing the cancer
2. radiation therapy. Using high-dose X-rays or other high-energy rays to kill or shrink cancer cells
3. CHEMOTHERAPY. Using drugs to kill or shrink cancer cells. Regional chemotherapy injects the anticancer drug directly into the tumor, while systemic chemotherapy carries the drug through the bloodstream.
4. liver transplantation. Replacing the diseased liver with a new, healthy liver from a donor

Some of the newer treatments include the following:

5. EMBOLIZATION. Embolization of the liver (blocking the blood flow to the tumors) without chemotherapy drugs
6. CHEMOEMBOLIZATION. Blocking the blood flow to the tumors and then injecting chemotherapy drugs to destroy them
7. CRYOSURGERY. Surgery to freeze and destroy cancer cells
8. hyperthermia. Using a special machine to heat the body to destroy cancer cells
9. RADIOFREQUENCY ABLATION. Using highly focused radio waves to destroy cancer cells

10. percutaneous ethanol injection (PEI). Injecting alcohol directly into the cancer cells to destroy them
11. biological therapy (immunotherapy). Using the body's immune system to destroy the cancer cells
12. hormone therapy. Using hormones to slow or stop the growth of cancer cells
13. gene therapy. Using genes to modify or destroy cancer cells

Some hospitals specializing in cancer therapy are taking innovative approaches to treat difficult cases. For example, a patient with HEPATOCELLULAR CARCINOMA (HCC), with tumors that are too numerous to be operated on, might first be given chemoembolization to shrink the tumors. When the tumors are small enough, a liver resection is performed to remove the tumors; then the operation is followed up by radiation therapy. The radiation therapy may be combined with special drugs that make cancer cells more susceptible to the radiation. Or else systemic or regional chemotherapy can be given following surgery. These are just a few possibilities, as the particulars depend on the patient's general health, the type of cancer, and many other factors.

The specific type of therapy can be a complex process best determined after consultations with oncologists (doctors who specialize in treating cancer) and hepatologists (liver specialists), as well as other physicians who may be involved in treatment. Issues to consider include the patient's general health status; the size, number, and location of the tumors; the stage the tumors are in; whether the tumors have recurred; the presence of liver cirrhosis or other chronic liver disease; and the patient's preferences.

Only 10 to 13 percent of patients diagnosed with hepatocellular carcinoma (HCC) are eligible for treatments intended to cure the condition, including surgery. For patients with metastatic colorectal carcinoma (from primary tumors in the colon or rectum), only about 5 percent qualify for surgery. Of these, 25 percent will be cured, provided that all the visible tumors can be completely removed. If the tumors are contained within one lobe of the liver, surgery may be the best treatment if the patient does not have any of the following conditions:

- ASCITES (accumulation of fluid in the abdomen)
- JAUNDICE (yellowing of skin and eyes)
- CIRRHOSIS (advanced scarring and distortion of the liver architecture)

The type of operation depends on the size of the tumor, how many tumors are present, and their location in the liver. The surgeon will remove as much liver tissue as necessary to eliminate all the tumors. The goal is to remove all the cancer with a margin of surrounding healthy liver tissue. If the liver is not damaged by scarring, up to approximately 80 percent of the organ can be safely removed. The remaining portion will be able to carry on the normal functions of the liver, and will eventually grow back almost to its original size.

Unfortunately, most liver cancer cannot be surgically removed. By the time cancer is discovered, the majority of cases are too advanced. If the cancer has spread beyond the liver to other organs or areas, surgery to remove tumors from the liver will not help the patient. Consequently, but for a few exceptions, surgery is reserved only for patients with primary liver cancer.

Second, the size, number, and location of the tumors in the liver will also determine whether surgery is possible. If there are too many tumors in the liver, or if the tumors are spread out over both lobes of the liver (the liver has a left and a right lobe), there will not be enough liver remaining to function and the patient will die of liver failure. When operating, the surgeon must remove some of the healthy liver tissue around the tumors; but if the tumors are too close to the bile ducts, or to the major blood vessels carrying blood in and out of the liver, removal of the tumors may damage the bile ducts or the blood vessels.

The third issue to consider is the health of the liver, quite apart from the cancer. It is not an easy matter to remove tumors if the liver itself is unhealthy or diseased, most typically from cirrhosis, because a cirrhotic liver cannot regrow or function properly. Surgery under those circumstances could lead to liver failure.

Treatments directed only at the liver tumors are called liver-directed therapy. Ablation techniques fall into the category of liver-directed therapy. Ablation is the removal or destruction of malignant tumors or tissue through hormones, drugs, radiofrequency, heat, and other methods. These include cryosurgery, thermal therapy, and radiofrequency ablation. Currently many studies are being conducted on ablation therapy because it can destroy liver tumors without resorting to extensive operations. It offers an alternative treatment to patients who cannot be operated on for liver resection (removal of a portion of the liver containing the tumors) for medical or other reasons. These liver-directed therapies can also be used in conjunction with surgery if the cancer cannot be completely removed through liver resection. When used together with surgery, doctors call them adjuvant therapies. Various ablation techniques, such as radiofrequency ablation, cryosurgery, and percutaneous ethanol injection can be given before or after liver resection.

As far as most doctors are concerned, the major drawback to ablation therapy is that its long-term outcome or effectiveness in prolonging the lives of patients has not been clearly demonstrated, at least not when used as the only treatment.

Ablation therapy should generally be reserved for patients with good liver function who meet the criteria for liver resection, other than advanced or non-liver-related medical conditions. In most cases, liver-directed therapy should not be considered for patients with metastatic cancer. In other words, the cancer cells should either not have spread beyond the liver or they should not have spread to the liver from other sites in the body. If they have, the preferred therapies are systemic—whole body approaches, such as systemic chemotherapy where the anticancer drug is circulated throughout the body through the bloodstream.

In the case of colorectal carcinoma (CRC), an aggressive cancer that originates in the colon or rectum, liver-directed therapy is almost never recommended because it does not increase survival time, and the symptoms are generally not severe enough to warrant palliative treatments—treatments effected only for the purpose of reducing the symptoms.

But in recent years, there have been more attempts at liver-directed therapy in selected patients with metastatic cancer, with some favorable results.

Liver transplantation involves the removal of the entire liver and replacement with a healthy liver. After a powerful antirejection medicine called cyclosporine was discovered in the 1980s, demand for liver transplantation has increased exponentially each year.

Meanwhile, surgery to replace a cancerous liver, which was one of the main indications for transplantation, declined sharply; many transplant centers stopped transplant surgeries altogether for patients with liver cancer. The reason is that cancer almost always comes back even after successful transplantation. But certain patients may be helped by liver transplantation. Transplant centers have become better at identifying such patients in the past decade, thanks to better diagnostic tests and better understanding of cancer. For certain patients who have small tumors and cirrhosis, liver transplantation may be a good option, but each individual must be thoroughly evaluated.

Liver transplantation may be considered if the following characteristics apply:

- Tumors are less than 5 cm in diameter.
- The cancer originated in the liver.
- The liver is functioning well.
- The patient is under 70 years of age.

To make sure that the tumors do not grow while the patient is waiting for a new liver, ablation therapy may be applied. The most commonly used therapies are chemoembolization, percutaneous ethanol injection, and radiofrequency ablation. Some hospitals are experimenting with using ablation therapy after transplant surgery.

Unfortunately, the prognosis is generally not good for the majority of patients with cancer. The overall survival rates for patients with liver cancer are not high. The five-year survival rate for patients with hepatocellular carcinoma is around 4 percent. The poor prognosis is because cancer is often not diagnosed until it has metastasized. Virtually no patients whose cancer has spread beyond the liver can live for very long; many die within months of diagnosis. Even when treatment cannot cure cancer, it can often help to relieve the pain and other symptoms caused by the cancer, and improve the quality of life.

Liver resection and liver transplantation have been shown to prolong survival rates in patients. The survival rate is higher among patients with normal liver compared to those who have chronic liver disease.

liver disease The LIVER is a remarkably resilient organ that can continue functioning and replace its own damaged tissue even after three-quarters of it has been removed. Because many liver cells share the responsibility for the same task, they can take over the function of the missing cells. The liver can even regenerate its original weight, as long as there is no permanent scarring of the tissues. Even so, there is a limit to this regenerative capacity.

In the front line of the body's defense system, the liver is vulnerable to many toxins and other agents that can potentially harm the body. The liver can be overworked, overstressed, and damaged by many factors. Virtually everything absorbed in the gut and the skin is sent first to the liver to be processed. Alcoholic beverages, recreational drugs, and certain medications and herbs can damage the liver. Other agents that can injure the liver include viruses, inflammatory disease, tumors, and auto-immune disorders.

A diseased liver is unable to carry on its numerous functions. And yet the liver may continue working for years without any obvious symptoms. It is not an organ prone to complaining; it will suffer in silence for years, rarely sending out early warning signs. Thus, by the time a patient develops a clinically abnormal liver function, the liver may be significantly compromised. The patient may already have advanced CIRRHOSIS (permanent scarring of the liver) or a significant destruction of the liver cells.

Symptoms and Diagnostic Path

Even at the end stage of liver disease, some people are asymptomatic—they experience no symptoms from the disease. If there are any symptoms, they are nonspecific. In other words, they do not indicate the type of liver disease or the severity of the problem. Feeling fine is no guarantee that the liver is healthy.

When symptoms are present, the patient may have one or several in varying combinations. Below are some general signs that are suggestive of a liver disorder.

Fatigue The body draws on glucose in the bloodstream for its energy needs. Because the liver is responsible for regulating the glucose level, one of the first things that happens when the liver is injured is getting tired easily for no apparent reason. This can happen with all types and stages of liver disease. Depression may also accompany the fatigue.

Flu-like symptoms Just as with the flu, there may be feelings of weakness all over, with achy joints and muscles, and decreased appetite. This condition may last for several days or several weeks. Although these symptoms occur more frequently in the acute stages of a liver disease, people with chronic liver disease may also experience it episodically during the course of the illness.

Fever Fever is most often experienced during the acute stage of a viral hepatitis, as well as in some medication-induced or alcoholic hepatitis. People with chronic liver disease do not generally experience fever.

Itching (pruritus) A person may experience itching all over the body or in specific areas, ranging in sensation from mild to extremely severe. It is one of the symptoms of PRIMARY BILIARY CIRRHOSIS, an inflammation of the bile duct in the liver. CHOLESTASIS—stagnation of BILE in the BILE DUCTS—can also cause itching. The itching might not be relieved by dermatological treatments or scratching. Retention in the body of unknown factors is most likely responsible for the itching, but the exact cause is not known.

Swelling in abdomen (ascites) and weight gain Unexplained weight gain and some distention in the abdomen may occur. These symptoms can be due to fluid retention caused by cirrhosis or other severe deteriorating liver disease.

Swollen ankles (pedal edema) The legs and ankles may become swollen as a result of fluid retention.

Bruising easily and bleeding (coagulopathy) The liver makes coagulation factors to help the blood clot and stop bleeding. But when the liver stops producing enough of these factors because it is diseased, there is a tendency to bleed excessively, called coagulopathy. Even engaging in normal daily activities, such as brushing the teeth or shaving, can result in bleeding. Unexplained bumps and bruises also occur more frequently. This is a condition most commonly seen in patients with cirrhosis.

Weight loss People suffering from chronic liver abnormalities sometimes experience unintentional weight loss.

Jaundice Liver disease may be suspected in a person with a current or past history of jaundice. In this condition the skin and the whites of the eyes acquire a yellow tint. The color is a result of bilirubin elevation.

Although jaundice is most often associated in people's minds with liver problems, one may have even a severe liver disease without ever experiencing jaundice. Conversely, there are many causes of jaundice that are not related to the liver.

An accurate diagnosis of liver disease has to be based on a combination of history, physical examination, laboratory tests, radiological tests, and liver biopsy. Patients should not expect a doctor to determine the presence of a liver disease just by showing the results of a few blood tests or describing some signs and symptoms.

Regular physical checkups provide a baseline for physicians from which to measure changes in an individual's general state of health, some of which may be subtle.

When a patient arrives at a clinic, the first order of business is filling out a form with questions about the patient's medical history. The patient should be prepared to provide a complete history and answer all questions as accurately and comprehensively as possible, even highly personal ones. These details are important in diagnosing suspected liver disease and in determining the nature and severity of the problem. Individuals need not fear breach of privacy because patient confidentiality is guaranteed by law. The patient must provide written consent before the doctor can release any information to a third party.

In addition to the usual questions about one's age, occupation, and symptoms, and a full medical, surgical, and anesthetic history, other information helpful in determining any abnormalities in the liver is as follows:

History of Liver Disease in the Family

- exposure to environmental toxins (pesticides, paint thinners, lead, etc.)
- alcohol consumption
- weight gain or loss in the past few months
- changes in appetite
- sexual history
- use of recreational drugs and needle sharing—even if only once, and a long time ago
- tattoos or body piercing
- received blood or blood products at any time
- military service
- recent consumption of wild mushrooms or seafood, in particular shellfish
- travel outside the United States
- bleeding problems
- vomiting of blood
- dark urine
- bloody or black bowel movements
- clay-colored feces
- unusual itching or rashes
- use of prescription and over-the-counter medications
- use of vitamins, supplements, and herbs

In addition to patient history, visual and other clues can aid the doctor's assessment of the patient's condition. Although many, or perhaps most, patients with liver disease appear to be completely normal on a physical checkup, some may show signs that indicate the presence of liver disease.

Liver palms Some individuals may develop a condition called liver palms (palmar erythema), in which the palms turn abnormally red. This is often associated with cirrhosis where, due to irreversible scarring and damage of its tissues, the liver fails to metabolize endocrine hormones properly. Various other liver diseases can also cause this condition.

Deputyren's contracture   The palms undergo a shortening and thickening beneath the skin, causing the fingers to become bent. The most common cause is alcoholic cirrhosis.

Reddish marks on the skin   Patients with chronic or severe liver disease may have enlarged blood vessels or small, reddish marks on the skin that resemble little spiders. They are called spider angiomatas, or spider, for short. They usually appear on the upper chest, back, arms, and shoulders. These marks turn white when pressure is applied to the center, then turn red again when the pressure is released.

Bone fractures   The liver helps to metabolize proteins. When the liver is too damaged to do so properly, muscles may waste away. This makes the individual more susceptible to bone fractures as the protective muscle lining progressively atrophies, rendering the bones more brittle.

Hormonal imbalances   Hormonal imbalances can occur in the late stages of liver disease. One reason for this is that the pituitary gland, which controls the hormones, becomes impaired. The liver may also fail to metabolize adequately circulating estrogens in the blood, as well as become less efficient in breaking down and building up cholesterol, from which estrogens and androgens (female and male hormones) are made. The result is an appearance of feminine characteristics in men. Men may experience breast enlargement (gynecomastia) and have to shave less often. Women too may discover less hair on their face and body, such as under the arms.

Confusion (encephalopathy)   Confusion, ranging from mild to severe, and other altered mental states can occur because of cirrhosis or severe liver deterioration. At its most severe, the patient may go into a coma. Behavioral changes include irritability. The mental dysfunction is due to the liver's inability to metabolize ammonia, the by-product of protein metabolism, and other nitrogen-containing toxins, which are damaging to the brain.

Liver tremors (astereixis)   A condition known as liver tremors or liver flap (astereixis) is often associated with encephalopathy. This is where the hands flap uncontrollably and drop when held up by the patient, palms out, like the hand of a police officer stopping traffic.

Physical examination   The head, eyes, skin, and abdomen are examined for abnormalities, such as yellow nodules or patches that often occur on the eyelids or other parts of the body. Percussion (drumming) of the liver area shows whether the liver feels hard, too big, or too small. A swollen spleen can also be an indication of liver disease.

Blood testing   Routine blood work panels usually include tests that reflect liver activity. These can at times uncover patients who otherwise have no symptoms of liver dysfunction. By themselves, however, blood tests are not sufficient to provide a complete clinical picture.

Liver panel   The liver panel is a battery of seven tests that help to detect the presence of liver disease or injuries. Four of the tests measure enzyme activity that may be elevated in some liver diseases.

The two enzymes that are measured on routine blood testing panels as indicators of possible liver disease are aminotransferases (ALT, also known as SGPT) and AST (also known as SGOT). They are present in hepatocytes, which are the primary liver cells.

ALT is found almost exclusively in the liver, and can provide a very rough estimate of liver cell deaths. It is good for detecting hepatitis, inflammation of the liver. AST is found not only in the liver but in other places as well, in particular the heart and skeletal muscles.

Blood tests measuring ALT and AST activities are often known as liver-function tests, but these tests do not actually assess the liver's functions. By measuring ALT and AST activities, they provide some indication of changes that may be occurring in the liver.

Two other enzymes also helpful in determining liver abnormalities are the cholestatic liver enzymes, alkaline phosphatase (ALP) and gamma-glutamyl transpeptidase (GGTP). Elevated ALP and GGTP activities suggest abnormality of large bile ducts.

In addition to the enzymes, the tests check for concentration of bilirubin and albumin, and measure the prothrombin time. An elevated concentration of bilirubin in blood is known as hyperbilirubinemia, and can indicate bile duct obstruction, severe acute liver damage, or advanced cirrhosis.

ALBUMIN is the main protein synthesized by the liver. How much albumin is present in the blood can show how well the liver is making this protein. The level may be decreased if there is a severe liver disease.

The liver produces blood-clotting factors. Prothrombin time (PT) measures the function of several blood-clotting factors. Severe liver disease can result in low levels of blood-clotting factors, which in turn increases the prothrombin time.

The physician must visualize the liver through imaging studies, which are taken by the radiologist. These will include the ultrasound examination, also known as sonogram. In some cases, the doctor may also request computerized axial tomography (CAT or CT scanning) or magnetic resonance imaging (MRI). These are all painless, noninvasive procedures.

Although advanced technologies like ultrasound, CT scans, and MRIs can be an excellent way to image the entire abdomen and assess the extent of liver tumors or gallbladders, they still fail to provide a complete picture of the inner workings of the liver. The liver may appear normal even if diseased. Generally, in chronic conditions, only a LIVER BIOPSY can accurately assess the condition of the liver. Thus, the biopsy remains the gold standard in diagnosing liver disease.

Pediatric Liver Disease

It is rare for children to acquire liver diseases that are seen in adults. Most cases of liver disease in children involve congenital or metabolic disorders. Some of the most common types of pediatric liver disease include the following:

- ALAGILLE SYNDROME. This is an inherited disorder. Children show poor growth within the first three months of life.

- ALPHA-1-ANTITRYPSIN DEFICIENCY. This is the most common hereditary liver disease in children. It may lead to HEPATITIS, inflammation of the liver, and CIRRHOSIS, scarring of the liver.

- BILIARY ATRESIA. This is a serious disease occurring in the very young infant. There is inflammation and obstruction of the bile ducts.

- galactosemia. This is a rare hereditary disease that usually appears in the first few days of life after the infant ingests breast milk or formula. The genetic disorder leads to a deficiency of a liver enzyme required to break down sugar (galactose) in milk. The earliest symptoms include vomiting, liver enlargement, and yellowing of the skin and eyes. If not treated, the infant will succumb to liver failure.

- hepatoblastoma. This is a malignant tumor of the liver that essentially occurs only in children, usually within the first three years of life. In children under five, it is more common in boys than in girls, and generally carries a poor prognosis. It is not associated with cirrhosis. There are approximately 100 new cases in the United States every year.

- kernicterus. This refers to bilirubin toxicity, and occurs when unconjugated bilirubin in the blood rises to toxic levels. Infants may be treated by phototherapy that helps the unconjugated bilirubin become increasingly water-soluble so that it can be easily excreted in the kidneys.

- NEONATAL JAUNDICE. In this condition, there is yellowing of the skin and eyes in a newborn. In most cases, jaundice disappears soon after birth, but if it persists, the infant may be treated with phototherapy.

- NEONATAL HEPATITIS. This inflammation of the liver occurs only in infants, usually between one and two months after birth. Symptoms include jaundice, failure to gain weight or grow, and an enlarged liver and spleen. The infant cannot properly absorb vitamins.

- Reye's syndrome. This is a rare complication of childhood respiratory infections. Symptoms include vomiting that begins three to seven days after the onset of flu or chickenpox, listlessness, staring, and drowsiness. It can cause fulminant hepatic failure.

- TYROSINEMIA. This is a severe liver disease in infants associated with a genetic inborn error of metabolism.

- type I glycogen storage disease. In this disease, there is either an absent or an abnormal activity of the enzyme glucose-6-phosphatase that helps maintain a normal blood glucose (sugar concentration) during fasting. Symptoms include failure to grow, an enlarged liver, and a distended abdomen. The patient is usually given a high-starch diet and continuous feedings.

liver donor   See LIVER TRANSPLANTATION.

liver enzymes   Enzymes are important proteins that catalyze, or speed up, chemical reactions within the body. Liver enzymes are any of the many enzymes that the liver produces, but the term "liver enzymes" most often refers to the routine blood tests done to assess the condition of the LIVER. Ongoing liver injury can also be monitored by measuring the enzyme levels in the blood.

Among the most sensitive and widely used enzymes are the two major aminotransferases—aspartate aminotransferase (AST or SGOT) and alanine aminotransferase (ALT or SGPT). Two other enzymes are often included as well: alkaline phosphatase (ALP) and gamma-glutamyl transpeptidase (GGTP).

Liver enzymes reside within liver cells, though they may not be confined to the liver. AST, for instance, is also in kidneys and the heart. The enzymes help the liver process food, vitamins, and other substances ingested by the body, and get rid of the resulting waste products. The laboratory tests measure the activities of these enzymes, and they are roughly equivalent to the amount of the enzymes in the bloodstream. A simple blood test can detect these liver enzymes, which leak into the bloodstream when the liver is injured. Therefore, an elevation of the enzymes may at times indicate that the liver is suffering from inflammation (HEPATITIS), injury, or disease. These enzymes can also reflect alcohol and drug use, as well as certain medications. In general, ALT and AST are elevated in most disorders where there is inflammation or destruction of liver tissues. These include chronic HEPATITIS B, HEP-ATITIS C, FATTY LIVER, and ALCOHOLIC LIVER DISEASE, among others. Elevations of ALP and GGTP suggest disorders of the BILE DUCT, though they can also be elevated in other LIVER DISEASES as well.

It should be emphasized that these blood tests provide only part of the picture. They fall far short of a definitive diagnosis as to whether there are abnormalities of the liver.

liver failure   Liver failure occurs when normal liver functions are severely impaired or stop altogether. It is an ominous condition, because the liver is responsible for so many important functions. When too many liver cells are damaged, the remaining cells cannot perform all the liver's functions. Food is not metabolized properly, toxins build up, and important chemical compounds are not produced. As a result, the patient's health fails rapidly. When enough liver cells die, the liver stops working, and encephalopathy—mental disorientation—follows. The patient becomes more and more confused, and may eventually go into a coma and die. Liver failure can also affect infants and children, and it occurs equally among men and women. It is estimated that each year approximately 2,000 people in the United States die of liver failure. The mortality rate can be as high as 80 to 90 percent without LIVER TRANSPLANTATION.

Acute liver failure is a sudden-onset liver failure without preexisting liver disease, and it is accompanied by altered mental status called HEPATIC ENCEPHALOPATHY. This abnormal mental functioning is believed to occur because the liver is no longer able to remove toxins, in particular, ammonia, from the blood. Advanced stages of acute liver failure are complicated by the bleeding disorder, COAGULOPATHY, as well as hepatic encephalopathy. Two subgroups of acute liver failure are commonly recognized, fulminant and subfulminant hepatic failure.

When the liver fails quite suddenly in individuals who appeared to be healthy and had no preexisting liver conditions, it is called fulminant hepatic failure (FHF). Its onset is quite rapid, and its course is short and severe. According to one definition of FHF, encephalopathy must occur within eight weeks after the illness begins, or at least two weeks after JAUNDICE (yellowing of skin and eyes) begins. But not everyone agrees on the definition. Some investigators use the criterion of a maximum of two weeks rather than eight for the occurrence of encephalopathy as the interval between the start of jaundice and encephalopathy.

If encephalopathy develops eight weeks to six months after the illness begins, or two weeks to three months after the beginning of jaundice, it is not FHF, but simply acute liver failure, sometimes also known as subfulminant hepatic failure. According to another definition, if there are other signs and symptoms of liver dysfunction, but no encephalopathy, then the condition should be described as acute liver failure.

The number-one cause of FHF is viral hepatitis, which accounts for about half the cases of FHF in the United States. Viral hepatitis is caused by hepatitis viruses A, B, C (rarely), D, or E. Hepatitis A virus (HAV) is a common cause of FHF in people of all ages. In areas where hepatitis B (HBV) is widespread, it is the most common cause of FHF. Women who are infected with HBV and give birth can pass it on to their infants, who may then suffer from liver failure. Chronic carriers of HBV, whether or not the hepatitis is manifested, who become infected with HEPATITIS D virus (HDV) can develop FHF. HEPATITIS E can also cause FHF, mainly in adolescents and young adults.

The second most common cause of FHF is overdoses of drugs or certain toxins. The most common type of drug overdose is acetaminophen (the main ingredient in Tylenol). Some 20 to 35 percent of cases are caused by acetaminophen overdose, and in some places, acetoaminophen may be the most common cause of FHF. Other drugs, such as isoniazid (to treat tuberculosis), can also cause liver toxicity. Eating poisonous mushrooms also results in FHF.

Other, less common causes of FHF include hemorrhage, heatstroke, heart failure, and severe dehydration. Certain metabolic abnormalities may cause liver failure. However, these metabolic conditions include preexisting liver disease, and, strictly speaking, they are not FHF. FHF can also be a result of WILSON'S DISEASE, an inherited disorder associated with neurological problems and very high BILIRUBIN levels in the blood. Reye's syndrome, an acute illness, is a rare cause of fulminant liver failure in children. FATTY LIVER of pregnancy, which most commonly occurs during the third trimester of pregnancy, is a potentially lethal disease and can also cause FHF. In many patients, though, the cause is often unknown.

It is important to find out the cause of the liver failure, if possible, because that makes a difference in the prognosis and the management of the illness.

Symptoms and Diagnostic Path
Here are some of the signs and symptoms of liver failure, which may not all be present in the same individual:

- abdominal pain
- anorexia (loss of appetite)
- acites (buildup of fluid in the abdomen)
- bruising and bleeding easily
- coma
- dark urine
- edema (swollen feet, ankles, and legs)
- encephalopathy (impaired brain function)
- light-colored stools
- fatigue and weakness
- fetor hepaticus (musty, sweet-smelling breath)
- fever
- itchy skin
- jaundice (yellow skin and eyes)
- nausea and vomiting

If the patient's medical history and a thorough physical examination reveal signs and symptoms of FHF, the doctor usually requests a number of tests to confirm the diagnosis and to determine the cause. They may include blood and urine tests, imaging studies such as ultrasound or computed tomography (CT), and a LIVER BIOPSY.

The presence of immunoglobulins (antibodies) against a particular type of viral hepatitis may indicate that the condition is caused by infection with that virus. Lab studies can confirm the diagnosis of viral hepatitis. The patient's blood sugar level may be low. LIVER ENZYME activities may be elevated, normal, or even decreased in patients with FHF. If the patient has a metabolic disorder, however, the enzyme levels are often very high. When hepatocytes (primary liver cells) die, the liver is unable to metabolize bilirubin sufficiently, and, therefore, direct and indirect bilirubin levels in the blood are almost always elevated. PROTHROMBIN TIME (PT), which measures how fast the blood clots, is prolonged, and the clotting time is a fairly good indicator of the severity of liver failure. The longer prothrombin time is a result of the inability of the failing liver to synthesize enough blood-clotting factors. Because the blood's poor clotting ability is not caused by vitamin K efficiency, administration of vitamin K does not normalize it.

Liver biopsy is often essential in diagnosis and in planning appropriate therapy. Although a biopsy can be useful, in rare cases the samples obtained may not be representative of the entire liver, and the results sometimes correlate poorly with the patient's prognosis. When a patient experiences end-stage liver disease and liver transplantation is considered, a biopsy is needed to prepare for the surgery. But excessive bleeding (coagulopathy) often occurs with liver failure, and the risk of a liver biopsy must be weighed against whatever benefits there may be in diagnosis and management. When there is a potential problem with excessive bleeding, a transvenous biopsy may sometimes be performed instead of the standard biopsy.

As the prothrombin time becomes longer and the platelet count gradually falls in cases of FHF, gastrointestinal bleeding can occur. The kidneys fail in up to 50 percent of FHF patients, and the lungs may also fail. The patient may have massive infection as well. There is always the danger of a coma as the encephalopathy progresses.

Another serious complication is brain swelling, which can lead to irreversible brain damage and, without liver transplantation, death. Brain swelling occurs in as many as 80 percent of patients. Thus, attention should be paid to early signs, which include increased muscle tone, seizures, agitation, slow response of the pupils of the eyes to light, and hypertension of the arteries. The patient's head should be elevated, and properly positioned, and manipulations should be avoided that increase intracranial pressure (pressure inside the cranium) to help prevent brain swelling. The intracranial pressure should be continually monitored, especially if the patient is in stage three or four of encephalopathy.

Bacterial and fungal infections frequently occur, both from the many invasive procedures required for treatment and from the liver failure itself. Pneumonia and urinary tract infections may develop. Sepsis (overwhelming infection) is common and is seen in slightly fewer than 80 percent of patients with advanced stages of coma. About 20 percent of the patients with sepsis have blood-borne bacterial or fungal infections.

Treatment Options and Outlook

Hospitalization is required as soon as FHF is diagnosed, and management of the illness is best undertaken in a center with a liver transplantation program. The patient should immediately be started on intensive care, and procedures for a transplant operation should get underway. For most patients, however, no therapy can regenerate the liver cells or reverse the injury. Medical treatment is usually directed at the specific cause of FHF, if known, and at controlling complications. Therefore, the type of therapy is based on the cause and the symptoms. The goals of therapy are to give supportive measures while waiting to see whether the liver recovers, usually with continuous monitoring. Vital functions should be maintained, and life-threatening complications should be identified and immediately treated. The side effects of liver failure may also be treated. The patient may receive some of the following treatments, alone or in combination:

- removing toxins normally handled by the liver
- removing extra fluid in the brain, legs, feet, and abdomen, using a procedure called paracentesis
- stopping any diarrhea
- stopping or lessening bleeding
- placing the patient on a special diet that may be high in calories
- administering vitamins
- kidney dialysis

Serious infections, such as septicemia, peritonitis, or pneumonia, are treated with appropriate antibiotics. If the underlying cause of liver failure is either viral or autoimmune hepatitis, appropriate medications are given to treat that specific condition. Acetaminophen overdose is treated with N-acetylcysteine. Generally, patients receive intravenous (IV) fluids to balance carefully fluids, electrolytes, and glucose (blood sugar) levels. The patient in a coma may have a breathing tube to help with breathing. Sometimes the patient may need total parenteral nutrition (nutrition given through a needle) to ensure adequate nourishment, especially if the patient is unable to eat. The patient may require nutritional supplementation, with the type and amount determined by the physician.

Liver damage cannot be reversed. If recovery of the liver appears unlikely, LIVER TRANSPLANTATION is the only effective mode of treatment and is considered no matter what the cause of the liver failure. The survival rate for patients who receive a liver transplant is higher than for those who do not. Thus, it is best to hospitalize the patient where there are facilities for liver transplantation.

In an acute emergency, living-related donor transplant may be performed if the patient has a relative willing to donate a segment of liver. This is particularly common with children. Today, instead of a traditional whole organ transplant of a liver from a deceased donor, there are other innovative approaches. These include AUXILIARY LIVER TRANSPLANTATION and XENOTRANSPLANTATION, as well as artificial and bio-artificial liver support devices. Recently, physicians have begun using liver-assist devices to support the patient's liver until it can recover or until a suitable donor organ is available for transplant.

If jaundice (yellowing of skin and eyes) occurs at least one week before the start of encephalopathy (mental impairment), the prognosis is poor. Usually patients with acetaminophen overdose or viral hepatitis A or B have a relatively short interval between jaundice and encephalopathy, and the prognosis is better than for patients with drug-induced liver injury or other types of hepatitis, where the interval between jaundice and encephalopathy is longer. Patients whose illnesses last longer than eight weeks before they start experiencing symptoms of encephalopathy have a higher likelihood of renal (kidney) failure. The chance of brain swelling increases with illnesses lasting fewer than four weeks before liver failure. No matter what the cause of the liver failure, the elderly experience a higher mortality rate.

Anderson, Kenneth, Lois E. Anderson, and Walter D. Glanze. *Mosby's Medical, Nursing, & Allied Health Dictionary, Edition 5.* St. Louis, Mo.: Mosby-Year Book, 1998, p. 50A5.

liver flukes   Flukes are parasitic flatworms (trematodes) that can infect various organs in larger animals. The word "trematode" is taken from a Greek word that means "having holes"; it refers to external suckers that adult flukes use to draw nourishment from their hosts. Flukes have complex life cycles that include hosts other than human beings. Infection in humans generally occurs in either the LIVER or the lungs, depending on the worm species. It is estimated that there are between 40 million and 100 million cases worldwide of human fluke infection, and liver-fluke infections are known in Europe, North America, the Middle East, China, Japan, and Africa.

Several species of liver flukes can infect humans, including *Opisthorchis viverrini, O. felineus,* and *Clonorchis sinensis. O. viverrini* is common in northeast Thailand, where at least one-third of the population is infected, and it is also common in Laos. *O. felineus* affects about 1.5 million people in Russia, and *C. sinensis* has infected several million people in the Republic of Korea, southern China, Hong Kong, Macao, and Vietnam. Infection usually occurs in children, and men may be more frequently and heavily affected than women. *Fasciola hepatica,* the sheep fluke, can also infect humans.

All flukes require a freshwater snail as an intermediate host. *O. viverrini, O. felineus,* and *C. sinensis* additionally require a freshwater fish or shellfish as a host, and *F. hepatica* requires an aquatic plant as a host. The life cycles are similar. Fluke eggs may be eaten by a certain type of freshwater snail. They then undergo asexual reproduction and produce free-swimming larvae, called cercariae, which can penetrate freshwater fish or crayfish and become encysted in skin or muscle tissue as metacercariae.

In the case of *F. hepatica*, the metacercariae attach themselves to plant surfaces. Infection occurs in humans and other mammals who eat uncooked or undercooked fish, plants, or animals that contain metacercariae. The cysts release metacercariae into the duodenum, and immature flukes migrate into the intestines and up through the ampulla of Vater to the biliary tree (passageways transporting BILE, the fluid produced by the liver) and mature in the small intrahepatic ducts (ducts within the liver). Adult liver flukes chronically infect the BILE DUCTS, pancreatic duct, or GALLBLADDER of humans and other mammals, and they eventually produce eggs, which are passed in the feces. In their adult stage, liver and lung flukes are symmetrical in shape, ranging in length between one-quarter inch and one inch, and look somewhat like long, plump leaves or blades of grass. The life span of flukes can be as long as 20 years, and infection can continue for two decades or longer.

These infections are caused by *Clonorchis sinensis*, the Chinese liver fluke, and *Opisthorchis viverrini*. The diseases are widespread, affecting more than 20 million people in Japan, China, Southeast Asia, and India. The life cycle of these liver flukes is similar to that of *F. hepatica* except that the metacercariae are encysted in freshwater fish rather than on plants. Dogs, cats, and other mammals that eat raw fish can be infected with *opisthorchiasis* and *clonorchiasis*.

Fascioliasis is the term applied to human infections by flukes of the genus *Fasciola*. The most common species is *F. hepatica*, the sheep liver fluke. *F. gigantica* is a similar species that can also cause infection in humans. *F. gigantica* is found in tropical regions and is much larger than *F. hepatica*, with lengths of 25 to 75 mm, widths of 15 mm, and eggs somewhat larger than those of *F. hepatica*. Other species of *Fasciola* are known to infect animals: *F. halli* and *F. californica* in cattle and sheep in the United States, *F. magna* in deer, *F. jacksoni* in elephants, and *F. nyanzae* in the hippopotamus.

Acute fascioliasis is much more common in sheep than in humans or other mammals. If a person ingests a large number of metacercaria (more than about 10,000) at once, the many migrating larvae cause a traumatic inflammation of the liver. Chronic fascioliasis is much more common in humans and other hosts than acute fascioliasis and occurs when fewer metacercaria are ingested.

Symptoms and Diagnostic Path

The symptoms of liver-fluke infection are the same, regardless of the type of worm present. Usually, fewer than 100 worms are present, and the patient has no symptoms. Only about 5 to 10 percent of those infected show clinically specific signs and symptoms, usually with heavier infestation. The severity of symptoms depends on the number of flukes present, which can be up to 21,000.

Symptoms of chronic fluke infection include malaise, loss of appetite, intermittent fever, diarrhea, pain in the right upper portion of the abdomen, and mild JAUNDICE. Blood tests may indicate anemia and eosinophilia. Apparently, *F. hepatica* is not fully adapted to human hosts, and sometimes infections occur in other organs, particularly the lungs and subcutaneous (under the skin) tissue.

The symptoms of acute fluke infection include abdominal pain, headache, loss of appetite, fever, anemia, and vomiting. Some patients develop hives, muscle pains, or jaundice. The liver capsule may rupture, causing peritonitis (inflammation of the lining of the abdominal cavity) and death.

A diagnosis of liver-fluke infection is usually made by examination of feces and detection of eggs. However, an acute syndrome may be difficult to diagnose because the fluke eggs do not appear in the patient's stool for several weeks after infection. In the United States and other developed countries, fluke infections are rare, and the stool samples may have to be sent to a laboratory with expertise in unusual diseases or conditions to identify the specific parasite. The patient's history, particularly travel or residence in an area known to have flukes, may also help identify the parasite. The number of eggs per gram of feces often is correlated to the number of adult worms present in the host, and light infections may not be detected. The eggs of the different species of worms responsible for fluke infections are indistinguishable by microscopic examination, but the types of flukes can be differentiated by examining the adult forms.

Blood tests may not provide good diagnoses, because they may not be specific for a particular species or because they may not distinguish between current and past infections. Patients with fluke infections usually have elevated serum alkaline phosphatase (ALP) and BILIRUBIN levels, and mildly to moderately elevated serum aminotransferase levels.

Imaging techniques, such as computed tomography scans (CT scans) or ultrasound scans of the abdomen can be useful in confirming a diagnosis of fluke infection. The number of worms correlates with the extent of abnormalities in the biliary tract within the liver observed in the scans.

If the infection is advanced, the bile ducts may be inflamed and obstructed, and eggs will not appear in the feces. Percutaneous aspiration (performed through the skin) of fluid or identification during surgery may lead to the discovery of flukes in the bile ducts or gallbladder.

Treatment Options and Outlook

Fluke infections can be treated with medications, including triclabendazole, praziquantel, bithionol, albendazole, and mebendazole. Praziquantel paralyzes the flukes' suckers, forcing them to drop away from the walls of the host's blood vessels. Bithionol is available in the United States only from the Centers for Disease Control (CDC). Depending on the species of fluke and the severity of infection, the course of treatment can vary from several days to several weeks. Most patients experience mild temporary side effects from these drugs, including diarrhea, dizziness, or headache. Cure rates vary from 50 to 95 percent.

Treatment for flukes is usually very effective in killing the parasites and also reverses biliary tract abnormalities. After treatment, dead flukes may appear in the stool or biliary drainage. If many worms are present, the dead flukes, surrounding debris, and/or stones may obstruct bile ducts, requiring endoscopic or surgical drainage.

Although flukes are found mainly in undeveloped regions, immigrants and travelers have brought them to the developed countries, including the United States. It is important to recognize these infections and their associated complications in travelers from areas where the worms are endemic.

In addition to treatment of infected individuals, new infections can be prevented or controlled by a combination of drug therapy, health education, and improved sanitation. Yet it seems difficult to convince people to change their traditional dietary patterns. Recommended sanitation measures include boiling or purifying drinking water, avoiding raw and undercooked fish, and not eating salads made from fresh aquatic plants. Pickling or smoking food does not kill cysts in fish or shellfish. Food should be cooked thoroughly in areas with fluke infestations.

Another control strategy is to interfere with the normal life cycle of the flukes, such as by controlling the population of the snails that are the intermediate hosts. It may be possible to drain some ponds. If livestock are spreading the flukes, they should be kept away from the ponds where the snails live. Also, livestock can be wormed.

At present, there are no effective vaccines against lung- or liver-fluke infections.

If a large number of worms are present, they may obstruct the bile ducts to cause cholelithiasis (stones), cholecystitis (acute or chronic inflammation), jaundice (yellowing of the skin and eyes), recurrent pyogenic cholangitis (inflammation of the bile duct, forming pus), and biliary abscesses. Biliary and gallbladder stones are more likely to occur in individuals infected with *Clonorchis* than with other flukes. If the infection lasts for a long time and is not treated, it can cause inflammation and periportal fibrosis (scarring surrounding the portal vein, the large vein that carries blood from the stomach and intestines to the liver), biliary hyperplasia (abnormal multiplication in the number of normal cells), and dysplasia (alteration in the size and shape of adult cells).

Adult *F. hepatica* flukes may migrate to other parts of the body. "Black disease" is a secondary infection by the bacterium *Clostridium oedematiens*, which grows in lesions produced by the young larvae migrating in the liver. In the Middle East, an acute throat irritation, *halzoun*, occurs when flukes are ingested in raw liver.

Hepatocellular carcinoma (primary cancer of the liver) and cholangiosarcoma (cancer of the bile ducts) are associated with liver-fluke infections, and they should be suspected in infected patients who experience weight loss, jaundice, epigastric pain (pain in the abdomen, just below the breastbone), or an abdominal mass.

Infection with liver flukes appears to increase significantly the risk of subsequently developing cholangiocarcinoma, or cancer of the bile ducts. Cholangiosarcoma is generally a rare type of tumor. The incidence of this type of cancer is significantly higher in areas where liver-fluke infection is prevalent. Indeed, the incidence of cholangiosarcoma in the region of Thailand where *O. viverrini* is found is about 40 times higher than the highest incidence outside Thailand. Furthermore, animal studies with hamsters, cats, dogs, fish, and rats have shown an increased rate of cholangiosarcoma in individuals infected with liver flukes of the species *O. viverrini* and *C. sinensis*.

Both hepatocellular carcinoma and cholangiocarcinoma have been reported to occur at a higher incidence in patients infected with *O. felineus* in northwestern Siberia. Both cholangiocarcinoma and hepatocellular carcinoma associated with infections of *C. sinensis* have been reported from China, Hong Kong, the Republic of Korea, and Japan and in immigrants to North America from China and Laos. Researchers are investigating the use of antibodies against *O. sinensis* and *O. viverrini* with follow-up ultrasound studies to identify individuals at high risk for cholangiocarcinoma. The incidence of cholangiocarcinoma in Thailand has been correlated with average levels of antibodies to *O. viverrini* and with fecal egg counts.

Apparently, liver flukes alone do not cause cancer. It is believed that the presence of flukes must be combined with other factors before cancer develops. One theory is that the parasites induce DNA damage and mutations due to the formation of carcinogens (cancer-producing substances) or free radicals. The cell damage from the fluke infection leads to fibrosis (scarring) of the bile ducts, abnormal, precancerous growths in the bile ducts, and proliferation of bile ducts, all of which play a critical role in the development of tumors. *O. viverrini* has been linked to mutations in a tumor suppressor gene. Also, people infected with *O. viverrini* tend to have increased levels of certain nitrogen compounds, related to carcinogens, in their urine. Studies in

hamsters showed that liver-fluke infection in combination with a substance that can lead to cancer in the liver (hepatocarcinogen) when added to the animals' drinking water or diet resulted in a high incidence of cholangiocarcinoma. Human diets in Thailand commonly contain substances converted in the stomach to the hepatocarcinogen used in the hamster study.

Most patients with liver flukes recover from the infections. However, patients with serious or long-lasting infections may have significant liver damage and be susceptible to other diseases. Infection does not cause an immune reaction that would prevent reinfection by the same or another species of flukes.

Goldsmith, Robert S. "Infectious diseases: Protozoal & helminthic." *Current Medical Diagnosis & Treatment 1998*, edited by Lawrence M. Tierney, Jr., et al. Stamford, Conn.: Appleton & Lange, 1998.

liver-function tests Liver-functions tests—also called a liver panel—are tests conducted on a blood sample when a physician suspects the possibility of LIVER DISEASE. The tests can vary, but in general they measure levels in the blood of enzymes and proteins associated with liver function or activities. The test results can indicate how well a liver is performing, and they may help pinpoint specific liver problems.

A doctor may order liver-function tests when a patient

- displays symptoms, such as JAUNDICE or fatigue, that suggest the possibility of a liver disorder

- has been exposed to HEPATITIS

- has a family history of liver disease

- has excessive alcohol intake

- is taking drugs or medication that can damage the liver

The tests conducted can vary depending on the specific nature of the doctor's suspicions. A liver panel, consequently, may measure any or all of the following:

- *total protein.* The total level of protein in the blood. An abnormal level, either high or low, may indicate any of a number of problems, including liver disorders, kidney disease, blood cancer, and malnutrition.

- *albumin.* A protein produced in the liver that helps maintain capillary pressure. A low level of ALBUMIN is a general indication of liver damage.

- *bilirubin.* A reddish brown pigment produced in the liver and excreted in bile. Abnormal levels of BILIRUBIN may indicate an obstructed bile flow or some other defect in the way the liver is processing bile.

- *prothrombin time.* How long it takes the blood to clot. Prothrombin is a protein made in the liver required for blood clotting. Liver damage or impaired bile flow can interfere with prothrombin production and affect the ability of the blood to clot.

- *transaminases.* Enzymes produced in the liver to help break down amino acids and manufacture proteins. The two transaminases are alanine aminotransferase (ALT) and aspartate aminotransferase (AST). If liver cells are damaged or dying, ALT and AST leak into the bloodstream. The ALT level is the best test for detecting hepatitis.

- *gamma-glutamyl transpeptidase.* An enzyme released by an injured liver, kidney, or pancreas

- *alkaline phosphatase (ALP).* An enzyme found in the bile. Elevated levels of ALP may indicate blocked BILE DUCTS, an injury to the liver, or certain types of cancer.

- *lactic dehydrogenase.* An enzyme released by a damaged liver, heart, lung, or brain

- *5-nucleotidase (5NT).* An enzyme released by the liver when it has been injured because of a blocked bile duct or other impairment of the bile flow

- *alpha-fetoprotein.* A protein released by the fetal liver or testes, indicating hepatitis or cancer.

- *mitochondrial antibodies.* Antibodies produced against mitochondria, small structures within cells. The presence of mitochondrial antibodies

may indicate CIRRHOSIS, hepatitis, or some other autoimmune disorder.

All these tests can help a clinician with diagnosis; however, it cannot be overemphasized that isolated laboratory test results have little meaning unless considered along with the patient's medical history and physical examination.

liver panel   See LIVER ENZYMES; LIVER-FUNCTION TESTS; LIVER PROTEINS.

liver proteins   The LIVER produces a number of proteins. Measuring the quantity of some of these proteins in the blood can help a doctor determine whether a serious liver disorder is present. Of particular interest are ALBUMIN, prothrombin (blood-clotting factors), and immunoglobulins (antibodies), all of which are primarily synthesized in the liver.

Albumin

Although albumin is only one of the many proteins synthesized by the liver, it has the highest concentration in the blood—about 65 percent of the protein in the blood—and the concentration is easy to measure. The protein is important in regulating fluid balance within the body, and it also transports small molecules, such as calcium and drugs, in the blood. The level of albumin in the blood, which reflects the protein-building capacity of the liver, can help physicians determine whether a patient has liver or kidney disease or whether insufficient protein is being absorbed by the body.

Liver cells secrete albumin and maintain the volume of blood in the arteries and veins. Thus, the protein is important in maintaining the oncotic pressure, the amount of blood in the veins and arteries. A normal range of albumin is generally from 3.5 to 4.5 grams per deciliter (g/dl), depending on the laboratory that does the testing. Albumin has a long half-life in the blood, and measured levels will not fall unless production is decreased for at least several weeks, and possibly a month or more. A low level of albumin is called hypoalbuminemia. It does not necessarily mean there is liver disorder. It may be caused by either expanded plasma volume or decreased albumin synthesis. Low albumin levels are not specific to LIVER DISEASE and may have other causes, including serious malnutrition; malabsorption syndromes, such as Crohn's disease; kidney disease; intestinal disorders; and extensive burns. If the albumin level becomes extremely low, fluid may leak out of blood vessels and into the surrounding tissues. When such a fluid leak occurs, it can cause swelling in the feet and ankles, known as edema. Edema occurs when levels drop below 2.5 g/dl.

A badly damaged liver, however, can no longer produce albumin, and a low albumin count may mean liver dysfunction, as might occur with CIRRHOSIS, moderate or advanced liver dysfunction, HEPATITIS, or liver tissue death (hepatocellular necrosis), among other conditions. Thus, patients with chronic liver disease and cirrhosis have an albumin level usually around 3 g/dl. Edema is common in patients with chronic liver disease, but less common in acute liver disease.

Blood-clotting factors The liver synthesizes most blood clotting factors including factors I (fibrinogen), II (prothrombin), V (proaccelerin), VII (proconvertin), IX (antihemophiliac, factor B, plasma thromboplastin component, christmas factor), and X (Stuart-Power Factor). Deficiency in one or more factors prolongs the time for formation of blood clots. The amount of clotting factors in the blood can decrease rapidly, within days or even hours after severe liver injury. In cases of severe liver disease, low levels of clotting factors may signal a need for an early liver graft.

Unlike the other clotting factors, factor V is not vitamin K–dependent, and measurement can help distinguish vitamin K deficiency from poor functioning of the liver. Serial measurement of factor V levels has been used to assess prognosis in sudden acute liver failure (fulminant hepatic failure). A factor V value of less than 20 percent of normal portends a poor prognosis without LIVER TRANSPLANTATION.

Prothrombin time (PT) The PROTHROMBIN TIME (PT) test measures how long it takes the blood to clot. The liver produces most of the blood-clotting factors, including I, II, V, VII, IX, and X. If the liver function is compromised significantly due to injury or disease, the liver does not create large enough quantities of the factors, and blood takes longer to clot. The prothrombin time—the time needed for blood to clot—normally is between nine and 11 seconds. An abnormally long prothrombin time may put one at risk for excessive bleeding.

Usually, the liver has to be significantly damaged before there is a marked increase in PT. After a severe injury, the clotting factors can decrease rapidly, sometimes within hours. As the liver heals, the PT returns to normal. In contrast, with chronic liver disease there may not be any noticeable change in PT until the liver has been severely damaged and scarred, as in cirrhosis.

Other possible causes of prolonged PT include certain bleeding disorders, blood-thinning medicines, and other medicines that can interfere with the test. Vitamin K is important for blood clotting, and a deficiency of this vitamin can also slow down PT. The deficiency is sometimes due to cholestatic liver disease, a stagnation of bile flow. Because blood-clotting factor V is not dependent on vitamin K, its measurement can help distinguish vitamin K deficiency from liver dysfunction.

Doctors may inject vitamin K to see whether the PT returns to normal. If it does, the liver is still functioning. If not, the patient may be suffering from COAGULOPATHY (tendency to bleed excessively) or a severe liver disease. Liver transplantation may have to be considered in case of liver failure.

Immune globulin Immune globulins (IG) are antibodies of the IMMUNE SYSTEM. Some of them are made by liver cells, and some are made by leukocytes, or white blood cells. Immune globulins are classified according to their structures into five types: IgA, IgD, IgG, IgE, and IgM. The most common is IgG, or gamma globulin, forming about 70 percent of the immunoglobulins in the blood. The variety of immunoglobulins present in the blood may increase in patients suffering from chronic liver disease or other conditions.

Platelet count Platelets are the smallest type of blood cells, and they are part of the primary mechanism for forming blood clots. The spleen stores platelets. In certain liver diseases, the spleen works overtime to compensate for the decreased functioning of the damaged liver and can become enlarged (splenomegaly). Normally, the spleen traps platelets, but this process becomes exaggerated in liver disease, and platelets become trapped within the sinusoids (small pathways) in the spleen. Thus, the number of platelets in the blood may decrease.

A normal platelet count is 15 to 450×10^3/microliter. A low platelet count, thrombocytopenia, is defined as a platelet count of fewer than 150×10^3/microliter. A low platelet count suggests liver disease but is not specific for it.

liver resection Liver resection is the surgical removal of a portion of the LIVER. It is done primarily to cut out different types of tumors. A segment of the liver may also be removed for LIVER TRANSPLANTATION when a living donor elects to donate part of his or her liver to a patient who needs a new liver. Such surgery is possible because the liver can regenerate up to 75 percent—perhaps as much as 80 percent—of its mass, as long as it does not have extensive scarring of its tissue, the hallmark of CIRRHOSIS.

Surgical resection is performed for HEPATO-CELLULAR CARCINOMA (the most common type of tumors that start in the liver), for colorectal metastases (cancer that spread from the colon and rectum), and sometimes for cancer that spread from other sites, such as the lungs. Surgical resection is the only treatment to date considered to be potentially curative of cancer, and against which all other treatments must be measured.

Liver resection is a major operation requiring an experienced and skillful surgeon. Not only is the liver partly covered by the rib cage, it is connected to the heart by many major blood vessels; therefore, surgery is a delicate task. Moreover, liver tissue tears easily. Not until the 1980s, with improvements in imaging studies such as ultrasound and advances in surgical techniques, has surgery to remove primary liver tumors became more common.

Proper surgical evaluation is essential if surgery is to be effective. Accordingly, the physician performs a thorough examination using blood tests and imaging studies to evaluate the patient and determine the best treatment options for that individual. Liver and kidney functions are checked, as well as hemoglobin (a substance inside red blood cells) levels and clotting factors that help stop bleeding. Aside from that, there is a chest X-ray and a pulmonary function test (PFT) to make sure the lungs are clear and in good condition electrocardiogram (ECG) to check for abnormalities in the heart, and an echocardiogram to determine how well the heart is pumping, as the strength of the heart is an important consideration in major surgery.

Every patient should first be considered for liver resection, since surgical removal of tumors is thought to offer the best chance for long-term survival. But not all patients can benefit from having their liver resected or withstand major surgery. Only about 20 percent of patients with LIVER CANCER are good candidates for liver resection. Patients who do not meet the criteria for resection may be referred for other, less invasive treatments. Newer approaches are constantly being developed to treat patients who cannot undergo this operation.

Patients who have the best prognosis if they undergo a resection are generally free of medical problems (except for their liver disease) that might limit their life expectancy. The liver function as measured by tests should be good, and it should be free of cirrhosis—or at least the cirrhosis cannot be at an advanced stage, with no associated complications, such as abdominal swelling or mental confusion. Cirrhotic patients are usually not good candidates for liver surgery because they do not have enough healthy liver tissue left to make surgery safe. If the surgeon cannot ensure that there is enough healthy liver remaining, the patient risks death from liver failure.

Other important factors are the size and location of the tumor. Surgeons today can work with several tumors, but ideally, there should be only a single tumor smaller than five centimeters in diameter. If there are multiple tumors, they should be confined to the liver, and not have spread to other sites. The tumor needs to be accessible as the surgeon can cut out a one-centimeter margin of healthy tissue around the tumor without risking injury to blood vessels or BILE DUCTS.

In recent years, physicians have obtained good results with patients whose original site of cancer was not the colon or rectum—the most common metastatic liver cancer—but only if the patients responded well to chemotherapy and if the tumors had not spread beyond the liver.

There are several different ways to resect a liver, including the following:

- segmentectomy—removing small segments of the liver
- lobectomy—removing one entire lobe of the liver. (The liver has a left and right lobe.)
- partial hepatectomy—partially removing the liver
- trisegmentectomy—removing of three-quarters of the liver
- wedge resection—removing only the immediate area around the tumor

Resecting segments of the liver, as in segmentectomy, allows the surgeon to treat multiple tumors, and helps to preserve more of the liver. This procedure may be followed by chemotherapy to kill miscroscopic tumors that may be present. Whether multiple tumors can be operated on depends on their locations.

When possible, physicians prefer doing a wedge resection because only small amounts of the liver need be removed. However, this procedure is limited to a tumor that is on the surface of the liver; if it is too deep within the liver, a wedge resection poses too much risk of injury to the blood vessels and can cause uncontrolled bleeding.

Procedure

Certain precautions must be taken before any surgery, particularly in regard to what is ingested into the body. Many people today are taking herbal remedies for various conditions, including kava kava for relaxation, garlic to fight infection, and Saint-John's-wort for depression. While herbs can be beneficial when taken properly, many popular ones can act as blood thinners or prolong the sedative effect of anesthesia. Therefore, the American Society of Anesthesiologists recommends that patients scheduled for surgery stop taking all herbal supplements at least two to three weeks before

their surgery, to ensure that the substances have cleared out of the body. Patients should provide the attending physician and the anesthesiologist with a complete list of all herbal remedies, as well as vitamins, supplements, and over-the-counter and prescription drugs. The anesthesiologist should also be informed in advance of any allergies the patient may have.

The operation is performed under general anesthesia. A very large cut—approximately 24 to 30 inches—is made across the abdomen. It starts under the armpit below the ribs on the right side, dips down to the middle, then curves up and continues to the opposite armpit. This cut, called a chevron incision, is vital to make the opening large enough to allow the surgeon complete access to the liver.

After controlling the blood flow in the targeted portion of the liver, the surgeon excises the tumor, leaving as much of the liver as possible, while making sure that the tumor is completely removed. A small margin of liver tissue—around half an inch—surrounding the tumors must also be cut out to make sure that any microscopic cancer cells that may be in the surrounding tissues are removed. An ultrasound gives the surgeon a closer look at the tumor to determine how much of the liver may need to be removed. The amount of liver removed can range from 3 percent to 80 percent, depending on the size and number of tumors. As surgical techniques become more advanced, surgeons can leave even more of the normal liver intact. The operation takes anywhere from two to six hours.

Although still somewhat controversial, there is a growing interest in surgery that does not require blood transfusions. Some surgeons have expertise in performing this so-called bloodless surgery with minor surgeries as well as for major operations like liver resection. The technique of bloodless medicine was initially implemented to treat Jehovah's Witness patients whose religious beliefs prohibit them from receiving blood or blood products; surgeons soon discovered the advantages this technique conferred and began using it on other patients as well. Before surgery, patients build up their own reserve of blood components. Surgeons then conduct the surgery to minimize blood loss.

This approach reduces the risk of infection and immunologic complications and leads to a lower mortality rate. Patients can also expect a shorter recovery time. But not all patients are suited for this type of operation.

After surgery, the patient is taken to a post-operation recovery room where nurses monitor progress. Discomfort at the site of the incision may persist for several weeks. It takes about six weeks for the incision to heal. The doctor can prescribe pain medication for relief. The patient should take no medication without first clearing it with the doctor, as almost all drugs have to be processed by the liver.

Usually, patients are encouraged to get out of bed and walk the day after the surgery, but strenuous activities should be avoided, and weights heavier than five pounds should not be lifted at least for six weeks.

Patients are discharged from the hospital within six to 10 days of the operation, but they can expect to feel more tired than usual for six to eight weeks afterward, and they may lose their appetite. This is normal; while patients can resume most normal activities, they must refrain from pushing themselves too hard, and they should try to eat a healthy, well-balanced diet to help the liver heal and regenerate. Food supplements may be taken under the advise of the physician. No alcohol should be consumed while recuperating from the surgery.

Although part of the liver will be gone after surgery, it will grow back almost to full size in just a few weeks after the resection; regrowth is quite fast initially. The scar from the surgery will remain, but it should fade over time and become less noticeable.

Risks and Complications

Liver resection can be performed with a low mortality rate, but this complex surgical procedure requires an experienced surgeon. The risk of death from liver resection is usually less than 2 percent—though in some cases it can be as high as 5 percent—but there is always a risk that the remaining liver will be unable to function, and the patient die of liver failure.

If there is considerable bleeding during the operation, the patient may be given a blood transfusion afterward. Should the bleeding continue, the patient must be returned to the operating room.

Other complications include the following:

- abscess
- ascites (fluid accumulation in the abdomen)
- bile leakage (greenish yellow fluid that aids in digestion)
- biliary fistula (abnormal passageway in the biliary system)
- bowel obstruction
- liver failure
- pneumonia
- renal (kidney) insufficiency
- wound infection

Contact the physician immediately for any changes for the worse and if there is fever, nausea, abdominal pain, redness, or swelling around the incision.

Outlook and Lifestyle Modification

Patients treated for hepatocellular carcinoma in Western countries have a five-year survival rate of about 27 percent to slightly under 50 percent. Patients with tumors fewer than five centimeters in diameter have higher survival rates than those with larger tumors, and patients without cirrhosis do better than those with cirrhosis.

Patients with colon cancer that spread to the liver have a survival rate of 22 percent to 60 percent. Survival is better for patients who have four or fewer tumors, and with tumors limited to the liver. Patients with primary tumors in the colon also fare better than those with rectal cancer.

When liver resection is successful, the tumor is completely removed and the cancer is stopped from growing and spreading. Unfortunately, however, there is a high risk of new tumors developing somewhere else in the liver, even if all visible tumors are removed at the time of surgery. They usually recur within two years after surgery, in about two-thirds of cases. The reason for this high recurrence is probably because residual microscopic tumor cells undetected at the time of the surgery continued to grow.

It is also possible to perform a liver resection using a laparoscope, a small, tube-shaped instrument with a light on the end to help the doctor view liver tissue for tumors. This procedure, called laparoscopic liver resection, is not yet widely accepted, primarily because bleeding is a possible complication during surgery. Because bleeding is more difficult to control during laparoscopic liver resection, if bleeding does occur, in about 80 percent of cases the laparoscopic procedure must be converted to open surgery. The benefits of laparoscopic procedures are that patients experience less discomfort and recover quicker, have shorter hospital stays, and return to full activities much sooner. Their scars are smaller because the incisions are smaller; there is much less internal scarring as well compared with standard open surgery.

A hand-access device is now available that allows the surgeon to insert the hand into the abdomen for the operation. This new device enables the surgeon to laparoscopically perform a wedge resection, which traditionally was done only as an open surgery.

According to the 2002 results of a multicenter European study published in the *Annals of Surgery*, laparoscopic liver resection of hepatocellular carcinoma is associated with higher incidences of bleeding, the need for blood transfusions, and postoperative complications. The same study concluded, however, that patients with hepatocellular carcinoma could probably be resected safely if they did not have cirrhosis of the liver, and as long as a surgical team experienced with laparoscopic surgery performed the technique. Surgeons should take care to obtain a one-centimeter margin of healthy tissue surrounding the tumor, as these margins were often missing in laparoscopic resection.

Despite improvements in imaging techniques, the report also emphasized the important diagnostic role that explorative laparoscopy ought to play in detecting and staging malignant tumors.

Although more studies are needed to evaluate this controversial technique, laparoscopic liver resection is feasible, and may become more common in the future.

Blumgart, L. H., and Y. Fong. "Surgical options in the treatment of hepatic metastasis from colorectal cancer." *Current Problems in Surgery* 5, no. 32 (May 1995): 333–421.

DiCarlo, I., and colleagues. "Liver metastases from lung cancer: Is surgical resection justified?" *Annals of Thoracic Surgery* 1, no. 76 (2003): 291–293.

Elias, D., J.-F. Ouellet, Bellon No., et al. "Extrahepatic disease does not contraindicate hepatectomy for colorectal liver metastases." *British Journal of Surgery* no. 90 (2003): 567–574.

Gigot, Jean-François M.D., et al. "Laparoscopic liver resection for malignant liver tumors: Preliminary results of a multicenter European study." *Annals of Surgery* 1, no. 236 (2002): 90–97.

Scheele, J., R. Stangl, A. Altendorf-Hofmann, and M. G. Paul. "Resection of colorectal liver metastases." *World Journal of Surgery* 1, no. 19 (January–February): 59–71.

Weber, J. C., et al. "Laparoscopic radiofrequency-assisted liver resection." *Surgical Endoscopy and other International Techniques* 17, no. 5 (August 2003): 87–95.

liver transplantation Transplantation is an operation that replaces a diseased organ with a healthy one, usually from another person. In the case of a liver transplant, either an entire LIVER or part of one can be transplanted. This treatment is for people whose livers have failed or been damaged through illness or injury.

Transplantation was once regarded as an experimental operation, but today it is a standard medical procedure. Liver transplantation is the second most common type of organ transplant in the United States; the most common organ transplant is a kidney. In the year 2002 alone, 5,329 operations were performed. Transplant patients can expect to lead a normal lifestyle and have an excellent quality of life.

During the 1950s and 1960s, liver transplant experiments were conducted on animals. The first human-to-human liver transplant was performed in 1963 by Dr. Thomas E. Starzl at the University of Colorado in Denver. The first, as well as a number of subsequent attempts, failed. Aside from the technical challenges of the operation itself, one of the biggest hurdles to successful transplantation has been rejection of the new organ by the recipient's immune system—the immune system recognizes the new organ as foreign tissue and tries to destroy it.

A breakthrough came in 1966 with the development of immunosuppressant drugs that treat organ rejection by suppressing the immune system. Immediately thereafter, in 1967, Starzl performed the first successful liver transplant on a girl with LIVER CANCER. She lived for 13 years before succumbing to recurring cancer.

In the early days, the survival rate was 30 percent in the first year. Subsequently, more effective IMMUNOSUPPRESSANTS were developed, further refinements were made to the techniques of liver transplantation, and methods for preserving donor organs were improved. With the introduction of cyclosporine, a highly effective immunosuppressant, success rates for liver transplantation reached 85 percent. Today, approximately 85 to 90 percent of patients survive for one year, and the five-year survival rate for patients at most centers is approximately 80 to 90 percent.

The demand for liver transplantation has been increasing. But the organs available have not kept pace with this demand. Thus, the shortage of available organs has led to the refinement in the past few years of various techniques for extending the usage of available organs, as well as the use of organs from live donors, usually from family members or relatives.

The several different types of transplantation procedures are defined by whether a whole liver or only a portion is transplanted, the source of the liver, and whether the patient's diseased or damaged liver is removed or left in place.

The standard and most common type of transplant uses the orthotopic approach, also called cadaveric whole transplant. The recipient's liver is removed and replaced with a whole liver taken from a brain-dead person.

In the heterotopic approach, also called an AUXILIARY LIVER TRANSPLANT, the patient's own liver is left intact, and a small portion of a donor's liver is placed next to it. The donor liver is usually attached very near the original liver, and the donor liver supports the patient's existing liver function. This procedure is often done when there is a possibility that the afflicted liver may recover. If the original liver recovers its functions, the donor liver shrivels away. (The patient may also be instructed to stop taking immunosuppressive drugs to allow the donor liver to be rejected.) If the original liver does not recover, it may shrivel away, leaving the donor liver to take its place.

In a living donor transplant, a lobe or section from the liver of a healthy living donor, usually family, relative or close friend, is given to a patient with a diseased liver. The liver has considerable ability to regenerate, and if the portions are large enough, the parts in the donor and in the recipient will each grow back to nearly normal liver size and regain full function. Patients have survived with only 15 to 20 percent of their original liver intact, as long as that portion was healthy.

In a SPLIT-LIVER TRANSPLANTATION, a donor liver is split into two parts and given to two separate people. New surgical techniques allow one liver to be used by two different recipients. Often, a smaller portion of the liver is given to a child or an infant, and the larger portion is given to an adult. The child needs only a small portion of an adult-size liver, while in the adult, the liver can grow to full size because of the liver's regenerative capacity. In recent years, surgeons have improved their techniques, and now donor livers can be split into two portions, each of which can be transplanted into an adult recipient.

XENOTRANSPLANTATION is an experimental procedure in which a liver from an animal is transplanted into the human body. Scientists became interested in using animal organs because of the shortage of human organs. And animal livers are resistant to infection by human viruses, such as hepatitis viruses. Therefore, an animal liver may eliminate viral replication in the transplanted organ, a problem that often happens with human donor organs in hepatitis patients. Most commonly, pig livers are used.

Obviously, liver transplantation entails a significant risk to the patient, and that risk must be weighed against the risks of disease progression and disability from the underlying liver disease. In general, a liver transplant is indicated if the patient develops life-threatening complications from the liver disease, or if all standard medical approaches have been exhausted and it appears that the patient will die within two years without a new liver.

A transplant may also be considered if the patient faces incapacitating symptoms and progressive disability that reduce quality of life to an unacceptable level, such as inability to work, social disability, and repeated hospitalizations. That means liver transplantation may be deemed the appropriate course for patients with liver failure, whether from acute or chronic liver disease. For instance, patients may show advanced JAUNDICE (yellowing of the skin and eyes), progressively elevated BILIRUBIN in their LIVER-FUNCTION TESTS, or recurrent mental confusion and impairment (encephalopathy) due to CIRRHOSIS, and these conditions cannot be adequately controlled by dietary measures.

Below are listed the common conditions that may necessitate a transplant surgery:

- progressive HEPATITIS, usually due to viral infection but may also be from alcoholic and autoimmune hepatitis

- abnormalities of the biliary system, such as primary sclerosing cholangitis

- BILIARY ATRESIA, the most common indication for transplantation in children

- liver damage from alcohol abuse

- PORTAL HYPERTENSION

- liver tumors

Once a patient is identified as a potential transplant recipient, it is usually better to refer her or him to an institute with transplantation capabilities earlier in the course of the disease, even though a donor organ may not be available immediately. A PRE-TRANSPLANT EVALUATION several years before the operation is necessary may be preferable to waiting until the operation becomes an emergency. It may be difficult for the patient to travel later, when he or she is seriously ill. Also, from the standpoint of the transplant team, early referral allows a more thorough evaluation. In addition, the patient can obtain nutritional support before the operation to forestall at least some of the severe loss of muscle and fat that occurs when advanced liver disease limits the patient's intake of nutrients.

Fulminant hepatic failure—severe and acute failure of the liver—requires immediate liver transplantation, possibly as an emergency measure.

Examples of such severe liver failure include situations when the patient has gone into a coma or has progressed to excessive bleeding (COAGULOPATHY) that cannot be corrected. Fulminant hepatic failure typically occurs during acute viral hepatitis, but it may also result from toxic reactions to some medicines, such as an overdose of acetaminophen (Tylenol) or from mushroom poisoning.

Liver transplantation is a very expensive operation, but expenses can be reduced if patients are referred early enough so that they are sufficiently healthy to wait for transplantation surgery at home rather than in the hospital. Whether insurance covers the cost of transplantation depends on the policy.

Improved technical skills and the availability of more powerful and effective immunosuppressive medication make transplants attractive for treatment of more disorders and more patients. Partly as a result of the success of liver transplants, worldwide demand for organs is increasing, and there is a severe shortage of available livers. According to data kept by the UNITED NETWORK FOR ORGAN SHARING (UNOS), which oversees the national system for organ sharing and has a contract with the federal government to manage transplant data and the allocation of livers, there were 17,327 candidates on the national waiting list as of September 2003. According to the Eurotransplant International Foundation, the second-largest organ procurement system in the world, the demand for donor organs is increasing by 15 percent yearly.

Most liver donations come from brain-dead human donors. Organs are screened to eliminate those with a poor chance of functioning in the transplant recipient. The liver cannot be used if the potential donor has had human immunodeficiency virus HIV, cancer, bacterial or fungal infection, or HEPATITIS B. The liver should have no more than 30 percent fat, because FATTY LIVERS do not function well when transplanted. Recently, some of the requirements have been relaxed to ease the shortage of available organs. For instance, livers of donors who had HEPATITIS C virus (HCV) may be used if the recipient has hepatitis C. Although donors under the age of 50 were preferred initially, recent studies show that age is generally not associated with higher rates of complications or death in organ recipients. Therefore, the donor's age is usually not relevant.

The donor liver has to be matched in size and blood type with the recipient. Preferably, the donor should be the same size or larger than the recipient. If the liver is too large, it can be reduced in size. Most people have natural antibodies in their blood that would destroy an organ from someone of a different blood type, so the donor and the recipient should have compatible blood types.

Procedure

The patient is asked to undergo preoperative tests and is given medications, including immunosuppressants to suppress the immune response to keep the body from rejecting the new liver. The patient may be given an enema to clean out the intestines. The patient is put to sleep with a general anesthetic. During the procedure, the patient is given IV fluids and sedatives, and tubes are inserted into the throat to assist with breathing and into the bile duct to help drain the bile. The bile duct is a small tube that carries bile made in the liver to the intestines.

A team of about 10 physicians, nurses, technicians, and assistants work together in the operating room. The surgeon makes a Y-shaped incision about a foot long from one side of the rib cage to the other to open the abdominal cavity. Special retractors hold the abdominal cavity open. The surgeons detach the diseased liver from the four main blood vessels and bile ducts between the liver and the intestine. A small cylindrical device called a stent is placed in a bile duct. This makes it possible for doctors to monitor the function of the new liver. The stent remains in place until approximately six weeks after the transplant.

A segment of the inferior vena cava, the largest vein in the body, which is attached to the liver and returns blood to the heart from the lower part of the body, is taken from the donor. The new healthy donor liver is inserted in the same anatomical location as that of the old liver. First, the veins are connected, followed by the artery and the bile duct, then the blood flow is restored. After making sure that the new organ is functioning properly, the clamps are removed and the surgeon closes the incision. The operation lasts anywhere from four to twelve hours.

Immediately after the operation, the patient is taken to the intensive care unit (ICU) and monitored closely. The patient is put on a respirator and will continue to receive IV fluids and medications to prevent rejection of the new liver, and will have a bladder catheter to drain urine. Other medications are given, such as those to fight infection. Some patients may need kidney dialysis for a few days. Care will be given to ensure that the bowels, fluid levels, and blood pressure all return to normal. Blood bilirubin concentration and liver enzyme activities will be closely monitored to see whether the new liver is functioning. Unless there are complications, the patient is moved from the ICU the following day to an inpatient floor of the hospital. There will be some pain during recovery, but the discomfort can be alleviated with medication.

The patient may stay in the hospital for anywhere between one to six weeks, although some patients stay much longer. After the operation, the patient receives nutrients delivered directly into the bloodstream intravenously. Soon, the patient transitions to a low-salt, low-potassium diet. Eventually, the patient should be able to resume a normal diet. The patient also will receive physical therapy.

Recovery time varies. Most patients can resume a normal life after receiving a new organ. Usually, the patient can return to normal activities, including work, about six months to a year after surgery. But, the time frame can vary considerably with individuals, and patients should talk to their doctors about what to expect.

Risks and Complications

One major complication of surgery is bleeding. Patients often have massive blood loss during surgery, possibly requiring transfusion of many units of red blood cells, fresh frozen plasma, and platelets. The most common complications after surgery are rejection of the transplanted liver and infection.

When one receives a whole or partial organ from another person, the recipient's body recognizes the foreign tissue and becomes sensitized against it. Rejection occurs when the body mounts an immune response to destroy and eliminate the foreign tissue from the body. Some degree of rejection is inevitable with every transplant. Patients can expect at least one episode of acute rejection—the body tries to destroy the transplanted organ—within the first year after a transplant. Rejection can usually be controlled with powerful and effective antirejection medications.

Because immunosuppressive agents, used to prevent organ rejection, block the body's immune defense, they also prevent the body from mounting an effective attack against bacteria and viruses. Therefore, patients are more vulnerable to infections of all kinds, including fungal, viral, and parasitic. Indeed, infection is the leading cause of death after transplantation. About half of patients experience infection, which usually appears during the first week after surgery. Such infections can be treated with the proper medication. Careful patient monitoring is important.

The body is also less resistant to cancer, including leukemias and lymphomas, due to the use of immunosuppressants. The patient may also develop pseudolymphoma, a kind of tumor often associated with Epstein-Barr infection. Reducing the dosage of the immunosuppressants may resolve the tumor.

Another, less frequent complication is the failure of the new organ to function. This is usually observed shortly after transplantation. The new liver may be damaged, or sometimes there is no apparent cause. Sometimes the new liver succumbs to infection or is rejected by the recipient. In addition, there may be problems with the lungs, kidneys, excessive bleeding, or operative techniques. If the complications are serious, the patient may need re-transplantation.

Other medical complications can occur. For instance, the original disease that inhabited the liver could return. This is often true of hepatitis viruses. Some relatively rare complications that can usually be controlled through medical or surgical interventions include high blood pressure (hypertension), blood clots in the main artery or vein to the liver (thrombosis), obstruction of the bile ducts, and bleeding in the gastrointestinal tract.

Outlook and Lifestyle Modification

Receiving a transplant involves a major lifestyle change that can cause patients and their families to experience anxiety, stress, and depression. They should not hesitate to seek help from a social worker or other counselor to deal with these changes. Professionals can help with various issues such as work, finances, marital conflicts, parent-child conflicts, and so forth, whether or not they are directly related to the transplantation.

During the late 1990s, Dr. Elmahdi Elkhammas and Dr. Mitchell Henry of the Ohio State University Medical Center developed a procedure that reduces the risks often associated with the highly complex transplant surgery. This new technique shaves about one hour and a half off the surgery time and reduces the amount of blood used by about 25 percent, compared with the traditional transplant procedure. The method involves rerouting of blood flow in the inferior vena cava, a major vein in the liver, which allows surgeons to perform some of the more intricate work before the donor liver is placed in the recipient's abdomen. According to Elkhammas, "We get the same excellent results by rerouting the blood flow. In addition, the patient spends less time under anesthetic and recovers more quickly, and we're able to save from three to five units of blood products per surgery." The decreased blood loss and time under anesthesia reduce the risk to the patient.

Researchers are also working on a nonsurgical approach, called the hepatocyte transplant. Small numbers of liver cells (hepatocytes) from a donor liver are infused into the recipient's liver, rather than transplanting an entire liver. There have been only limited attempts and the procedure is still in early clinical stages, but it looks promising for treatment of acute liver failure.

Pediatric Liver Transplantation

Many advances have occurred in the field of liver transplantation in the past 30 years, raising the five-year survival rate of infants and children from a low of 20 percent before 1980 to a high of nearly 80 percent today. The first successful liver transplant on a child was performed in 1967, but transplant operations remained rare because mortality remained quite high. Another problem was the often debilitating side effects from the high-dose immunosuppressants the patients had to take to counter organ rejection. These included serious infections, growth retardation, and cataracts. New medications such as cyclosporine made it possible to reduce the dosage and thus substantially reduce the side effects. These improvements have made liver transplantation today an appropriate treatment for end-stage liver disease for both pediatric and adult patients.

As liver transplants have become more successful, the greatest hurdle for infants and children awaiting a new liver has become the lack of suitable organs for transplantation, a shortage even more critical than that for adults, particularly for infants weighing less than 10 kilograms. It is estimated that some 25 to 50 percent die while waiting for transplantation because appropriate donors cannot be found. The time period varies greatly on the pediatric patient's relative state of health and underlying disease process.

Many advances of the past 30 years, such as innovative surgical techniques, the procurement of organs, and infection control and immunosuppressive medications, have greatly increased the odds for survival. Innovative surgical techniques that have vastly increased the number of donor organs for children (as well as small adults) include cut-down liver transplantation, split-liver transplantation, and partial transplantation from living related donors. These three procedures evolved by utilizing the principle that as long as there was sufficient mass and certain components of the liver such as the bile duct, the organ could function.

Cut-down, or reduced-size liver transplantation makes it possible to use an adult liver that may weigh 10 times more than the infant's liver. Since the adult donor's large hepatic artery (blood vessel that carries blood from the heart to the liver) can be used, it also reduces the risk of forming a blood clot within the artery (thrombosis), which can lead to graft failure.

Split-liver transplant allows a single liver to be divided into two lobes and given to two recipients. The smaller, left lobe is given to the child.

The liver's ability to regenerate and grow back to its full size has made it possible for family and relatives to donate a section of their liver to the child with minimal risks and complications. The advantages of using a living-related donor are the timeliness of the surgery and the quality of the graft. Since there is no need to wait for a suitable donor organ, the transplantation can be done electively, rather than as an emergency when severe, irreversible complications of the liver may already have developed. A graft from a living donor generally ensures good quality (sometimes cadaveric livers can be compromised in quality), and in theory at least the parent or relative and child have a similar tissue type, which reduces the risk of acute and chronic organ rejection.

Postoperative risks to the donor are minimal, as the volume of the organ removed is rarely more than 30 to 40 percent when the recipient is a child. Either a full lobe or only the left lateral segment is taken.

The most common indication for liver replacement in infants and children is biliary atresia, an inherited disorder that causes obstruction in bile flow. Transplantation can also restore the health of patients with metabolic disorders such as ALPHA-1-ANTITRYPSIN DEFICIENCY and Crigler-Najjar syndrome.

In young infants with biliary atresia, an operation called a Kasai portoenterostomy is performed to replace the missing external biliary system with a segment of the infant's own intestine. This surgery may correct the problem, though in most cases it is not completely successful and the patient needs a transplant, either immediately or when older.

The doctor may recommend that children complete a basic immunization series before the transplantation because the immune system will be chronically suppressed with medication. Parents will want to explore the best course of action for their child.

New medications have made it less likely that the patient will suffer from organ rejection or infections, the two main complications of transplantation. Advances are expected in the use of ARTIFICIAL AND BIO-ARTIFICIAL LIVERS, animal livers, and gene therapy, though they remain controversial.

Broelsch, C. E., P. F. Whitington, J. C. Edmond, et al. "Liver transplantation in children from living related donors." *Annals of Surgery,* 1991.

Cox, Kenneth L. "Recent advances in pediatric liver transplantation." *Western Journal of Medicine,* 158, no. 2 (February 1993): 178(1).

Dickson, E. Rolland, Lynne S. Evans, Raymong S. Koff, Seymour M. Sabesin, Byers W. Shaw, and Erik Lenk. "Who's a liver transplant candidate?" *Patient Care* 21, no. 4 (September 30, 1987): 83.

Fackelmann, K. A. *Science News* 136, no. 23 (December 2, 1989): 358(1).

Kocoshis, Samuel A., Andreas Tzakis, Satoru Todo, Jorge Reyes, and Bakr Nour. "Pediatric liver transplantation: History, recent innovations, and outlook for the future." *Clinical Pediatrics,* 32, no. 7 (July 1993): 386(7).

Macleod, A. M., and A. W. Thomson. "FK 506: An immunosuppressant for the 1990s?" *Lancet* 337, no. 8732 (January 5, 1991): 25(3).

McCarthy, M., and M. L. Wilkinson. "Recent advances: Hepatology." *British Medical Journal* 318, no. 7193 (May 8, 1999): 1,256–1,259.

"New technique reduces time, risk for liver transplants." Reported by Ohio State University Medical Center. Oct. 31, 2001. Available online. URL: http://www.sciencedaily.com. Accessed in April 2004.

Polsdorfer, J. Ricker. "Liver transplantation." *Gale Encyclopedia of Medicine.* Vol. 1. Farmington Hills, Mich.: Thomson Gale, 1999, p. 1,797.

Van Thiel, D. H., R. R. Schade, T. E. Starzl, et al. "Liver transplantation in adults." *Hepatology* (1982): 637–640.

liver tumors　A physician examining a liver using radiological studies (imaging studies such as ultrasound and CT scan) often finds abnormal masses in the liver, which may be seen as "lesions," or "spots" in the liver. These liver masses are otherwise known as liver tumors. They are liver cells that have proliferated into abnormal growths that serve no function in the body.

Advances in radiological techniques have made the discovery of such liver masses more probable. They may be detected accidentally in the course of evaluating the patient for a non-liver-related condition. At other times, the tumors may be discovered because the patient has symptoms of possible liver disease.

It may also be that patients visited the clinic for their regular cancer screening. Doctors often recommend that people who have a higher risk for developing liver cancer should be screened every six months to a year.

Many people become frightened at the mention of tumors, but liver tumors are not necessarily fatal. Tumors can be benign or malignant.

BENIGN LIVER TUMORS are not cancerous. The growth of the cells in the tumor, cyst, lump, tissue, or cells is under control and these tumors will not spread to nearby tissue or to other parts of the body. There are many types of benign tumors; the most common are hemangioma, hepatic adenoma, and focal nodular hyperplasia. Hemangiomas rarely cause symptoms and do not require treatment. Adenomas are much more rare, but can be seen in women who have been taking contraceptive pills or receiving high-dose hormone replacement therapy. They usually disappear when the pills or hormones are discontinued.

Malignant tumors are cancerous and potentially fatal. All cells of the body are constantly growing and dividing, replacing dead and damaged cells. Normally, this process is orderly and controlled. But for various reasons this mechanism occasionally fails, and some cells continue to divide and to grow, turning into a tumor.

Broadly, malignant tumors can be categorized into two different types of LIVER CANCER: primary liver cancer and metastatic liver cancer. In primary liver cancers, the cancer starts within the liver tissue itself. Sometimes cancer cells that originated in another organ or area of the body break away and travel to other parts of the body through the bloodstream or lymphatic system. The cancer is said to have metastasized then. Cancer cells spread most often to the liver because the liver acts as a filtration system for the blood. Metastatic liver cancer is cancer that started somewhere else in the body and spread to the liver. Anyone discovered to have cancerous growths requires a thorough medical examination to determine the type of cancer so the appropriate treatment can be given.

Whenever tumors are found in the liver, it is necessary to conduct further testing to determine the exact nature of the mass. Taking a comprehensive medical history of the patient and blood tests cannot determine whether a tumor is benign; nor are radiological scans sufficient for that purpose. When a diagnosis is uncertain, the doctor may take some tissue sampling—LIVER BIOPSY—to make a diagnosis. A biopsy carries the risk of increased bleeding because many tumors have an abundant supply of blood vessels. Using extra-fine needles can reduce such a risk. If the tumor happens to be malignant, there is a risk, though very small, that the needle may break the tumor and "seed," or spread, it into other parts of the liver.

Sometimes surgery to remove the tumor may be necessary if it cannot be confidently determined that the tumor is benign, or if the doctor believes there is a likelihood that it could turn malignant later.

See also HEPATOCELLULAR CARCINOMA.

Diagnosing Liver Tumors

A diagnosis of liver tumors starts with the doctor checking the patient's history for risk factors. There may be no symptoms at this point, but the doctor gives a physical examination first and pays close attention to the condition of the patient's abdomen. Pressing around the liver area with the patient lying flat on the examination table, the doctor may detect that the liver, and sometimes the spleen, is enlarged. The liver is swollen and hard, and there may be soreness or tenderness in the area. The doctor may be able to feel an abnormal mass or a swelling in the abdomen, caused by an accumulation of fluids. Sometimes it is possible to feel masses or lumps in the liver. Another possible sign of liver tumor is an abnormal sound, a rubbing noise called bruit, when the doctor uses a stethoscope to listen to the blood vessels near the liver. The pressure of the tumor on the vessels makes this noise. Not all these signs will be present, however.

Chest X-rays may be taken to find out whether the tumor has spread from the lungs in the event that malignant tumors are discovered.

No simple tests can positively identify liver tumors, especially in early cases, and the tests must be interpreted in context with various diagnostic modalities, including the following:

- blood tests
- diagnostic imaging (radiological tests)
- liver biopsy or laparoscopy

The most widely used blood test, called ALPHA-FETOPROTEIN (AFP), is generally used to diagnose primary liver cancer. AFP is a tumor marker that is often elevated in patients with hepatocellular carcinoma (HCC). It is only rarely elevated in CHOLANGIOCARCINOMA, a cancer of the bile ducts within the liver.

AFP testing is the cornerstone of screening methods because it can be measured simply and inexpensively. However, the values can be raised in cases of cirrhosis or viral hepatitis, even in the absence of cancerous cells. Conversely, tumors smaller than five centimeters in diameter often do not cause any elevations in AFP. Thus, AFP does not catch every patient with HCC; it detects only about two-third of patients. Some doctors have begun to use an additional blood test called DES-GAMMA-CARBOXYPROTHROMBIN (DCP).

Other tumor markers include carcinoembryonic antigen (CEA) and carbohydrate antigen 19-9 (CEA 19-9).

CEA is most sensitive for liver cancer that has spread from the colon or rectum. An estimated 75 to 90 percent of these patients have an elevated CEA. Only 10 percent of patients with intrahepatic cholangiocarcinoma—bile duct cancer—have elevated levels of CEA. A rapidly rising level of CEA suggests that the cancer may have spread to the liver.

CA19-9 levels are often elevated in patients with intrahepatic cholangiocarcinoma, in contrast to AFP, which is elevated in HCC.

Noninvasive diagnostic imaging techniques Many noninvasive techniques are available today to image the liver to diagnose tumors. They can generally identify tumors more than one centimeter in diameter (about three-eighths of an inch). These imaging techniques have improved considerably in the past few decades, in some cases avoiding unnecessary surgery.

Ultrasound (sonography) is often the first choice for a diagnosis because it is inexpensive and well tolerated by patients. It is useful for detecting the location and number of tumors. The drawback, however, is that it is very operator-dependent; the skill of the operator can affect its accuracy.

Tumors as small as 0.5 to 1 cm may be detected by ultrasound. Ultrasound can also detect the number of tumors and location and indicate how close they are to blood vessels. If they are too close, they may be difficult to remove surgically.

A more in-depth analysis of the liver can be obtained through computed tomography and magnetic resonance imaging.

Computed tomography (CT) scanning works best in providing an overview of the entire abdomen. It is the standard imaging technique for viewing the liver. Although it is not as sensitive as ultrasound, it is useful for assessing the extent of the tumors within the gallbladder or bile duct. The CT scan can also be conducted with the injection of an iodinated material that is soluble in fat into the blood vessels. Precancerous growths and cancers tend to take up and store this material more than normal cells do. Injection of this contrast material increases the sensitivity of CT scanning for cancerous cells.

Magnetic resonance imaging (MRI) is safe and gives detailed images, allowing liver lesions to be more precisely defined. It is better at imaging liver tumors that have a great deal of blood flow. But the MRI does require longer imaging times and the quality of the image is less consistent than that of the CT.

The MRI is generally considered to be superior to CT in investigating liver disease. But both the CT scan and the MRI scan can accurately show the relationship of the tumor or tumors to the major blood vessels entering and leaving the liver, as well as the bile ducts and other important structures inside the liver. It is important to determine this in order to determine whether the tumors can be safely removed.

Magnetic resonance cholangiopancreotography (MRCP) provides a detailed view of the bile ducts and is useful for examining tumors in the ducts. The positron emission tomography (PET) scan is effective at detecting diseases that may exist outside the liver. Therefore, it is especially useful in patients who are suffering from metastatic cancer that spread from other places in the body. The PET is more sophisticated at viewing sites outside the liver than the CT scan and the MRI, which are not good at identifying small tumors that may have spread to the lymph nodes or other places in the body.

Although imaging studies are useful in locating abnormal tissue in the abdomen, and differentiating between cancerous cells and normal tissue or some benign tumors, they cannot distinguish between cancer originating in the liver or spreading from another site. Because each radiologic examination has its own advantages and disadvantages, a combination of tests is used at times.

Invasive diagnostic techniques   To make the definitive diagnosis of cancer, a sample of tissue must be removed and examined under a microscope to determine whether any cancer cells are present. This is the only way to confirm that an abnormality in the liver is cancer. The LIVER BIOPSY may be performed with a CT or ultrasound to guide the doctor in locating the tumor. Normally, CTs or ultrasounds are not needed to do a biopsy, but they may be used when there are tumors and the doctor needs to select the best site for a tissue sample. A biopsy is done only if the doctor feels the tissue can be removed safely. There is the risk of excessive bleeding, as well as a small risk of "seeding" a cancer—spreading the cancer cells along the course of the biopsy needle.

In a procedure called laparoscopy, an instrument called a laparoscope may be used. This small, tube-shaped instrument with a light at the end helps the doctor view the area and remove a small piece of liver tissue to be examined for the presence of cancer cells. An incision is made in the abdomen for this.

Ultrasound can also be performed using a laparoscope if malignancies are suspected after a radiological examination. It is used to evaluate the malignancies and to determine the stage they are in.

Another application of ultrasound is with open surgery (intraoperative sonography). This allows the sonographic probe to come into direct contact with the liver surface, allowing detection of tumors as small as three millimeters, and providing exact anatomic resolution.

A device called an endoscope may be used to examine the interior lining of a body cavity, such as the stomach, colon, or BILE DUCTS.

To examine the bile ducts more closely, they may be injected with a dye. This requires a needle to be inserted into the bile ducts within the liver. This procedure is called cholangiography.

An examination called a catheter angiography may also be performed to determine whether the cancer originated in the liver (primary liver cancer) or spread from another part of the body (metastatic liver cancer). The doctor has to visualize the blood vessels. To do so, the blood vessels are dyed so that they can be seen on an X-ray. The dye is injected through a catheter (tube) inserted into the main blood vessel carrying blood to the liver.

It is not easy to detect liver cancer in its early, most treatable, stage. In fact, it is possible that blood tests will show minimal abnormalities, even when half or more of the liver is consumed by cancer. Accordingly, it is extremely important that an evaluation be made on the strength of multiple diagnostic modalities and a careful assessment of the patient's medical history.

Okuda, H., T. Nakanishi, K. Takatsu, et al. "Clinico-pathologic features of patients with hepatocellular carcinoma seropositive for alpha-fetoprotein-L3 and seronegative for des-gamma carboxyprothrombin in comparison with those seropositive for des-gamma-carboxyprothrombin." *Journal of Gastroenterological Hepatology* 17 (2002): 772–778.

medications for treating chronic hepatitis B As many new medications are being developed for HEPATITIS B, health care providers have a wider choice when they need to switch their patients to different medications, either because of side effects or drug resistance. Currently, about half of patients being treated for chronic hepatitis B acquire drug resistance after two to three years. Researchers are working on a new test that may help to predict which patients may be more likely to develop drug resistance, according to the type of hepatitis B virus that infects them.

Conventional Interferon

INTERFERON therapy (IFN) was found to be effective for chronic HBV patients in 1988. Interferon is also commonly used to treat HEPATITIS C. Only interferon-alpha 2b (Intron A) is approved for the treatment of hepatitis B in the United States. Interferon is a naturally occurring protein produced by the body's white blood cells to help combat infection. Interferon has two functions: it stimulates the body's immune system into eliminating the virus, and it affects the ability of viruses to divide in liver cells.

Many types of interferon are produced by the body, including beta interferon and gamma interferon. For treatment of HBV, dosage is usually 5 million units daily, or 10 million units three times per week for four to six months. The drug is given by injection, self-administered by the patient. The injection is subcutaneous, going just under the skin; it does not need to go deep into the muscle, as with a flu shot. Therapy is usually from four to six months.

Treatment with IFN has been shown to suppress HBV reproduction and improve long-term outcome and survival rate, reducing the risk of disease progression and complications. Therapy is intended to reduce liver inflammation and convert the infection from B e antigen positive (HBeAg+) to B e antigen negative (HBeAg–). This reversal is called seroconversion. About one-third to one-half of patients will be able to clear the B e antigen from their blood.

Studies indicate that many patients experience fewer liver-related complications as a result of taking IFN. One Canadian study suggests that treating with IFN alone (monotherapy) may delay or prevent LIVER CANCER in patients with advanced scarring of the liver, but in general, this is not the recommended treatment approach. With other medications available today, other drugs or combinations of drugs are usually preferred.

IFN therapy is usually not as effective for people who acquired hepatitis B at birth (as is the case for many Asians) or for those with mutant strains of HBV.

The biggest drawbacks of IFN are the medication's side effects, which some patients find difficult or intolerable, and the inconvenience of having to inject the drug three times a week. Side effects include flu-like symptoms such as fever, chills, headaches, muscle or joint aches, tiredness, and weakness. In some cases patients may need to discontinue the treatment because the side effects become too difficult to manage. The doctor may recommend other medications then. For instance, lamivudine (see below) has almost no side effects and is well tolerated by patients, especially those who have CIRRHOSIS with associated complications. A number of studies have shown an improvement in liver function with lamivudine. In general, cirrhotic patients, even if they have only mild complications from the extensive liver scarring, should not be treated with IFN, as they may experience adverse effects. Adefovir is another drug that patients may try if IFN does not work.

Patients who have high levels of HBV DNA and low alanine aminotrasferase (ALT) values when they begin treatment are usually not as responsive to treatment as patients with lower HBV DNA levels and higher ALT values. Unfortunately, even in patients who have been selected according to criteria that predict a good outcome, response rates for the most part are disappointing. It appears that the majority of patients with chronic hepatitis B do not respond to treatment with interferon.

Treatment with Pegylated IFN

A newer version of interferon, pegylated interferon, seems to offer advantages over standard interferon. Pegylated IFN was developed through a process that produces a drug with a prolonged half-life, which means that it stays in the body longer without losing its effectiveness. The Food and Drug Administration (FDA) has approved Schering-Plough's pegylated interferon product, Peg-intron (peginterferon alfa-2b), as well as Roche's Pegasys. Available studies cannot clearly show whether one brand of pegylated interferon is more effective than the other.

One of the advantages of pegylated IFN is that because it stays in the body longer, patients need only one injection a week instead of the customary three with conventional IFN, and that it does not require dosing by body weight.

A second advantage is that pegylated IFN seems to be more effective than conventional IFN. Studies suggest that more patients are able to convert from B e antigen positive to B e antigen negative than those treated with conventional IFN. In addition, even patients who have a more-difficult-to-treat HBV infection—such as those who have lower ALT levels and high levels of HBV DNA—appear to respond better than they do with conventional IFN.

Side effects reported by patients are about the same as for conventional IFN.

Treatment with Lamivudine

Lamivudine (3'-thiacytidine) is an antiviral agent that was initially evaluated as a treatment for AIDS patients infected with human immunodeficiency virus (HIV). Because HBV uses reproductive mechanisms similar to HIV, drugs developed for HIV are often effective. Lamivudine (LVD; LAM) is a nucleoside drug. These drugs slow viral reproduction. Unlike interferon, nucleosides do not have any direct effect on the immune system.

Experts often recommend lamivudine as the first line of therapy, and it is suggested that treatment continue until HBV DNA is no longer detectable in the blood. The usual dosage is 100 milligrams orally once a day. Treatment may last from three months to a year.

One study showed that after 12 months of taking 100 milligrams of lamivudine daily, the seroconversion rates (from detectable amounts of the B e antigen in their blood, to no detectable B e antigen in the blood) ranged from 17 to 21 percent. Other studies have shown higher response rates. But in almost all cases, after patients stopped taking the medication, about half reverted to pre-treatment status. In other words, B e antigen could be found in the blood again.

The main advantage of lamivudine is that it has few side effects, and it is thus much easier for patients to continue the therapy. It is also easier for patients to administer because it is taken orally rather than by injection, as with interferon. Therefore, unlike interferon, lamivudine is well tolerated by most people. Another advantage is that lamivudine can be used by patients with advanced cirrhosis.

Hepatitis B carriers undergoing immunosuppressive or cancer chemotherapies, especially when corticosteroids are included, tend to have flares and reactivation of HBV replication, because their immune systems are suppressed. Administration of LVD has been reported to reduce the frequency and severity of the hepatitis flares and to improve survival.

Lamivudine is now being used before and after LIVER TRANSPLANTATION to prevent recurrent infection in the liver graft. LVD is given alone or with hepatitis B virus immunoglobulin.

One big drawback is that long-term therapy is often necessary to maintain response to the drug. It is also associated with a high rate of viral resistance, particularly when used over a long period of time. This resistance is due to a mutation in the virus called the YMDD variant.

It was reported at the November 2003 conference in Boston for the American Association for the Study of Liver Diseases that the incidence of lamivudine resistance increases from 13 to 52 percent in the first year, 32 percent after two years, and to 67 percent at four years of therapy. At the same time, when these mutations occur, HBV DNA reappears in the blood, and ALT values are elevated again. Long-term follow-up studies also showed that over time, any initial benefit is negated when patients develop LVD-resistant mutants.

Fortunately, the YMDD variant is thought to be less harmful than the original hepatitis B virus, called the wild type HBV. Despite the emergence of the YMDD variant, some experts believe that patients may be better off continuing their treatment with the drug. If they discontinue the drug, their symptoms can worsen because the more aggressive wild type HBV, which had been suppressed by the drug, will become predominant again.

On the other hand, two recent reports from Asia suggest that discontinuation of LVD does not result in more "flares," and that stopping LVD may be a reasonable option. However, if patients have irreversible scarring of the liver (cirrhosis) or immunosuppression (their immune system is suppressed, either by immunosuppressive medication or because of an illness like AIDS), they should be switched to a newer medication called adefovir dipivoxil before getting off LVD.

Adefovir Dipivoxil

Adefovir dipivoxil is an oral antiviral drug. The newest of the approved drugs, it is becoming widely prescribed and is often the first line of therapy recommended by experts. It is taken for at least one year. The recommended dose of ADV for adults with normal kidney function is 10 mg daily orally. The dosing interval should be increased in patients with renal insufficiency.

The drug helps to reduce significantly levels of HBV DNA. In one study, HBV DNA became undetectable in 70 percent of patients, and ALT levels became normal. It was shown to be effective in suppressing not only the standard HBV virus (wild-type HBV), but also lamivudine-resistant HBV mutants.

The drug is also effective in chronic hepatitis B patients who have the mutant form of the virus with negative B e antigen (HBeAg–), for which neither interferon nor lamivudine works well.

In one trial of 184 patients who were HBeAg negative, after two years of treatment more than half the patients had undetectable levels of HBV DNA and normal ALT levels. This study was included in a review of hepatitis B treatments by Anna S. F. Lok and Brian J. McMahon in the March 2004 issue of *Hepatology*. They also reported on studies that show that HBeAg-positive patients treated with 30 mg or 10 mg doses of ADV had a higher proportion of patients with histologic response (cells and tissues are examined under a microscope), HBeAg loss, normalization of ALT, and reduction of HBV DNA.

Another benefit is that, like lamivudine, ADV has minimal side effects, though kidney problems have been reported with long-term use. Since it is taken orally instead of by injection like interferon, it is easier for patients to take.

ADV resulted in a significant reduction of serum HBV DNA in 72 percent of patients with lamivudine-resistant HBV after five months of therapy. High ALT and low HBV DNA predicted a faster response to treatment.

At the November 2003 conference in Boston for the American Association for the Study of Liver Diseases, investigators concluded that treatment with a 10 mg daily dosage significantly reduced HBV DNA, and improved laboratory results and survival rates. It also appeared to stop inflammation and keep liver scarring from progressing. Moreover, it was an effective treatment for liver transplant patients both before and after surgery who had initially failed lamivudine therapy. This was true even for patients who had developed viral mutations after treatment with lamivudine.

The drawback is that the rate for seroconversion—where B e antigen no longer becomes detectable in the blood—tends to be low. In one study only 12 percent of patients experienced seroconversion after 48 weeks, and 21 percent after 100 weeks. In addition, a longer-term study showed that, just as with lamivudine, resistant mutant strains develop with adefovir after 96 weeks of therapy. The rate of their emergence may be slower than for lamivudine. The resistant mutant appears to be susceptible to treatments with lamivudine and entecavir, another new medication.

When patients stop taking the medication, viral rebound can occur. That means that the virus, which had been successfully kept from reproducing wildly, is now rapidly multiplying again.

Entecavir

The nucleoside analogue entecavir (ETV) is an oral antiviral drug with activity against both regular (wild-type) and lamivudine-resistant HBV.

ETV, given in doses of 0.5 and 1.0 mg, has been shown to have superior antiviral activity in patients who did not respond to lamivudine. The medication was more potent, as defined in terms of ALT levels, HBeAg status (whether the B e antigen was present in the blood or not), and YMDD mutations.

At the November 2002 conference for American Association for the Study of Liver Diseases, researchers reported in their studies on the good results they had with entecavir. Their findings indicate that treatment with entecavir caused rapid reduction of HBV DNA in the patients' blood. So far, they have not noted any development of resistance to entecavir. In terms of side effects or adverse affects and the number of patients discontinuing the drug because of them, entecavir appeared to be comparable to lamivudine. Most common side effects were headache, rhinitis, fatigue, and abdominal pain.

New medications   LDT (Telbivudine) and ACH-126, 443 are two new HBV drugs in early development. LDT is from Idenix Pharmaceuticals; its dosage is 400–600 mg per day. ACH-126, 443 is by Achillion Pharmaceuticals. So far, studies show that this oral drug is readily absorbed by the body, there were no apparent drug-related adverse events, and animal studies showed no significant toxicity even at high doses.

Many other new HBV drugs are currently on the horizon. Many are nucleoside analogues, a class of drugs that interfere with the virus's ability to make enzymes. The nucleoside analogues include the following:

- Emtricitabine (FTC) by Gilead Sciences
- Telbivudine (LdT) by Idenix
- Clevudine (L-FMAU) by Gilead Sciences
- Valtorcitabine by Idenix
- Amdoxovir (DAPD) by Triangle Pharmaceuticals
- Racivir by Pharmasset
- MCC 478 by Eli Lily

There are also immune stimulants:

- HE 2000 by Hollis-Eden
- Zadaxin by SciClone
- Theradigm by Epimmune

COMPARISON OF THREE APPROVED TREATMENTS OF CHRONIC HEPATITIS B			
Indications	**IFN alfa**	**Lamivudine**	**Adefovir**
HBeAg+, normal ALT	not indicated	not indicated	not indicated
HBeAg+, chronic hepatitis	indicated	indicated	indicated
HBeAg–, chronic hepatitis	indicated	indicated	indicated
Duration of treatment			
HBeAg+, chronic hepatitis	4–6 months	≥1 year	≥1 year
HBeAg–, chronic hepatitis	1 year	1 year	1 year
route	subcutaneous	oral	oral
side effects	many	negligible	potential nephrotoxicity
drug resistance	–	0%, year 1 / –70%, year 5	none, year 1 / –3%, year 2
cost*	high	low	intermediate

abbreviations: ifn- alfa interferon alfa; hbeag, hepatitis b e antigen

*based on treatment duration of 1 year

Source: Lok, Anna S. F., and McMahoun, Brian J. "Hepatitis B: Update of recommendations." *Hepatology* 39, 3 (March 2004): 857–861.

Baffis, Vicki, and colleagues. "Use of interferon for prevention of hepatocellular carcinoma in cirrhotic patients with hepatitis B or hepatitis C virus infection." *Annals of Internal Medicine* 131, no. 9 (November 1999): 696–701.

Benhamou, Yves, and others. "Significant and sustained efficacy of adefovir dipivoxil (ADV) after four years of treatment in chronic hepatitis B (CHB) patients with lamivudine-resistant (LAM-R) HBV and HIV coinfection." Abstract 1. Digestive Disease Week. May 15–20, 2004. New Orleans.

Buti, M., and others. "Efficacy and safety of adefovir for the treatment of patients with chronic hepatitis B (CHB) resistant to lamivudine in Spain." Abstract 422. 39th annual meeting of the European Association for the Study of the Liver (EASL). April 14–18, 2004. Berlin, Germany.

Editors. "Pegasys more effective than current hepatitis B treatments in new study." *Biotech Business Week* (November 24, 2003): 88.

Schiff, E. R., and others. "Entecavir 1.0 Mg is consistently superior to Lamivudine at 48 weeks across multiple baseline HBV disease characteristics in Lamivudine-refractory patients." Abstract 442. 39th EASL. April 14–18, 2004. Berlin, Germany.

Shen, H., and others. "Combination therapy with lamivudine and famciclovir for chronic hepatitis B infection." *Clinical Gastroenterology and Hepatology* 2, no. 4 (April 2004): 330–336.

neonatal hepatitis   Neonatal hepatitis is an inflammation of the LIVER that occurs exclusively in early infancy. It is also sometimes called giant cell of newborns or idiopathic neonatal hepatitis. Most cases occur within a month to two after birth, with symptoms such as JAUNDICE (yellowing of the skin and eyes) and an enlarged liver and spleen. The infant fails to grow properly, as it cannot absorb vitamins required for normal growth.

The cause is unknown in many cases of neonatal hepatitis. Many cases can be attributed to rare, inherited errors of metabolism or to infection before or shortly after birth by a virus transmitted by the mother, such as HEPATITIS A or HEPATITIS B.

Symptoms and Diagnostic Path
A LIVER BIOPSY is performed for diagnosis if no virus has been identified as the cause. In this procedure, a small tissue from the liver is taken to be examined under a microscope.

Neonatal hepatitis must be distinguished from BILIARY ATRESIA, another infant LIVER DISEASE, as treatment approaches are completely different. Infants with neonatal hepatitis have normal, intact BILE DUCTS, in contrast to those who have biliary atresia. In both diseases, the infant presents with jaundice and an enlarged liver.

Prognosis depends on the underlying cause of the disease. Some infants may have permanent liver disease, while others recover with little or no scarring to their liver. If the disease becomes chronic, the infant will not be able to digest fats or absorb fat-soluble vitamins; A, D, E, and K. This in turn leads to poor bone and cartilage development and a tendency to bleed, among other problems. Because the liver is unable to eliminate toxins in the bile, persistent itching and skin eruptions may result.

Treatment Options and Outlook
There are no specific treatments for neonatal hepatitis. Formulas with more easily digested fats are given, while vitamin supplements and medications may be prescribed.

If neonatal hepatitis was caused by the hepatitis A virus, it should resolve itself within six months, but hepatitis B or HEPATITIS C viruses tend to cause chronic liver disease. If the infant develops CIRRHOSIS, a liver transplant may ultimately be needed.

Infants who developed neonatal hepatitis as a result of infection by cytomegalovirus (opportunistic virus that causes cellular enlargement), rubella (measles), or viral hepatitis may be contagious to others.

Funato, Tadao, et al. "Quantitative evaluation of cytomegalovirus DNA in infantile hepatitis." *Journal of Viral Hepatitis* 8, no. 3 (May 2001): 217–222.

neonatal jaundice   Many newborns develop a yellow discoloration of the skin and the whites of the eyes. These hallmarks of JAUNDICE are a common occurrence in human infants. The cause of the jaundice is elevated blood concentrations of BILIRUBIN, a by-product of the breakdown of red blood cells. This condition is called hyperbilirubinemia.

Hyperbilirubinemia may be caused by abnormalities of the LIVER, an increased rate of bilirubin production, or a decreased rate of conjugation, or conversion of the BILE from a fat (lipid)-soluble form to a water-soluble form. Bilirubin must be conjugated to be excreted in the urine and stool.

If it is not excreted, it can be reabsorbed into the body.

There are mainly two reasons that newborns commonly develop hyperbilirubinemia. One is primarily due to the immaturity of the LIVER ENZYME system. An infant's liver cannot yet process the bilirubin as fast as a mature liver. The liver must turn the bilirubin into a water-soluble form before it can be eliminated. The immature liver causes a delay in eliminating the bilirubin. This is not a liver disease; it normalizes as the infant grows older.

The second reason is that newborns have a high volume of red blood cells; moreover, these deteriorate more quickly than other cells, which increases their turnover rate. Bilirubin in the blood is carried to the liver, processed and excreted from the body as a waste product. The body has to process this excess of red blood cells and bilirubin, and the large amount contributes to the yellowish discoloration of the skin and eyes. Jaundice due to the above reasons is known as physiologic jaundice because hyperbilirubinemia occurs universally in newborns. This is a normal condition, not a disorder. Bilirubin accumulates in the blood of all newborns, and the discoloration is caused by a natural process of the breakdown of red blood cells. The total concentration of bilirubin in the blood usually peaks at 5 to 12 mg/dL on the second or third day after birth.

But sometimes other factors cause jaundice in infants, such as an incompatibility of blood types, e.g., ABO incompatibility and Rh incompatibility. This results in the rapid breakdown of red blood cells. Jaundice can also be caused by certain enzyme deficiencies, or structural abnormalities in red cells.

Infants can be expected to develop physiologic jaundice usually on the second or third day after birth. This is normal. But if jaundice occurs fewer than 24 hours after birth, it is considered abnormal—nonphysiologic, or pathologic. This may happen, for instance, if the infant's intestine is absorbing more of the bilirubin than normal. Jaundice is also considered nonphysiologic if total bilirubin levels exceed 15 mg/dL in a full-term infant or 10 mg/dL in a preterm infant.

An excessive absorption of bilirubin slows down the excretion of bilirubin from the stool. There are three possible causes. It could be the result of a deficiency of intestinal bacteria that metabolize bilirubin. Another cause may be poor feeding. The third cause may be a genetic defect, GILBERT'S SYNDROME, or a deficiency in a certain enzyme (uridine diphosphate glucuronosyltransferase) necessary for conjugating bilirubin.

According to the American Academy of Pediatrics, in the United States approximately 60 percent of the 40 million term newborns in the first week are clinically jaundiced. Of premature babies, the rate may be as high as 80 percent in the first three days after birth. The condition, although transient, accounts for up to 75 percent of readmissions to the hospital in the first week after birth. There is controversy regarding when treatment should begin, and the adverse consequences of neonatal jaundice.

Symptoms and Diagnostic Path

The initial symptoms of a rise in bilirubin level can be subtle and therefore easy to miss. These can include increased drowsiness, poor feeding, and decreased amounts of urine and stool. There may be orange spots on the diaper caused by uric acid crystals, a sign of dehydration. If the infant's cries become more high-pitched than normal, it may indicate early neurological damage.

Treatment is not necessary in most cases, particularly in physiologic jaundice. The jaundice should disappear within a week or two. However, treatment may be necessary if pathology is suspected. For instance, persistently high concentrations of bilirubin can be highly dangerous. They are neurotoxic and disrupt some cellular processes. An Rh factor or ABO blood incompatibility between the mother and the infant can cause jaundice to appear within the first 24 hours after birth. Doctors are still unable to predict with consistency which infants will proceed from benign jaundice to a much more serious form of neonatal jaundice, called kernicterus.

Kernicterus can be life-threatening. The high bilirubin levels can cause brain damage in infants. When this happens, treatment cannot be delayed. The afflicted infant may suffer from neurologic impairment, such as hearing loss, a paralysis of upward gaze, seizures, and a low IQ. The damage is caused by excessive amounts of bilirubin, which although a natural by-product of the body, can be toxic to the central nervous system and, under certain circumstances, can cause detrimental neurologic effects. As yet, investigators have an incomplete understanding of how bile toxicity may affect vulnerable brain cells and cause brain damage. It appears that concentrations in which bilirubin becomes harmful can vary, depending on the geographic location or the ethnicity of the patient.

Following the introduction of exchange transfusion and phototherapy (therapy with lights) to treat hyperbilirubinemia, kernicterus was rarely seen. Unfortunately, it appears to be making a comeback. This serious condition can affect even apparently healthy babies. It may be due to a change in risk profile caused by the early discharge of infants without prompt medical follow-up.

Testing includes blood typing (ABO and Rh) and a serum screen for unusual isoimmune antibodies. There should be a follow-up of all newborns who were discharged from the hospital fewer than 48 hours after birth. The infant should also be examined if there is dark urine or light-colored stool. A measurement should be made of direct serum bilirubin. If jaundice continues beyond three weeks, the doctor will take urine samples for bilirubin and the measurement for total and direct serum bile obtained.

Studies suggest that the following infants have a higher risk of hyperbilirubinemia, with total serum bile levels greater than or equal to 20 mg/dL:

- birth in the hospital
- male
- Asian race
- gestational age between 36 and 38 weeks
- older maternal age
- family history of jaundice
- family history of liver disease
- family history of thyroid gland abnormalities

Treatment Options and Outlook

Treatment is aimed at preventing progression to kernicterus, where bilirubin may deposit in the brain, causing central nervous system damage and even death. The focus is on decreasing levels of bilirubin through a standard treatment for neonatal jaundice called phototherapy. The therapy is also known as Bililight, or Bilirubin Reduction Light. The therapy uses light to convert bilirubin into a form that is readily excreted. Lights are placed over the infant's bed. The light is absorbed by the bilirubin just under the infant's skin. The light changes the structure of the bilirubin, converting it into lumirubin, which is water-soluble. How fast bilirubin is excreted depends on the wavelength of light used and its dose. Standard fluorescent white light is most commonly used for phototherapy.

During the light therapy, masks are placed over the infant's eyes to protect them from the bright light. The baby's position is moved frequently to assure maximum exposure, and to ensure that all the areas of the skin are exposed to the light.

American Academy of Pediatrics, Provisional Committee for Quality Improvement and Subcommittee on Hyperbilirubinemia. "Management of hyperbilirubinemia in the healthy term newborn." *Pediatrics* 94, no. 4 (October 1994): 558–565.

Melton, Kristin, M.D., and Henry T. Akinbi, M.D. "Neonatal jaundice: Strategies to reduce bilirubin-induced complications." *Postgraduate Medicine* 106, no. 6 (November 1999): 167–178.

Palmer, Heather, Sudhakar Ezhuthachan, Christine Newman, Brenna Pradell-Boyd, Jeffrey M. Maisels, and Marcia A. Testa. "Management of hyperbilirubinemia in newborns: Measuring performance by using a benchmarking model." *Pediatrics* 112, no. 6 (December 2003): 1264(10).

Zepf, Bill, M.D., P. A. Dennery, et al. "Neonatal hyperbilirubinemnia." *New England Journal of Medicine* 344 (February 22, 2001): 581–590.

occupational liver disease On-the-job exposure to infections or toxic substances contributes to the incidence of many diseases. Occupation-related infections, however, tend to be underrecognized and underreported, even though according to some studies they may be responsible for as many as 860,000 illnesses and more than 60,000 deaths each year.

LIVER DISEASE related to exposures on the job can be particularly difficult to pin down. The reasons are many. Because liver disease is often asymptomatic, it can go unsuspected by affected workers. When finally diagnosed, a liver disease may not be suspected for an occupational cause, especially if the patient also engages in risky behavior such as heavy drinking or drug use. Contributing to the difficulty is the fact that liver abnormalities often cannot be detected except through biopsy, a procedure that cannot be administered on a routine basis in an industrial setting.

A few occupational diseases and their workplace associations are well known and highly publicized, while others remain obscure. Repetitive motion syndrome (RMS), commonly called carpal tunnel syndrome, for example, has become well known through its association with the operation of computers. Somewhat less well represented in the public consciousness are the associations of RMS and similar conditions—De Quervain's tendonitis, cervical strain, and thoracic outlet syndrome—with many jobs involving repetition and awkward postures, including supermarket checking, meat packing, and industrial assembly.

Still more obscure are the occupational causes of diseases whose workplace associations can be established only through careful research. Case reports have suggested, for example, that exposure to organic solvents may cause or contribute to fatty liver disease (FLD). That suggestion is borne out in a study conducted at Linkoping University in Sweden. The study compared the clinical records of 30 male patients, aged 20 to 59, diagnosed with FLD to those of 120 males randomly selected from the general population in the same geographical area. The study's conclusions suggest that males with a moderate exposure to solvents for at least one year are about four times more likely to develop FLD than the general male population. The same study seems to show that those with heavy exposure are almost eight times as likely to develop FLD. Some consider the connection firmly established, but that study and others that are highly suggestive stop short of claiming to be conclusive. The case is not yet proven and awaits the accumulation of further evidence.

Health care workers are particularly susceptible to occupational-related diseases, especially to outbreaks of airborne infections. The health care field is known to have suffered outbreaks of more than 15 infectious diseases—including tuberculosis, chicken pox, measles, and influenza—with infection rates of up to 40 percent. The risk of outbreaks, which is high and unavoidable, is faced daily.

In the recent past, it was relatively common for health workers to contract HEPATITIS B in the course of their duties. HBV, widely known as a sexually transmitted disease, can also be transmitted through contact with any bodily fluid of an infected person, be it blood, saliva, urine, or semen. That health care workers would be at risk of contracting HBV is predictable, but they are not the only ones at risk. Anyone in an occupation in which there is risk of coming in contact with body fluids or tissue is at risk of contracting HBV.

Police officers, especially drug-enforcement officers, often suffer needle-stick injuries while performing their duties. One report, based on an anonymous questionnaire distributed to 1,738 members of the San Diego, California, police department, indicates that 30 percent of respondents had suffered one needle-stick injury, and 27 percent had experienced two or more such injuries. A similar survey conducted in the Denver, Colorado, police department indicates similarly high rates of potentially harmful incidents, including contact with nonintact human tissue, human bites, and lacerations from contaminated equipment. As many as 10 percent of those who become infected from such incidents become chronic sufferers.

The risk of contracting HBV has been mitigated in recent years by the development of an HBV vaccine, and epidemiological studies have suggested a number of prevention strategies. Prevention guidelines published by the British Liver Trust and the World Health Organization include those below:

- vaccination against HBV
- blood tests for all "at-risk" workers
- treatment of any body fluid as though it is infected
- waterproof dressings to cover all open wounds or abrasions
- proper use of appropriate personal protective equipment, such as face masks during mouth-to-mouth resuscitation

Chemical Exposure

Chemically induced occupational liver damage may be a much larger problem than anyone suspects. Of the thousands of industrial chemicals in use, only a few have been adequately tested for hepatotoxicity. The list of agents that are or may be toxic to the liver is still growing.

It can take years of research to confirm the toxicity of a chemical. Vinyl chloride is a case in point. Its role in serious liver disease among PVC workers was confirmed only after the chemical had been used extensively for more than 40 years. Such experience teaches the need to intensify research into occupation-related liver toxicity.

Part of that intensification must be the development of noninvasive and convenient-liver-function tests, or a liver panel. Liver disease is often asymptomatic, and routine testing may be the only certain way of detecting it. Causes of many liver diseases, such as CIRRHOSIS, are still largely unknown. Evidence linking liver disease to occupational chemical exposure is still largely circumstantial, and further study is the only way finally to establish or dismiss those apparent links. Precise causal factors are complicated as well. Experiments on animals, for example, suggest that liver disease sometimes results from exposure to multiple chemical agents in combination, while exposure to one or another of those same agents may not be toxic. The onset of liver disease can also be exacerbated by a combination of chemical exposure and alcohol consumption.

The following table lists 20 industrial chemicals known to cause acute liver injury when handled improperly. A worker who uses one of the listed solvents in an enclosed space without proper ventilation or respiratory protection, for example, runs the risk of illness or death from liver disease. The table is organized by the Chemical Abstract Service (CAS) registry number. The CAS number is a unique identifier of chemical agents that indicates, for example, that acetone and dimethyl ketone are actually the same substance.

INDUSTRIAL CHEMICALS ASSOCIATED WITH ACUTE LIVER INJURY AS THE PRIMARY TOXIC EFFECT		
CAS#	Chemical Name	Other Chemical Names
62-75-9	N-Nitrosodimethylamine	Dimethylnitrosamine DMNA NDMA N,N-Dimethylnitrosamine
78-87-5	Propylene dichloride	1-2-Dichloropropane
109-99-9	Tetrahydrofuran	Diethylene oxide 1,4-Epoxybutane Tetramethylene oxide THF

INDUSTRIAL CHEMICALS ASSOCIATED WITH ACUTE LIVER INJURY AS THE PRIMARY TOXIC EFFECT		
CAS#	Chemical Name	Other Chemical Names
106-93-4	Ethylene dibromide	1,2-Dibromoethane
		Ethylene bromide
		Glycol dibromide
101-77-9	4,4'-Methylene-dianiline	MDA
		4,4'-Diaminodiphenylmethane
		para, para'-Diaminodiphenylmethane
		Dianilinomethane
		4,4'-Diphenylmethanediamine
		4,4' Methylene bis (2-chloraniline)
		diaminodiphenylmethane
		DDM
118-96-7	2,4,6-Trinitrotoluene	1-Methyl-2,4,6-trinitrobenzene
		TNT
		Trinitrotoluene
		sym-Trinitrotoluene
		Trinitrotoluol
79-46-9	2-Nitropropane	Dimethylnitromethane
		iso-Nitropropane
		2-NP
56-23-5	Carbon tetrachloride	Tetrachloromethane
68-12-2	Dimethylformamide	Dimethyl formamide
		N,N-Dimethylformamide
		DMF
79-27-6	Acetylene tetrabromide	Symmetrical tetrabromoethane
		TBE
		Tetrabromoacetylene
		Tetrabromoethane
		1,1,2,2-Tetrabromoethane
79-34-5	1,1,2,2-Tetrachloroethane	Acetylene tetrachloride
92-52-4	Diphenyl	Biphenyl
		Phenyl benzene

INDUSTRIAL CHEMICALS ASSOCIATED WITH ACUTE LIVER INJURY AS THE PRIMARY TOXIC EFFECT		
CAS#	Chemical Name	Other Chemical Names
107-06-2	Ethylene dichloride	1,2-Dichloroethane
		Ethylene chloride
		Glycol dichloride
127-19-5	Dimethyl acetamide	DMAC
		Acetic acid, dimethylamide
		Dimethyl acetamide
		Acetdimethylamide
		Dimethylacetone amide
		Dimethylamide acetate
558-13-4	Carbon tetrabromide	Carbon bromide
		Methane tetrabromide
		Tetrabromomethane
1321-64-8	Pentachlorona-phthalene	Halowax 1013
		1,2,3,4,5-Pentachloronaphthalene
1321-65-9	Trichlorona-phthalene	Halowax
		Nibren wax
		Seekay wax
1335-87-1	Hexachlorona-phthalene	Halowax 1014
1335-88-2	Tetrachlorona-phthalene	Halowax
		Nibren wax
		Seekay wax
2234-13-1	Octachlorona-phthalene	Halowax 1051

These 20 chemicals in the table represent only those chemicals known to cause liver injury directly. An additional 156 chemicals may cause liver injury as a secondary effect. Many of those chemicals are associated with elevated levels of LIVER ENZYMES, an indicator of liver injury. Those chemicals include a number of agents with long biological half-lives—such as heavy metals, polychlorinated biphenyls (PCBs), and chlorine-containing pesticides—which may cause liver injury only after prolonged periods of chronic exposure.

Other chemicals are known to cause liver injury in animals and humans after ingestion, though it is possible that those same chemicals could cause liver damage through inhalation or absorption through the skin.

Role of the Family Physician

Any effort to increase recognition of occupational diseases must involve family physicians. Patients with illnesses that may be work-related often seek initial care from their family physician, whose recognition of the links may determine the diagnostic tests performed and the treatments recommended. Early detection of an occupation-related illness can prevent it from progressing into more dangerous and less treatable forms, and may help other workers in similar situations avoid similar problems.

Family physicians wishing to increase their own awareness of the possible links between occupation and disease, and to help patients increase their awareness as well, may consider developing skills in taking occupational histories, and should routinely provide access to occupational health resources.

Occupational Histories

An occupational history is the single most important method of recognizing links between illness and occupation. It should consist of a standard set of questions asked of every patient. In a busy practice, a set of screening questions and a self-administered questionnaire may be the most efficient method of gathering the necessary information.

Screening questions help lay the groundwork for more detailed occupational histories. The answers to screening questions can indicate whether a more detailed investigation of occupational history might be productive. The screening questions should be geared to gathering answers to just a few key questions:

- What type of work does the patient do?

- Does the patient think his or her health problems might be work-related?

- Do the symptoms display any environmental differences? Are the symptoms different when the patient is at home than when the patient is at work?

- Has the patient been exposed, currently or in the past, to chemicals, dusts, metals, radiation, noise, or repetitive work?

- Do any of the patient's coworkers experience similar symptoms?

If the answers to one or more screening questions suggest a connection between the patient's health problems and the patient's job, the completion of a comprehensive occupational history is indicated. Much of the history can be self-administered, and the completed history should be part of the patient's chart, where it can be available for review and periodic updating.

A complete occupational history should encompass all jobs the patient held during his or her lifetime, including military service, and should include all the following information:

- employer names and addresses

- dates of employment

- job titles

- major job duties

- known exposures to hazards

It is particularly important for the patient to list both job titles and job duties. Job titles by themselves are often meaningless or, worse, misleading. Two workers with the same job titles may experience vastly different exposures, depending on their specific duties.

Exposure information should be exhaustive and detailed. The patient may not be aware of all the information required, so the physician should review the form and ask for additional details about jobs that appear relevant to the patient's current symptoms. Complete exposure information includes information on both the types of exposure and the assessments of the likely dosages.

Types of exposure include metals, chemicals, dusts, physical exposures (repetitive motion, noise, radiation, etc.), biological agents, and psychological elements such as stress. All possible exposures need to be known, even indirect ones. Patients who work in an industrial setting may not be directly exposed to hazards, for example, but can still be affected by exposures that occur within close proximity.

An assessment of the dosage can be a complex investigation that may have to include any or all of the following elements:

- concentration of chemical agents used
- frequency of handling chemical or biological agents
- presence and operating efficiency of exposure controls, including operable doors and windows, walls and partitions that affect air flow, and local exhaust ventilation systems such as a vacuum apparatus attached to a machine or exhaust slots on a tank
- use of personal protective equipment such as respirators, gloves, and earplugs. Information may include:
  - frequency of use. Does the patient use the protective equipment consistently?
  - fit. Does the equipment, especially respirators, fit correctly?
  - appropriateness. Is the equipment appropriate for the exposure hazard?
  - maintenance. Is the equipment stored and maintained properly?

Some of the necessary information can be obtained from the employer. The Occupational Safety and Health Administration (OSHA) mandates access to such information through its Hazard Communication and Access to Medical Record Standards. Any such contact, however, requires the patient's permission. If the patient is reluctant to grant that permission, the patient can make the request personally either directly to the company or through a union representative.

A company's usual response is a material safety data sheet (MSDS). It identifies hazardous materials used on the work site and explains the health hazards of each one. Its scope is limited, however, and it can be viewed with some skepticism. It includes only those substances that OSHA considers harmful; substances whose health effects are unknown or unproven may not be mentioned. The MSDS also focuses on acute effects, and often does not cover chronic exposures at low levels.

Quantitative data are sometimes provided, but those data, too, may be less than definitive. Data on the concentration of a substance in the air, for example, may be inaccurate due to the limitations of monitoring techniques. It is possible as well that OSHA's permissible exposure limit, or PEL, is set too high. If a patient's history points consistently to an occupational exposure, contradictory data provided under OSHA rules is not by itself a sufficient reason to dismiss the connection as unlikely. In that situation, information regarding differing symptoms at work and at home and symptoms of coworkers can be important indicators.

Information about leisure activities and hobbies can be important as well. Smoking, excessive use of alcohol, and drugs, for example, may exacerbate illness that is otherwise work-related. Some recreational activities can also contribute to an exposure, as when a patient is exposed to similar stresses—dust or noise, for example—both on the job and in recreational activities.

Occupational Health Resources

Family physicians often refer patients to clinics that specialize in occupational medicine. Such clinics can provide valuable information about the probable health effects of exposure, diagnostic tests that can be employed, and recommendations on whether a patient should return to work. Many clinics have a multidisciplinary approach, using teams of health professionals, industrial specialists, and social workers to address occupational illnesses comprehensively. Some clinics can provide workplace evaluations in addition to education and help accessing available benefit systems.

Lists of clinics and specialists in occupational medicine can be obtained from the Association of Occupational and Environmental Clinics (AOEC) and the American College of Occupational and Environmental Medicine (ACOEM). Additional resources include the National Institute for Occupational Safety and Health (NIOSH), and OSHA. OSHA is a particularly important resource. A physician who believes that a serious hazard is not being addressed may ask OSHA to intervene. Most states provide offices similar to OSHA.

A number of computerized databases are available by subscription or through medical libraries or regional poison control centers. Micromedex, Silver Platter, and the Canadian Center for Occupational Health and Safety are some commonly used CD-ROM systems. The Internet also contains useful Web sites related to toxic exposures.

Organizations that may be helpful include the following:

- Association of Occupational and Environmental Clinics (AOEC)

- American College of Occupational and Environmental Medicine (ACOEM)

- National Institute for Occupational Safety and Health (NIOSH)

- Occupational Safety and Health Administration (OSHA)

    (The local OSHA office is listed in the telephone book. Find it in the federal government listings, under Department of Labor.)

- poison control centers. Poison control centers across the country can be consulted for information on a variety of hazards and treatment of overexposures.

Bastian, P. G. "Occupational hepatitis caused by methylenedianiline." *American Journal of Industrial Medicine* 35, no. 2 (February 1999): 132–136.

Chen, J. D., J. D. Wang, S. Y. Tsai, and W. I. Chao. "Effects of occupational and nonoccupational factors on liver-function tests in workers exposed to solvent mixtures." *Archives of Environmental Health* 52, no. 4 (July–August 1997): 270–274.

Dossing, M., and J. Sonne. "Drug-induced hepatic disorders: Incidence, management and avoidance." *Drug Safety* 6 (December 1994): 441–449.

Fiorito, A., F. Larese, S. Molinari, and T. Zanin. "Liver function alterations in synthetic leather workers exposed to dimethylformamide." *American Journal of Industrial Medicine* 32, no. 3 (September 1997): 255–260.

Grant, Martyn. "Marty Grant offers an overview of the disease and examines the worker groups at most risk from infection." *Safety and Health Practitioner* 22 (June 2004): n.p.

Harrison, R., G. Letz, G. Pasternak, and P. Blanc. "Fulminant hepatic failure after occupational exposure to 2-nitropropane." *Annals of Internal Medicine* 107, no. 4 (October 1987): 466–468.

Hoet, Perrine, Mary Louise M. Graf, Mohammed Bourdi, Lance R. Pohl, Paul H. Duray, Weiqiao Chen, Raimund M. Peter, Sidney Nelson, Nicolas Verlinden, and Dominique Lison. "Epidemic of liver disease caused by hydrochlorofluorocarbons used as ozone-sparing substitutes of chlorofluorocarbons." *Internal Archives of Occupational and Environmental Health* 56, no. 1 (1985): 1–21.

Lundberg, I., and M. Hakansson. "Normal serum activities of liver enzymes in Swedish paint industry workers with heavy exposure to organic solvents." *British Journal of Industrial Medicine* 42, no. 9 (September 1985): 596–600.

Lundqvist G., U. Flodin, and O. Axelson. "A case-control study of fatty liver disease and organic solvent exposure." *Internal Archives of Occupational and Environmental Health* 72, no. 1 (January 1999): 19–25.

Redlich, C. A., A. B. West, L. Fleming, L. D. True, M. R. Cullen, and C. A. Riely. "Clinical and pathological characteristics of hepatotoxicity associated with occupational exposure to dimethylformamide." *Gastroenterology* 99, no. 3 (September 1990): 748–757.

Redlich, Carrie. "Occupational Liver Disease." *Western Journal of Medicine* 152, no. 2 (February 1990): 176.

Rees, D., N. Soderlund, R. Cronje, E. Song, D. Kielkowski, and J. Myers. "Solvent exposure, alcohol consumption and liver injury in workers manufacturing paint." *Scandinavian Journal of Work and Environmental Health* 19, no. 4 (August 1993): 236–244.

Sepkowitz, K. A. "Occupationally acquired infections in health care workers. Part I." *Southern Medical Journal* 90, no. 9 (September 1997): 872–877.

Tomei, Francesco, Angiolino Iaviocoli, Bruno Papaleo, and Tiziana Paola Baccolo. "Liver damage in pharmaceutical industry workers." *Archives of Environmental Health* 50, no. 4 (July–August 1995): 293.

Wrbitzky, R. "Liver function in workers exposed to N,N-dimethylformamide during the production of synthetic textiles." *Annals of Internal Medicine* 125, no. 10 (November 15, 1996): 826–834.

Zimmerman, H. J., and J. H. Lewis. "Chemical- and toxin-induced hepatotoxicity." *Archives of Internal Medicine* 8 (April 28, 1997): 913–919.

organ procurement organization (OPO) An organ procurement organization is a not-for-profit agency that is responsible for the details of organ procurement. Specifically, an OPO identifies organ donors; retrieves, preserves, and transports organs; and maintains data about organ donors. An OPO is also responsible for educating medical staff and the general public about organ donation. An OPO might be based in a hospital, or it might be independent of hospitals.

One may contact an OPO directly for any of the following reasons:

- to obtain general information on how to become an organ and tissue donor
- to obtain a donor card
- to research a speech or an educational project about organ donation

- to contact the family of the donor of an organ
- to contact the recipient of a loved one's organs and tissues
- to obtain a speaker for an organization or school
- to find out how to help promote organ donation

For more information, contact the following:

Association of Organ Procurement Organizations
1364 Beverly Road
Suite 100
McLean, VA 22101
(703) 556-4242
(703) 556-4852 (fax)
http://www.aopo.org

painkillers and the liver Many Americans—perhaps upwards of 30 percent—regularly use over-the-counter pain medication to relieve headache, arthritis pain, and back pain. Commonly used painkillers include acetaminophen, aspirin, and ibuprofen. In general, such medications are not toxic to the liver when used as directed.

There are exceptions, however, and when used improperly any painkiller can be toxic to the LIVER. Before taking pain medication, it is important to consider dosage, existing liver conditions, and other substances recently consumed, including both medication and alcohol.

Acetaminophen

Acetaminophen, also called paracetamol, is best known under the brand name Tylenol. It is both an analgesic (painkiller) and an antipyretic (fever reducer). Unlike other painkillers, acetaminophen does not upset the stomach, and when first introduced in 1955 quickly became a popular alternative to aspirin and similar drugs. When taken in small doses, under four grams a day, acetaminophen is also quite safe for the liver. In fact, it is the preferred painkiller for patients with LIVER DISEASE.

Acetaminophen does have its dangers, however, and can be deadly when taken in excessive dosages or combined with alcohol.

Acetaminophen overdose is the most common cause of drug-induced LIVER FAILURE in the United States. The drug can cause liver failure when taken in large quantity over a short period of time. A single dose of acetaminophen of more than seven grams is considered poisonous to the average adult. Four grams per day, or about eight pills in 24 hours, is generally considered safe. But individuals with liver disease should limit their consumption to under two grams per day. Two grams is the equivalent of one extra-strength 500-milligram (mg) Tylenol tablet or capsule every six hours, or two every 12 hours.

Alcohol taken in conjunction with acetaminophen significantly increases the risk of liver failure. For that reason, people who drink and also take acetaminophen regularly are advised to restrict their acetaminophen intake to one or two grams per day.

People who take acetaminophen for pain relief can overdose accidentally by taking other medications that also contain acetaminophen. It is an active ingredient in more than 200 over-the-counter drugs, including Nyquil and other cold medications. Consequently, it is important that people taking acetaminophen for pain relief carefully read the labels of any other medications they intend to take, to avoid ingesting too much of the drug.

Certain drug interactions can also be a problem. Omeprazole (Prilosec), phenytoin (Dilantin), and isoniazid (INH) can all increase the risk of liver damage when taken in combination with acetaminophen. Those who take acetaminophen and also take other drugs should consult a physician about possible drug interactions. It is especially important for patients with liver disease to confer with their hepatologist (liver specialist) before taking any over-the-counter medication, particularly when they also use acetaminophen.

Aspirin and Ibuprofen

Aspirin and ibuprofen are nonsteroidal anti-inflammatory drugs (NSAIDs). Like acetaminophen, NSAIDs are both analgesic and antipyretic, but also reduce inflammation.

NSAIDs have long been known to have potential for causing injury to the liver, and many stronger NSAIDs have had to be withdrawn from the market. Aspirin doses in excess of 2,000 mg per day, for example, have been known to be hepatotoxic, and there are reports of ibuprofen causing severe liver injury in patients with hepatitis C.

Ibuprofen (Motrin or Advil) is often used by chronic HEPATITIS C patients to combat joint pain. Although ibuprofen has a low liver toxicity at the recommended dosage, it has been known in some cases to cause an elevation of liver enzymes, sometimes as much as tenfold.

NSAIDs also have other effects that can be harmful to patients with liver disease. They increase blood-clotting time and interfere with blood coagulation. The effect can last for as long as seven days after stopping the drug. Since interferon treatments can also disrupt blood coagulation, patients undergoing interferon therapy must use aspirin and other NSAIDs with care, if at all. For similar reasons, patients taking corticosteroids such as prednisone, or anticoagulants such as coumadin, are advised to avoid NSAIDs.

NSAIDs can also cause salt and water retention. They may worsen associated conditions such as leg swelling and ascites (fluid accumulation in the abdomen) and counteract the effects of diuretics.

Older women are particularly susceptible to the toxic effects of NSAIDs, and are generally advised to avoid all NSAIDs. Similarly, patients with liver disease—especially advanced liver disease—are also advised to avoid using NSAIDs. Most doctors recommend taking acetaminophen in dosages of fewer than two grams instead of NSAIDs.

physician selection   See FINDING A SPECIALIST in APPENDIX I.

porphyria   The liver plays a role in synthesizing a group of pigments, called porphyrins, that are intermediate products formed during the process of synthesizing heme, the iron-containing part of hemoglobin (the iron-bearing component of red blood cells). The multistep process of forming heme requires several enzymes and includes steps that occur in the liver and other steps that occur in the bone marrow.

Porphyria is a group of conditions in which one of several possible hereditary genetic defects interferes with the production of one or more of these enzymes. The faulty enzyme production may be caused by either dominant or recessive genes, depending on which step of the heme synthesis chain is affected. If any of the enzymes is abnormal, it can inhibit the process of heme formation, causing a buildup of an intermediate porphyrin. Some metabolites of porphyrins are toxic, and when they accumulate in the body, they can cause abnormal sensitivity to light, abdominal pain, and nerve damage, including paralysis. Excess porphyrins may be excreted in the urine and stool.

Hepatic porphyria occurs when the genetic defects relate to the part of heme synthesis that occurs in the liver. Several different conditions are considered to be hepatic porphyrias. The most common are porphyria cutanea tarda (PCT) and acute intermittent porphyria. These are different diseases, with different symptoms, different diagnostic tests, and different treatments. Rarer forms of porphyria may be misdiagnosed.

One characteristic symptom of hepatic porphyria is urine with the color of port wine. Hepatic porphyria may include skin manifestations, sudden attacks of pain, and other neurological symptoms. Symptoms may first occur during childhood, but the most common age of onset is between 20 and 40 years. The symptoms range from acute—appearing severely and rapidly—to latent, where the patient has an enzyme deficiency but no symptoms. Attacks may develop over hours or days, and they may last from days to weeks. They may be triggered by drugs, such as barbiturates, tranquilizers, birth control pills, and sedatives; chemicals; fasting; smoking; drinking alcohol; infections; emotional and physical stress; menstrual hormones; and exposure to the sun. The disease is more common in women than in men, and the attacks may be related to the patient's menstrual cycle.

Symptoms and Diagnostic Path

The symptoms of porphyria fall into two major groups. Treatment is available for both types of symptoms.

Acute porphyrias affect the nervous system; symptoms include abdominal, chest, back, and/or muscle pain; muscle numbness, tingling, cramping, or paralysis; vomiting; constipation; and personality changes or mental disorders. The symptoms are intermittent.

Cutaneous porphyria occurs when excess porphyrins are transmitted by blood from the liver to the skin. The porphyrins react to light and cause skin irritation. Symptoms of cutaneous porphyria include blisters, itching, and swelling of skin that is exposed to sunlight, as well as sensitivity of the skin to trauma. Crusting and scarring may occur and heal slowly.

Porphyria is diagnosed through blood, urine, and stool tests. Diagnosis may be difficult because the range of symptoms is common to many disorders and interpretation of the tests may be complex. Porphyria cutanea tarda (PCT) can be diagnosed by testing the blood plasma, urine, and stool for porphyrins. While most porphyrias cause high levels of porphyrins in the plasma, increased concentrations in urine and stool are characteristic of PCT. The urine of a person with PCT is often reddish or brownish and will glow pink under a fluorescent light.

Since porphyria or a predisposition to develop porphyria is hereditary, it may be desirable to test children and other blood relatives of affected individuals.

Treatment Options and Outlook

Each form of porphyria is treated differently. Treatment may involve administering heme, giving medicines to relieve the symptoms, or drawing blood. People who have severe attacks may have to be hospitalized.

PCT is the most easily treated porphyria. The main treatment removes blood to lower the amount of iron in the patient's system. Typically, a pint of blood is withdrawn every one to two weeks, and this procedure is repeated five or six times. Low doses of the antimalaria medications chloroquine or hydroxychloroquine may be prescribed to remove excess porphyrins from the liver. Patients are usually advised to avoid alcohol consumption.

Seizures may occur in acute intermittent porphyria and other hepatic porphyrias. The seizures may not respond to treatment with conventional antiseizure medications.

PCT can cause liver damage, including CIRRHOSIS. There is evidence that porphyria patients have a significantly higher risk of developing LIVER CANCER (hepatocellular carcinoma) than the normal population.

Andant, C., H. Puy, J. Faivre, and J. C. Deybach. "Acute hepatic porphyrias and primary liver cancer." *New England Journal of Medicine* 338, no. 25 (June 18, 1998): 1,853–1,854.

Bonkowsky, H. L., P. R. Sinclair, S. Emery, and J. F. Sinclair. "Seizure management in acute hepatic porphyria: Risks of valproate and clonazepam." *Neurology* 30, no. 6 (1980): 588–592.

Kauppinen, R., and P. Mustajoki. "Acute hepatic porphyria and hepatocellular carcinoma." *British Journal of Cancer* 57, no. 1 (1988): 117–120.

portal hypertension Hypertension, or high blood pressure, can occur inside veins in the abdominal organs. The vein is a blood vessel that carries the blood from other parts of the body. The primary vein that carries blood from the abdominal organs to the LIVER is the portal vein. When this vein clots or if scar tissue from disease compresses the vein, the blood backs up and the blood pressure in the vein rises. The resulting condition is called portal hypertension. It may be thought of as a type of high blood pressure from which the liver suffers.

Medically, portal hypertension may be defined as a portal pressure gradient of 12 millimeters of Mercury (mmHg) or greater. Normal portal pressure is 5 to 10 mmHg.

Blood flows to the liver from two different sources, the hepatic (liver) artery and the hepatic portal vein. Blood goes to the liver because toxic substances must be neutralized, and the liver must process every food and compound the body ingests. The portal vein carries the blood from the entire gastrointestinal (GI) tract, containing nutrients from the intestines, into the liver.

The portal system of veins includes all the veins from the lower esophagus (muscular digestive tube extending from the mouth to the stomach), stomach, large and small intestines, spleen, pancreas, GALLBLADDER, and part of the rectum. These veins merge to form the large portal vein of the liver, which supplies up to 75 percent of the blood flow to the liver. The portal vein is about eight centimeters in length. The superior mesenteric vein and the splenic vein join behind the neck of the pancreas to form the portal vein. (The superior mesenteric vein carries blood from the small intestines. The splenic vein is formed from several small veins on the surface of the spleen.)

After entering the liver, the portal trunk divides into two branches. The right branch of the vein enters the right lobe of the liver, and the left branch enters the left lobe, turning into tiny channels called sinusoids, which are small blood vessels running through the liver. Blood drains back into the general circulation, leaving the liver through the hepatic vein.

Two main causes of portal hypertension are recognized; the most common cause is an increased resistance to the blood flow, and the other is an increase in the volume of the blood.

An increased resistance to blood flow is usually caused by LIVER DISEASE, which slows down the flow, increasing the pressure inside the large portal vein. In Western countries, the most frequent cause of this type of portal hypertension is CIRRHOSIS, or advanced scarring of the liver. Cirrhosis can be caused by an infection of the liver, by drinking too much alcohol, or by ingesting harmful chemicals. In the case of alcoholic liver disease, the main liver cells (hepatocytes) may also swell, contributing to the increased blood pressure.

Cirrhosis damages the cells of the liver. As the liver cells die, scar tissue forms; the buildup of this scar tissue prevents the blood from flowing properly through the liver. The scarring distorts the structure of the liver and causes the central veins to become narrowed and constricted, further restricting the blood flow. The liver's capacity to regenerate itself can, in certain instances, be detrimental. The liver's attempt to replace the dying cells results in the growth of nodules, which are small masses of tissue or clusters of cells. These nodules most likely also contribute to the compression of the veins, although nodules can be present in the liver without clinical evidence of portal hypertension.

The liver may also attempt to bypass the obstructions by creating alternative routes or passageways for the blood, known as collateral shunts or collaterals. The blood can then be redirected and circulated to the rest of the body. This, however, can create its own drawbacks and complications, such as mental confusion and agitation or tremors.

The blood circulating through the liver must be returned to the heart. If the blood cannot flow normally through the portal vein, the body may attempt to divert the flow into other veins, as happens in about 80 to 90 percent of patients with portal hypertension. This results in an increased amount of blood flowing through these blood vessels, causing them to become swollen, because they are not designed to handle such high-pressure blood flow. They turn into varices, or varicose veins, which have thin walls and can break open easily and bleed. BLEEDING VARICES are serious and sometimes fatal.

Although cirrhosis is by far the most common cause of portal hypertension in industrialized nations, in other parts of the world, particularly tropical and subtropical climates, the predominant cause is schistosomiasis, or flukes of the genus *Schistosoma.*

In children, the most common cause of portal hypertension is thrombosis of the portal vein. Thrombosis is the formation of an aggregation of blood factors that frequently cause an obstruction in the blood vessels.

Although portal hypertension caused by an increase in blood flow through the portal vein is rare, it can at times be a contributing factor in cirrhosis. There may be a blockage in the splenic or portal vein, or impaired blood flow in the vein that drains out of the liver. Occasionally, increased blood flow is an important factor in enlarged spleens (splenomegaly).

The causes of portal hypertension fall into roughly three categories based on the location of the block to the blood flow: prehepatic, intrahepatic, and posthepatic. Prehepatic refers to the portion of the portal vein that flows into the liver; intrahepatic is the vein running within the liver; and posthepatic is the part of the vein draining the liver. Some overlap exists with this method of classification, and classification systems may differ somewhat.

Major posthepatic causes of portal hypertension are right-sided heart failure, constrictive pericarditis, and BUDD-CHIARI SYNDROME (BCS). The prehepatic causes of portal hypertension include portal vein thrombosis (PVT) and portal compression or obstruction by biliary and pancreatic neoplasms (abnormal growth) and metastases (cancerous growth that has spread to other parts of the body). The most common intrahepatic cause is cirrhosis.

It was believed that the anatomic abnormalities causing portal hypertension were permanent, but recent evidence suggests that major factors contributing to this condition are potentially reversible. This is significant because it suggests that drugs can be used at least partially to treat portal hypertension. The potentially reversible factors include the ability of the sinusoidal lining cells to contract, the body's production of vasoactive substances—which influence the dilation or constriction of blood vessels—as well as various systemic factors that affect certain minute arteries known as splanchnic arterioles.

In the United States, the frequency of portal hypertension is related to cirrhosis, which is most commonly caused by alcohol-induced liver disease. The exact worldwide incidence of portal hypertension is not known, but in Africa, the Middle East, and the Far East, cirrhosis, which is often responsible for portal hypertension, is linked to the prevalence of hepatitis B and hepatitis C. In India and Japan, non-cirrhotic idiopathic (of unknown origin) portal hypertension is more common.

Symptoms and Diagnostic Path

Portal hypertension is asymptomatic; signs and symptoms usually arise from complications of the disorder. The body redirects the impeded blood flow, bypassing the liver by developing collateral vessels that directly connect the portal blood vessels to the general circulation. Thus, poisons and wastes in the blood that normally are filtered and removed by the liver can build up in the body, causing complications such as mental confusion (encephalopathy) and agitation or tremors (shaking). Varicose veins in the esophagus (esophageal varices) are quite fragile and can easily rupture and bleed, sometimes massively. Varices may also develop in the rectum and bleed, though this occurs much less frequently. Bleeding most frequently occurs in patients with cirrhosis of the liver, and mostly from the varices in the lower esophagus. Rarely does bleeding occur when the portal pressure is less than 12 mmHg. Typically, patients suddenly present with hemorrhaging of the upper gastrointestinal tract. Bleeding is a serious complication, as it causes deterioration of the liver functions and may lead to death from liver failure. Sometimes renal (kidney) failure is also possible.

The spleen, which drains its blood supply into the portal vein, can often become enlarged. This is one of the most common findings with portal hypertension. Often, the spleen is enlarged from the normal 300 grams or fewer to between 500 and 1,000 grams.

When blood is under high pressure, some of its liquid portion is squeezed through the vessels and pools in the abdominal cavity. The massive accumulation of fluid expands the abdomen, a condition known as ASCITES. Kidneys can also retain sodium and water, causing even more fluid to be accumulated.

Portal hypertension can also cause the liver to shrink and atrophy because of the lack of certain hormones, mainly insulin and glucagons, which are responsible for maintaining the normal structure and function of the liver. Coma and death can result in serious cases.

Some common symptoms include the following:

- abdominal swelling (ascites)
- blood in vomit
- blood in stool
- dark stool
- encephalopathy (mental impairment)
- enlarged spleen (splenomegaly)
- hemorrhoids
- peptic ulcers
- variceal bleeding

The buildup of pressure in the stomach can also lead to bleeding, known as portal hypertensive gastropathy. This causes upper-intestinal bleeding and dark stools.

In addition to the above, other conditions usually associated with liver disease may also appear:

- asterixis (abnormal small, involuntary movements)
- gynecomastia (development of mammary glands in men)
- JAUNDICE (yellowing of the skin and eyes)
- muscle wasting
- palmar erythema (mottling or reddening of the palms)
- spider angiomas (abnormal collection of blood vessels near the surface of the skin)
- testicular atrophy

An evaluation consists of taking a complete medical history, a physical examination, imaging studies, and, in some patients, portal pressure measurements. Once a diagnosis is confirmed, the doctor attempts to determine the cause of the illness and assess its severity before deciding on the course of treatment.

A medical history helps determine the cause of portal hypertension and, secondarily, the presence of the complications of portal hypertension. The doctor checks to see whether the patient has ever had blood transfusions, a history of alcohol abuse or intravenous drug use, a personal or family history of jaundice, pruritus (itching all over the body), or hereditary liver diseases (such as WILSON'S DISEASE).

A physical examination may reveal an enlarged spleen, which can be felt through the abdominal wall. Portal hypertension is unlikely to be present if the spleen is not enlarged, although the size of the spleen does not necessarily correlate with the severity of portal hypertension. Ascites, one of the indications of portal hypertension, can be detected by noting abdominal swelling from fluid accumulation, and hearing a dull sound when tapping (percussing) the abdomen.

The doctor may also elect to measure the diameter of the portal vein. To do so, the patient must fast for a minimum of four hours. When portal hypertension is not present, the diameter of the portal vein is around 13 mm. The test measuring the portal vein has a sensitivity of only 45 to 50 percent, although its specificity is 100 percent. The sensitivity of the test can be increased to 81 percent if the diameters of the splenic vein and superior mesenteric vein are also measured. Sensitivity indicates the ability of a test to detect disease correctly, while the specificity of a test relates to its ability to avoid incorrectly identifying as abnormal things that are normal. When developing tests, scientists generally try to strike a balance between sensitivity and specificity.

As clinical evidence is usually sufficient for a diagnosis of portal hypertension, and as all the various measurement techniques are invasive and entail some risk, physicians rarely measure the portal pressure. In fact, measurements generally are not necessary, since the portal hypertension can be inferred if the blood going to the portal vein has been diverted to collateral vessels, and if the patient suffers from enlarged spleen, abdominal swelling, and possibly mental confusion. In select patients, however, a measurement may be required.

One measurement technique involves wedging a catheter—a long, tubular device—into a small hepatic vein branch. The portal pressure can be determined by comparing the pressure in the wedged hepatic vein with values in the nonwedged hepatic vein. This method is effective except in cases of presinusoidal portal hypertension.

Catheter ANGIOGRAPHY is the X-ray study of the blood vessels. It is performed to image blood vessels to determine whether they are narrowed or blocked altogether. A contrast medium, or dye, is used to highlight the vessels, after which a rapid succession of X-ray imaging is taken to show blood flow. Unlike a conventional X-ray, it is an invasive procedure in which a catheter passes through an artery leading to the body area of interest. This procedure is not suitable for patients who are allergic to the contrast medium or have blood-clotting problems, kidney disease, or kidney injury. Pregnant women are also advised to avoid this procedure.

A splenoportograph, a variation of an angiogram, may be performed. A contrast medium is injected directly into the spleen to view the splenic and portal veins. Patients undergoing an angiogram are required to stop eating eight hours before the procedure. It is best to abstain from water as well, though a small amount of water may be permissible.

Invasive angiographic techniques have their place when much more specific examinations for the evaluation of portal hypertension, such as surgery, are indicated.

Today many catheter angiographic studies have been replaced by noninvasive, rapid, and highly sensitive and specific tests, such as computed tomography (CT) angiography and magnetic resonance (MR) angiography, which do not require a catheter to be inserted. New techniques such as ultrasound (US), computed tomography (CT), computed tomography angiography (CTA), and magnetic resonance angiography (MRA) are now available, and are expected to further limit the use of angiographic methods. A CT scan can look for and examine any collateral vessels. An ultrasound scan may be used to examine the blood flow in the portal blood vessels and to detect the presence of fluid in the abdomen. In the evaluation of the liver and portal hypertension, the modalities of choice are ultrasound techniques (US), such as duplex ultrasound (US) or spectral Doppler imaging.

The duplex ultrasound combines Doppler and conventional ultrasound. The ultrasound scan can examine the structure of the blood vessels and the blood flow, and detect the presence of fluid in the abdomen, while Doppler measures the speed of blood flow and produces color-coded images to indicate where the blood flow is severely blocked.

Under normal conditions, as the blood flows through the portal vein toward the liver (called hepatopetal) flow there are fluctuations in the velocity of the blood flow in the portal vein. But in portal hypertension, these fluctuations disappear and there is a continuous flow. When there is a further increase of pressure in the portal vein, the blood begins to flow in a biphasic, or to-and-fro direction. Finally, the direction of the blood flow is reversed (hepatofugal.)

Treatment Options and Outlook

Treatment is directed at the cause of the portal hypertension. Treatment mainly involves prevention of further injury to the liver. Medication may be given to keep the blood vessels from breaking open, but because of its side effects, it is not appro-

priate for everyone. Bleeding from broken blood vessels must be treated immediately. Since bleeding from esophageal varices is a medical emergency, and the most lethal complication of portal hypertension, the first step is to stop the bleeding. After confirming that the bleeding is from the varices, the veins may be blocked off. Drugs such as propranol or vasopressin may be given to reduce the pressure in the portal vein. Transfusions may be given to replace lost blood. If medication does not stop the bleeding, surgery may be necessary to redirect the blood flow away from the liver. An operation called portal vein shunting can be considered in certain patients. The operation allows blood from the portal vein to be redirected.

Patients should be evaluated for LIVER TRANSPLANTATION as it is an effective treatment—perhaps the definitive treatment—for portal hypertension. But liver transplantation is recommended only for patients who cannot be managed successfully with invasive methods, such as shunt surgery. Liver transplantation is probably not indicated in patients who still have good liver function and whose liver is producing all the necessary proteins.

The mortality rate depends on the underlying cause of portal hypertension. The bleeding of esophageal varices as a complication of cirrhosis is the most life-threatening condition in portal hypertension. The majority of cirrhotic patients—almost 90 percent, according to some estimates—develop varices, and approximately 30 percent of varices bleed. The first episode of bleeding is estimated to carry a mortality rate of 30 to 50 percent. Surgery does not appear to change the mortality rate.

D'Amico, G., L. Pagliaro, and J. Bosch. "Pharmacological treatment of portal hypertension: An evidence-based approach." *Seminar Liver Disease* 20, no. 3 (2000): 399.

Vorobioff, J., J. E. Bredfeldt, and R. J. Groszmann. "Hyperdynamic circulation in portal-hypertensive rat model: A primary factor for maintenance of chronic portal hypertension." *Seminar Liver Disease* 19, no. 4 (1999): 475–505.

post-transplantation care   Under optimal circumstances, the patient may be released as early as a week or two after the liver transplant operation. The patient still needs to keep in close contact with the transplant team. Patients from out of state may therefore wish to remain close to the transplant center for at least a month after surgery in case of complications. Patients must also be closely monitored to see how well their new liver is functioning and to make necessary adjustments in medications and dosage. Generally, visits of once or twice weekly to the transplant center are recommended in the first month, then are gradually tapered off. Although patients will always need periodic checkups, these will decrease in frequency as their health improves and their condition stabilizes. After a period of time, to be determined on an individual basis by the attending physician, they can visit a liver specialist or other doctors instead of the transplant center.

Taking Precautions

When the patient finally goes home he or she will be required to take body temperature, weight, blood pressure, and pulse measurements on a regular basis. Although the risk of infection is greatest in the first few weeks after surgery, the risk is never entirely gone, so the patient must take an active role in managing health. It is advisable during recovery to avoid large crowds and people with infections or illnesses, and to wash hands frequently, particularly after exposure to crowds of people. Vitamins and supplements may be recommended for patients with poor nutritional status.

Transplant recipients should not be given live virus vaccinations. They should instead consider passive immunization with immune globulins.

The doctor should be notified immediately if the patient experiences infection, swelling, rashes, discharges, bruises, black stools, persistent pain, or other physical changes.

Aside from infection, the most immediate risk after transplantation is rejection of the new organ. This danger is most acute during the first year but, as with infection, the risk always remains, so the patient must watch for any signs and symptoms of rejection. If they occur, the transplant center or the primary care physician should be contacted without delay.

Before a transplant patient is discharged from the hospital, the hospital staff will teach the patient how to obtain required medications, take blood pressure measurements, and use a thermometer. After discharge, the patient will be asked to monitor the blood pressure, temperature, and weight. Some of the medications prescribed for transplant patients can cause hypertension (high blood pressure), which can lead to strokes. Thus, it is very important for the patient to monitor the blood pressure regularly.

The patient will be expected to return to the transplant clinic or doctor's office for follow-up visits and blood tests.

Transplant recipients should contact the transplant center to reorder medications, review laboratory results, and raise medical questions or concerns as they arise. If the patient is nauseated or vomiting and cannot take medications, the transplant center should be contacted immediately to arrange for intravenous administration, if necessary. The transplant center should also be contacted for persistent diarrhea or constipation.

Because transplant recipients must take medications on a regular basis, it is a good idea to have at least a week's supply of each medication and to obtain refills as needed.

Many medications, including those available over the counter, interfere with immunosuppressive medications, such as cyclosporine. Thus, transplant recipients should consult their transplant center or doctor before taking any medications, including ibuprofen (e.g., Advil or Motrin), aspirin or aspirin products (e.g., Alka-Seltzer or Bufferin), or cold medications or cough syrups that contain alcohol. If another physician prescribes a new medication, the transplant patient should check with the transplant service before taking it.

The antirejection drugs taken by transplant patients suppress the immune system, so transplant recipients must take precautions to avoid infections. Such steps include those below:

- washing hands often, especially after contact with children or pets
- avoiding contact with bodily waste from animals, such as cat litter and bird droppings

- avoiding crowds for the first few weeks after receiving the transplant
- making sure that water and food are safe
- avoiding contact with sick people
- practicing safe sex

Patients should check with their transplant team before having dental work, because dental work can cause infections. The transplant physician will probably prescribe an antibiotic to be taken before the dental work is performed.

If the patient or someone close to the patient plans to be vaccinated, check first with the transplant team. Many vaccines contain live viruses that can be transferred to people with suppressed immune systems.

Organ rejection is always a concern for transplant recipients, but there are different types of rejection, with different levels of severity. The sooner rejection is detected, the more likely it will be reversible. Most rejections can be treated with medications.

To prevent rejection, medications must be taken as prescribed. In addition, patients should eat well, exercise, and keep their appointments with their transplant clinic. Patients should discuss any health changes with the transplant team and also check with the team before taking over-the-counter medications. In addition, patients should inform their primary care doctors of any changes in their medications made by the transplant team.

Rejection of the New Organ

The symptoms of organ rejection include the following:

- abdominal discomfort
- cough or sore throat
- diarrhea
- fever
- general malaise
- jaundice (yellowing of skin and eyes)
- less urine
- redness or drainage of a wound
- pain or tenderness over the transplant site
- pulse rate change
- vomiting
- weight gain

Taking immunosuppressants   To prevent the body from rejecting the new organ, transplant patients must take antirejection medications called IMMUNOSUPPRESSANTS, which suppress the body's immune response. Acute, or sudden, rejection can sometimes lead to chronic rejection, in which there may be a gradual loss of organ function. This is an ongoing concern for transplant recipients. However, powerful new immunosuppressive agents have improved the odds tremendously for transplant patients' survival. Rejection rates have dropped from the 15 to 20 percent range to as low as 2 percent in many transplant centers. The drawback is that many side effects are associated with immunosuppressants. Besides that, the heightened risk of infection is inevitable, given the nature of the drugs. Doctors try to balance the twin threats of infection and rejection by adjusting the type, combination, and dosage of drugs; to do so, they monitor blood levels frequently, as well as perform LIVER BIOPSIES. Enough variety of medications is available today that adjustments can be made to fit the unique needs of each patient.

Steroids are usually administered as part of the arsenal of antirejection medication, but the trend today is to stop their use as soon as possible so that side effects can be minimized. Similarly, to control side effects as well as the risk of infection, investigations are now being conducted to examine the possibility of discontinuing all immunosuppressants. But until doctors can be confident that all medication can be stopped safely, patients can expect to be on a lifelong regimen of immunosuppressants.

Patients should remember that they are immune-suppressed and recognize that sexual relations can expose them to various infectious diseases. They should be especially careful if their partners have sores or open wounds. On the other hand, good sexual relationships are important in recovery, and there is no reason that patients cannot enjoy them. Counselors may be consulted about sexual concerns. Support groups are available for transplant patients.

Most transplant patients can lead a normal life after receiving a new liver. They can, for the most part, resume their previous work. Their chance for leading a happy, productive life is significantly improved after transplantation.

Travel Transplant recipients may need to make special arrangements when they travel. They should carry an adequate supply of medications for the trip or carry written prescriptions for refills, because prescriptions cannot be telephoned across state lines. Medications should not be packed in checked luggage, in case the luggage gets lost. Patients who expect to receive test results from their transplant team should make sure the team can contact them with the information. The transplant team also can provide the names of transplant centers near the travel destination or destinations, in case the recipient needs blood tests or help during the trip.

Medic-Alert tags Transplant recipients should consider wearing a Medic-Alert bracelet or necklace indicating that the wearer has had a liver transplant and the location of the facility where the transplant was performed. The tag should also indicate that the wearer is taking immunosuppressant drugs and any other health problems the recipient may have, such as asthma, diabetes, allergies, or hypertension. It is also a good idea to carry a wallet card at all times with the same information.

Emotional and psychological issues Liver disease and liver transplants can have a major impact on the recipient's life, and the transplant recipient may have to deal with significant emotional and psychological issues, including financial concerns. The transplant recipient can take actions to maintain a positive attitude, such as being as active mentally and physically as possible. It may be helpful to write down goals and track progress toward reaching the goals. Joining a support group may provide information and help. The transplant team may be able to provide options for payments if the ongoing cost of medications or loss of income creates significant financial worries. The patient may be able to learn new job skills at home or through a vocational rehab program.

pregnancy A pregnant woman can suffer from LIVER DISEASES. Whether she can have successful, uncomplicated pregnancies depends on the illness and on her health condition. Generally, if the woman does not have other complicating factors, she should be able to have healthy children without further damaging her LIVER. However, some liver disease may adversely affect pregnancy and childbirth. A woman with CIRRHOSIS often suffers from amenorrhea (lack of menses) and hence may have difficulty conceiving, particularly if she is already suffering from complications of cirrhosis. Women with cirrhosis who do become pregnant may have an increased risk of serious complications during pregnancy.

AUTOIMMUNE HEPATITIS (AIH), which generally affects young women of childbearing age, can cause menstruating to stop. But if the woman receives appropriate treatment, menstruation should return and she should be able to become pregnant.

Women with ALCOHOLIC LIVER DISEASE are also often infertile. Moreover, their infants are at high risk for developing abnormalities.

Some liver diseases are unique to pregnancy, such as INTRAHEPATIC CHOLESTASIS OF PREGNANCY and FATTY LIVER of pregnancy. Intrahepatic cholestasis of pregnancy is a condition during pregnancy in which the bile flow within the liver is impaired. Fatty liver of pregnancy is serious and often fatal, but fortunately very rare. Occurring during the last three months of pregnancy, it is characterized by a sudden onset of symptoms such as JAUNDICE (yellowing of skin and eyes), ASCITES (accumulation of fluid in the abdomen), and fulminant hepatic failure. A diagnosis must be made by liver BIOPSY. If diagnosis is confirmed, an emergency cesarean section may have to be performed.

preparing for surgery Millions of Americans undergo surgery every year. All surgeries have risks and benefits that patients must be familiar with before deciding whether the procedure is appropriate. An uninformed patient may experience a longer and more difficult recovery, and the surgery may not have been necessary in the first place.

It is important to discuss feelings, questions, and concerns with the physician before the surgery. If the physician's responses are confusing, ask more questions. The physician should supply written instructions, if necessary, and provide sources to consult for more information.

Some patients may find it helpful to write their questions down ahead of time and to take notes of the discussion to help them review the information before making a final decision. A well-informed patient tends to be more satisfied with the outcome of a procedure.

The following important topics should be discussed.

- the operation being recommended. The physician should clearly explain the surgical procedure, including the steps involved, and provide illustrative examples. The patient should ask whether there are different methods for performing the operation and why the physician favors one over another.

- why the procedure is necessary. Surgery may be performed to relieve or prevent pain, to diagnose a problem, or to improve body function. The physician should explain why the procedure is being recommended and how it may improve the patient's medical condition.

- other treatment options. In some cases, medication or nonsurgical treatments, such as lifestyle changes, may be as beneficial as surgery. The physician should clearly explain the benefits and risks of those options so the patient can make an informed decision about whether the surgery is really necessary. Sometimes it is better to wait and monitor the condition over time. If the condition improves or stabilizes, surgery can sometimes be postponed. Of course, after a period of monitoring the physician may determine that surgery is still the best option.

- the benefits of the surgery, including patient longevity. The benefits of some surgical procedures last only a short time and may necessitate a second operation. Others may last a lifetime. The physician should outline the specific benefits of the surgery and how long those benefits typically last.

- published information available about the procedure. The physician should provide information on published studies and comparative statistics concerning the possible outcomes of the procedure. Published studies allow the patient to make an informed decision and have realistic expectations about its probable outcome.

- risks and possible complications. Surgery always carries risks, and it is important to weigh the benefits against the risks. The physician should outline the possible complications, such as infection and bleeding, and possible side effects. The patient should also ask about ways to manage any pain that may follow the procedure.

- the consequences of not having surgery. What will happen if the procedure is not performed? Will the condition worsen, or might it resolve itself?

- the physician's experience in performing the procedure. A physician who is thoroughly trained and experienced in performing the procedure can minimize the risks. Point-blank questions about the physician's experience with the procedure—including credentials and additional certifications, the number of times he or she has performed it, his or her record of success, and the complications encountered—are both reasonable and acceptable. Additional information regarding the surgeon's expertise with the procedure can be obtained from a primary care physician, a local medical society, or a health insurance company.

- physicians who can provide a second opinion. Many health plans now require patients to obtain a second opinion before undergoing elective surgery. The physician should be able to supply the names of other qualified individuals who perform the procedure.

- where the surgery will be performed. Where a surgery is done is often as important as who is doing it. To lower costs, many procedures are done on an outpatient basis or in ambulatory care centers, while others need to be performed on an inpatient basis. The physician should explain why he or she recommends one setting over the other, and should provide information on his or her affiliations with accredited health care facilities.

- the type of anesthesia to be administered. The physician should explain whether a local, regional, or general anesthesia will be administered and why that type of anesthesia is being recommended. The patient should also ask who will be administering the anesthesia—both anesthesiologists and nurse anesthetists are highly qualified to administer anesthesia—and ask to meet with that person before the operation to discuss concerns. Anesthesia and anesthesiologists are discussed below.

- expectations during recovery. The patient needs to know what to expect in the first few days following surgery, as well as in the weeks and months afterward. How long will hospitalization last and what limitations will apply? Will any special supplies or equipment be needed upon discharge? Knowing the answers to those questions ahead of time may help the patient to recover more quickly.

- the costs of the operation. Health plans vary in their coverage of different procedures. The physician should be able to supply specific information on the costs and health plan coverage.

Determining Costs

Fees should be discussed before surgery. Fees may include, but are not limited to, the surgeon's fee, separate billing for other services such as an assisting surgeon or the anesthesiologist, and hospital fees.

It is important to determine what portion of the costs the insurance or health plan will pay. If anticipated costs present a problem, it is advisable to discuss other financial solutions with the physician.

Obtaining a Second Opinion

Asking another physician or surgeon for a second opinion is an important step in ensuring that the recommended procedure is the best option. A second opinion can help in the formulation of an informed decision about the best treatment for the condition, the risks and benefits of surgery, and possible alternatives.

Many health plans now require, and will pay for, a second opinion on certain nonemergency procedures. Medicare may also pay for a second opinion. A patient can request a second opinion even if his or her health plan does not require it.

Patients who decide to get a second opinion should check their health plan to see whether it is covered. The primary care physician or hospital can provide names of qualified physicians. The second physician must have all relevant medical records to avoid repeating tests and procedures that have already been performed.

In the case of emergency surgeries, there may not be time to obtain a second opinion. The necessity of getting a second opinion should always be weighed against the severity and urgency of the medical condition.

Anesthesia and Anesthesiologists

During surgery, patients are given some form of anesthesia—medicine administered for the relief of pain and sensation. There are three different types of anesthesia: local, regional, and general. The type used depends on the type of surgery and the patient's medical condition.

Local anesthesia is given to stop temporarily the sense of pain in a particular area of the body. A patient remains conscious during a local anesthetic. For minor surgery, a local anesthetic can be administered by injection to the site. When a large area must be numbed, or if a local anesthetic injection will not penetrate deeply enough, physicians may resort to regional anesthetics.

Regional anesthesia numbs only the portion of the body that will be operated on. Usually an injection of local anesthetic is given in the area of nerves that provide feeling to that part of the body. There are several forms of regional anesthetics. They include spinal anesthetics, epidural anesthetics, and brachial plexus anesthetics.

- A spinal anesthetic is an injection of an anesthetic agent directly into the spinal canal in the lower back, causing numbness in the lower body. It is often used for lower abdominal, pelvic, rectal, or lower-extremity surgery.

- An epidural anesthetic involves continually infusing drugs through a thin catheter that has been placed into the space outside the spinal fluid in the lower back, causing numbness in the lower body.

It is commonly used for labor and childbirth and for surgery of the lower limbs.

- A brachial plexus is a local anesthetic injected into the area containing the bundle of nerves that supply the upper extremity, causing numbness in the arm.

General anesthesia causes a patient to be unconscious during surgery. The medicine is either inhaled through a breathing mask or tube, or administered through an intravenous line (thin plastic tube inserted into a vein), usually in the forearm. A breathing tube may be inserted into the windpipe to maintain proper breathing during surgery. Once the surgery is complete, the anesthetic is stopped and the patient wakes up in the recovery room. In most cases sleep is induced by injection through the intravenous line.

The medical doctors trained to administer and manage anesthesia during surgical procedures are called anesthesiologists. They are also responsible for managing and treating changes in critical life functions—breathing, heart rate, and blood pressure. Anesthesiologists immediately diagnose and treat any medical problems that might arise during and immediately after surgery.

Before surgery, the anesthesiologist evaluates the patient's medical condition and formulates a plan that takes that patient's physical condition into account. It is vital that the anesthesiologist know as much about the patient's medical history, lifestyle, and medications as possible. Particularly important information the anesthesiologist needs to know includes the following:

- reactions to previous anesthetics. If the patient has ever had a bad reaction to an anesthetic drug, the anesthesiologist needs to know exactly what the reaction was and what the specific symptoms were. As much detail as possible is needed, such as feelings of nausea on awaking, the amount of time it took to wake up, and so on. Any problems related to anesthesia in the patient's family history are also useful to know about.

- current herbal supplements. Some herbal products commonly taken by millions of Americans can cause changes in heart rate and blood pres-

sure, and may increase bleeding. The herbs gingko biloba, for conditions associated with aging; garlic, to help prevent colds, flu, and other infectious diseases; ginseng, to increase energy levels and resistance to stress; and ginger may lead to excess blood loss by preventing blood clots from forming. In addition, Saint-John's-wort, a popular herb used for mild to moderate depression, and kava kava, another popular herb used for depression and mood elevation, may prolong the sedative effect of the anesthetic. The American Society of Anesthesiologists advises patients planning to have surgery to stop taking all herbal supplements at least two to three weeks before surgery to rid the body of those substances.

- known allergies. Discussing any known allergies with the anesthesiologist is very important. Some anesthetics trigger cross-allergies, particularly in persons who have allergies to eggs and soy products. Allergies to both foods and drugs should be identified.

- recent and current prescription and over-the-counter medications. The surgeon and anesthesiologist should know about prescription medications and over-the-counter medications being taken, or taken in the recent past. Some prescription medications such as coumadin, a blood thinner, must be discontinued for some time before surgery. Physicians also need to be aware of personal medical regimens, such as dietary supplements or a daily aspirin to prevent heart attack. Substances used in those regimens may prolong bleeding and interfere with anesthetics.

- cigarette smoking and drinking frequency. Cigarette smoking and alcohol can affect the body just as strongly as many prescription medications. The effect of cigarettes and alcohol on the lungs, heart, liver, and blood can change the way an anesthetic drug works. Before surgery the surgeon and anesthesiologist should be told about past, recent, and current consumption of those substances.

- street drug usage (such as marijuana, cocaine, amphetamines, heroin, and others). It is crucial that the physician know about past, recent, and current consumption of street drugs. Patients are often reluctant to discuss illegal drug consumption, but they should realize that a physician's only interest in this information is to learn enough to provide the safest anesthesia possible. Medical discussions with a physician are confidential, and patients who withhold information about illegal drugs may be endangering their lives.

To gather the necessary information, the anesthesiologist conducts a preoperative interview, either in person or over the telephone. During the interview, the anesthesiologist reviews medical history, discusses the information mentioned above, discusses anesthetic choices, and provides information about what to expect during surgery.

If the patient and the anesthesiologist have not personally met during the preoperative interview, they will meet immediately before surgery to review medical history and the results of any medical tests previously conducted. By that time the anesthesiologist will have a clear understanding of the patient's anesthetic needs.

Preoperative Paperwork

Before surgery, the patient may be asked to sign an informed consent form, which states in detail that the patient understands everything involved with the surgery. The consent must be read carefully before signing, and any questions should be discussed with the physician.

In surgeries where significant risks are involved, hospital staff may encourage the preparation of "advance directives." Advance directives are legal documents that state a patient's preference in treatment and resuscitation, and are used to guide treatment if the patient is unable to participate in treatment decisions. There are two types of advance directives: the living will and the Durable Power of Attorney for Healthcare.

A living will is a document that states a patient's wishes in the withholding or withdrawing of life support when suffering from an incurable and terminal condition.

A Durable Power of Attorney for Healthcare is a document that designates another person to make health care decisions if the patient is unable to make them. The designated person also has the

power to make the final decision about cessation of treatment.

Parental consent is required for any diagnostic procedure or surgery on a preadolescent child. "Emancipated adolescents," however, may consent to their own medical care. An emancipated adolescent is someone who is married, attends college away from home, has a child, or is in military service.

Sometimes an adult patient cannot make decisions about medical care due to accidental unconsciousness, confusion due to old age, or severe illness. In those instances, a family member will be asked to make any necessary medical decisions.

After a patient is diagnosed and surgery is recommended, most insurance companies require "precertification" from the physician's office before allowing a patient to undergo the procedure. Patients should check with their insurance carrier on the appropriate steps to take. Some insurance companies also require patients to pay a co-payment for the hospital stay.

Preparing for Surgery

Preparations for surgery depend on the diagnosis. The physician will provide information on how to prepare. General anesthesia, however, may require the patient to do any or all of the following:

- stop drinking and eating for a certain period of time before the time of surgery
- bathe or clean, and possibly shave the area to be operated on
- undergo various blood tests, X-rays, electrocardiograms, or other procedures
- take an enema the evening before surgery, to empty the bowels

Regardless of the surgical procedure, patients should observe the following:

- not wear makeup the day of surgery
- not wear nail polish
- not wear contact lenses
- leave valuables and jewelry at home

- advise the medical staff of dentures or other prosthetic devices

Often, to make their experience more comfortable and efficient, patients are advised to bring the following:

- loose-fitting clothes to wear
- Social Security number
- insurance information
- Medicare or Medicaid card

Checklist for surgery The decision to have surgery is a very important one. The patient needs to be fully informed and prepared for the procedure, as well as for any special needs following surgery. Preparation will affect the outcome and the results. The following is a checklist to help prepare for surgery:

- Make a list of questions to ask regarding the type of surgery recommended.
- Determine whether the surgical procedure is desirable.
- Obtain a second opinion, if desired or necessary.
- Check insurance or health plan coverage of the planned procedure.
- Obtain costs from physicians and from the hospital or outpatient facility.
- Schedule the surgery.
- Prepare lists of prescription medications, over-the-counter medications, herbal supplements, and illegal substances used currently or in the recent past, and review with the anesthesiologist and surgeons.
- Schedule preoperative laboratory tests.
- Arrange for a preoperative interview with the anesthesiologist.
- Follow all instructions during the weeks and days preceding surgery.
- Discontinue indicated prescription or over-the-counter medications and herbal supplements before surgery, as directed by the surgeon or physician.

- Arrange for necessary home care and equipment following surgery.
- Sign all informed consent forms and other legal forms before surgery.
- Quit smoking to help in the recovery process.

Getting ready On the day of the surgery, the patient can expect some or all of the following to occur:

- changing into a hospital gown
- receiving an identification bracelet
- having an intravenous line inserted in the forearm for anesthetics and other medications
- being transported on a stretcher to the operating room

Postoperative discomfort and complications The amount and character of discomfort following surgery depends on the type of surgery performed. Some typical discomforts include:

- nausea and vomiting from general anesthesia
- soreness in the throat caused by a tube placed in the windpipe for breathing during surgery
- soreness and swelling around the incision site
- restlessness and sleeplessness
- thirst
- constipation and flatulence

Sometimes complications occur after surgery. Individuals experience complications differently. Specific treatment for any postsurgical complications are based on the following:

- patient's age, overall health, and medical history
- extent of the disease
- type of surgery performed
- patient's tolerance for specific medications, procedures, or therapies
- patient's opinion or preference

The following are the most common complications, as defined by the American Medical Association:

- shock. Shock is a dangerous reduction of blood flow throughout the body, most often caused by reduced blood pressure. Treatment may include any or all of the following:
    stopping any blood loss
    maintaining an open airway
    keeping the patient flat
    reducing heat loss with blankets
    intravenous infusion of fluid or blood
    oxygen therapy
    medication

- hemorrhage (bleeding). Rapid blood loss—from the site of a surgery, for example—can lead to shock. Treatment of rapid blood loss may include infusions of saline solution and plasma preparation to help replace fluids.

- infection. When bacteria enter the site of surgery, an infection can result and may spread to other organs and tissue through the bloodstream. Treatment of wound infections may include antibiotics and draining of any abscess.

- deep-vein thrombosis. Sometimes blood clotting occurs within deep-lying veins. Large blood clots can break free and clog an artery to the heart, leading to heart failure. Treatment depends on the location and the extent of the blood clot, and may include anticoagulant medications (to prevent clotting), thrombolytic medications to dissolve clots, or surgery.

- pulmonary (lung) complications. Pulmonary complications can arise within 48 hours of surgery from lack of deep breathing. This may also result from inhaling food, water, or blood, or pneumonia. Symptoms may include wheezing, chest pain, fever, and cough (among others).

- urinary retention. Temporary urine retention, or the inability to empty the bladder, may occur after surgery. Caused by the anesthetic, urinary retention is usually treated by the insertion of a catheter to drain the bladder until the patient regains bladder control.

reaction to anesthesia. Although rare, allergies to anesthetics do occur. Symptoms can range from light-headedness to liver toxicity.

Recovery Immediately after surgery, the patient will most likely spend time in the recovery room with tubes attached to the body to enable the attending physician to monitor blood pressure, drain secretions (such as urine and drainage around the liver), and administer medications. In the days that follow, the doctor will evaluate progress by checking the patient's vital signs, diet, and activity level. Recovery time depends on the type of surgery performed, the patient's state of health, and willingness to take an active role in getting well.

pre-transplant evaluation Before physicians can recommend LIVER TRANSPLANTATION, they must make sure that they have exhausted all other treatments and that a transplant is in the best interest of the patient. Unless it is an emergency, such as drug overdose, poisoning, or other cases of acute LIVER FAILURE, the patient has to undergo a thorough pre-transplant evaluation, after which he or she will be placed on a waiting list for an available LIVER.

Selecting the appropriate candidate for liver transplantation is crucial to its success. First, a hepatologist (liver specialist) makes an assessment of the patient's stage within the disease, its expected progression, surgical risks, and the probable consequences of not performing the transplant. If the doctor determines that transplantation is the best option, the patient is referred to a transplantation center to be evaluated further by a transplant team. These centers have doctors with special expertise in treating patients with end-stage CIRRHOSIS or severe and acute liver failure, as well as surgeons whose subspecialties are performing liver transplants and other liver surgeries. They will review all the records and the laboratory data, as well as psychosocial evaluations, to make sure the patient can comply with the rigorous instructions for post-transplant care and accept a lifelong course of immunosuppressive medication. The evaluation may take one to two days.

The patient and family members will be introduced to the transplant team, consisting of this core group:

- transplant surgeon
- hepatologist
- anesthesiologist (to give anesthetics for the operation)

Other team members will provide various additional aspects of care for the transplant patient. These team members may include a variety of specialists:

- transplant coordinator—usually a registered nurse who coordinates various events related to the surgery, including locating the donor liver and contacting the patient
- infectious disease consultant—makes sure the patient has no dormant infection that could flare up while the immune system is suppressed
- psychiatrist or psychologist—provides insight and support for the patient and family members regarding feelings and issues related to the transplant
- physical therapist—helps the patient become stronger and may recommend an exercise plan suited to the patient's condition
- dietitian or nutritionist—gives advice about diet before and after transplant and helps the patient avoid weight gain that may result as a side effect of certain immunosuppressive drugs
- social worker—helps link the patient to services and people in the community for assistance with recovery after leaving the hospital and may also advise about Medicare, Medicaid, and other insurance coverage if there is not a separate financial counselor
- pharmacist—advises patient and family regarding immunosuppressive medications and other drugs that the patient will need before and after surgery

Comprehensive testing assesses the patient's overall health status and identifies potential problems that could occur during transplantation.

Therefore, the patient will be expected to undergo a number of procedures. Normally, there is a chest X-ray and pulmonary (lung) function tests to check the patient's lungs and respiratory tract and an electrocardiogram (EKG or ECG) to make sure the heart is healthy. There will also be one or more imaging studies, such as an ultrasound, computed axial tomographic (CAT) scans, or magnetic resonance imaging (MRI), to determine the size and shape of the liver and whether there are blockages in the BILE DUCTS and major blood vessels. Additional tests will probably be ordered, for example, to check for intestinal and kidney abnormalities. If the patient has LIVER TUMOR, a total body bone scan is performed to make sure it has not spread to the bones.

Some conditions are absolute contraindications for transplantation, because a successful outcome is unlikely. These conditions include HIV infection, active abuse of alcohol or recreational drugs, cancer existing outside the liver, severe heart or lung disease, irreversible brain dysfunction, multiple-organ failure, and inability to adhere to instructions for post-transplant medication and care.

Several other relative contraindications for transplantation may exist. These conditions do not necessarily exclude patients, but they are not optimal for a transplant. It is certainly desirable to intervene before such complications develop. Examples of relative contraindications are advanced age (age 70 or older), advanced malnutrition, morbid obesity, renal (kidney) insufficiency, having received a portosystemic shunt to reduce portal pressure in the liver, or a blood clot in the portal vein of the liver.

After the transplant team decides that transplantation is the best option for the patient, he or she is placed on the waiting list for a new liver. The surgery, its risks, and possible complications will be explained to the patient and family. Normally, patients are advised to boost their nutritional intake and improve their health status as much as possible before the operation.

The hepatologist continues to monitor the patient's condition during the waiting period. If the candidate has a living relative who can donate a portion of liver, the surgery can be scheduled to fit the needs of both the donor and the recipient. Because there is a shortage of donor livers, however, if the candidate must rely on a donor liver from a stranger, he or she should expect to wait for a period ranging from weeks to years. The length of the wait depends on many factors, and the average transplant candidate remains on the list for up to two years.

After a donor liver has become available, it must be transplanted within 12 to 18 hours. Thus, while on the transplant list, the candidate is required to carry a pager or cell phone. As soon as an organ becomes available, the transplant team calls the candidate, who should then stop eating or drinking immediately and go to the hospital as quickly as possible. The transplant surgeon will examine the donor liver to make sure it is in acceptable condition before surgery can begin.

prevention   See HEPATITIS C; HEPATITIS C METHODS OF TRANSMISSION.

primary biliary cirrhosis   Primary biliary cirrhosis (PBC) is a chronic LIVER DISEASE that destroys the BILE DUCTS in the LIVER. The defining characteristic of PBC is inflammation of the liver's smallest bile ducts.

Primary biliary cirrhosis is considered to be a cholestatic liver disease—characterized by CHOLESTASIS, or failure of bile flow. The name "primary biliary cirrhosis" is actually not an accurate description of the disease because CIRRHOSIS may not be present until the disease is quite advanced. A more descriptive name is "nonsuppurative cholangitis," which means "inflammation without pus." This long-term illness progresses slowly. The good news is that patients may continue to lead active, productive lives for many years.

Liver cells excrete BILE, which is carried by a system of tiny ducts that merge into the common bile duct that leads into the small intestine. Bile aids in digestion, particularly of fats, and provides the brown color of stools. When PBC damages the ducts, bile accumulates in the surrounding liver tissue, causing additional damage. Bile may also back up into the bloodstream, causing various symptoms. Eventually, PBC leads to cirrhosis and, possibly, to LIVER FAILURE.

PBC occurs in all races, at about the same prevalence, although there may be a higher rate of occurrence in people from northern Europe. It accounts for almost 2 percent of deaths worldwide from cirrhosis. About 20 to 150 people per million have PBC, and about four to 15 cases per million people are diagnosed each year. Patients are generally between the ages of 20 and 80 when diagnosed, and most often between the ages of 40 and 60. Ninety to 95 percent of PBC patients are women. The disease seems to be diagnosed more frequently than previously, probably due to better diagnostic tests.

The cause of PBC is unknown. Because autoantibodies are generally present in PBC patients, it appears to be an autoimmune disease. This view is supported by the fact that PBC patients often suffer from allergies or other autoimmune diseases, where the body's IMMUNE SYSTEM attacks a part of the body as if it were foreign tissue. Other causes or triggers, however, such as infectious agents and toxins, have not been completely excluded.

There appears to be a genetic susceptibility to PBC; first-degree relatives (parents, siblings, and children) of PBC patients have about a 1,000 times greater chance of developing the disease than the general population. However, the disease does not follow a simple recessive or dominant inheritance pattern, and it may affect only one of a pair of identical twins. Thus, there seem to be additional triggering events or factors. Tainted well water, certain types of infections (e.g., Epstein-Barr virus), and certain medications, such as INTERFERON and the antipsychotic chlorpromazine, have been suggested as possible triggers. PBC is not related to alcohol consumption or chronic viral hepatitis.

Symptoms and Diagnostic Path
PBC patients may have no symptoms. Indeed, 48 to 60 percent of patients have no symptoms when they are diagnosed, and it is not unusual for patients to go more than 10 years without experiencing symptoms. Often, the disease is identified after abnormal blood test results are found during a routine examination. A high level of the liver enzyme ALKALINE PHOSPHATASE may lead to more detailed testing and a diagnosis of PBC. When

symptoms are present, they are often the result of long-standing cholestasis, or accumulation of bile in the blood stream.

The most common symptoms of PBC are fatigue and pruritis, or severe itching, without a skin rash. About 78 percent of PBC patients experience fatigue, which may have causes other than PBC. Itching, experienced by 65 percent of PBC patients, is caused by retention of unknown bile substances. The discomfort ranges from mild to debilitating, and it is often worse at night.

In addition, high cholesterol levels may lead to formation of cholesterol deposits under the skin surface, with bumps that may appear on the eyelids, palms, soles, elbows, knees, ankles, wrists, or buttocks. These bumps usually are not painful. The skin may become darker, resembling a tan, due to accumulation of melanin. The patient may have diarrhea and lose weight from malabsorption of fat and other nutrients. Osteoporosis, or loss of calcium from the bones, may be present. In later stages, characteristic symptoms of liver disease may occur, such as weakness, JAUNDICE, abdominal swelling, bleeding from esophageal varices (varicose veins in the digestive tube), and HEPATIC ENCEPHALOPATHY (mental confusion and impairment).

Patients with PBC often suffer from other conditions, including a variety of autoimmune diseases. There is a fairly high rate of rheumatoid arthritis and thyroid dysfunction, usually hypothyroidism, in PBC patients. Common symptoms of hypothyroidism include coarse dry skin and hair, loss of energy, weight gain, and sensitivity to cold. Sjögren's syndrome, in which the tear and salivary glands fail to function properly, is another autoimmune disease that causes dry eyes and mouth. Another associated condition is celiac sprue, in which sensitivity to gluten causes malabsorption of nutrients from intestine; this results in diarrhea and abdominal distention. Iron deficiency anemia may occur and lead to weakness and a tendency to become fatigued easily. CRST (pronounced "crest") syndrome results in calcium deposits in the skin, pain in or thickening of the skin of toes and fingers, and small red skin lesions. Dermatomyositis is an inflammation and rash on the face, neck, chest, arms. A fairly large

percentage of PBC patients also develop gallstones. Kidney and lung disorders also are more common in PBC patients than in the general population.

Many patients are referred for evaluation for PBC based on an elevated serum (blood) ALKALINE PHOSPHATASE (ALP) level. They may not have symptoms at the time they are referred. PBC exhibits many of the same indicators as other liver diseases, and a diagnosis is based on the patient's medical history, physical examination, blood test results, imaging studies, and histological (microscopic examination of tissue) results. Most often, the patient is a middle-aged woman who complains of itching and fatigue in the earlier stages, or jaundice in the later stages. Patients may have signs and symptoms of cirrhosis and liver failure.

A physical examination may disclose an enlarged liver and spleen, a tender liver, a dark skin tone, jaundice, and finger clubbing, where the tips of the fingers are enlarged and rounded. About 20 percent of PBC patients have xanthalasmas, or yellow cholesterol nodules, around the eyes. Xanthomas, another type of cholesterol deposit, may be observed in the creases of hands, arms, legs, elbows, or knees. The patient may have severe scratch marks from trying to relieve itching. Other indicators of PBC include spiderlike skin lesions (spider nevi) and red palms.

The following table summarizes blood test results observed in PBC patients.

Test	Results
CBC	normal in early stages, may be anemic later due to gastrointestinal blood loss from varices, congestion of the stomach lining due to portal vein pressure, or enlarged spleen
platelet count	normal in early stages, may be low if cirrhosis is present
prothrombin time (PT)	blood clotting ability; normal until cirrhosis develops; may be elevated if patient is not absorbing vitamin K
albumin	normal until cirrhosis develops
alkaline phosphatase (ALP)	enzyme present in bile ducts, markedly elevated in almost all patients

Test	Results
bilirubin	bile pigment, usually normal in early stage but increases as disease progresses
gamma-glutamyltranspeptidase	enzyme present in bile ducts, markedly elevated in almost all patients
alanine aminotransferase (ALT)	enzyme made in liver, normal or moderately elevated
serum aspartate aminotransferase (AST)	enzyme made in liver, normal or moderately elevated
serum bilirubin	normal early in disease, increases as disease progresses
serum cholesterol	elevated in 75% of patients, and can be extremely high
total gamma-globulin	normal until cirrhosis develops
serum IgM	type of antibody, elevated in 90% of patients
immunoglobulin	elevated in about 90% of patients
antimitochondrial antibody (AMA)	autoantibody against mitochondria, present in 90% of patients; level does not correlate with severity of disease or prognosis; also found in some patients with autoimmune and drug-induced hepatitis. May have false positives
antinuclear antibodies	present in 50% of patients; found in normal individuals and patients with autoimmune disorders

Imaging studies may be performed to look for or rule out other causes of the patient's symptoms. An X-ray of the bile ducts may show obstructions with other causes. A sonogram may reveal gallstones.

A LIVER BIOPSY is used to determine both the existence of PBC and the progression of the disease. PBC is classified into four stages, determined by examination of the biopsy samples:

- Stage I—Asymmetrical destructive features are seen in the bile ducts. The bile ducts are attacked by white blood cells.
- Stage II—There are fewer normal bile ducts and more small, abnormal bile ducts than in a nor-

mal liver. There may be evidence of inflammation in tissues surrounding the bile ducts.

- Stage III—Few, if any, bile ducts are present, and there is progressive scarring, or fibrosis.
- Stage IV—established cirrhosis, with regenerating nodules surrounding liver cells. Although the biopsy may not provide a cause of the cirrhosis, an absence of bile ducts suggests PBC.

The liver tissue of a PBC patient may not be uniform. Thus, a biopsy may indicate more than one stage of the disease. Also, sampling variations may result in different stages at different times in the same patient. Generally, there is a gradual progression over years from stage I to stage IV. However, similar features may be seen with other liver diseases, and the biopsy results are considered along with other test results and physical observations.

Because serum IgM is usually elevated in PBC, and AMA is almost always present, the lack of these characteristics suggests that the diagnosis could be incorrect. Also, a PBC diagnosis in a male should be checked carefully, due to the rare occurrence of this disease in men.

Treatment Options and Outlook

Treatment of PBC focuses on managing the symptoms and delaying liver damage. The following areas need to be considered:

Nutrition. PBC progresses slowly, and medical treatments are oriented toward maintaining good nutrition, relieving symptoms, and attempting to slow the progress of the disease as much as possible.

Because the flow of bile acid from the liver to the intestines and general liver function are impaired in PBC patients, nutrients are often not absorbed properly. Diarrhea may add to this problem. Severe deficiencies may result in night blindness and difficulty with adapatation to darkness (vitamin A), osteoporosis (vitamin D and calcium), frequent nosebleeds, bleeding gums, and bruising (vitamins E and K). Osteoporosis, or loss of bone, leads to pain and fractures, and it is particularly common among PBC patients. Thus, it is important for these patients to receive adequate nutrition. Vitamin and mineral supplements are often recommended.

The diet should be well balanced and include at least 1,200 milligrams (mg) of calcium per day to prevent osteoporosis. Also, if blood levels of vitamin D are below normal, a vitamin D supplement may help the body to absorb calcium from the intestine. Recent tests have shown that S-adenosylmithionine (SAMe) may be beneficial. A patient who is having diarrhea and losing weight may be told to restrict dietary fat. An addition of medium-chain triglyceride oil and pancreatic enzyme supplements to the diet may be helpful. The patient may try one or both.

If edema or swelling is present, reducing salt intake and perhaps taking diuretics (fluid pills) may help.

Itching. Perhaps the most distressing symptom of PBC is itching. If the itching is mild, it might be alleviated with warm baths, emollients, alcohol sponges, or antihistamines, such as Benadryl. If these approaches do not work, Questran (cholestyramine) or cholestipol hydrochloride may be prescribed. These drugs are taken orally and bind bile acids, allowing them to be excreted from the intestines rather than absorbed into the blood. Steroids, such as prednisone or methyltestosterone, may be helpful. In more severe cases, rifampin, cimetidine, phenobarbital, or morphine antagonists, such as naloxone, nalmefene, and naltrexone, may bring relief. Phototherapy, or exposure to UVB light, may help. In severe cases, plasmapheresis may be tried. In plasmapheresis, blood is drawn from the patient, plasma is removed from the blood, and the blood is reinfused. Sometimes, fresh frozen plasma or albumin (protein in the blood) is added before the blood is reinfused. However, this procedure is expensive and is considered to be a last resort. If the itching is truly intolerable, a liver transplant may be required.

Maintaining or improving liver function. Although there is no cure for PBC, several drugs improve blood test results for liver function. Recent research suggests that they may also reduce liver damage. In early stages of the disease, the most common treatment seems to be ursodeoxycholic acid (UDCA, ursodiol, Actigall, or Urso [URSO]),

cholchicine, or methotrexate. Often a combination of these drugs is prescribed.

Ursodeoxyucholic acid is a bile acid that alters the makeup of bile in the liver and seems to reduce liver damage. It appears to decrease the incidence of major complications, such as esophageal varices, and may extend the period before a transplant is necessary. In addition, it may decrease the severity of itching and fatigue. Eighty percent of patients experience some benefits from this drug, and the results tend to be better if it is taken earlier in the course of the disease. The minimal side effects include diarrhea, decreased white blood cell count, elevated glucose levels, elevated creatinine, peptic ulcers, and skin rashes.

Colchicine is an anti-inflammatory drug that has been used for many years to treat gout, and it seems to slow the progression of PBC by inhibiting liver fibrosis. Although laboratory test results may improve, colchicine does not significantly improve symptoms. The main side effect is diarrhea.

Methotrexate is an immune suppressant. It brings improvement in liver enzyme levels, fatigue, and itching. However, it may have serious side effects; one study reported a severe but reversible lung inflammation in 14 percent of patients. It also decreases the body's ability to fight infections.

A number of other drugs have been studied for use in treating PBC, particularly anti-inflammatory agents and IMMUNOSUPPRESSANTS (medications that suppress the immune system). Many of these drugs appear to have harmful side effects that outweigh their benefits. In particular, corticosteroids are probably not effective and may increase osteoporosis. Most recent studies indicate that tacrolimus may be beneficial. Prednisone and azathioprine (Imuran) are not effective, and they accelerate osteoporosis. Cyclosporin probably has no significant benefits, and it can cause high blood pressure and kidney dysfunction. Chlorambucil is toxic to bone marrow. Maltolate has not been shown to be effective. D-penicillamine, a copper-binding drug, was shown to be ineffective and possibly toxic in several studies.

LIVER TRANSPLANTATION. Liver transplantation is now an accepted treatment for end-stage liver disease, including advanced PBC. PBC shows slow progress, and it is possible to plan ahead for a transplant. The optimum time for referral to a transplant center is when the patient's BILIRUBIN concentration reaches 4 mg/dl.

Transplantation may eliminate symptoms, such as itching, that cannot be controlled by any other method, as well as bleeding from varices and encephalopathy (mental confusion) that occur with end-stage liver disease. If the new liver functions well, osteoporosis may reverse over a 12- to 18-month period. PBC may recur in the donor liver, and it may be difficult to differentiate from rejection. The risk of recurrent PBC in transplant recipients can be influenced by the choice of immunosuppressant agents.

PBC is a slow, progressive disease. Depending on when the diagnosis is made in the course of the disease, the time between diagnosis and end-stage liver disease ranges from several months to 20 years. Patients who are asymptomatic when diagnosed generally live for 10 to 17 years. If they are already symptomatic at the time of diagnosis, the life expectancy is seven to 12 years. Many patients lead active, normal lives and remain symptom-free for ten or more years after diagnosis. Most patients die of cirrhosis and liver failure, if an unrelated cause of death does not occur first.

In general, high bilirubin levels and the development of PORTAL HYPERTENSION (blood backed up in the portal area of the liver) indicate a poor prognosis. Of the laboratory tests, the serum bilirubin concentration is the best prognostic indicator. Life expectancy, without a liver transplant, is about two years when the serum bilirubin concentration reaches 6 mg/dl. Transplantation is a standard treatment for advanced PBC, and it can extend the patient's life significantly. A great deal of research currently underway is aimed at discovering the cause, preventing damage to the bile ducts and liver, improving symptoms, and prolonging life.

Related Disorders

A number of other disorders are related to PBC or may coexist with PBC. Many of these disorders are autoimmune diseases.

- thyroid dysfunction—About 20 percent of PBC patients are hypothyroid, meaning that their thyroid function is low. The standard treatment is oral hormone replacement therapy. Hyperthyroidism, or an overactive thyroid, is less common, and it may be treated with medication, surgery, or radiation.

- Sjögren's syndrome—Also called dry gland syndrome, this autoimmune disease is characterized by dry eyes and a lack of saliva production. Artificial tears, drinking fluids, and sucking on sugarless candies are helpful. The drug pilocarpine (Salagen) may be helpful.

- metabolic bone disease—PBC patients are at risk for developing hepatic osteodystrophy, characterized by painful, hairline rib and vertebral fractures. About 25 percent of PBC patients develop osteoporosis. Osteomalacia, a softening of bones due to mineral loss, may also occur. Vitamin D and calcium supplements may help treat these diseases. Liver transplantation improves osteoporosis after about 12 months.

- cholesterol deposits in skin—Ten to 20 percent of PBC patients develop cholesterol deposits in the skin as a result of extremely high cholesterol levels in the blood. These deposits can form around the eyes, joints, and buttocks. Usually they are treated with drugs that control cholesterol levels, such as cholestyramine, or with plasmapheresis. Surgical removal often leads to regrowth.

- iron deficiency anemia—This condition usually results from bleeding. The treatment is to manage the bleeding. It the small intestine has been damaged by celiac sprue, a gluten-free diet may be recommended.

- CRST syndrome—This results in calcium deposits in the skin, pain in or thickening of the skin of toes and fingers, and small red skin lesions. Raynaud's syndrome, where fingertips turn blue and become numb when exposed to cold or emotional stress, is part of CRST syndrome. Moisturizers help with thickened skin, and antibiotics are prescribed if skin ulcers become infected. Calcium channel blockers may be prescribed for Raynaud's syndrome.

- dermatomyositis—An inflammation and rash on the face, neck, chest, and arms. Steroids may bring relief. The patient may be referred to a rheumatologist.

- scleroderma—A thickening and hardening of skin and some internal organs due to excessive collagen deposits

- vitiligo—Another autoimmune disease, characterized by smooth, nonpigmented patches of skin.

- kidney disorders—about 20 percent of women with PBC have recurrent urinary tract infections. These infections are often asymptomatic and do not require antibiotics. Other kidney diseases occur but are not common.

- lung disorders—PBC patients have a higher than normal incidence of SARCOIDOSIS, in which granulomas, or nodules with a variety of inflammatory cells, form in the lungs, skin, liver, lymph nodes, and bones. Sarcoidosis resembles PBC, and the two diseases may coexist.

- diarrhea—Diarrhea may be caused by medications, celiac sprue, or maladsorption of fat.

- gastrointestinal pain—The pain intensity does not correlate with the severity of PBC, and it may disappear without treatment.

- gallstones—PBC patients have a 30 to 40 percent risk of developing gallstones. If symptoms develop, they are generally treated by surgical removal of the gallbladder.

- celiac sprue—PBC patients are about 10 times more likely to suffer from celiac sprue than the general population. Patients do not tolerate gluten, a protein found in grains. Avoiding grains helps relieve the symptoms

- autoimmune hepatitis (AIH)—This may have symptoms that overlap with those of PBC, including the presence of AMA (antimitochondrial antibody) in the blood. Patients with overlapping symptoms usually respond well to conventional treatment for AIH.

- hepatitis A and B—It may be desirable to screen PBC patients for HEPATITIS A and B, and then, if they are not infected, to vaccinate them to prevent additional liver damage from a viral infection.

- liver cancer—The risk of developing liver cancer after a diagnosis of PBC is between 2 and 6 percent for women, and higher for men.

- heart disease—Despite the high cholesterol levels seen in about 75 percent of PBC patients, they do not face a higher risk of heart disease. Usually, the HDL, or "good" cholesterol, level is high, and it cannot be reduced with diet.

Bach, N., and F. Schaffner. "Familial primary biliary cirrhosis." *Journal of Hepatology* 20, no. 6 (June 1994): 698–701.

Neuberger, J., et al. "Immunosuppression affects the rate of recurrent primary biliary cirrhosis after liver transplantation." *Liver Transplantation* 10, no. 4 (2004): 488–491.

primary sclerosing cholangitis (PSC) Primary sclerosing cholangitis (PSC) is a chronic, slowly progressing disease in which the BILE DUCTS, both inside and outside the LIVER, become inflamed and scarred. The inflammation of the bile ducts is called cholangitis. Ducts in the pancreas and GALLBLADDER may also be affected. Eventually, the bile ducts become blocked, preventing bile drainage from the liver, and liver cells become damaged. Bile may also enter the bloodstream. In the end stages, cirrhosis develops, leading to liver failure.

Worldwide, PSC occurs in about three out of 100,000 people. PSC usually begins between the ages of 30 and 60, but it can arise during childhood. About 70 percent of patients are male, and the mean age of diagnosis is around 40 years. Years may pass before the patient has symptoms or is diagnosed with the disease.

The cause of PSC is unknown, but it is generally believed to be an autoimmune disease, and genetic factors may be present. Many patients do not have symptoms when they initially visit a doctor, and the diagnosis is made only after blood tests show abnormal results, particularly elevated levels of serum alkaline phosphatase. When present, the main symptoms of PSC are itching, fatigue, and JAUNDICE. Chills and fever may result from bacterial cholangitis.

PSC may occur without other coexisting diseases, but about 70 percent of patients suffer from inflammatory bowel disease, particularly ulcerative colitis or Crohn's disease. It is often associated with bacterial infections of the bile ducts, or bacterial cholangitis, and an increased risk of developing CHOLANGIOCARCINOMA—cancer of the bile duct.

Primary sclerosing cholangitis is defined by the following characteristics:

- alkaline phosphatase levels more than 1.5 times the upper limit of the normal range of values for six months
- abnormal bile ducts inside and outside the liver
- liver biopsy results consistent with PSC, and that exclude other forms of chronic liver disease
- no evidence of secondary causes of cholangitis

The cause of PSC is unknown, but many researchers suspect that it is an autoimmune disease. Because about 70 percent of PSC patients also have inflammatory bowel disease, there may be a genetic link between the two diseases. Other possible causes include infectious agents, toxins, and recurrent infections of the bile ducts. There may be a relationship between genetic factors and an unknown virus or bacteria.

PSC is not related to viral hepatitis, alcohol consumption, or smoking. For reasons not completely understood, previous tonsillectomy may decrease the risk of developing PSC.

Symptoms and Diagnostic Path

At first, PSC progresses slowly, and there may be no symptoms for many years. Usually the first indications are abnormal blood test results, particularly elevated alkaline phosphatase, when tests are ordered for some other reason, such as ulcerative colitis or Crohn's disease.

When PSC symptoms develop, they may be intermittent or continuous, and they may worsen gradually. They have two causes: bile is not draining properly through the bile ducts, and the liver is not functioning properly. The common early

symptoms include fatigue and discomfort in the right upper abdomen.

Fatigue is reported in about 75 percent of patients. About 70 percent of patients develop itching when bile seeps into the bloodstream. Blockages of the bile ducts may cause jaundice, seen in about 60 percent of patients. About 40 percent of patients experience loss of appetite and weight loss. In about 35 percent of patients, bacterial cholangitis causes episodes of fever, chills, and upper abdominal tenderness. Eventually, patients develop cirrhosis and its complications, and ultimately, liver failure may develop.

PSC may be suspected because of the patient's medical history, particularly if there is a history of inflammatory bowel disease, and from abnormal blood tests for alkaline phosphatase and gamma-glutamyltranspeptidase (GGTP). Some patients may seek help because they are already experiencing symptoms, such as itching, jaundice, fever, weight loss, signs of CIRRHOSIS complications, or bacterial cholangitis. The patient will probably be referred to a gastroenterologist (digestive disease specialist) or a hepatologist (liver disease specialist). A PSC diagnosis is usually based on the combination of symptoms, blood tests, and imaging of the bile ducts.

Blood tests check how well the liver is functioning and look for antibodies that may be related to the disease. The accompanying table summarizes blood test results seen in PSC patients.

serum alkaline phosphatase	elevated in 99 percent of PSC patients
gamma-glutamyl-transpeptidase (GGTP)	almost always elevated in PSC patients
serum aminotransferase	elevated in 95 percent of PSC patients
serum bilirubin	elevated in 65 percent of PSC patients
serum albumin	normal early in disease, decreases later
prothrombin time	normal early in disease, increases later; may be due to poor vitamin K absorption

serum copper	abnormal in 50 percent of PSC patients
serum ceruloplasmin	abnormal in 75 percent of PSC patients
urine copper	abnormal in 65 percent of PSC patients
bilirubin	normal or slightly elevated early in disease, markedly elevated later; large fluctuations may occur
serum IgM	elevated in about 50 percent of patients
blood gamma globulin	elevated in about 30 percent of patients
antineutrophil cytoplasmic antibodies (ANCA)	present in about 50 percent of patients
antismooth muscle antibodies	may be present
antinuclear antibodies	may be present

The most reliable test for diagnosing PSC is an X-ray obtained with a procedure called ENDOSCOPIC RETROGRADE COLANGIOPANCREATOGRAPHY (ERCP). The patient is sedated, and a flexible, lighted endoscope is threaded through the mouth and into the small bowel. A thin tube is then threaded through the endoscope and into the bile ducts, and a dye is injected to highlight the bile ducts. An X-ray is then taken. Images of the bile ducts may also be obtained with magnetic resonance imaging (MRI) or by laparotomy, a surgical procedure. PSC is diagnosed if the bile ducts have multiple constrictions and enlarged areas both inside and outside the liver.

Liver biopsies are not usually used to diagnose PSC, but they may help confirm the diagnosis and determine the extent of damage from the disease and whether the patient has cirrhosis.

In diagnosing PSC, it is important to rule out secondary causes of sclerosing cholangitis, such as drugs, bile duct cancers, and past biliary tree surgery. AIDS patients may have similar damage caused by cytomegalovirus (CMV) or *Crytosporidia*. Usually, these secondary causes can be ruled out by considering the patient's medical history, physical examination, and laboratory tests. An ultrasound scan may be ordered to exclude other diseases.

Treatment Options and Outlook

There is no cure for PSC, but treatments are available to maintain liver function and alleviate symptoms and complications

Liver function The immunosuppressive drug Ursodiol (Actigall or Urso or ursodeoxycholic acid) changes the bile composition in the liver. It improves laboratory test results, and it may increase survival time or the time before referral for a liver transplant. Other immunosuppressants have been prescribed, including prednisone, azathioprine, cyclosporine, methotrexate, and choleretic. Colchicine may help prevent fibrosis of the liver. D-penicillamine may help control abnormal copper levels.

Fatigue The most common symptom of PSC is fatigue. Patients may need to limit their daily activities. Exercise may be helpful, and energy supplements may help as well.

Nutrition Many PSC patients can follow a normal diet, at least until they have more severe symptoms. Many patients do not absorb and use fat-soluble vitamins properly, and the doctor may recommend supplements of vitamins A, D, and K.

Some patients have difficulty digesting fat because of the decreased bile flow out of the liver. As a result, they may have a type of diarrhea, called steatorrhea, in which the stools are bulky, pale, and difficult to flush. There may also be nausea. A low-fat diet often improves the diarrhea and abdominal discomfort associated with it. The doctor may prescribe medium-chain triglycerides (MCT), fats that are easier to digest. These patients may need to consult a dietician to make sure they receive proper nutrients and sufficient calories to maintain energy levels. A dietician may also help manage the effects of cirrhosis and other complications of advanced liver disease, such as fluid retention and encephalopathy (mental confusion). A low-salt diet, possibly in combination with diuretics (water pills), can alleviate swelling of the abdomen and feet from fluid retention.

Many herbal and Chinese remedies can interfere with other medications, in addition to possibly adding to the work of a liver that already is not functioning well. PSC patients should check with their doctors before taking any medication their doctors have not prescribed.

Alcohol and tobacco Chronic liver diseases, such as PSC, may interfere with liver function, including its ability to break down alcohol and drugs. The patient may be advised to limit alcohol consumption. Most doctors also advise PSC patients to avoid smoking.

Bleeding PSC patients have an increased risk of bleeding. They should inform their dentists and other health care providers that they have PSC. In addition, they may want to avoid medicines, such as aspirin, that can promote bleeding.

Itching When bile accumulates in the bloodstream, intense itching (pruritis) occurs. Itching can be treated with Questran or cholestyramine, which bind bile in the intestine and prevent absorption into the blood. Other drugs prescribed for itching include rifampicin and naltrexone.

Dry mouth and eyes PSC patients sometimes suffer from dry mouth and dry eyes. Sucking on lozenges and artificial tears help alleviate the discomfort.

Surgery Sometimes the doctor may recommend an endoscopic or surgical procedure to dilate the major bile ducts. The doctor inserts a tiny tube into the duct through an endoscope, and a balloon at the end of the tube is inflated to expand the duct. A stent, or section of plastic tubing, may be placed inside the duct to keep it open. This procedure should be done by an experienced physician.

Other surgical treatments for PSC include reconstruction of the biliary tract and proctocolectomy, or removal of diseased intestine, for ulcerative colitis.

Liver transplantation If PSC progresses to the point where the liver begins to fail, liver transplantation may be considered to prolong and improve the quality of the patient's life. A transplant may be suggested if there are complications of cirrhosis, such as bleeding esophageal varices, ascites, encephalopathy, and severe inability of the liver to synthesize proteins. A very high level of bilirubin in the blood may also indicate that a transplant is appropriate. A patient with recurrent bacterial cholangitis may also be referred for transplant.

PSC is a slowly progressing disease, and the patient can plan for elective transplant surgery. Survival rates are as high as about 90 percent after one year and 75–80 percent after five years, with a good quality of life after recovery from the surgery. PSC rarely recurs after transplantation. However, PSC patients appear to have an increased risk of rejecting the new liver, even years after the transplant.

PSC patients are subject to the same complications as with other chronic liver diseases. Portal hypertension can lead to variceal bleeding, ascites (abdominal swelling), and encephalopathy. Surgical procedures can control bleeding from esophageal and peristomal varices. Spontaneous bacterial peritonitis can also occur.

Chronic bile duct obstruction, or cholestasis, can cause fatigue, pruritis (itching), diarrhea, fat-soluble vitamin deficiencies, and metabolic bone disease, such as osteoporosis.

Complications specific to PSC include bacterial cholangitis, biliary stone disease, obstruction of the major bile ducts, and cholangiocarcinoma (bile duct cancer).

PSC is a progressive disease that ultimately leads to cirrhosis and liver failure. The course of the disease is usually slow, but it may be unpredictable. There may be no symptoms for many years, or the symptoms may remain stable, intermittent, or progress gradually. Liver failure may occur after seven to 15 years of the disease. The median time to death or liver transplant is about 10 years from diagnosis.

PSC patients usually have recurrent bouts of bacterial cholangitis, and many develop cholangiocarcinoma, a cancer of the bile ducts.

Related Disorders

Inflammatory bowel disease Many PSC patients also suffer from inflammatory bowel disease, including Crohn's disease and ulcerative colitis; this suggests that there may be a common cause for the two conditions. Indeed, inflammatory bowel disease precedes PSC in about 75 percent of PSC patients. There is speculation that an inflamed colon allows toxins or infections to reach the bile ducts and cause inflammation there. The bowel disease may be asymptomatic, mild, or severe, and its presence does not seem to affect the course of PSC.

Bacterial cholangitis Bacterial cholangitis, or infection of the bile ducts, is common in PSC patients. This type of infection may be life-threatening, and it is treated aggressively with broad-spectrum antibiotics, often in a hospital setting. The doctor may order prophylactic (preventive) treatment with ciprofloxacin (Cipro), which becomes concentrated in the liver.

Cancer PSC patients have a risk of 0.5 to 1 percent of developing each year cholangiocarcinoma, or cancer of the bile ducts. This form of cancer is the major cause of death in PSC patients who do not undergo a liver transplant. Cholangiocarcinoma is usually suspected in patients who have had PSC for some time and whose condition becomes worse. PSC patients are also at risk for other hepatobiliary cancers. One study found that a large proportion of PSC patients developed hepatobiliary malignancies within one year after receiving the diagnosis of PSC.

Cholangiocarcinoma is usually diagnosed with an ERCP or computed axial tomography (CAT) scan. These patients have a poor prognosis, since this type of cancer does not respond well to chemotherapy or radiation. Also, the presence of this type of cancer will probably prevent approval of the patient for a liver transplant.

Some researchers believe that PSC predisposes patients to several other types of gastrointestinal cancers, including pancreatic and colon cancers. The risk of developing colorectal cancer (a tumor involved in both the colon and the rectum) is 10 times higher in PSC patients, probably linked to the high frequency of ulcerative colitis and Crohn's disease in these patients. One study found that the risk of developing pancreatic cancer is 14 times higher in PSC patients than in the general population. There may be some overlap between pancreatic carcinoma and cholangiocarcinoma.

Doctors usually recommend colonoscopies at regular intervals for a PSC patient who also has inflammatory bowel disease, both to check for colitis and to look for malignancies in the colon. It is not clear whether PSC patients are more susceptible to colon cancers than other patients with inflammatory bowel disease.

Autoimmune hepatitis (AIH) Signs of PSC are present in about 6 percent of AIH patients, and more often in children. These patients typically have a poor response to treatment with steroids.

Osteoporosis PSC patients are at risk for osteoporosis because they tend not to absorb and use nutrients properly. The usual treatment is to correct any vitamin deficiencies and take calcium supplements. For postmenopausal women, estrogen replacement therapy may help.

A number of other disorders are found at increased frequency in PSC patients. These include inflammatory bowel disease, celiac sprue, sarcoidosis, chronic pancreatitis, rheumatoid arthritis, retroperitoneal bibrosis, thyroiditis, Sjögren's syndrome, autoimmune hepatitis, systemic sclerosis, lupus erythematosus, vasculitis, Peyronie's disease, membranous nephropathy, bronchiectasis, autoimmune hemolytic anemia, immune thrombocytopenic purpura, histiodytosis X, cystic fibrosis, and eosinophilia. Many of these are autoimmune diseases.

Bergquist, A., A. Ekbom, R. Olsson, et al. "Hepatic and extrahepatic malignancies in primary sclerosing cholangitis." *Journal of Hepatology* 36 (2002): 321–327.

Florman, S., et al. "The incidence and significance of late acute cellular rejection (7,000 days) after liver transplantation." *Clinical Transplantation* 18, no. 2 (May 2004): 152–155.

Schrumpf, E., and K. M. Boberg. "Hepatic and extrahepatic malignancies and primary sclerosing cholangitis: there is an increased risk of pancreatic carcinoma in patients with primary sclerosing cholangitis." *Gut* 52, no. 2 (February 2003): 165(1).

prothrombin time (PT) The prothrombin time (PT) test measures how long it takes a person's blood to clot. The time needed for blood to clot normally runs between nine and 11 seconds. An abnormally long prothrombin time may put one at risk for excessive bleeding.

The LIVER produces most of the blood-clotting factors, including I, II, V, VII, IX, and X. When liver function has been significantly compromised through injury or disease, the liver does not create enough factors, and it takes the blood longer to clot.

Usually the liver has to be significantly damaged before there is a marked increase in PT. After a severe injury, the clotting factors can decrease quite rapidly, sometimes within hours. As the liver heals, the PT returns to normal. In chronic liver disease, there may be no noticeable change in PT until the liver has been considerably damaged and scarred, as in CIRRHOSIS.

Other possible causes of prolonged PT include lack of vitamin K, certain bleeding disorders, blood-thinning medicines, and other medicines that can interfere with the test.

Vitamin K deficiency can slow down PT because the vitamin is important for blood clotting. The deficiency is sometimes due to cholestatic liver disease, in which there is a stagnation of bile flow. Because blood-clotting factor V is not dependent on vitamin K, its measurement can help distinguish vitamin K deficiency from liver dysfunction.

Doctors may inject vitamin K to determine whether the PT returns to normal. If it does, the liver is still functioning. If not, the patient may be suffering from coagulopathy (tendency to bleed excessively) or a severe LIVER DISEASE. LIVER TRANSPLANTATION may have to be considered in case of LIVER FAILURE.

psychological help   See DEPRESSION.

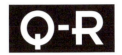

quasispecies See HEPATITIS C.

radiofrequency ablation (RFA) Radiofrequency thermal ablation or radiofrequency ablation (RFA) is a therapy for treating cancer by using alternating current radiofrequency to heat and destroy tumors in the LIVER. RFA is a medical procedure that has been used for decades. It can be used on patients who have inoperable cancer, both liver lesions that started in the liver (primary) and lesions that spread from other areas of the body (metastatic).

There are different kinds of thermal therapy that use various methods such as microwave, laser, or high-intensity focused ultrasound to heat and ablate, or cut out, tumors from an organ. With RFA, a special needle is inserted into the tumor, and heat is generated through agitation caused by alternating electrical current (radiofrequency waves) moving from the needle into the tissue. The resulting heat causes the tumor cell to coagulate—to thicken and become jellylike. Cells that coagulate cannot continue to grow, and they die. The dead cells are eventually reabsorbed into the body, and the tumors are replaced by scar tissue that shrinks over time.

Radiofrequency ablation is most commonly performed for the primary liver cancer, HEPATO-CELLULAR CARCINOMA (HCC), and colon and rectal cancer that metastasized to the liver (CRC). Recent advances have made it possible to ablate larger volumes of tissue, and tumors seven centimeters in diameter have been successfully destroyed; in the future, it may be possible to treat even larger lesions.

Radiofrequency ablation is also used to treat cancer in the bone, kidney, heart, prostate, breast, brain, lymph nodes, and ganglia. The Food and Drug Administration (FDA) has approved the use of RFA to treat liver cancer, but treatments for some of the other conditions are still considered experimental.

LIVER RESECTION is considered the gold standard in the treatment of cancer against which all other modalities must be measured. A great deal of data are available to support the effectiveness of surgery in treating cancer. The reality, however, is that most cancer cases are inoperable for various reasons, for instance, if there are small liver lesions that are too difficult or too widespread to surgically remove the portion of the liver containing the tumor. And for patients with cancers that have metastasized from the colon or rectum—in fact, most any cancer that has spread from other parts of the body—liver resection is usually contraindicated. Or, as not uncommonly, the tumors may have been surgically removed but grown back. CHEMOTHERAPY may also have failed to keep the tumors under control. For these and other patients, RFA may be an effective therapy.

RFA is not considered a cure for cancer—though preliminary studies show promising results—but it can be used to prepare otherwise inoperable patients for surgery. Doctors can destroy small tumors that are too spread out or in locations that are too difficult for surgery. Reducing the tumor load may push the cancer back into an earlier stage, based on the CANCER STAGING criteria, which measure the progression of cancer. An earlier stage of cancer is more amenable to treatment, and a patient formerly considered ineligible for surgery can now be operated on.

Procedure

First, the doctor makes a careful assessment to determine whether the patient will benefit from RFA.

RFA is generally performed on patients who are not considered good candidates for surgery. The tumors usually have to be limited to the liver. In the case of colorectal metastasis (cancer that has spread from the colon and rectum), the tumors must not have spread to other organs. However, RFA can be used to relieve the symptoms of patients for whom the tumors have spread to other parts of the body. Even if the cancer is considered incurable, RFA can help patients enjoy a better quality of life by reducing the tumors and thus diminishing symptoms.

There is a limit to the volume of tumor tissue that can be eliminated by RFA. The procedure works best on tumors that are smaller than five centimeters in diameter. And ideally, patients should have no more than three tumors that are no greater than four centimeters in size. However, recent developments have made it possible to treat larger masses, and some doctors are reporting good results with tumors as large as seven centimeters. Technical advances may eventually permit even larger tumors to be treated effectively.

As with surgery, RFA cannot eliminate microscopic-size tumors, although unlike surgery, it can destroy many small ones. It also cannot prevent cancer cells from growing back.

Patients are expected to abstain from all food and drink after midnight before the procedure the following day. The doctor will instruct them to stop taking aspirin 10 days before the procedure, as well as any blood thinner medications they may be taking. They should make sure their doctor is aware of any other medications or herbal remedies they may be taking. Also, an arrangement with a family member or a friend should be made for the patient to be accompanied home if RFA is performed on an outpatient basis.

Many U.S. insurance companies pay for radiofrequency ablation if it is used to treat liver tumors. Patients should check with their insurance carriers ahead of time to make sure their insurance plan covers the procedure, and take care of the paperwork.

RFA can be done percutaneously (inserting the needle through the skin), laparoscopically (using a lighted scope inserted through an incision), or in an open surgical procedure. General anesthesia is not necessary if the procedure is done through the skin; all that is needed is sedation, which is administered through an IV needle. The patient may fall asleep during the procedure, depending on how deep the sedation is.

To prevent discomfort during the procedure, the patient is also given pain medication, and local anesthetic will be injected where the incision is to be made in the skin, to numb the area.

For smaller tumors, doctors prefer the less invasive percutaneous method because it can be done on an outpatient basis; the patient goes home the same day or the following day, after overnight observation. Recovery time is also shorter.

Drawing on new research suggesting that larger tumors can be more successfully removed using a surgical approach, some surgeons are opting for open surgery. For this, general anesthesia is required. Even if an open surgery is required, RFA is still less invasive than liver resection in which a portion of the liver must be removed along with the tumor.

The equipment basically consists of three components: needle electrodes, an electrical generator, and grounding pads. The needles come in different versions to suit the patient's needs and condition. Most commonly used needles include the coaxial umbrella, which is a needle within a needle that opens like an umbrella inside the tumor; the internally cooled probes, which are cooled with liquid (to prevent overheating), and multiple probes.

The electrode needle, which is about 15 grams, is inserted into the tumor while guided by and monitored by imaging methods. The imaging technique most commonly used is ultrasound, followed by computed tomography scan and magnetic resonance imaging. The patient is monitored for routine cardiovascular and respiratory functions to ensure safety during the procedure. Each ablation session may last between 10 to 30 minutes, depending on the particular equipment used and the size and location of the tumors. If there are many tumors, several sessions may be needed.

Electrical current in the range of radiofrequency waves is passed between the needle electrode and the grounding pads placed on the patient's skin. The patient becomes like an electrical circuit. The alternating radiofrequency energy heats the electrode inside the tumor, and the heat, reaching more than 113 degrees Fahrenheit, spreads from the inside out—like a microwave—to destroy the tumor. Tumor cells are believed to be more susceptible to heat than normal cells; thus, radiofrequency ablation is able to destroy tumors safely and a very small surrounding rim of healthy liver tissue. The margin of normal tissue next to the tumors has to be burned to ensure that no single tumor cell remains. The physician creates a sphere of dead tissue ranging in size from three to five and a half centimeters. In large tumors, the surgeons may make several overlapping spheres, using multiple placements of the needle. Most patients feel little or no pain during the procedure. If the cancer comes back, it usually recurs at the edge of the treated area, and can usually be retreated. It is rare for bleeding to occur because the heat closes off the small blood vessels.

After the procedure, the patient remains in a recovery room until he or she is completely awake and ready to go home. In more complicated cases, or if an open surgery was performed, the patient is hospitalized. The patient receives more medication for pain and possible nausea. Fewer than 2 percent of patients continue to have pain a week after RFA.

To make sure that all the tumors are destroyed, the doctor conducts a CT scan of the liver after the procedure, either the same day or several days later. Sometimes, because of inflammation in the treated area, it may be difficult to differentiate between inflamed tissue and remnants of a tumor. In time, the affected area will heal and the patient will be ready for the first CT scan after the ablation. After that, patients can expect to have a CT scan every three months to check for new tumors.

One of the greatest benefits is that radiofrequency ablation offers patients a treatment alternative when surgery may not be possible. For instance, the needles used for the ablation can be placed in locations that cannot be reached in surgery. Additional benefits are that RFA can treat multiple liver tumors and the procedure can be repeated if the tumor regrows or recurs, or if the treatment had been incomplete. If RFA is done through the skin, the patient can go home the same day; with laparoscopic RFA, the patient generally goes home after an overnight hospital stay.

Patients who had open surgery with general anesthesia take longer to recover.

RFA is a safe, well-tolerated, minimally invasive technique with few complications. Hospital admission is not required for treating smaller tumors. Recovery is quicker than would be for liver resection; patients can usually resume normal activities within a few days.

RFA expands treatment options for patients. Because it does not exclude conventional treatments, it can be an adjunct to treatments such as surgery, radiation therapy, chemotherapy, alcohol ablation, and chemoembolization.

According to a report presented at the 29th annual scientific meeting of the Society of Interventional Radiology, combining two least invasive treatments for liver cancer is as effective as surgery for treating a solitary tumor (hepatocellular carcinoma) up to seven centimeters in diameter. The study combined embolization—blocking the blood supply to the tumor—with radiofrequency ablation. The study shows that combining treatment modalities can effectively treat patients and allow them to live as long as they would with surgical resection, but without the trauma.

Risks and Complications

The greatest risk is that the organs and tissues near the liver, including the GALLBLADDER, BILE DUCTS, colon, and diaphragm, may become injured and require surgical correction. But complications like that occur in only about 3 to 5 percent of all cases. The likelihood of injury depends partly on the location of the tumor. The closer the tumor is to important structures, the greater the possibility of damage. For example, the bile ducts may become injured, and this can cause biliary obstruction, where bile flow is impeded. Another possibility is what physicians call the "heat sink effect" in tumors close to major blood vessels. The blood that flows through these vessels is cooler than the tissue being cooked, and its "cooling" effect could impede the heating of the tumor cells. As a consequence, the areas close to these blood vessels may not be adequately treated, or become the site for a new growth.

Patients may experience low-grade fevers following the procedure. Some bleeding has also been reported, but it usually stops on its own. If the bleeding is severe, surgery or some other procedure may be needed. There may also be inflammation in a nearby organ, such as the gallbladder, but that should subside in a few weeks. There is also a low risk of infection, skin burn, abnormal heart rhythms, and collapse of the lung. Additionally, RFA can cause shoulder pain, usually of brief duration, but occasionally longer. Pain medication can help until the pain completely disappears. A small number of patients may be ill for a few weeks after the procedure.

Overall, few complications have been reported in the use of RFA.

Surgeons have been experimenting with radiofrequency ablation–assisted liver resection to reduce blood loss during surgery. Patients losing too much blood during surgery may experience a higher rate of complications after the operation. Moreover, patients' long-term survival time may be somewhat shortened.

Studies have reported that, with the use of RFA, it is possible to resect the liver without resorting to blood transfusions, or at least to perform a virtual bloodless surgery. The heat probe is used on healthy liver tissue to coagulate the margins of resection during liver resection. However, RFA requires a longer time for the operation.

Editors. "Combination of minimally invasive treatments as effective as surgery." *Cancer Weekly* 9, no. 16 (May 4, 2004): 128.

Ronnie, T. P., et al. "Effectiveness of radiofrequency ablation for hepalocellular carcinomas larger than 3 cm in diameter." *Archives of Surgery* 139, no. 3 (March 2004): 281–287.

Stella, M., A. Percivale, M. Pasqualini, A. Profei, N. Gandolfo, G. Serafini, and R. Pellicci. "Radiofrequency-assisted liver resection." *Journal of Gastrointestinal Surgery* 7, no. 6 (September–October 2003): 797–801.

Weber, J. C., G. Navarra, L. R. Jiao, J. P. Nicholls, S. L. Jensen, and N. A. Habib. "New technique for liver resection using heat coagulative necrosis." *World Journal of Surgery* 21, no. 3 (March–April 1997): 254–259.

sarcoidosis Sarcoidosis is a chronic autoimmune disease that causes inflammation of body tissues. This inflammation causes cells to build up into small lumps called granulomas. The symptoms of sarcoidosis may appear suddenly, or the condition may progress gradually. Symptoms can vary widely and depend on the tissues affected. It often affects several body sites at the same time. Some people have no symptoms—in these individuals, a physician may see signs of the disease in an X-ray taken for another reason, such as a chest X-ray taken during a routine exam.

Sarcoidosis usually affects the lungs and lymph nodes first, but it can spread to any part of the body, including the LIVER. The disease may go away quickly or may have symptoms that come and go for years. Sarcoidosis can affect anyone, but it is more common in people between 20 and 40 years of age. The cause of sarcoidosis is unknown and may include a family history of the disease or an environmental trigger (being exposed to something that may cause the disease to start). Sarcoidosis is not contagious.

Sarcoidosis often causes granulomas to form in the liver. If symptoms occur because of these granulomas, they can include pain in the upper-right portion of the abdomen, fatigue, itching, fever, and liver enlargement. Nausea, vomiting, and JAUNDICE (yellowing of the skin and eyes) may also occur.

Tests may be done to learn whether sarcoidosis is affecting the liver. Blood tests, imaging tests (such as a CT scan), or a liver biopsy may be needed. Fortunately, the disease seldom causes permanent liver damage. Treatment of sarcoidosis solely due to liver involvement is usually not necessary. Often, the physician may monitor blood tests over time to make sure the liver is tolerating the disease. If severe or bothersome symptoms occur, or if liver function is affected, drug treatment may be necessary. Most drugs used to treat sarcoidosis are immunosuppressants, such as steroids. There have been rare cases of sarcoidosis where liver transplantation was necessary.

For more information about sarcoidosis, please contact the following:

Sarcoidosis Research Institute
3475 Central Avenue
Memphis, TN 38111
(901) 327-5454
http://www.sarcoidosisresearch.org

serum protein electrophoresis Serum protein electrophoresis is a blood test that analyzes the proportion of different types of protein in the blood. Other names for the test are lipoprotein electrophoresis and serum lipid protein.

Serum is the clear yellowish fluid that oozes from a blood clot after the blood has coagulated. It contains a large variety of proteins, which are formed from amino acids and perform a wide variety of functions in the body. Measuring the relative concentrations of certain proteins in serum can provide vital clues to liver function and helps in the diagnosis of LIVER DISEASE.

Electrophoresis is the laboratory technique used to detect the protein levels. The technique exposes the blood serum to an electric current that causes the proteins to form a series of bands indicating the relative proportions of the protein levels. Four major types of protein are measured in this way: ALBUMIN, alpha globulins, beta globulins, and gamma globulins.

Albumin, produced in the liver, is essential to maintaining internal pressure in the capillaries, which helps prevent fluid from building up in the tissues. Albumin normally constitutes about 60 percent of the proteins in the blood; the remaining 40 percent consists of the globulins, which are produced by liver cells and the IMMUNE SYSTEM to help fight infection. The globulins can be roughly divided into four types: alpha-1, alpha-2, beta, and gamma globulins. Gamma globulins include the antibodies (immunoglobulins) IgA, IgD, IgE, IgG, and IgM.

The accompanying table shows the normal levels of proteins in the blood:

Element	Normal Range (grams per deciliter)
total protein	6.4–8.3 g/dL
albumin	3.5–5.0 g/dL
alpha-1 globulin	0.1–0.3 g/dL
alpha-2 globulin	0.6–1.0 g/dL
beta globulin	0.7–1.2 g/dL
gamma globulin	0.7–1.6 g/dL

The results of the serum protein test may indicate any of a number of conditions, depending on which proteins show abnormal levels. For example;

- Abnormally low levels of total protein may indicate malnutrition or nephrotic syndrome, a condition characterized by excessive fluid in the tissues and large amounts of albumin in the urine.
- High levels of alpha-1 globulins may mean acute and chronic inflammatory disease; low levels may indicate ALPHA-1-ANTITRYPSIN DEFICIENCY.
- Elevated levels of beta globulins are typical of bleeding (COAGULOPATHY) disorders.
- Elevated levels of gamma globulin (IgG) may indicate chronic liver disease or the presence of AUTOIMMUNE HEPATITIS. Elevated IgM can mean primary biliary cirrhosis.

Some drugs can affect the measurement of total protein in the blood. Those drugs include the following:

- corticosteroids (synthetic hormones often used to stop transplant rejection)
- neomycin (a broad-spectrum antibiotic)
- isoniazid (for treating tuberculosis).

The serum protein electrophoresis is an informative test that can provide valuable clues to a physician confronted with a patient with possible liver disease.

sexual transmission See HEPATITIS B; HEPATITIS C METHOD OF TRANSMISSION.

shock liver Shock liver is injury and death of hepatocytes (liver cells) caused by an inadequate supply of blood or oxygen to the liver. The name "shock liver" is derived from the condition of "shock," when the blood flow, and therefore blood pressure, in the body is reduced significantly. Also called ischemic hepatitis or hepatic ischemia, shock liver is a relatively uncommon condition, occurring in an estimated 0.16 to 0.50 percent of patients admitted into intensive care units.

Hepatocytes rely on a constant supply of blood and oxygen in order to function correctly. When blood flow to the liver is insufficient or when the blood circulating through the liver is oxygen-deficient, hepatocytes do not receive enough oxygen and die through a process called cell necrosis (cell death). While cell death is serious, the condition actually has few, if any, symptoms associated with it and rarely causes severe, lasting damage if recognized and treated quickly. Individuals with shock liver may feel weak or light-headed, although these feelings are caused by the low blood pressure, not the damage to the liver cells themselves. Occasionally, symptoms of nausea, vomiting, and liver enlargement and tenderness are present.

Shock liver is secondary to the condition that causes a patient's low blood pressure (hypotension), diminished blood supply to the liver, or hypoxemia (lack of oxygen in the blood). These conditions include heart failure, respiratory failure, heatstroke, sepsis (serious bacterial infection), severe burns, dehydration, and heavy bleeding (hemorrhage). Blood clots or other conditions that create narrowing or blockage in the hepatic artery or portal vein (blood vessels in the liver) may also cause shock liver, although this is less common.

Symptoms and Diagnostic Path

Diagnosis of shock liver requires liver-function tests to determine blood levels of the liver enzymes aspartate aminotransferase (AST) and alanine aminotransferase (ALT), as well as identifying the underlying cause of hypotension or oxygen deprivation to the liver (e.g., heart failure, sepsis). Because hepatocytes release ALT and AST as they die, patients with shock liver have very high levels of these enzymes in their blood, sometimes as high as 50 times the normal level. Another liver enzyme, LDH, is also often quite elevated. A patient's ALT and AST levels usually rise one to three days following the acute (sudden) episode of decreased blood or oxygen supply. Enzyme levels return to normal fairly quickly, usually within a week to 10 days. Because these signs are present in multiple liver disorders, additional tests may be run to exclude other causes of liver damage.

Treatment Options and Outlook

Treatment of shock liver does not involve treatment for the liver itself, but rather of the condition that caused the reduced blood flow or oxygen supply. For example, when sepsis is the underlying condition, antibiotics are used to treat the infection, or when dehydration is the culprit, fluids are given to reverse the hypovolemia (low blood volume caused by dehydration). Once the underlying condition is addressed, the blood and oxygen supply to the liver are restored and stabilized, and the shock liver state gradually resolves.

Death from shock liver is uncommon. The condition is normally self-limiting when the underlying cause of the shock liver is treated. But if left untreated, shock liver may develop into fulminant hepatic failure, a serious condition that can be fatal. In these cases, an emergency LIVER TRANSPLANTATION may be warranted. Kidney failure may accompany shock liver because the same condition or conditions causing reduced blood or oxygen supply to the liver cause reductions to the kidneys as well.

splenomegaly (enlarged spleen)   See HEPATOMEGALY.

split-liver transplantation   Split-liver transplantation is an innovative technique developed as an attempt to ease the shortage of donor organs. Conventional whole-organ LIVER TRANSPLANTATION has become such a safe and effective procedure that the pool of patients waiting for new organs continues to expand, widening the existing gap between the availability of donor organs and transplant candidates. UNITED NETWORK FOR ORGAN SHARING (UNOS) reports that there are three times as many patients listed for liver transplantation in the United States as there are available cadaveric donor livers. Currently more deaths occur in potential recipients before receiving a transplant than in patients in the first year after the operation.

In split-liver transplantation, a LIVER from a deceased donor is split into the left and right lobe so that it can be used for two recipients, an adult and a child. This procedure essentially doubles the size of the donor pool by transplanting one liver into two recipients. An adult receives the larger right side of the liver, and the smaller left side is implanted into a child or a small adult.

This technique for splitting a liver is derived from a procedure called reduced-size transplantation, first performed in 1984. Because only a limited number of organs of the appropriate size could be found for infants and children, surgeons began cutting down cadaveric livers that were too large for their pediatric patients. Then the unused portion of the liver was discarded. To make more economical use of a scarce resource, surgeons refined their techniques, and in 1988, they succeeded in separating the two lobes of a donor liver into two viable organs.

Because of the architecture of the liver, it is easier to create two unequal portions than to cut it in half. Eventually, increased expertise led to new techniques that enabled surgeons to split the donor liver more evenly so that one organ could be transplanted into two adult patients.

Initial results were extremely disappointing, however, and the split-liver technique was not widely used. It was reported that in the early 1990s, only 50 percent of patients and grafts survived the first year. Fortunately, major advances have been made in the last 10 years or so, improving the odds considerably. Today, patient survival rates are comparable to those for conventional whole-liver transplants.

spontaneous bacterial peritonitis (SBP)   Peritonitis is an inflammation (irritation and swelling) of the lining of the abdomen. This lining, called the peritoneum, is a thin, two-layered membrane that covers both the abdominal wall and the abdominal organs. Fluid may accumulate between the layers of the peritoneum (in the peritoneal cavity, or space). This condition is called ASCITES. Ascites is not a normal finding. It usually occurs in people who have liver or kidney failure, but ascites can also be caused by other illnesses, such as congestive heart failure. Sometimes, bacteria can infect this fluid. This condition is called spontaneous bacterial peritonitis (SBP).

SBP can happen to anyone who has ascites, but it is most common in patients who have CIRRHOSIS, extensive scarring, of the LIVER. In some cases of SBP, it may never be known how the fluid became infected. Other times, the source of the infection is obvious, such as with patients receiving peritoneal dialysis. A weakened immune system or any type of advanced LIVER DISEASE can increase the likelihood of SBP. Most people who get SBP are adults; children rarely get it.

Symptoms and Diagnostic Path
Symptoms of SBP can be so minor as to escape notice, especially in its early stages. Up to one-third of SBP cases have no symptoms at all. This makes SBP particularly dangerous; if not treated quickly and aggressively, SBP can be life-threatening. It can also lead to serious complications such as kidney failure or gastrointestinal bleeding.

When symptoms occur, they often include fever, chills, new or worsening abdominal pain, gastrointestinal distress (such as diarrhea, nausea, or constipation), changes in mental activity, dizziness or fainting, and ascites that does not respond to diuretics. There may also be decreased urine output, which can be a sign of new or worsening kidney failure.

To determine whether there is an infection of the peritoneal fluid, a paracentesis must be done. This procedure removes the excess fluid from the abdomen. Sometimes the physician can discover that an infection is present just by the appearance of the fluid removed. The fluid can be analyzed in the laboratory to find out for sure whether there is an infection, what type of bacteria is causing it, and what medicine will be most effective in treating it. Blood tests, such as a white blood cell count and a blood culture, may also be done.

Treatment Options and Outlook
Treatment with an antibiotic such as cefotaxime can begin right away, even before the laboratory results come back. Other medicines may be administered to lessen the chance of complications such as kidney failure and gastrointestinal bleeding. A hospital stay may be required.

steatosis   See FATTY LIVER.

superinfection and coinfection   Superinfection occurs when an individual already infected with one organism is later infected with either the same or another organism. The infectious organisms may be viruses or bacteria, and the second infectious agent may have developed resistance to antibiotic or antiviral drugs used to treat the first infection. In some cases, the first infection is benign. Coinfection, in contrast, occurs when an individual is concurrently infected with two different viral or bacterial organisms. Some patients may become infected with HEPATITIS B at the same time they are infected with HEPATITIS D.

Superinfection
Patients with chronic hepatitis B (HBV) infections may develop superinfections with other hepatitis viruses, such as HEPATITIS C (HCV) or hepatitis D (HDV). If these chronic hepatitis B patients are super-infected with hepatitis C or hepatitis D, this can lead to severe and/or progressive liver disease.

Patients with chronic hepatitis B who become super-infected with acute hepatitis C tend to suffer from a clinically severe course during the acute phase. When hepatitis C turns chronic—as it does in the majority of individuals—the long-term prognosis is much worse than in patients who have only active hepatitis B infection or who are also infected with hepatitis D. They are at increased risk for developing CIRRHOSIS and liver cancer, HEPATOCELLULAR CARCINOMA, (HCC). On the other hand, hepatitis B patients with hepatitis C superinfection may clear hepatitis B surface antigen (HBsAg) earlier than patients who have only active hepatitis B.

Liau, Yun Fan, et al. "Impact of acute hepatitis C virus superinfection in patients with chronic hepatitis B virus infection." *Gastroenterology* 126, no. 4 (April 2004): 1,024–1,029.

Coinfection with HCV and HBV

Sometimes people become infected with both hepatitis B virus (HBV) and hepatitis C virus (HCV). This is referred to as coinfection. If the HBV infection is active—the patient tests positive for hepatitis B antibodies—the hepatitis B virus appears to suppress the replication of hepatitis C viruses. However, if the HBV infection is not active—the patient tests negative for hepatitis B antibodies—but has evidence of viruses for both hepatitis B and hepatitis C in the blood, the patient is likely to have more severe liver damage from hepatitis C. LIVER BIOPSIES of coinfected patients whose HBV infections are inactive tend to show more FIBROSIS than biopsies from patients infected only with HCV. In addition, coinfected patients with inactive HBV tend to have poorer responses to treatment with INTERFERON and an increased risk of developing liver cancer. This risk is greatly magnified in coinfected patients who also consume excessive alcohol.

Treatment of coinfected patients If a coinfected patient has both viruses in an active state but does not have CIRRHOSIS, or advanced liver scarring, it may be possible to treat both infections. Because HBV is more easily transmitted to others than HCV, it may be desirable to treat HBV first, for public health reasons. Interferon treatment regimens may be effective against both viruses. Patients with HBV and HCV coinfection and cirrhosis will probably be referred to a specialty center.

Coinfection with HIV and HCV

It is estimated that 200,000 to 300,000 people in the United States have both human immunodeficiency virus for AIDS (HIV) and hepatitis C (HCV). This condition, referred to as HIV/HCV–coinfection, is a growing public health problem. Because of the high rate of coinfection, U.S. public health guidelines recommend that all HIV-infected persons be screened for hepatitis C. Related concerns are for all HIV-positive persons to prevent HCV infection, and those already HCV-infected to reduce or minimize liver disease.

HIV/HCV–coinfection is not the only issue at stake. Because of similar routes of transmission—contaminated blood and body fluids—it is possible for a person also to be coinfected with HIV and hepatitis B (HBV), or even all three at once: HIV, HCV, and HBV. Approximately 9 percent of HIV-positive individuals are coinfected with HBV, compared with between 25 to 30 percent coinfected with HCV.

HIV and hepatitis C are both blood-borne viruses that can replicate rapidly, though it is easier to treat HCV than HIV. Both viruses are most efficiently spread through direct blood-to-blood transmission, putting people who share needles at greater risk for acquiring both HIV and HCV. Among those who acquired HIV through percutaneous exposure (through the skin by puncture), the rate of HCV coinfection is extremely high—estimated to be between 50 and 90 percent for injection drug users. Another group likely to be HIV and HCV coinfected are hemophiliacs and those who received repeated blood product transfusions before 1987, when such products were not yet heat-treated to inactivate pathogens. Some people also contracted HCV from blood transfusions before 1990. The rate of HIV/HCV coinfection is also high among prison inmates.

HCV is not as easily spread through sexual activity as HIV. According to the Centers for Disease Control and Prevention (CDC), patients who became HIV-positive through sexual activity have HCV infection rates similar to those for other adults in the general population, estimated to be about 3 to 5 percent. But because HIV and HCV coinfected people tend to have higher HCV viral loads (the amount of virus in the blood), the risk of sexual or perinatal transmission (from mother to child during pregnancy or childbirth) of hepatitis C is greater if the individual also has HIV. Recent data suggest that 5 percent or fewer of HCV-infected mothers transmit the virus to their infants, but if the women also have HIV, then the transmission rate of HCV may triple.

Coinfection is associated with higher viral loads of HCV, more rapid progression to HCV-related liver disease, and a higher risk for cirrhosis, scarring of the liver. HCV infection in HIV-positive patients is regarded as an opportunistic infection, and was included in the 1999 USPHS/IDSA Guidelines for the Prevention of Opportunistic Infections in Persons Infected with Human Immunodeficiency Virus. Hepatitis C is not, however, considered to be an AIDS-defining illness.

HIV-positive patients coinfected with hepatitis B may also progress more rapidly to symptomatic liver disease and cirrhosis, and there is a higher risk of serious liver damage.

The effect of HCV and HBV on the progression of HIV is less clear; some studies have indicated that they may not accelerate HIV disease progression, while others find that the presence of HCV could negatively influence the course of HIV infection.

It appears that individuals with HIV are more likely to be infected with HCV genotype 1, which is associated with a more aggressive disease course than the other genotypes. Accordingly, some researchers believe that individuals infected with genotype 1 progress more rapidly to AIDS or death, but this point is still debated.

In the past, most people with HIV were expected to die from AIDS, and less attention was paid to other long-term conditions like chronic hepatitis C, particularly because it is a slow-progressing disease. Now that better treatments such as highly active antiretroviral therapy (HAART) has dramatically reduced opportunistic illnesses and mortality, more HIV-positive people infected with HCV in the 1970s or 1980s are beginning to develop advanced liver disease or experience liver failure. The result is that an increasing number of patients with HIV are being hospitalized for HCV-related complications or are dying from liver failure caused by HCV. In response, investigators are putting greater effort into learning the characteristics of HIV coinfection with viral hepatitis.

The general consensus today is that most HIV/HCV–coinfected people can be treated for hepatitis C. In a departure from past practices, HIV-positive individuals diagnosed with hepatitis C are being evaluated and considered for treatment just like anyone else. Patients considered candidates for HCV treatment are those at greatest risk for hepatitis C progression.

As with those infected with hepatitis C alone, the most effective treatment for HIV/HCV–coinfected people is a combination of pegylated, or long-acting, interferon and ribavirin. Standard interferon can be also be used, but it appears less effective than the long-acting version.

For most cases, experts recommend that HIV and any opportunistic illnesses be controlled first before beginning HCV treatment. For example, if an individual has advanced HIV disease, low CD4 counts, other opportunistic illness(es), and is severely immnosuppressed, hepatitis C treatment should not be undertaken before the CD4 cell count is raised and the HIV and other illnesses controlled. (A CD4 cell count assesses the health of the immune system by measuring the number of immune system cells that have CD4 receptors.) On the other hand, if the HIV infection is relatively new, and there is little immune system impairment but advanced hepatitis C, it may be preferable to treat hepatitis C first. Such treatment decisions must be made on an individual basis.

Response rates to treatment may be lower than in individuals with HCV alone, but the findings are somewhat contradictory. It may be that an individual's HCV genotype has more bearing on response rates than HIV infection.

Some studies have found that coinfection with HCV seemed to increase the likelihood of progression to AIDS and death. Furthermore, immune recovery after starting with HAART seems to be impaired in coinfected persons whose rate of recovery of CD4 cells was not as high as those who had HIV alone.

Yet other, recent studies suggest that HIV-positive patients may do as well as those with HCV alone, if their HIV disease is well controlled and they have relatively high CD4 cell counts. These patients achieve good results and side effects are similar to those patients without HIV. It is recommended that coinfected patients who are not receiving HCV therapy be monitored regularly for progression of liver disease. Liver biopsies may be repeated every three years or so.

The impact of HIV treatment on hepatitis C and vice versa is not clearly understood at this time. It appears that HAART increases hepatitis C viral load in patients; however, some studies show that it continues to increase only in patients with low CD4 cell counts.

Bini, E., et al. "Safety and efficacy of interferon alfa-2B and ribavirin combination therapy for the treatment of hepatitis C in patients coinfected with HIV." Abstract 653. 52nd annual meeting of the American Society for the Study of Liver Diseases. November 9–13, 2001. Dallas, Texas. Available online. URL: http://www. thebody.com/confs/aasld2001/other.html. Dowloaded on February 1, 2005.

Greub, G., et al. "Clinical progression, survival, and immune recovery during antiretroviral therapy in patients with HIV-1 and hepatitis C virus coinfection: The Swiss HIV Cohort Study." *Lancet* 356 (2000): 1800–1805.

Sherman, Kenneth, M.D., et al. "Hepatitis C virus prevalence among patients infected with human immunodeficiency virus: A cross-sectional analysis of the US adult AIDS clinical trials group." *Clinical Infectious Diseases* 34, no. 6 (March 15, 2002): 831–837.

———. "HCV and HIV: A tale of two viruses." *Reviews in Gastroenterological Disorder* 4, suppl. 1 (2004): 548–554.

Staples, C. T., Jr., D. Rimland, and D. Dudas. "Hepatitis C in the HIV (human immunodeficiency virus) Atlanta V.A. (Veterans Affairs Medical Center) Cohort Study (HAVACS): The effect of coinfection on survival." *Clinical Infectious Diseases* 29 (July 1999): 150–155.

thyroid diseases Thyroid disorders are sometimes associated with LIVER DISEASE. Patients with chronic liver problems may also have thyroid disorders, and patients undergoing thyroid drug therapies may develop liver problems. Similarly, patients undergoing interferon treatment may develop thyroid problems. Most commonly, thyroid complications are associated with AUTOIMMUNE HEPATITIS, HEPATITIS C, and PRIMARY BILIARY CIRRHOSIS.

About Thyroid Diseases

The thyroid is a butterfly-shaped gland at the base of the neck, in the area of the Adam's apple, straddling the lower part of the larynx and the upper part of the trachea. The pituitary gland secretes hormones, and the gland responds by producing thyroid hormones. These hormones regulate the metabolism of cells throughout the body.

Thyroid disorders are divided into the following four broad categories:

- production of too much thyroid hormone (hyperthyroidism)
- production of too little thyroid hormone (hypothyroidism)
- thyroid cancer
- noncancerous thyroid disease

Symptoms of thyroid disorders resemble those of certain psychiatric conditions. Hyperthyroid individuals may show signs of nervousness, poor concentration, emotional instability, and depression, in addition to physical symptoms such as heat intolerance, palpitations, weight loss, weakness, and shortness of breath. Hypothyroid symptoms include memory impairment and psychosis, as well as fatigue, hair loss, and dry skin.

Thyroid disorders are readily diagnosed through blood tests, and are easily treated with thyroid medication.

Thyroid Disorders and Liver Disease

Thyroid hormone levels play an important part in liver function, just as the liver plays an important role in metabolizing thyroid hormone. Consequently, relationships between thyroid function and liver function should come as no surprise.

Associations between liver disease and thyroid abnormalities have been noted in both clinical and laboratory studies. Patients with chronic liver disease may also have thyroiditis (thyroid inflammation), hypothyroidism, or hyperthyroidism, or may test abnormal for thyroid function. As liver inflammation resolves, thyroid test results often improve.

Patients with autoimmune hepatitis (AIH) commonly display either hyperthyroidism or hypothyroidism. AIH patients who are prone to develop other autoimmune disorders—as many as one-third of all AIH patients—are more likely to develop a thyroid disorder than patients without that disposition.

About 5 percent of hepatitis C patients also display symptoms of thyroid disorders, both hypothyroid and hyperthyroid. Those symptoms may develop or worsen in response to INTERFERON therapy, though they often diminish or disappear altogether when interferon therapy is discontinued.

Up to 20 percent of people with PRIMARY BILIARY CIRRHOSIS (PBC) also have some kind of thyroid dysfunction. Hypothyroidism is a more common problem in patients with PBC, but hyperthyroidism has also been observed.

These thyroid-liver associations can be problematical. Primary thyroid abnormalities can cause abnormal LIVER-FUNCTION TESTS, and vice versa, leading to errors in patient care. Most researchers advise that the possibility of primary thyroid dysfunction be considered in any case of unexplained abnormalities in liver-function tests. It is also advisable that patients who suffer from AIH, or who are undergoing interferon treatments, be monitored for thyroid complications.

toxic hepatitis   See DRUG-INDUCED HEPATITIS.

transfused blood   See HEPATITIS B; HEPATITIS C.

transfusion-transmitted virus (TTV)   In 1997, a new virus was discovered in Japanese patients with HEPATITIS and LIVER DISEASE. The virus was named transfusion-transmitted virus, or TTV, because it appeared to be spread via blood transfusions. The virus contains a single strand of DNA, and several variations have been found. Further research has found the virus worldwide, in healthy people as well as those with liver disease. In some countries, close to 100 percent of the population is infected.

It is not clear whether the virus causes disease in humans or whether it might be linked to any liver diseases. In one study, DNA from TTV was detected in almost half of a group of patients with fulminant non-A-G hepatitis and another group with chronic liver diseases of unknown causes. Thus, the virus may play a role in the development of some types of liver disease. However, TTV alone does not appear to cause hepatitis.

Transmission of TTV is believed to occur via blood transfusions. But the widespread occurrence suggests that it can also be transmitted in other ways than exposure to blood and blood products, such as through oral ingestion and vertical transmission (from a mother to her child during childbirth).

One study in Scotland found evidence of the virus in about half of a variety of blood products that were tested. Treating blood products with heat or detergents designed to kill viruses does not remove the virus from the blood products, but the treatments may reduce the likelihood of infecting the recipients of the products.

TTV has not been linked to any specific human disease, and there are no known treatments for those infected with the virus.

Ikeda, H., et al. "Infection with an uneveloped DNA virus (TTV) in patients with acute or chronic liver disease of unknown etiology and in those positive for hepatitis C virus RNA." *Journal of Hepatology* 2 (February 1999): 205–212.

transplantation   See LIVER TRANSPLANTATION.

transplant immunology   See LIVER TRANSPLANTATION.

transvenous intrahepatic portosystemic shunt (TIPS)   A transvenous intrahepatic portosystemic shunt (TIPS) is a shunt, or bypass, placed between the portal vein, which drains blood from the intestines into the liver, and the hepatic vein, which carries blood from the liver to the heart. The procedure is performed to manage complications of PORTAL HYPERTENSION—abnormally high blood pressure in the portal vein—such as bleeding of the varices and ASCITES (abdominal swelling). It is performed only when other methods have proven ineffective.

The procedure is usually performed by an interventional radiologist. Guided by ultrasound and fluoroscope, the radiologist inserts a small catheter (a narrow tube) into a vein in the neck, and advances it to the liver. A tract is created between the portal vein and the hepatic vein, and a stent—a small, collapsible metal tube—is placed in the tract to join the two veins. The effect is to allow some of the blood being drained from the intestines to be shunted directly into the vein that drains the liver, thereby lowering the pressure in the portal vein.

The main complication of a TIPS procedure is HEPATIC ENCEPHALOPATHY, a syndrome commonly observed in patients with CIRRHOSIS. It is sometimes characterized as mental confusion, but it can be more profound than that; the term also implies personality changes and intellectual impairment. About 25 percent of patients who undergo a TIPS procedure develop or experience worsening of the syndrome, caused because blood shunted into the hepatic vein has not been detoxified by the filtering action of the liver.

Another complication of a TIPS procedure is the potential that the shunt will eventually become blocked and have to be replaced. About 50 percent of shunts become blocked within one year, though they have been known to be effective for periods of up to three years.

Because of those complications, the primary use of a TIPS procedure is to rescue a failed endoscopy (using a hollow tube with a light at the end) or as a temporary bridge to an eventual liver transplant.

type I glycogen storage disease   See LIVER DISEASE.

tyrosinemia   Tyrosinemia is a genetic disorder of metabolism that often results in severe LIVER DISEASE. With tyrosinemia, the body cannot break down an amino acid—a building block of protein—called tyrosine. Tyrosine, found mostly in animal and plant food sources, is one of 20 common types of amino acids.

In humans, the LIVER is primarily responsible for metabolizing tyrosine. When tyrosine fails to be metabolized properly, toxins that build up in the liver and kidneys ultimately damage these organs, causing serious health problems.

Tyrosinemia is an autosomal recessive hereditary disorder, meaning a child may inherit the disease if both parents are carriers of it. When two carriers of the disease have a child, there is a one-in-four chance that the child will be born with the disease.

Symptoms and Diagnostic Path

Infants born with tyrosinemia may become ill quickly, sometimes showing symptoms within the first months of life. Infants with this type of tyrosinemia, often called acute tyrosinemia, may have a distended abdomen caused by an enlarged liver and spleen. They may have difficulty gaining weight, bleed easily, have jaundiced skin, and have edema (swelling) in the lower extremities. Early development of symptoms may be related to a poorer prognosis.

Sometimes symptoms of tyrosinemia have a slower onset and are, at least initially, less pronounced. This type of tyrosinemia, often called chronic tyrosinemia, is characterized by symptoms that manifest later in childhood. Symptoms may include liver and spleen enlargement, fluid in the abdomen resulting in abdominal distention, poor weight gain, and recurring vomiting and diarrhea.

Both forms of tyrosinemia may lead to CIRRHOSIS (advanced scarring of the liver), HEPATOCELLULAR CARCINOMA (liver cancer), LIVER FAILURE, kidney failure, severe bleeding, rickets (soft, weak bones), and nervous system problems that can lead to respiratory failure.

Diagnosis of tyrosinemia is based on a variety of blood and urine tests. Liver function, serum albumin (level of albumin, a protein in the blood), and clotting factors may be abnormal. BILIRUBIN and transaminase levels in the blood may be elevated. The metabolite succinylacetone—a substance produced in the process of metabolism—found in blood or urine, and abnormal blood levels of the enzyme fumarylacetoacetase (FAH) contribute to the conclusive diagnosis of tyrosinemia. Fumarylacetoacetate hydrolase (FAH) is essential in metabolizing tyrosine. If it is absent, toxic metabolic products accumulate in the body's tissues, leading to injury of the liver and kidneys.

For couples at high risk of being carriers of the disease, genetic testing can be done to determine the risk of passing the illness to their children. During pregnancy, testing amniotic fluid or performing a chorionic villus sampling (CVS) can determine whether the fetus has tyrosinemia. CVS is a type of procedure in which fetal cells are obtained for the testing of genetic disorder.

Treatment Options and Outlook

There is no cure for tyrosinemia, and the disease has a high fatality rate if left untreated. Individuals with tyrosinemia are often placed on diets low in the amino acids phenylalanine, methionine, and tyrosine. This means they must also restrict intake of proteins such as meats, dairy, nuts, and beans, since those items contain tyrosine. However, dietary measures alone cannot prevent progression of the disease. LIVER TRANSPLANTATION has traditionally been the only chance for long-term survival for those with tyrosinemia. A new treatment utilizing the drug 2-(2-nitro-4-trifluoromethylbenzoyl)-1,3-cyclohexanedione (NTBC), coupled with dietary restrictions, has so far shown to improve the prognosis of the disease.

Al-Dhalimy, M., K. Overturf, M. Finegold, and M. Grompe. "Long-term therapy with NTBC and tyrosine-restricted diet in a Murine model of hereditary tyrosinemia Type I." *Molecular Genetics and Metabolism* 75, no. 1 (January 2002): 38–45.

Grompe, M. "The pathophysiology and treatment of hereditary tyrosinemia type 1." *Seminary Liver Disease* 21, no. 4 (November 2001): 563–571.

Holme, E., and S. Lindstedt. "Diagnosis and management of tyrosinemia type I." *Current Opinion in Pediatrics* 6 (December 1995): 726–772.

———. "Nontransplant treatment of tyrosinemia." *Clinical Liver Diorders* 4 (November 2000): 805–814.

Kvittingen, E. A. "Hereditary tyrosinemia type I—An overview." *Scandinavian Journal of Clinical Laboratory Investigations Supplement* 184 (1986): 27–34.

Paradise, K., A. Weber, E. G. Seidman, J. Larochelle, L. Garel, C. Lenaerts, and C. C. Roy. "Liver transplantation for hereditary tyrosinemia: The Quebec experience." *American Journal of Human Genetics* 47, no. 2 (August 1990): 338–342.

van Spronsen, F. J., Y. Thomasse, G. P. Smit, J. V. Leonard, P. T. Clayton, V. Fidler, R. Berger, H. S. Heymans. "Hereditary tyrosinemia type I: A new clinical classification with difference in prognosis on dietary treatment." *Hepatology* 20, no. 5 (November 1994): 1187–1191.

United Network for Organ Sharing (UNOS)   The United Network for Organ Sharing manages the U.S. system for donating and transplanting organs. UNOS is a private, nonprofit organization based in Richmond, Virginia. It operates the Organ Procurement and Transplantation Network (OPTN), under contract to the U.S. Department of Health and Human Services.

The Organ Transplant Act (OTA) of 1984 established the OPTN and specified that it be operated by a private, nonprofit organization under federal contract. UNOS won the contract in 1986 and has managed OPTN ever since.

By law, all transplant centers and organ procurement organizations that receive Medicare funds must belong to OPTN. Other members include independent laboratories, medical and scientific organizations, professional organizations, voluntary health and patient advocacy organizations, and members of the public with an interest in organ donation and transplantation.

In general, the purpose of OPTN is to help obtain an adequate supply of donated organs and to help distribute the available organs efficiently and equitably. More specifically, the OPTN's responsibilities are to do the following:

1. facilitate the organ matching and placement process
2. develop consensus policies for recovering, allocating, and transporting organs
3. collect, manage, and disseminate scientific data on organ transplantation
4. develop and maintain a national organ transplant waiting list
5. educate professionals and the public about organ donation and transplantation

For more information, visit the UNOS Web site: http://www.unos.org.

vaccines for viral hepatitis The Centers for Disease Control and Prevention (CDC) Advisory Committee on Vaccination Practices recommends that all people with chronic LIVER DISEASE receive vaccinations for viral hepatitis.

Hepatitis A

Two vaccinations, equally effective, are available today against HEPATITIS A. The Food and Drug Administration (FDA) approved HAVRIX in 1995 and VAQTA in 1996. The injections are usually given in two doses six to 12 months apart. Within one month, 95 to 99 percent of the recipients develop immunity to hepatitis A. Protection lasts 10 to 20 years.

Before 1995, an injection of IMMUNE GLOBU-LIN (IG) was the only way to obtain protection. Immune globulin is made from human plasma pooled from many people with hepatitis A, and sterilized and tested negative for other infectious diseases.

IG continues to be used for people who have been recently exposed to HAV, as it confers immediate protection against the virus. IG must be administered within two weeks of exposure to HAV. The effect of IG is only short term, lasting no more than three to five months.

Travelers to areas where hepatitis A is endemic should have their first vaccine dose at least three weeks before departure. To ensure protection, they may also choose to receive immune globulin.

Children over the age of two can be vaccinated. IG can be given to children under the age of two who are at risk for HAV infection.

Universal vaccination against HAV is not recommended because the risk of infection is low in the United States. However, individuals at risk for the infection are advised to be vaccinated. In states with consistently high rates of infection, routine vaccination of children over the age of two is mandated. These include Alaska, Arizona, California, Idaho, Nevada, New Mexico, Oklahoma, Oregon, South Dakota, Utah, and Washington.

Hepatitis B

The vaccine for HEPATITIS B was licensed in 1982. It has been heralded as the vaccine that can prevent LIVER CANCER because it can prevent both infection and complications related to the infection. Chronic hepatitis B often progresses to CIRRHOSIS, or advanced liver scarring, and liver cancer.

Adults receive three shots: the initial dose, the second dose one month later, and the third dose six months after the initial injection. Approximately 90 percent of adults and 95 percent of children enjoy complete protection against hepatitis B for 10 years, or possibly a lifetime. Side effects, if any, are similar to those for hepatitis A vaccination.

Everyone with risk factors for hepatitis B should receive the vaccination. It is also highly recommended for anyone with chronic liver disease. In particular, patients with chronic hepatitis C suffer a far greater risk of developing liver cancer if they also become coinfected with hepatitis B.

All newborns in the United States are routinely vaccinated against hepatitis B, as mandated by the Advisory Committee on Immunization Practices (ACIP) in 1991. All pregnant women are screened for antibodies to hepatitis B surface antigen (HBsAg). If the mother tests negative, the infant should receive both a hepatitis B vaccination and hepatitis B immune globulin (HBIG) within 12 hours of birth. At age one to two months, the second dose of hepatitis B vaccine is given, and the third dose at six months. HBIG is made from plasma pooled from people with antibodies against hepatitis B surface antigen (HBsAb, or anti-HBs). It is approved by the FDA. Like IG for hepatitis A, HBIG provides immediate but temporary protection after accidental exposure to infectious blood or body fluids. It must be administered within two weeks of contact. It is more than 90 percent effective.

It is recommended that all children ages 11 to 12 should be vaccinated if they were not vaccinated at birth.

There has been some controversy regarding the safety of HBV vaccines. Critics contend that the vaccines may be linked to such illnesses as multiple sclerosis, diabetes, and sudden infant death syndrome. In response, the U.S. Congress held hearings to investigate the issue. Officials from the U.S. Centers for Disease Control and Prevention (CDC) testified that HBV vaccine is absolutely safe and no evidence exists to show that it could be a trigger for various illnesses.

Combined hepatitis A and B vaccination   A combination vaccination for hepatitis A and B, TWINRIX, is available for patients who need inoculations against both infections. It is as efficient as single-agent vaccines. This three-dose combination vaccination is ideal for those who have to travel at short notice to regions with a high prevalence of hepatitis A and B, as it confers protection against both viruses in two months after the initial dose, thus accelerating the vaccination schedule. There is a reduced dose format for children between the ages of one and 18, TWINRIX JUNIOR.

The combination vaccine simplifies immunization schedules, allowing for fewer shots than if the two were administered separately. The convenience also makes it more accessible to people who have indications for both A and B hepatitis, and simplifies routine immunization. (See hepatitis A and hepatitis B.) Those not at risk for both hepatitis infections do not need the combination.

The following persons should be considered for the combination vaccine:

- travelers to areas in which hepatitis A and hepatitis B are endemic, including certain parts of Africa, Asia, and the Americas

- people who live in areas where both hepatitis A and B are endemic

- people with chronic liver disease, including chronic hepatitis C

- users of illicit injection and/or oral drugs

- men who have sex with other men

- hemophiliacs who receive transfusions of clotting factors

- people who require additional doses of both hepatitis A and hepatitis B vaccine

Additionally, individuals with hepatitis C who are not already immune to either or both hepatitis A and B should be vaccinated by a combination or single-agent vaccine. Patients can be tested for immunity with a simple, inexpensive blood test.

Hepatitis C

No vaccination is available against HEPATITIS C, and immune globulin is also ineffective against the virus. Unlike other viral infections, most patients do not develop immunity against hepatitis C because the virus constantly changes to new forms. Antibodies produced against the original virus do not work against these mutated forms; this makes it extremely daunting to create a vaccine. A further challenge to the development of a vaccine is the existence of more than six strains of hepatitis C. An effective vaccine would need to offer protection against all the variants.

Investigators are trying different approaches to create a vaccine that circumvents these obstacles to immunization. For example, the Center for Vaccine Development at Saint Louis University School of Medicine has been testing an experimental vaccine developed by Chiron Corporation that uses bioengineered versions of proteins on the surface of the virus.

Hepatitis D

No vaccination exists for HEPATITIS D, but preventing hepatitis B ensures against infection because the hepatitis D virus needs the B virus to replicate. Individuals already infected with hepatitis B should protect themselves against further infection by avoiding high-risk behaviors. (See HEPA-TITIS D.)

Hepatitis E

There is no vaccine against HEPATITIS E, but recombinant vaccines are currently being prepared.

Centers for Disease Control and Prevention. "Hepatitis B national immunization program." Modified February 11, 2003. Available online. URL: http://www.cdc.gov/nip/vacsafe/concerns/hepB. Downloaded on November 8, 2004.

Centers for Disease Control and Prevention. "Prevention of hepatitis A through active or passive immunization: Recommendations of the Advisory Committee on Immunization Practices (ACIP)." *MMWR* no. RR-12 (1999): 1–38.

Centers for Disease Control and Prevention. "Recommendations for prevention and control of hepatitis C virus (HCV) infection and HCV-related chronic disease." *MMWR* no. RR-19, 47 1(998): 1–39. Available online. URL: ftp://ftp.cdc.gov/pub/Publications/mmwr/rr/rr4719.pdf. Downloaded on November 8, 2004.

viral hepatitis   See HEPATITIS; HEPATITIS A; HEPATITIS B; HEPATITIS C; HEPATITIS D; HEPATITIS E.

viral load   See HEPATITIS C.

viruses   See HEPATITIS; HEPATITIS A; HEPATITIS B; HEPATITIS C; HEPATITIS D; HEPATITIS E.

wellness lifestyle   See LIFESTYLE AND CHRONIC
HEPATITIS C.

Wilson's disease   Wilson's disease—also called
hepatolenticular degeneration—is an inherited
metabolic disorder that causes copper to accumulate in body tissues.

In this hereditary disease, a deficiency of the protein ceruloplasmin causes abnormal copper accumulations in the LIVER and other organs. Wilson's
disease most often affects the liver, brain, kidneys,
and cornea. The copper accumulations cause liver
dysfunction and neurologic or psychiatric symptoms. If untreated, it can cause LIVER FAILURE, movement and speech disorders, psychiatric problems,
and, eventually, death.

Wilson's disease affects between one in 30,000 and
one in 40,000 people worldwide, and about 6,000
people in the United States. The disease appears to
occur in all races and ethnicities. The defective gene,
ATP7B, that causes Wilson's disease is located on
chromosome 13. About one in 100 people are carriers for the gene, which is autosomal recessive. Thus,
both parents of an affected child must be carriers of
the defective gene, and both males and females can
be affected. Carriers do not have any symptoms of
the disease and need no treatment. Occasionally,
Wilson's disease occurs as a spontaneous mutation,
rather than passing from both parents to their child.

More than 200 different mutations of the
ATP7B gene have been identified, so there is no
simple genetic test available for screening for the
disease. However, there are tests that can be used
to diagnose Wilson's disease. It has been recommended that all siblings and children of Wilson's
disease patients should be tested for the disease,
as well as other relatives who have symptoms or

laboratory test results that indicate liver or neurological damage.

In about half of Wilson's patients, the liver is
the only organ affected. The liver damage may be
difficult to distinguish from infectious hepatitis or
infectious mononucleosis without proper diagnostic blood tests.

Copper is an essential mineral for humans. It is
present in most foods, and most people consume
more copper than they need. Normally, the liver
processes copper that is consumed, and any excess
processed copper passes into the GALLBLADDER in
BILE. The copper is released from the gallbladder
into the small intestine with bile, and from there it
is normally excreted with digestive waste products.

Wilson's disease patients do not process copper properly in the liver, and they do not release
excess copper properly into the bile. Therefore, the
mineral builds up in the liver, beginning at birth.
Eventually, the excess copper causes liver damage.
As a result of copper-related liver damage, copper
may be released into the bloodstream and deposited in other organs, often in the kidneys, brain,
and eyes. Copper accumulation in the brain causes
neurological damage that results in speech impairment, swallowing difficulties, tremors, and muscle
stiffness. If left untreated, severe brain damage,
liver failure, and death occur. A sudden release of
copper into the blood can cause hemolytic anemia,
a type of anemia that results from chemical poisoning of red blood cells.

Symptoms and Diagnostic Path

Patients with Wilson's disease may not have any
symptoms of illness. If symptoms do occur, they
usually appear between the ages of six and 20,
most often during the teenage years. But patients
as young as three and as old as 60 have been diag-

nosed with the disease. The average age at which neurological symptoms appear is 21. Symptoms can be observed in the eyes, liver, central nervous system, urinary system, or musculoskeletal system. If patients are not treated, they will develop symptoms and eventually die.

About half of Wilson's patients have symptoms of liver disease. The symptoms may resemble those of more common disorders, such as viral hepatitis or infectious mononucleosis, with JAUNDICE (yellowing of the eyes and skin), ascites (abdominal swelling), vomiting blood, and abdominal pain. Patients may have acute hepatitis, chronic active hepatitis, cirrhosis, or FULMINANT HEPATITIS (a severe form of liver inflammation). The LIVER DISEASE may occur in episodes at intervals of months to years. If untreated, all patients eventually develop CIRRHOSIS, advanced scarring of the liver.

The first symptoms of Wilson's disease are neurological in between one-third and one-half of patients, and these symptoms may appear without symptoms of liver disease. Neurological symptoms may include hand tremors (shaking), uncontrollable movements of the limbs, muscle rigidity, drooling, difficulty swallowing, speech and language problems, and headache. Usually there is no change in the patient's intelligence.

In about one-third of Wilson's disease patients, the first symptoms are psychiatric, such as depression, irritability, severe insomnia, inability to concentrate, inability to cope, increased anger, and inappropriate behavior. Patients may have difficulty completing tasks in school or at work. Signs of mental illness may appear, such as homicidal or suicidal behavior, depression, and aggression.

Other symptoms are also associated with Wilson's disease. Kidney damage may reduce the filtering capacity and function or be associated with kidney stones. Severe osteoporosis, or loss of bone density, occurs at abnormally young ages in some Wilson's patients. Female patients may have irregular or no menstrual cycles, infertility, or multiple miscarriages.

Because Wilson's disease can cause severe liver damage, it is important to diagnose the condition as early as possible, preferably before the patient has symptoms. However, Wilson's disease is rare, and it may not be diagnosed early. Therefore, any

time a person has recurring liver disease and unexplained neurological symptoms, the possibility of Wilson's disease should be investigated.

Even if the patient does not have symptoms, tests can either rule out or diagnose Wilson's disease. The most common tests include those below:

- slit lamp eye exam for Kayser-Fleischer rings. These are rusty brown, golden brown, or greenish rings around the cornea. About half of patients with liver symptoms have Kayser-Fleischer rings, but rings may be present in patients with other types of liver disease.

- blood test for levels of serum ceruloplasmin, a copper-binding protein. About 80 percent of patients have serum ceruloplasmin levels of less than 20 mg/dL. The test results may not be reliable for women who are pregnant or taking birth control pills or for infants less than six months old.

- blood tests for liver enzyme levels. Early in the course of the disease, liver enzyme levels may be only slightly higher than normal. As the disease progresses, blood enzyme levels will indicate a fatty degeneration of the liver.

- 24-hour urine copper test. Most patients with Wilson's disease have abnormally high levels of copper in their urine.

- LIVER BIOPSY with tissue analysis for elevated copper levels. All patients with Wilson's disease have elevated copper levels in their livers.

- genetic testing may be useful in diagnosis. It is most useful in finding Wilson's disease in relatives of a patient who has been diagnosed.

Other signs that might be observed by a doctor include swelling of the liver and spleen; fluid buildup in the lining of the abdomen; anemia; low blood platelet and white blood cell counts; high levels of amino acids; protein, uric acid, and carbohydrates in urine; and softening of the bones.

Treatment Options and Outlook

Patients being investigated or treated for Wilson's disease should be cared for by specialists in Wilson's disease or by their primary physicians in consultation with such specialists.

Wilson's disease can be treated, with the goals of both preventing additional copper buildup and removing excess copper from the patient's body. With treatment, the progress of the disease can be stopped, and often the symptoms can also be improved. If the disease is discovered early enough, the patient can enjoy normal health. However, the treatment must be continued for the rest of the individual's life. If treatment is stopped, the patient will die.

Several drugs are used to treat Wilson's disease, and sometimes more than one is prescribed.

- Zinc acetate (Galzin) blocks absorption of copper in the intestinal tract, helping to eliminate accumulated copper and prevent new accumulation. The drug works slowly, taking four to eight months to remove accumulated copper from the body. It may be given to asymptomatic patients and to patients who have already been treated with other drugs. Zinc acetate has relatively few side effects.

- Penicillamine (Cuprimine or Depen) binds copper in a way that increases the rate at which copper is excreted in urine. It may take as long as a year to obtain the maximum effect. Some symptoms, particularly neurological symptoms, may become worse during the first few months of treatment. Both short-term and long-term side effects have been observed with penicillamine.

- Trientine (Syprine) functions in a similar way to penicillamine, causing increased urinary excretion of copper. It appears to have less of a tendency to increase neurological symptoms than penicillamine.

- Tetrathiomolybdate is another copper-binding drug that is currently under investigation for treatment of Wilson's disease. It may avoid the neurological deterioration seen with penicillamine.

With each of these medications, the patient should be monitored to make sure the medication is taken as directed, to check for side effects, and to make sure the dosage is correct. In addition, patients may be advised to take vitamin B6 (pyridoxine) supplements and to avoid foods with high copper contents, such as liver, shellfish, nuts, chocolate, dried fruit, and mushrooms.

Patients with severe hepatitis or liver failure may be candidates for LIVER TRANSPLANTATION. The long-term transplant survival rate is about 80 percent.

The most common complication of Wilson's disease is anemia due to a deficiency of copper. Most often, anemia occurs in patients who have taken zinc for many years and follow a vegetarian diet.

If a patient develops fulminant hepatitis, a sudden release of copper into the bloodstream can cause life-threatening hemolytic anemia, which occurs when copper poisons red blood cells.

The prognosis for most Wilson's disease patients is excellent if they are treated for the condition. If the disease is not treated, patients become severely disabled, losing, for example, the ability to walk, talk, and eat, and they usually die before reaching the age of 50.

If the liver disease progresses or is accompanied by complications, such as cirrhosis (advanced liver scarring) or variceal bleeding, a liver transplant may be recommended.

Steindl, P., P. Ferenci, H. P. Dienes, G. Grimm, I. Pabinger, C. Madl, T. Maier-Dobersberger, A. Herneth, B. Dragosics, S. Meryn, P. Knoflach, G. Granditsch, and A. Gangl. "Wilson's disease in patients presenting with liver disease: a diagnostic challenge." *Gastroenterology* 113, no. 1 (July 1997): 212–218.

Strand, S., W. J. Hofmann, A. Grambihler, H. Hug, M. Volkmann, G. Otto, H. Wesch, S. M. Mariani, V. Hack, W. Stremmel, P. H. Krammer, and P. R. Galle. "Hepatic failure and liver cell damage in acute Wilson's disease involve CD95 (APO-1/Fas) mediated apoptosis." *Natural Medicine* 4, no. 5 (May 1998): 588–593.

Wachter, Kerryi. "Tetrathiomolybdate may have potential for initial Wilson's disease therapy. (Preventing neurologic damage)." *Internal Medicine News* 36, no. 10 (May 15, 2003): 12.

xenotransplantation Because there is such a shortage of organs, researchers have turned to xenotransplantation as a possible source of unlimited organs. Xenotransplantation is defined as the transplanting, implanting, or infusing of living cells, tissues, or organs from one species to another.

Taking the LIVER of an animal and transplanting it to a human patient is a highly experimental and controversial procedure. If it does ever become widely available, it would have a major impact on the lives of transplant candidates by cutting down the wait for new organs, which can be months or sometimes years. But there are many obstacles to overcome before animal livers or any other organs can be used for transplantation. Experiments in xenotransplantation conducted in the early 1900s all failed because of the human body's rejection of animal organs. In the early 1990s, three attempts at liver xenotransplants—one from a pig, and two from baboons—were unsuccessful. Recipients of whole animal organs usually live only a few months, at best about nine months. The only successes are limited to the transplant of animal cells such as porcine islet cells (one of the endocrine cells) and fetal neuronal cells (a cell constituting the nervous tissue).

The cross-species barrier is a difficult one to transcend. The liver from a pig (the most promising source so far because the pig liver functionally resembles a human liver) is instantly rejected because the IMMUNE SYSTEM detects certain proteins on the surface of pig cells to be foreign. Current immunosuppressive drugs are not powerful enough to stop this intense reaction against such foreign proteins from animal tissue.

One way to inhibit acute rejection by the human body is to clone pigs that lack these foreign proteins or to create genetically modified pigs that possess human genes for cell membrane proteins. But some scientists object on grounds that these proteins could act as a receptor for viruses, specifically variants of porcine endogenous retrovirus (PERV), which could mutate to infect human cells. Others feel that the risk is small.

Aside from safety concerns, there are religious objections, ethical issues, high financial costs, and other as yet unexplored issues that need to be resolved before xenotransplantation can become a routinely accepted medical procedure.

Buhler, L., S. Deng, J. O'Neil, H. Kitamura, M. Koulmanda, A. Baldi, J. Rahier, I. P. Alwayn, J. Z. Appel, M. Awwad, D. H. Sachs, G. Weir, J. P. Squifflet, D. K. Cooper, and P. Morel. "Adult porcine islet transplantation in baboons treated with conventional immunosuppression or a non-myeloablative regimen and CD 154 blockade." *Xenotransplantation* 9 (2002): 3–13.

Cooper, D. K. C. "Clinical xenotransplantation—How close are we?" *Lancet* 326 (2003): 557–559.

Horvath-Arcidiacono, Judith A., et al. "Human natural killer cell activity against porcine targets: Modulation by control of the oxidation-reduction environment and role of adhesion molecule interactions." *Cell Immunology* 222, no. 1 (August 2003); 35–44.

Ravelingien, A., F. Mortier, E. Mortier, I. Kerremans, and J. Braeckman. "Proceeding with clinical trials of animal to human organ transplantation: A way out of the dilemma." *Journal of Medical Ethics* 30, no. 1 (February 2004): 92(6).

United Network for Organ Sharing, 2002. Available online. URL: http://www.unos.org. Accessed April 2004.

APPENDIXES

APPENDIX I
MEDICAL ISSUES, PROCEDURES, AND TESTS

clinical trials

Clinical trials are carefully controlled research studies using human volunteers to test the safety and effectiveness of new drugs and treatments.

The studies also monitor side effects and compare the new drug or treatment to existing ones. To compare the effectiveness and value of a potential new drug or therapy, scientists give the treatment under investigation to a group and compare their reactions to a control group that receive no treatment, or an existing treatment.

In the United States, the process of developing new drugs and treatments is regulated by the Food and Drug Administration (FDA). Normally, experiments are first conducted in the laboratory and then with specially bred animals. If a treatment looks promising, human clinical trials are then allowed. Clinical trials are normally conducted in three phases. Phase I looks at toxicity and an appropriate range of doses using a relatively small number of patients. It is usually conducted among a small group of 20 to 80 people. Phase II considers how effective the drug is and uses a larger number of patients, from 100 to 300. Phase III involves an even larger number of patients—from 1,000 to 3,000—to obtain more detailed information about the treatment's effectiveness. After the three phases are finished and the drug or treatment has been marketed, more studies are done. These are Phase IV studies, which look at various populations to determine the effect of the new drug or treatment and monitor any side effects for long-term use.

Many large hospitals recruit volunteers for clinical trials. These trials give patients, particularly those who have not benefited from existing treatments, an opportunity to receive new therapies that are not yet on the market. Volunteers are given a thorough physical examination to ensure that they are suitable for the trials, and they are carefully monitored throughout the study. Individuals wishing to participate in clinical trials may ask their doctors. For more information, they may also contact the National Cancer Institute's Cancer Information Service (http://www.cancer.gov/clinicaltrials).

complementary and alternative medicine

Complementary and alternative medicine (CAM) is defined by the National Center for Complementary and Alternative Medicine (NCCAM), a component of the National Institutes of Health (NIH), as "a group of diverse medical and health care systems, practices, and products that are not presently considered to be part of conventional medicine."

Today there is an increasing interest in therapeutic practices outside the conventional health care paradigm. When such practices are used as a supplement to allopathic medicine, they are referred to as complementary medicine, while alternative medicine is used in place of allopathic medicine. However, the terms are often used interchangeably.

Complementary and alternative medicine may include such healing modalities as acupuncture, homeopathic remedies, chiropractic, aromatherapy, massage, and vitamin therapy. They may have biomedical explanations; some are now widely accepted, while others are considered questionable at best.

Nearly half of the U.S. population today uses CAM. These therapies are sought out for a diversity of medical and psychological conditions, such as arthritis, cancer, insomnia, depression, back pain, and acquired immunodeficiency syndrome (AIDS). Patients with liver disease are just as likely as the rest of the population to seek out alternative forms of treatment, according to a report published in the September 2002 issue of the *American Journal of Gastroenterology.* A survey of 989 patients with liver disease revealed that 39 percent have tried some form of complementary and alternative therapy, compared with 41 percent for the general population. Most of the patients used alternative treatments mostly for conditions besides liver disease, such as fatigue or depression.

Similar findings were reported at the 55th meeting of the Annual American Society of the Study of Liver Diseases, in November 2004 in Boston, where the results of a survey conducted by the outpatient clinic of Vancouver Hospital was presented. According to this survey, 59 percent of patients who had been recently diagnosed with hepatitis C used CAM therapies, the most common being milk thistle, an herb often used to treat liver conditions. The most popular reasons given for the use of CAM therapies were to improve the quality of life, boost the immune system, and slow disease progression. The authors of the survey report that the majority of patients felt that "CAM therapies had improved their energy levels, reduced stress, and gave them a sense of control over the illness whereas only 43.9 percent felt that CAM therapies improved liver function."

The survey also found that CAM users were more likely to delay or decline conventional treatment. Moreover, patients tended to consult friends or family instead of physicians for information about CAM, and to rely on anecdotal information for their decision making. This may be because physicians trained in Western medicine often lack knowledge about CAM or do not support their patients in seeking alternative treatment modalities when conventional ones fail to bring desired results. The reluctance to seek out allopathic doctors may also reflect the high cost of conventional medical care in the United States, where a significant percentage of people lack health insurance. It is best if physicians can disseminate reliable CAM information and

help patients make sound choices. To this end, more clinics and hospitals in the United States are beginning to offer what they call "integrative medicine." NCCAM defines integrative medicine as a health care system that combines mainstream medical therapies and CAM therapies "for which there is some high-quality scientific evidence of safety and effectiveness."

Mulkins, A. L., et al. "Complementary and alternative medicine: A survey for people diagnosed with hepatitis C." Abstract 418. 55th annual meeting of the American Association for the Study of Liver Diseases. October 29–November 2, 2004. Boston. Available online. URL: http://www.hivandhepatitis.com/2004icr/aasld/docs/hcv/110804_a.html. Downloaded on January 25, 2005.

Strader, Doris B., Bruce R. Bacon, Karen L. Lindsay, Douglas R. La Brecque, Timothy Morgan, Elizabeth C. Wright, Jeff Allen, M. Farooq Khokar, Jay H. Hoofnagle, and Leonard B. Seeff. "Use of complementary and alternative medicine in patients with liver disease." *American Journal of Gastroenterology* 97, no. 9 (September 2002): 2,391.

computed tomography

Computed tomography (CT) is a medical imaging technique that uses X-rays to produce images of the body's internal organs. Where a conventional X-ray produces only outlines of bones and organs, however, a computerized axial tomography (CAT) scan can visualize selected cross sections, or "slices," of the patient's body, can obtain those cross sections at virtually any angle, and can construct three-dimensional models of internal organs. CT is the most commonly used technique for imaging the liver.

The biggest advantage of CT is that it can visualize a wide variety of tissue types, including lungs, bone, soft tissue, and blood vessels. The disadvantages of CT include the dangers associated with exposure to X-rays and the possibility of allergic reaction to the iodine-based contrasting agents that are often used to facilitate CT imaging.

X-rays are essentially the same as visible light, but they have more energy. The high energy of X-rays allows them to pass unimpeded through most of the soft tissues of the human body, while more solid structures block them, wholly or partially. A conventional X-ray image, then, is a shadow picture; an X-ray "light" is directed toward one side of the body, and a frame of film on the other side captures the shadows of structures that block that light.

The disadvantage of conventional X-rays is that structures not in the direct path of the light cannot be imaged. For example, if a small bone is situated directly behind a larger one, only the shadow of the larger bone is captured. To make the smaller bone visible, either the patient or the X-ray source must be moved or angled to a more advantageous position. That is the basic idea behind a CT scan: It can move the X-ray source and the patient relative to each other, allowing it to capture an image of an entire cross section of the body.

HOW A CT SCANNER WORKS

A typical CT scanner looks like a square donut standing on its side. The "donut hole" is an opening generally 24 to 28 inches (61 to 71 cm) in diameter. The X-ray detection units—the functional equivalent of film in a standard X-ray machine—and the X-ray tubes are arranged around the inside surface of the hole, on a movable ring. (In an alternative design, the X-ray source and detection units remain stationary, and a reflector revolves and directs the X-rays as required.) The patient lies on a platform that can be moved into and out of the opening. The simplest CT scan involves moving the table into the opening until the appropriate portion of the patient's body is situated directly in line with the X-ray source, and then rotating the ring in a full circle as the X-ray source is repeatedly activated. The detection unit opposite the source detects areas of light and darkness, and feeds that data into a computer. The computer assembles the data into an image of a thin cross section of the patient's body. In each 360-degree scan, typically involving about 1,000 snapshots or "profiles," the computer acquires one slice.

A CT scanner is controlled by a battery of computers. A main computer, called the host, orchestrates the operation of the entire system. Another dedicated computer assembles the data from the X-ray detectors into images. The movement and angling of the patient table are controlled by other microprocessors. A workstation that includes a keyboard, mouse, monitor, and other controls allows the technician to control and monitor the process.

The earliest CT scanners had only one X-ray source and one detection unit, and the only allowable movement of the platform was in and out of the opening. The newest scanners may have as many as 16 X-ray sources, and the platform can be moved in and out of the opening, raised or lowered, and angled as needed. The extra X-ray sources allow images to be taken much more quickly, and the range of motion of the platform allows for much more complex images.

GETTING A CT SCAN

To prepare for a CT scan, a patient should wear comfortable, loose-fitting clothing without metal fasteners such as zippers or snaps. Since the image can be affected by metal objects, hairpins, jewelry, eyeglasses, hearing aids, and any detachable dental work, such items may have to be removed. In some cases, the patient may be asked to abstain from eating or drinking anything for an hour or longer before the exam. Women should always inform their doctor or X-ray technologist if there is any possibility they are pregnant.

The procedure begins with the patient lying on the CT table. Pillows may be provided to help support the body and hold it in a suitable position during the scan. As the scan begins, the table moves slowly into the scanner. Depending on the area of the body being examined, the motion of the table may not be clearly discernible.

A CT scan of the gastrointestinal tract may require the use of a contrast material to enhance the visibility of certain tissues. The material might have to be swallowed, or it might be administered by enema. Before administering the material, the radiologist will ask the patient to identify any history of the following:

- allergies, especially to medicines or iodine
- diabetes
- asthma
- heart problems
- thyroid conditions
- kidney problems

All those conditions indicate a higher risk of reaction to the contrast material or potential problems eliminating the material from the body after the exam.

A CT scan usually takes anywhere from five minutes to half an hour, depending on the nature of the exam. When the exam is over, the patient might be asked to wait for the images to be examined in case additional images are needed.

The scan causes no pain. The patient is usually alone in the room during the scan, although the technologist can see, hear, and speak with the patient at all times. In pediatric patients, a parent may be allowed in the room but is required to wear a lead apron to prevent radiation exposure.

RISKS OF CT SCANNING

A CT scan involves exposure to radiation in the form of X-rays, though the benefits of a scan are generally considered to outweigh by far the potential for harm. The effective radiation dose of a CT scan is about the same as an average person receives from background radiation during a three-year period. For safety, the abdomen and pelvis are shielded during a CT scan, except in cases where the abdomen and pelvis are the body parts being scanned.

CT scans are not usually given to pregnant women. If contrast material is administered as part of the scan, nursing mothers should always wait 24 hours before resuming breast feeding.

In rare cases, there may be serious allergic reaction to the contrast material, but radiology departments are well equipped to handle any such problems.

USES OF CT SCANNING

CT is unique among current radiological techniques in its ability to image a combination of soft tissue, bone, and blood vessels. Conventional X-ray images of the head, for example, show only the dense bone structures in the skull. Magnetic resonance imaging (MRI) is an excellent choice for imaging soft tissues and blood vessels, but is not as good at imaging the bones of the skull. CT images, however, can be selectively "windowed" to show soft tissue, bone, and blood vessels as needed.

CT is one of the most widely used radiological tools for studying the chest and abdomen. It is often the preferred tool for diagnosing diseases of the bowel and colon, and for visualizing the liver, spleen, pancreas, and kidneys. CT is also widely used as a diagnostic tool for many types of cancer, because it allows a physician to verify the presence of a suspected tumor and to measure its size, precise location, and involvement with nearby tissue.

A CT scan often involves the administration of a dye containing iodine ("contrast material") to enhance the scan. The dye makes blood vessels and other structures more visible in the scan pictures. Contrast material may be used to detect tumors, evaluate blood flow, or locate areas of inflammation. For scans of the chest, pelvis, and spine, the dye is injected into the bloodstream or in the area surrounding the spine. For abdominal scans, the dye is administered orally. Depending on the purpose of the scan, pictures may be taken both before and after the contrast material is administered.

For investigation of the liver, a "helical" or "spiral" CT scan is often preferred. In order to acquire a high-quality CT image, the patient must hold his or her breath during the scan. In a conventional CT scan, an X-ray is taken of a single slice, then there is a delay to allow the patient to breathe before the next slice is imaged. A helical CT scan, however, involves high-speed scanning accompanied by continuous movement of the patient table, allowing images of several slices during a single breath hold, a strategy that was unavailable with older CT technology. The advantages of helical scanning include shorter examination times, improved visibility of blood vessels, and better enhancement of organ tissue.

Compared with other modern imaging technologies such as MRI, CT is relatively inexpensive and more widely available, and requires fewer controls on the environment. The super-strong magnets used in MRI technology, for example, require that no material containing iron be brought into the imaging room. CT has no such restriction.

Those characteristics make CT the preferred imaging technique in emergency room and trauma center settings. All trauma centers have CT scanners. The scanners can help evaluate trauma victims for internal bleeding, inflammation, infection, and the presence of foreign objects such as glass or metal fragments.

CT is also used, in conjunction with contrast materials, to evaluate blood flow through the blood vessels and organs.

LIVER SCANNING

CT scanning of the liver is an accurate method of determining the site and extent of injuries to the liver and the surrounding area. A technique called multiphase helical scanning is now considered the standard for liver CT scans. The technique uses helical scans and the timed injection of contrast material to increase the sensitivity of the scan and make it more specific to the liver. CT scans not enhanced with contrast material are of limited value in liver trauma but can be useful for diagnosing bleeding into the peritoneum.

The CT criteria for staging liver trauma, based on the American Association for the Surgery of Trauma (AAST) liver injury scale, are as follows:

- grade one—subcapsular hematoma (a blood-filled swelling just beneath the liver's encapsulating tissue) less than one centimeter in maximum thickness, capsular avulsion (tearing away of the encapsulating tissue), superficial laceration of the liver less than one centimeter deep, and isolated blood tracking around the portal vein

- grade two—parenchymal laceration (a cut in the liver) one to three centimeters deep and parenchymal or subcapsular hematomas one to three centimeters thick

- grade three—parenchymal laceration more than three centimeters deep and a parenchymal or subcapsular hematoma more than three centimeters in diameter

- grade four—parenchymal/subcapsular hematoma more than 10 centimeters in diameter, destruction or devascularization (interruption of blood supply due to obstruction or destruction of blood vessels) of one lobe

- grade five—global destruction or devascularization of the liver

- grade six—hepatic avulsion (tearing away of the liver)

For tumors, multiphase helical scanning can detect small tumors that were missed on regular-contrast CT scans or ultrasound examinations of the liver. Normally, the liver receives about 75 percent of its blood from the portal vein and 25 percent from the hepatic artery, while hepatic tumors, whether primary or secondary, receive most of their blood supply from the hepatic artery. Consequently, with hepatic arterial injection, tumors enhance to a greater degree than normal liver tissue.

A CT angiogram is similar to the CT scan but uses a contrast dye injected into the superior mesenteric artery, one of the arteries that supply the liver. The X-rays detect the dye as it flows through the bloodstream, outlining the blood vessels in the liver and the flow of blood through the organ. Computer analysis generates images and stores them for further study.

Unlike CT scans, most CT angiograms are done in a hospital setting. A local anesthetic is administered, and a catheter is inserted into a blood vessel in the groin. The tip of the catheter is positioned near the liver, and an injection of contrast material is made. Shortly after the injection, a CT scan is performed. This test provides very detailed information on the number and location of liver tumors. Typically, the test takes two to three hours to perform and requires a hospital stay of six to eight hours for observation.

magnetic resonance imaging

Magnetic resonance imaging (MRI) is a medical imaging technique that uses a strong magnetic field instead of X-rays to produce images of the body's internal organs. The main advantages of MRI are that it does not use ionizing radiation (X-rays) and it can produce almost any view of virtually any portion of the body without having to move the patient. Its main disadvantages are its high cost and it cannot safely image patients who have pacemakers or who have orthopedic hardware, such as screws, plates, or artificial joints, in the area to be scanned. In addition, some MRI machines, particularly older models, are not well tolerated by patients who suffer from claustrophobia—fear of enclosed spaces.

OVERVIEW OF MRI

MRI exploits a property of atoms called magnetic resonance. That property has to do with how atoms behave in a magnetic field, and how they react to radio waves.

An atom consists of a nucleus surrounded by electrons, which have a negative electrostatic charge. The nucleus itself consists of neutrons, which have no electrostatic charge, and protons, which have a positive charge. The nucleus spins in much the same way that a top spins: it does not remain perfectly straight but wobbles as it spins.

When atoms are placed in a magnetic field, the protons in the nuclei tend to line up along that field. About half of the atoms line up with the protons facing one end of the magnetic field, and about half line up facing the other end. There are always a few, however, that do not line up with the magnetic field at all. The number of exceptions is related to the magnetic moment of the atom, which is simply a measure of the atom's tendency to align with a magnetic field. The larger the magnetic moment, the stronger the tendency and the fewer the exceptions.

When atoms are aligned inside a magnetic field and bombarded by a radio frequency (RF) wave, the exceptional atoms that have not aligned with the field absorb the radio wave energy—that is, they "resonate"—and spin in a different direction. In fact, they all spin "in phase," which means that they wobble at precisely the same rates and in the same directions at the same time. When the radio wave is turned off, the atoms slowly begin to "relax," eventually returning to their original spins. In doing so, they give off the energy they previously absorbed.

Each different type of atom absorbs RF energy at a specific frequency, and gives off energy at a different specific frequency. For example, a hydrogen nucleus absorbs and gives off energy at different frequencies than a carbon nucleus. In addition, the relaxation time of an atom—the time it takes for the nucleus to return to its original spin—varies from a few hundred milliseconds to a few seconds, depending on its environment. A hydrogen nucleus in water relaxes slowly; a hydrogen nucleus in fat relaxes very quickly. In the jargon of radiology, the relaxation time is called T1.

At the same time that the atoms are slowly relaxing, they are also slowly dephasing: their wobbles are gradually becoming more varied, eventually returning to their entirely random motion relative to one another. Like relaxation time, the time it takes to dephase depends on the type of tissue. The dephase time is called T2, and its characteristics are slightly different from those of T1.

All these properties of atoms allow an MRI machine to take "pictures." The machine begins by generating a strong magnetic field and transmitting an RF signal at a specific frequency. Most MRI machines use the frequency of hydrogen because it is the most abundant atom in the body and has a large magnetic moment. Then, by analyzing the characteristics of T1 or T2, the computer attached to the MRI machine can generate images of different types of tissue.

THE MRI MACHINE

MRI machines vary greatly in size and shape, with newer models generally being smaller, lighter, and of more open design. Typically, however, an MRI machine might be a cube about seven feet wide by seven feet tall by 10 feet long. A tunnel or tube, called the bore, runs through the machine from front to back. A patient lies on the back on a table that slides into the bore. Whether the patient slides in head first or feet first, as well as how far into the bore the patient is carried, depends on the type of examination to be conducted. Once the body part to be examined is in the center of the machine, the scan can begin.

The necessary magnetic field is generated by electromagnets in the top and bottom of the machine. An electromagnet consists of coils of wire wrapped around a cylindrical core: when electricity passes through the wire, a magnetic field is generated. Most MRI machines use superconducting magnets. In a superconducting magnet, the wire is bathed in liquid helium at a temperature of about 450 degrees below zero. At that temperature, the electrical resistance of the wire is reduced to zero, which reduces the power requirements of the machines and makes them more economical to operate.

The magnets in an MRI machine generate a very powerful field. MRI magnets are rated in either tesla units or gauss units. One tesla is equal to 10,000 gauss. Most of the MRI machines in use today use magnets rated in the range of 0.5 to 2.0 teslas, or 5,000 to 20,000 gauss. Considering that the magnetic field of the earth is about 0.5 gauss, the weakest MRI machine in general use generates a magnetic field that is 10,000 times as strong as the earth's magnetic field. Despite the strength of that field, however, there are no known biological hazards, though most facilities prefer not to scan pregnant women. There is little research on the effects of magnetic fields on a developing fetus, and facilities prefer to err on the side of caution.

In addition to the main magnets, an MRI machine has other, less powerful magnets called gradient magnets. These are rated in the range of 180 gauss to 270 gauss. While the main magnets bathe the patient in a stable and very strong magnetic field, the gradient magnets alter that field at specific points, which allows the operator to pick out specific areas to be imaged.

In addition to the magnets, every MRI machine must have a source for generating an RF pulse. RF pulses are usually applied through coils that conform to the shape of the body part being scanned. MRI machines come with many different coils designed for specific parts of the body: head, neck, shoulders, wrists, and so on. The coils also function as detectors, detecting the signals given off by protons as they relax and dephase.

The entire system is controlled by a computer. The computer controls the patient table, the gradient magnets, and the RF coils, receives data picked up by the coils, and generates the scan images.

An MRI scan begins when the patient is suitably positioned inside the bore. First, the main magnetic field is established. Then an RF pulse specific to hydrogen is generated, and at the same time the gradient magnets are activated by rapidly switching them on and off. When the RF pulse is switched off, the hydrogen protons begin to relax, and the signals they give off are picked up by the coil. The coil sends those signals to the computer system, which analyzes them and uses the data to generate images.

For some MRI scans, contrast material is injected into the area to be scanned. While the basic purpose of MRI contrast material is essentially the same as that of contrast materials used in X-rays and computed tomography (CT) scans, the MRI contrast works in a fundamentally different way. X-ray and CT contrast materials work by blocking the X-ray photons and preventing them from reaching the film or photon detector. MRI contrast material works by altering the local magnetic field in the tissue being scanned. Normal and abnormal tissue react to that alteration in different ways, affecting the signal given off by the relaxing and dephasing protons. Those minor differences are picked up by the RF detector, allowing the computer to image many different types of tissue abnormalities.

USES OF MRI

MRI is ideal for a large number of conditions. It is especially useful for diagnosing, evaluating, and visualizing the following:

- bone tumors and cysts
- early stages of a stroke
- herniated discs in the spine
- infections in the brain, spine, or joints
- masses in soft body tissues
- multiple sclerosis
- shoulder injuries
- tendonitis
- torn ligaments in the wrists, knees, and ankles
- tumors of the pituitary gland and brain

ADVANTAGES AND DISADVANTAGES

MRI is particularly sensitive to liver tissue and can image blood vessels in the liver without the need of contrast material. In centers with the newest equipment, it is well recognized that MRI is superior to CT for the investigation of liver diseases. The greatest advantages of MRI over CT include:

- imaging patients with suspected liver tumors with high blood flow. The most important tumor in this category is primary liver cancer (hepatocellular carcinoma or hepatoma)

- evaluating patients with liver metastases (cancer that spread to the liver)

- distinguishing between benign and malignant lesions of the liver. In this category, patients with known primary tumors such as colon cancer often have liver lesions.

There are distinct advantages in using MRI over other imaging technologies. It does not use ionizing radiation, and its contrast materials have a low incidence of side effects. It can also image in any plane without moving the patient because the gradient magnets allow the operator to isolate specific parts of the body.

There are drawbacks to MRI as well. The strength of the magnetic field necessitates careful precautions. Any metal object near the MRI machine can become a dangerous projectile when the machine is turned on. For that reason both patients and operators are carefully screened for the presence of metal objects. The strength of the magnetic field also makes MRI unsuitable for scanning patients who have metal implants, such as shunts, embedded in soft tissue. People who have pacemakers cannot be scanned, and cannot even go near an MRI machine. Aneurysm clips in the brain are particularly dangerous because the magnet can move them, causing tears in the artery that the clip was meant to repair. An aneurysm is a balloonlike bulge or weakening of an artery wall that grows thinner and weaker and may cause bleeding. The surgeon places a tiny clip to stop or prevent an aneurysm from bleeding.

Orthopedic hardware firmly embedded in bone is usually safe, as are staples over which scar tissue has formed. The presence of metal objects in the area of the scan, however, can disturb the magnetic field and cause distortions in the images.

MRI also requires that the patient hold very still for long periods. MRI exams often last up to 90 minutes or more, and even a slight movement in the part being scanned can distort the image. MRI is thus often unsuitable for patients who are unable to remain still for extended periods.

Claustrophobia (fear of enclosed spaces) can also be a problem, especially with older machines. The bore of the machine is extremely confining, and patients with claustrophobia or other severe anxiety states often cannot tolerate it. The size of the bore can also make MRI unsuitable for very large patients, who simply do not fit into the machine.

MRI machines are also very noisy. Rising electric current in the gradient magnets is opposed by the main magnetic field. This causes a continual, rapid hammering. The stronger the main field, the louder the noise. In many facilities, patients are given earplugs or stereo headphones to help them cope with the noise.

Finally, MRI machines are extremely expensive to purchase, and consequently the exams are quite costly.

For many patients, however, the benefits of MRI more than outweigh its disadvantages, and as the technology progresses, newer models mitigate some of the drawbacks. Many newer models, for example, have a more open design and a shorter bore, and claustrophobia is thus less of a factor. Small MRI machines designed for specific body parts are also being developed. MRI machines that can be placed directly on specific body parts, such as an arm, knee, or foot, are already in use in some facilities.

State-of-the-art MRI systems can overcome long examination times and inconsistent image quality by using short scan sequences while the patient holds his or her breath. A routine MRI examination of the liver, for example, typically includes non-contrast-enhanced T1 and T2 images in at least two planes: transverse (across the liver from side to side) and coronal (up and down the liver from back to front). More T1 images are then acquired after the administration of a contrast agent. This type of MRI protocol is best performed on one of the more powerful MRI systems.

Since MRI is less widely used than CT for the investigation of liver disease, there is also greater variability in performing and interpreting MRI studies compared with CT. MRI is, however, unsurpassed in diagnosing benign liver tumors that do not require further investigation or treatment, and in diagnosing small malignant tumors.

positron emission tomography

Positron emission tomography (PET) is a medical imaging technique that uses radioactive isotopes to produce images of the body's organs and tissues. PET images differ from other imaging techniques such as computed tomography (CT) and magnetic resonance imaging (MRI) in that PET images reflect organ and tissue function rather than physical structure.

THE BASICS OF PET

The nucleus of an atom is composed of protons and neutrons. The number of protons in the nucleus determines the nature of any given material. Oxygen, for example, has eight protons in its nucleus. Any atom with eight protons in its nucleus is some form of oxygen. Similarly, fluorine has nine protons in its nucleus, and any atom with nine protons in its nucleus is some form of fluorine.

The number of neutrons in the nucleus determines the form, or "isotope," of the material. The most common form of oxygen, for example, has eight protons and eight neutrons in its nucleus, and is called 16-O. Another isotope of oxygen, however, 18-O, has eight protons and 10 neutrons.

The ratio of neutrons to protons affects the stability of the nucleus. A nucleus with too few or too many neutrons is unstable and subject to decay. That decay is called radioactivity, and an isotope that is radioactive is called a radioisotope.

Radioactivity can also result from an imbalance between protons in the nucleus and the electrons surrounding the nucleus. Normally, an atom has the same number of electrons as protons, and its nucleus is electrically neutral. If there are too many protons, the nucleus is unstable because it has a positive charge. To stabilize, the nucleus must shed that charge by converting one of its protons to a neutron. The conversion causes the charge formerly held by the proton to be given off as a particle called a positron.

A positron is a form of antimatter. It is identical to an electron but has a positive instead of a negative charge. Once emitted from an atom, a positron does not travel far before it collides with an electron in a nearby atom. That collision annihilates both the positron and the electron, and produces energy in the form of two photons, called gamma rays, traveling 180 degrees apart. Those photons easily pass through the body. When detected, the 180-degree separation of the two photons is termed a coincidence line. The detection of coincidence lines allows the PET scanner to form its images.

Positron-emitting radioisotopes, called tracers, are prepared in a cyclotron by bombarding a target material with protons. A typical procedure, for example, uses the oxygen isotope 18-O as a target. A bombarding proton is taken into the nucleus, ejecting a neutron in the process, to form an isotope of fluorine, 18-F. That isotope has nine protons but only the eight electrons that were in the original oxygen atom, making it a positron-emitting radioisotope.

Once the tracer has been prepared, it is attached to a natural body compound. The most commonly used compound is glucose, but water and ammonia may also be used. When the material is injected into the body, the tracer collects in various areas of the body, and the gamma rays from the decay of the nuclei can be detected with a PET scan.

HOW A PET SCAN WORKS

PET scans, usually done on an outpatient basis, may require special preparation. The patient usually is asked not to eat for at least four hours before the test, but is encouraged to drink a lot of water. Patients on certain medications may be required to alter their usual medication patterns. Diabetic patients may be given specific dietary guidelines designed to control glucose levels. Because PET involves radioactive substances, women who are, or might be pregnant, should inform their doctors.

The first step in a PET scan procedure is administering a tracer to the patient, either by injection or inhalation. In general, it takes 45 minutes to an hour for the tracer to be distributed through the body and to collect in the organs or tissues to be scanned.

The PET scanner itself looks much like a CT scan machine: a square doughnut standing on its side, with a table that carries the patient into the doughnut hole. Nine rings of gamma ray detectors are arranged around the inside of the doughnut hole. As the gamma rays from the decay of the radioisotope are detected, the photons are converted to electrical signals. Those signals, in turn, are fed into a computer that interprets them as an image.

The image that results from a PET scan, however, is unlike similar images from a CT or MRI scan. Where a CT or MRI scan shows the physical structure of an organ, a PET image shows the functioning of an organ. That is because the distribution of the tracer in organs or tissues depends on how the organ handles the tracer biochemically. Healthy tissue, for example, uses glucose for energy to function; consequently, a tracer attached to glucose will show up on a PET scan. Cancerous tissue, however, uses glucose at a much higher rate than normal tissue, and results in a much higher concentration of the tracer. The PET computer interprets that higher concentration as a brighter area. Thus, in a PET image cancerous tissue shows up as brighter than normal tissue.

USES OF PET

At present, PET scanning is used primarily to evaluate patients with cancer, cardiac illness, and diseases of the brain.

For cancer patients, PET can be used to

- distinguish benign from malignant tumors
- stage cancer by showing metastases anywhere in the body
- evaluate the progress of cancer therapies and treatment

For patients with cardiac illness, PET can be used to

- determine after a heart attack whether the heart muscle would benefit from surgery
- evaluate heart muscle functioning in patients with coronary artery disease or diseases of the heart muscle.

For patients with diseases of the brain, PET can be used to

- provide an early and accurate diagnosis of Alzheimer's disease
- locate tumors in the brain and distinguish tumor from scar tissue
- locate the focus of seizures for some patients with epilepsy
- assess tumor and other sites in the brain for delicate surgery

The role of PET scanning for the liver is still being established, but its use has been approved for evaluating metastatic colorectal cancer (cancer that has spread from the colon and rectum). PET scans of the liver using the 18-F isotope attached to glucose are useful for evaluating the response of liver metastases (cancer that spread to the liver) to therapy, and can be used to detect the presence of tumors in treated lesions. Some centers recommend that a PET scan be performed for all patients with metastatic colorectal cancers before a surgical intervention.

ADVANTAGES AND DISADVANTAGES

The main advantage of a PET scan is that, because it images body functions instead of body structures, it can help physicians detect biochemical changes that suggest disease long before anatomical changes occur. Thus, a PET scan can diagnose some diseases before their effects are apparent on a CT or MRI scan.

The ability to image functioning, however, can also be a disadvantage in some situations. A PET scan can give false results if the patient's chemical balances are not normal. If the patient has eaten anything within several hours before the test, for example, blood sugar or insulin levels may adversely affect the scan results.

Also, the structural information available from PET scans is relatively limited compared with CT and MRI scans. That often makes PET best used as part of a larger diagnostic workup, perhaps including CT or MRI scans for providing information on tissue structures. Perhaps partially in recognition of that limitation, PET manufacturers in 2000 began to produce machines that combine PET and CT in a single scanner, allowing both types of scans to be taken in the same procedure.

PET does use radioactive tracers, but the isotopes used are short-lived and the exposure is low. In general, tracers used in PET scanning give about the same radiation exposure as two X-rays. Because of the radioactivity, however, it is important for patients who are pregnant or breast feeding to weigh carefully the benefit expected of the scan against the potential of exposing the fetus or infant to radiation. In addition, because the tracers decay so quickly, they must be produced in a laboratory near the radiology center, and the examination must begin at the scheduled time.

Insurance coverage can also be a problem for some PET procedures. PET is an expensive and relatively new modality, and some of its uses are still considered to be experimental. Patients should check with their insurance providers to make sure any proposed PET scans are included in their coverage.

ultrasound

Ultrasound—also called sonography or US—is a radiological technique that uses sound waves instead of X-rays to produce images of the body's internal organs. The advantages of ultrasound are that it is a relatively safe, relatively inexpensive, and noninvasive method of obtaining pictures of what is occurring in the body at any given time, and it produces high-resolution pictures of cysts (fluid-filled sacs). Its main disadvantages are that it may produce poor images in patients who are large or obese, in patients who have excessive amounts of bowel gas, and in patients with cirrhosis. In some cases, it may also have trouble distinguishing lesions in the liver from normal liver tissue.

Ultrasound is based on the same sonar technology used by ships at sea and by fish detectors designed for anglers. Sonar directs a controlled sound over a given area. When the sound waves strike an object, they echo back toward the sonar device. The echoes, when analyzed electronically, can indicate the object's distance away, its size and shape, and even its internal consistency (solid, fluid, or mixed).

A medical ultrasound scanner consists of a computer to modulate the generation of sound and analyze the echoes, a video display screen to show the images, and a hand-held transducer probe. The transducer probe is typically about the size of a bar of soap or a cell phone. In essence, it acts as both a speaker and a microphone, though its technical aspects are more sophisticated than either of those terms implies. When the radiologist or sonographer passes the probe over the body, it emits high-frequency sound waves that are inaudible to the human ear and directs them into the body. At the same time, it picks up the returned echoes and converts them to electronic impulses, which pass through a cord to the computer. The computer interprets the electronic signals as visual images of the internal organs and displays those images on the video screen.

A typical ultrasound device sends and receives millions of sound pulses each second, and the transducer probe can be moved along the body and angled differently to obtain different views of the internal organs. The frequency of the sound waves directed into the body determine how deeply the waves penetrate and the resolution of the image. There are also different kinds of probes. While the most typical probe is designed to move across the surface of the body, probes of special design can be inserted into various orifices of the body—rectum, vagina, esophagus—to get closer to the organ being scanned and to provide a more detailed image.

Because the probe is continually sending and receiving sound waves and echoes, the images produced are "real-time" images, a computer term indicating that the images are updated continually, for as long as the computer receives data. Consequently, the images can show movement in the organs as they occur. That is, a typical ultrasound scan is less like taking a still photograph and more like shooting a motion picture. In fact, an entire session can be recorded on videotape or compact disc. That characteristic enables physicians to record and review processes as they occur, and expands the utility of ultrasound beyond the simple visualization of static objects.

Compared with many other radiological techniques, ultrasound is relatively inexpensive, simple, readily available, quick, and well tolerated by patients. Those characteristics make it the preferred technique in a large number of situations.

Ultrasound imaging is used extensively for evaluating the kidneys, liver, gallbladder, pancreas, spleen, and blood vessels of the abdomen. Because it does not use ionizing radiation, such as X-rays, it is widely used in obstetrics and gynecology to perform such functions as

- assessing the size and position of the fetus
- checking the sex of the baby
- monitoring fetus development (by making several scans over a period of time)
- detecting tumors of the ovaries and breasts

It has also been used in cardiology to see inside the heart as an aid in identifying abnormalities in structure or function, and in urology to help detect prostate cancer.

Ultrasound is often one of the first tests ordered during the CANCER STAGING process. In liver surgery, it may be the first choice for screening and follow-up because it is relatively mobile and can be taken to the bedside. In patients with liver tumors, ultrasound can be used to locate a tumor, measure its size, and determine whether it is a solid tumor or a cyst. It is also considered more accurate than the computed tomography (CT) scan and magnetic resonance imaging (MRI), which have largely been discarded in cancer screening.

Because it provides real-time images, it is also used often to guide the needle during needle biopsies (using a needle to obtain a tissue sample). In obstetrics, ultrasound is particularly useful in guiding the needle during amniocentesis (taking a sample of the amniotic fluid) to avoid harming the fetus—a process that once trusted to luck. Real-time imaging is also useful in placing catheters.

Improvements in the original ultrasound technology—three-dimensional ultrasound and Doppler ultrasound—have increased its utility.

The typical ultrasound device, seen in most doctors' offices, produces a two-dimensional image, or "slice," of the object being scanned. In the last several years, however, the technology has advanced to the point where three-dimensional imagery has become possible. Three-dimensional images give the radiologist, the physician, and the patient a much better view of the organ in question, and is especially useful for

- examining the prostate and detecting tumors
- searching for masses in the colon and rectum
- detecting lesions in the breasts
- assessing the development of a fetus, and especially in detecting abnormalities in facial or limb development
- visualizing blood flow in an organ or in a fetus

Another specialized development is Doppler ultrasound. The so-called Doppler effect, named after the Austrian physicist who first described it, is an apparent change in the frequency of a wave when the source and the observer are moving relative to each other. Expressed in a more practical way, the Doppler effect is what makes the pitch of a train whistle seem to become higher and then lower as the train approaches, passes, and moves away. The effect is measurable, and is related to how fast the train is moving.

The same effect can be observed in an ultrasound scan. When a moving object is scanned, the echoes return at a lower frequency when the object is moving away from the probe, and at a higher frequency when it is moving toward the probe. How much the frequency changes depends on how fast the object is moving. That characteristic makes it possible for the computer to calculate the object's speed.

The primary use of Doppler ultrasound has been in examining the blood vessels. Images produced by Doppler ultrasound can help a physician see and evaluate blockages to the flow of blood, such as blood clots, and plaque buildup inside the blood vessels. Doppler ultrasound can also be used to calculate the rate of blood flow through the heart and the major arteries. Data on the speed and volume of blood flow often helps a physician determine whether a patient is a good candidate for a procedure such as angioplasty (insertion of an inflated balloon inside an occluded artery).

PROCEDURE

For a standard ultrasound procedure, little preparation is usually needed. Depending on the type of scan, however, a patient may be asked to eat or drink nothing for the preceding 12 hours. Other scans may require the bladder to be full.

In the usual procedure, the patient is placed on an examining table and a clear gel is spread on the area that will be examined. The gel lubricates the skin and prevents the formation of air pockets between the probe and the body. The radiographer or sonographer then presses the probe firmly against the skin and sweeps it over the area of interest, repeating as necessary until all the images of interest are captured.

There may be some discomfort from the pressure applied to the probe as it is guided over the skin, especially if the images to be gathered require that the patient have a full bladder, but in general the process is completely painless.

A full ultrasound examination usually takes fewer than 30 minutes. When it is over, the patient may be asked to wait while the images are reviewed, but often the images will have been reviewed as they were received, and the patient is released immediately.

Results from the examination are sent to the referring physician, who may discuss the results with the patient during an ensuing office visit. Some facilities may provide results and images that can be accessed over the Internet.

Ultrasound is sometimes performed surgically. That procedure, called intraoperative ultrasound, can be done with open surgery, or it can be done laparoscopically. (A laparoscope is a slender, hollow tube used to perform minor surgery on organs inside the abdominal or pelvic cavity.) Either procedure can bring the ultrasound's transducer probe into direct contact with an organ such as the liver, making it possible to detect lesions as small as three millimeters. It also provides precise anatomical resolution, making it possible to visualize clearly the proximity of lesions to blood vessels and to the hilum (the area where ducts, nerves, and blood vessels join with the organ).

Intraoperative ultrasound is often done during surgical procedures on the liver because it can identify all the lesions within the liver. Laparoscopic ultrasound is an important tool in staging liver malignancies and evaluating liver tumors.

RISKS AND COMPLICATIONS

There are no known anatomical risks with a standard ultrasound procedure. There is no exposure to harmful radiation or to high magnetic fields. There was at one time concern about the possibility of cavitation (formation of low-pressure bubbles) when dissolved gases come out of solution due to local heating caused by sound waves, but no study on either humans or animals has borne out those concerns.

Because the generated sound waves are reflected by air and gas, ultrasound is not the preferred method for imaging the bowel. A barium exam or a computed tomography (CT) scan is usually preferred.

Ultrasound also has difficulty penetrating bone and cannot see beyond the surface of bony structures. For visualizing bone, magnetic resonance imaging (MRI) or some other imaging technology is preferable.

In general, results of standard ultrasounds are more variable than those of other imaging technologies. The results of ultrasound tests done on the liver, for example, are highly dependent on the experience and level of interest on the part of the radiographer or sonographer performing the procedure. The results are also highly dependent on the quality of the equipment, as well as on the general physical condition of the patient. Ultrasound may not work well on obese patients or those with excessive amounts of air in hollow organs or in the part of the lungs overlying the liver. In such cases, ultrasound may not always detect all tumors.

financing health care

Patients diagnosed with liver disease or chronic liver conditions face lifelong medical costs. The cost of regular examinations, liver-function tests, periodic liver biopsies, antiviral medicines such as interferon, and liver transplants taxes resources. If health insurance proves inadequate, the patient may be forced to seek help from unaccustomed places.

As of this writing, patients requiring interferon therapy, for example, may spend in the neighborhood of $500 per month—perhaps more, depending on dosage and specific therapy options—for injections, blood tests, and doctor visits. Traditional health insurance may not cover all those costs. Financial assistance for interferon treatments, however, is available from the pharmaceutical company. There are qualifying restrictions for such assistance; patients in the United States and Canada who might have trouble affording treatment can contact Schering for information.

Patients requiring transplants have the highest costs. The cost of liver transplantation varies widely, but at the time of this writing, the average is about $150,000, not including pre- and postoperative care. Usually the hospital has an expert in financing transplantations who can offer advice and assistance in exploring available options, which include public fund-raising campaigns, grants or services from charitable organizations or patient advocacy groups, assistance from community organizations, and help from faith-based groups.

GOVERNMENT HEALTH INSURANCE

Under certain circumstances, government health insurance may be available in the form of Medicare, Medicaid, or veterans benefits.

Medicare is a two-part program. Part A covers hospitalization, and is available at no cost to U.S. citizens and permanent residents 65 or older. People who receive certain disability benefits, or who have chronic kidney disease, may also qualify. Part B covers physician services, prescriptions, and some outpatient services. It is optional and requires the payment of a monthly premium.

People already receiving Social Security or Railroad Retirement benefits automatically get Medicare Part A beginning the month they turn 65. Others should contact their local Social Security office for eligibility and enrollment information. People with low income may qualify for state aid to help pay Medicare premiums and other medical expenses, and should call their county social services department to find out whether they qualify.

Medicaid pays for medical assistance to individuals and families with low incomes and limited resources. Eligibility requirements and available services vary from state to state. Interested individuals should contact their county social services department for information.

Veterans may qualify for Veterans Administration (VA) health benefits. The basic eligibility requirement is veteran status, which simply means service in the U.S. military and a discharge under other than dishonorable conditions. Specific eligibility requirements, however, are more complex than that, and not every honorably discharged veteran is guaranteed access to the program.

DISABILITY INSURANCE

Patients with chronic liver disease such as HEPATITIS C may find themselves unable to function as well as they did at home or on the job. This can be the case if hepatitis C has progressed to the stage of CIRRHOSIS (irreversible scarring of the liver), and the condition is worsening. Patients who are too sick to work may

have a variety of options for receiving their regular paycheck for a limited period of time, and for receiving disability payments for longer periods.

Some companies offer paid disability leave for short periods, or allow their employees to use accumulated sick leave. A disability leave may require extensive documentation or consultation with a company-approved physician. Patients who need disability leave from their job, or think they may need it in the future, should talk to their company's medical benefits representative.

Regardless of whether employer-sponsored disability leave is available, having to take extended time off from work does not necessarily mean losing one's job. The Family and Medical Leave Act of 1993 allows eligible employees to take up to 12 weeks of unpaid leave each year because of serious health problems, or to care for a family member who has a serious health problem. Eligibility is determined by a complex formula that includes whether the employer is covered by the act, how long the employee has been working for the company, and how many hours the employee worked over the 12 months preceding the beginning of the leave. Employers covered by the act are required to make "reasonable accommodations" for employees with serious illnesses.

Interested individuals should contact the Wage and Hour Division of the Department of Labor's Employment Standards Administration.

The Americans with Disabilities Act (ADA) also provides some protection for people with disabilities. It applies not only to access issues such as wheelchair ramps and accessible restrooms, but also to a company's employment, attendance, and leave policies.

The Social Security Administration offers two programs for disabled people: Social Security Disability Insurance (SSDI) and Supplemental Security Income (SSI).

Generally speaking, SSDI is for any eligible worker or immediate family member who has a physical or mental impairment expected to prevent her or him from working for at least one year or to result in death. SSDI benefits last until the covered individual is able to return to work.

An SSDI claim must be filed with the Social Security Administration and takes about 90 days to investigate. The agency's investigation includes obtaining a host of medical and personal records, including the names of all the doctors and hospitals that provided treatment; lists of medications; medical records from therapists, doctors, and clinics; laboratory test results; copies of W-2s or federal tax returns; and so on. A person filing an SSDI claim should have as many personal and medical records on hand as possible, to help speed up the claim process.

SSI is a need-based supplementary income program. It is for the aged (65 or older), blind, or disabled person who is unable to work and has little or no income. People who receive SSI often receive additional money from the state, and often qualify for other aid as well, such as Medicaid or food stamps. Interested individuals should contact the Social Security Administration and their local public welfare office for information. Have Social Security number handy when calling.

FINANCIAL ASSISTANCE FOR CANCER CARE

Aside from the physical and emotional toll, cancer can impose heavy economic burdens on patients and their families. Health insurance may pay a portion of the costs, but it may not be enough, and some people lack insurance altogether. For these individuals, some resources are available, through some government-sponsored programs and others.

Patients should not hesitate to discuss their financial concerns with their health care providers, who may help make some arrangements.

The Centers for Medicare & Medicaid Services (CMS) (formerly the Health Care Financing Administration—HCFA) has 10 regional offices, in Boston, New York, Philadelphia, Atlanta, Chicago, Dallas, Kansas City (Missouri), Denver, San Francisco, and Seattle. Contact

Central Office
7500 Security Boulevard
Baltimore, MD 21244-1850
(877) 267-2323 (toll-free)
(410) 786-3000 (local)
(866) 226-1819 (toll-free for the
   hearing-impaired)
(410) 786-0727 (local for the hearing-impaired)
http://www.cms.hhs.gov

Medicare
http://www.medicare.gov
(800) MEDICARE (633-4227)

Veterans Health Administration
Central Office:
810 Vermont Avenue NW
Washington, DC 20420
(877) 222-8387
(202) 273-5400
http://www.va.gov
   For questions about eligibility and to obtain more specific information on the provisions of the act, contact

The President's Committee on Employment of People with Disabilities Information Line (Job Accommodation Network)
(800) 232-9675

ADA Technical Assistance Center
(800) 949-4232

Social Security Administration
Office of Public Inquiries
Windsor Park Building
6401 Security Boulevard
Baltimore, MD 21235
(800) 772-1213
(800) 325-0778 (for the hearing-impaired)
   For financial assistance based on a sliding scale for patients who have difficulty paying for interferon, contact Schering:
(800) 521-7157, ext. 147 (U.S.)
(800) 363-3422 (Canada)

U.S. Department of Labor
Wage and Hour Division of the Department of
   Labor's Employment Standards Administration
Frances Perkins Building
200 Constitution Avenue NW
Washington, DC 20210
(866) 487-9243
(877) 889-5627 (for the hearing-impaired)
http://www.dol.gov
http://www.dol.gov/esa
   For resources on financial assistance for cancer care, contact the following:

American Cancer Society (ACS)
(800) 227-2345
http://www.cancer.org

The AVONCares Program for Medically Underserved Women
(800) 813-HOPE (4673)
http://www.cancercare.org

finding a specialist

Managing liver disease can be a complicated undertaking. When treating a patient with a liver disorder, a primary care physician may suggest that the patient see a hepatologist or a gastroenterologist. A hepatologist is a physician whose medical specialty is treating liver problems. A gastroenterologist is a physician who has specialized in disease of the digestive system, including the liver. A hepatologist or a gastroenterologist has years of specialty training, besides basic medical training. Either specialist can work with a primary care physician to choose the correct treatments, manage medicines, and decide what tests and monitoring are needed to stay at optimum health.

The first step in choosing a hepatologist or a gastroenterologist is to consult with the primary care physician. Patients must make sure they understand why they need to see a specialist if they are being referred to one by their physician. Patients should do the following when getting a recommendation for a specialist from their doctor:

- If possible, obtain a list of specialists with whom the physician has worked in the past, as good communication between the primary care physician and the specialist is essential.

- Ask how often the physician has worked with each specialist in the past, and what he or she thought of the experience.

- Request the name of more than one hepatologist (or gastroenterologist) to choose from in the patient's geographical area.
- State a gender and/or age group preference.

Patients are also encouraged to check with a national organization—such as the American Liver Foundation—or local support group related to the illness. A support group is full of members who are being treated for the same liver problem, and the members will likely have valuable opinions on hepatologists or gastroenterologists from a patient's point of view.

WHAT TO LOOK FOR WHEN CHOOSING A SPECIALIST

When choosing a physician of any specialty, ask questions. A professional physician should have no problem if the patient wants to ask questions or meet together before making decisions. In fact, the office staff should be willing to provide the patient with a list of the hepatologist's credentials over the phone. Some questions to ask are:

- Is the hepatologist/gastroenterologist accepting new patients? Does the physician accept the patient's health insurance? (It is advisable to verify this with the insurance company.)

- What education does the physician have? Any special residencies, internships, fellowships, or other additional training?

- How long has the physician been specializing in hepatology or gastroenterology? How long has the physician been practicing medicine?

- What board certifications does the physician hold? Board certification means that the physician has passed a structured educational program and has proven his or her competencies in a particular area of medicine.

- How much experience does the hepatologist/gastroenterologist have in managing patients with the patient's particular liver disorder?

- Is it difficult to get an appointment? Is someone on-call for the physician during evenings and weekends, in case of an emergency?

It is recommended that patients or their families verify the physician's qualifications by doing one of the following:

- Make a call to the medical licensing board in the physician's state to determine whether the physician has had any complaints or disciplinary actions.

Or

- Contact the county clerk's office to find out whether the physician has any malpractice lawsuits against him or her.

FEELING COMFORTABLE WITH THE SPECIALIST

It is important to have a physician who is skilled and knowledgeable. Not feeling comfortable when communicating with the physician and the office staff can be detrimental to one's health in the long run. Indeed, studies have shown that patients with HEPATITIS C who have problems communicating with their physicians respond less well to medical treatment than those who enjoy good rapport.

It is therefore important for the patient to take some time when choosing a hepatologist or any other specialist. Credentials alone cannot determine whether a physician is a good match for a patient. The best way to tell is for the patient first to make an appointment with the physician and ask himself or herself the following questions:

- Is the office staff friendly and helpful?
- Does the physician take time to answer questions and address concerns?
- Is it possible to communicate openly with the doctor?
- Does the doctor inspire confidence in her or his ability to deal with the particular illness the patient is presenting?
- Does the doctor appear competent and concerned with the patient's well-being?

Although it is true that doctors do not have time to chat for extended periods, they should still let the patient ask more than a few questions and should be comfortable explaining the risks and benefits of any test or treatment they recommend. The physician should be actively involved in deciding what is best for the patient's health.

If the answer to any of these questions is no, it is probably to the patient's benefit to find a doctor who inspires more trust.

APPENDIX II
ORGANIZATIONS FOR LIVER AND RELATED CONCERNS

General

American Association for the Study of Liver Disease (AASLD)
1729 King Street, Suite 200
Alexandria, VA 22314-2720
(703) 299-9766
http://www.aasld.org

American College of Gastroenterology (ACG)
P.O. Box 342260
Bethesda, MD 20827-2260
(301) 263-9000
http://www.acg.gi.org

American Gastroenterological Association (AGA)
4930 Del Ray Avenue
Bethesda, MD 20814
(301) 654-2055
http://www.gastro.org

American Liver Foundation
75 Maiden Lane, Suite 603
New York, NY 10038-4810
Helpline (24 hours, 7 days a week):
    (800) 465-4837 or (888) 443-7222
(212) 668-1000
http://www.liverfoundation.org

American Medical Association (AMA)
515 North State Street
Chicago, IL 60610
(800) 621-8335
http://www.ama-assn.org

British Liver Trust
Portman House
44 High Street
Ringwood BH24 1AG
United Kingdom
+44 1425 463080
http://www.britishlivertrust.org.uk
For publication orders: publications@
    britishlivertrust.org.uk

Canadian Liver Foundation
2235 Sheppard Avenue East, Suite 1500
Toronto, ON M2J 5B5
Canada
(800) 563-5483
http://www.liver.ca

Center for Proper Medication Use
P.O. Box 13329
Philadelphia, PA 19101-3329
(215) 895-1131

CenterWatch-Clinical Trials Listing Service
Thomson Center Watch
22 Thomson Place, 47F1
Boston, MA 02210-1212
(617) 856-5900
http://www.centerwatch.com

Children Affected by AIDS Foundation
Los Angeles Office:
6033 West Century Boulevard, Suite 280
Los Angeles, CA 90045
(310) 258-0850
Chicago Office:
70 East Lake Street, Suite 430
Chicago, IL 60601

(312) 580-1150
http://www.caaf4kids.org

Children's Liver Alliance

(formerly the Biliary Atresia and Liver Transplant
    Network, Inc.)
3835 Richmond Avenue, Suite 190
Staten Island, NY 10312-3828
(718) 987-6200

Children's Liver Association for Support Services (CLASS)

27023 McBean Parkway #126
Valencia, CA 91355
(877) 679-8256 (toll-free)

Children's Liver Disease Foundation

36 Great Charles Street
Birmingham B3 3JY
United Kingdom
+44 (0) 121 212 3839
Fax: +44 (0) 121 212 4300
http://www.childliverdisease.org

Falk Foundation

Liver Diseases
Dr. Falk Pharma
+49 (761) 15 14 -0
http://www.falkfoundation.com

Food and Drug Administration (FDA)

MEDWATCH
5600 Fishers Lane
Rockville, MD 20857
(888) 463-6332
http://www.fda.gov

Genetic and Rare Diseases Information Center

P.O. Box 8126
Gaithersburg, MD 20898-8126
(888) 205-2311
(888) 205-3223 (TTY)
http://rarediseases.info.nih.gov/html/resources/
    info_cntr.html

Immunization Action Coalition

1573 Selby Avenue, Suite 234
St. Paul, MN 55104
(651) 647-9009
Fax: (651) 647-9131
http://www.immunize.org

Latino Organization for Liver Awareness (LOLA)

P.O. Box 842
Throggs Neck Station
Bronx, NY 10465
(888) 367-LOLA
http://www.lola-national.org

National Digestive Diseases Information Clearinghouse (NDDIC)

2 Information Way
Bethesda, MD 20892-3570
(800) 891-5389
http://digestive.niddk.nih.gov

National Health Information Center (NHIC)

P.O. Box 1133
Washington, DC 20013-1133
(800) 336-4797
(301) 565-4167
http://www.healthfinder.gov

National Institute of Allergy and Infectious Diseases (NIAID)

AIDS Clinical Trials Information Service
6610 Rockledge Drive, MSC 6612
Bethesda, MD 20892-6612
(800) 874-2572

National Institute of Diabetes and Digestive and Kidney Diseases (NIDDK)

1 Information Way
Bethesda, MD 20892-3560
(301) 654-3810
http://www.niddk.nih.gov

National Institutes of Health (NIH)

Office of Communications and Public Liaison
Building 31, Room 9A04, 31 Center Drive,
    MSC 2560
Bethesda, MD 20892-2560
http://www.nih.gov

National Organization for Rare Disorders (NORD)

55 Kenosia Avenue
P.O. Box 1968
Danbury, CT 06813-1968
(800) 999-6673 (voice mail only)
(203) 744-0100
http://www.rarediseases.org

Alpha-1-Antitrypsin Deficiency (AIAD)

Alpha 1-Antitrypsin Deficiency (AIAD) or AIAD Related Emphysema
National Jewish Medical and Research Center
1400 Jackson Street
Denver, CO 80206
800-222-LUNG
http://www.nationaljewish.org/medfacts/alpha1.html

Alpha 1 National Association
275 West Street, Suite 210
Annapolis, MD 21401
(401) 216-6916
http://www.alpha1.org

Alpha-1 Foundation
2937 SW 27th Avenue, Suite 302
Miami, FL 33133
(877) 228-7321 (toll-free)
(305) 567-9888
Fax: (305) 567-1317
http://www.alphaone.org

AlphaNet, Inc.
2937 SW 27 Avenue, Suite 305
Coconut Grove, FL 33133
(800) 577-2638
http://www.alphanet.org

American Lung Association
61 Broadway, 6th Floor
New York, NY 10006
(800) LUNG-USA
http://www.lungusa.org/diseases/luna1ad.htm

Autoimmune Liver Disorders

American Autoimmune Related Diseases Association (AARDA)
National Office:
22100 Gratiot Avenue
Detroit, MI 48021
(586) 776-3900
http://www.aarda.org
Washington Office:
750 17th Street NW
Suite 1100
Washington, DC 20006

(202) 466-8511
(800) 598-4668 (literature requests)

Cancer

Allegheny General Liver Cancer Program
320 East North Avenue
Pittsburgh, PA 15212-4772
(412) 359-6738
(412) 359-6288
http://www.livercancer.com

AMC Cancer Research Center
AMC Cancer Research Center Information
    and Counseling Line
1600 Pierce Street
Denver, CO 80214
(800) 321-1557
(303) 233-6501
http://www.amc.org

American Cancer Society
1599 Clifton Road, NE
Atlanta, GA 30329
(800) 227-2345
http://www.cancer.org

American Institute for Cancer Research (AICR)
1759 R Street NW
Washington, DC 2000
(800) 843-8114
http://www.aicr.org.

Cancer Care, Inc.
275 Seventh Avenue
New York, NY 10001
(800) 813-HOPE
http://www.cancercare.org

Cancer Hope Network
Two North Road
Chester, NJ 07930
(877) HOPENET
http://www.cancerhopenetwork.org

Cancer Information Service of the National Cancer Institute
(800) CANCER
(800) 638-6070 (Alaska)
(800) 524-1234 (Hawaii)

Candlelighters Childhood Cancer Foundation
National Office
P.O. Box 498
Kensington, MD 20895-0498
(800) 366-2223
(301) 962-3520
http://www.candlelighters.org

Colorectal Cancer Network (CCNetwork)
P.O. Box 182
Kensington, MD 20895-0182
(301) 879-1500
Fax: (301) 879-1901
http://www.colorectal-cancer.net

**National Cancer Institute
(National Institutes of Health)**
9000 Rockville Pike
Bethesda, MD 20892
(800) 422-6237
(800) 332-8615 (for the hearing-impaired)
http://www.cancer.gov

Hemochromatosis

American Hemochromatosis Society, Inc. (AHS)
4044 West Lake Mary Boulevard
Unit #104, PMB 416
Lake Mary, FL 32746-2012
(888) 655-4766
(407) 829-4488
http://www.americanhs.org

Canadian Hemochromatosis Society
272-7000 Minoru Boulevard
Richmond, BC V6Y 3Z5
Canada
(877) 223-4766 (toll-free in Canada only)
(604) 279-7135
Fax: (604) 279-7138
http://www.cdnhemochromatosis.ca

The Haemochromatosis Society
Hollybush House
Hadley Green Road
Barnet, Herts EN5 5PR
England
Phone/Fax: +44 0208 449 1363
http://www.ghsoc.org

Hemochromatosis Foundation, Inc.
P.O. Box 8569
Albany, NY 12208

(518) 489-0972
Fax: (518) 489-0227
http://www.webmd.com/hw/blood-disorders/
shc29hem.asp

Iron Overload Diseases Association (IOD)
433 Westwind Drive
North Palm Beach, FL 33408-5123
(561) 840-3512
http://www.ironoverload.org

Hepatitis

CDC Hepatitis Hotline
(404) 332-4555 (voice mail for requesting faxed
information)

**Centers for Disease Control and Prevention
(CDC)**
Hepatitis Branch, Mailstop G37
Atlanta, GA 30333
CDC Hepatitis Hotline: (888) 443-7232
CDC Public Inquiries: (800) 311-3435
http://www.cdc.gov/ncidod/diseases/hepatitis

Hepatitis B Foundation
700 East Butler Avenue
Doylestown, PA 18901-2697
(215) 489-4900
Fax: (215) 489-4920
http://www.hepb.org

The Hepatitis C Foundation
1502 Russett Drive
Warminster, PA 18974
(215) 672-2606

Hepatitis Education Project
4603 Aurora Avenue North
Seattle, WA 98103
(206) 732-0311
http://www.scn.org/health/hepatitis/index.htm

Hepatitis Foundation International (HFI)
504 Blick Drive
Silver Spring, MD 20904-2901
(800) 891-0707
http://www.hepfi.org

**Hepatitis Information Network Educational
Events (HepNet)**
3535 Trans-Canada Highway
Pointe Claire, QC H9R1B4

Canada
http://www.hepnet.com/events.html

Hepatitis Prevention Programs
1573 Selby Avenue, Suite 234
St Paul, MN 55104
(651) 647-9009
Fax: (651) 647-9131
http://www.hepprograms.org

Massachusetts Department of Public Health
Bureau of Communicable Disease Control
State Laboratory Institute
305 South Street
Jamaica Plain, MA 02130
(617) 983-6550
Fax: (617) 983-6925
Hepatitis C Hotline: (888) 443-HepC
http://www.mass.gov/dph/cdc/masshepc

National HCV Prison Coalition
HCV Prison Project
Phyllis Beck, Director
P.O. Box 41803
Eugene, OR 97404
(541) 607-5725
Fax: (541) 607-5684
http://www.hcvinprison.org

Projects in Knowledge
Care & Counsel III
Helping patients stay the course on treatment
   for hepatitis C
Overlook at Great Notch
150 Clove Road
Little Falls, NJ 07424
(973) 890-8988
http://www.projectsinknowledge.com

National Reye's Syndrome Foundation
P.O. Box 829
426 North Lewis
Bryan, OH 43506-0829
(800) 233-7393
(419) 636-2679 or (419) 636-9897
http://www.reyessyndrome.org

Primary Biliary Cirrhosis

PBCers Europe
http://members.tripod.com/pbcfunchat

PBC Foundation
54 Queen Street
Edinburgh EH2 3NS
Scotland
+44 131 225 8586
Fax: +44 131 225 7579
http://www.pbcfoundation.org.uk

APPENDIX III
TRANSPLANTATION AND RELATED ORGANIZATIONS

American Liver Foundation
75 Maiden Lane, Suite 603
New York, NY 10038
(800) 465-4837
http://www.liverfoundation.org

American Red Cross Tissue Donation
American Red Cross
2025 E Street NW
Washington, DC 20006
http://www.redcross.org/donate/tissue

American Society for Artificial Internal Organs (ASAIO)
World Headquarters
P.O. Box C
Boca Raton, FL 33429-0468
(561) 391-8589
Fax: (561) 368-9153
http://www.asaio.com

American Society of Transplantation
15000 Commerce Parkway, Suite C
Mt. Laurel, NJ 08054
(856) 439-9986
http://www.a-s-t.org

American Society of Transplant Surgeons (ASTS)
1020 North Fairfax Street, Suite 200
Alexandria, VA 22314
(888) 990-2787
http://www.asts.org

British Organ Donor Society (BODY)
Balsham, Cambridge CB1 GDL
United Kingdom
http://users.argonet.co.uk/body

California Transplant Donor Network (CTDN)
1611 Telegraph Avenue, Suite 600
Oakland, CA 94612
(888) 570-9400
(510) 444-8500
Fax: (510) 444-8501
http://www.ctdn.org

Center for Liver Disease and Transplantation (CLDT)
Columbia University Medical Center
Presbyterian Hospital Building
622 West 168th Street, 14th floor
New York, NY 10032-3784
(212) 305-0914
(800) 227-2762 (24/7 referrals hotline)
(877) 548-3763 (toll-free referrals)
http://hora.cpmc.columbia.edu/dept/liverMD

CenterSpan
http://www.centerspan.org
webmaster@centerspan.org

Children's Liver Alliance
(formerly Biliary Atresia and Liver Transplant
    Network, Inc.)
3835 Richmond Avenue, Box 190
Staten Island, NY 10312
Voice mail and fax: (718) 987-6200
OrganTrans@msn.com

Children's Liver Association for Support Services
27023 McBean Parkway #126
Valencia, CA 91355
(877) 679-8256 (toll-free)

Phone/Fax: (661) 263-9099
http://www.classkids.org

Children's Organ Transplant Association
2501 COTA Drive
Bloomington, IN 47403
(800) 366-COTA
http://www.cota.org

Coalition on Donation
700 North 4th Street
Richmond, VA 23219
(804) 782-4920
http://www.donatelife.net
coalition@donatelife.net

Columbia University Medical Center
Presbyterian Hospital Building
622 West 168th Street
14th floor
New York, NY 10032-3784
(212) 305-0914

Donate Life
U.S. Department of Health and Human Services
The official Web site for organ and tissue
    donation/transplantation
http://www.organdonor.gov/

First Family Pledge
http://www.cherubs.org/Web%20Pages/pledge.html

International Liver Transplantation Society
15000 Commerce Parkway, Suite C
Mt. Laurel, NJ 08054
(856) 439-0500
http://www.ilts.org
ilts@ahint.com

**International Transplant Nurses Society
(ITNS)**
1739 East Carson Street, Box 351
Pittsburgh, PA 15203
(412) 343-ITNS
http://www.itns.org

LifeNet
5809 Ward Court
Virginia Beach, VA 23455
(800) 847-7831
(757) 464-4761
http://www.lifenet.org

Living Bank–Organ and Tissue Donor Registry
P.O. Box 6725
Houston, TX 77265-6725
(800) 528-2971
(713) 528-2971
http://www.livingbank.org
info@livingbank.org

Living Donors Online
International Association of Living Organ
    Donors, Inc.
705 Cheswich Overlook
Marietta, GA 30067
http://www.livingdonorsonline.org

Matching Donors
http://www.nationalmatchingdonorsregistry.com

National Foundation for Transplants
1102 Brookfield Road, Suite 200
Memphis, TN 38119
(800) 489-3863
Local: (901) 684-1128
http://www.transplants.org

National Transplant Assistance Fund
475 West Chester Pike, Suite 230
Newtown Square, PA 19073
(800) 642-8399
http://www.transplantfund.org

National Transplant Society
3149 Dundee Road, Suite 314
Northbrook, IL 60062
http://www.organdonor.org

Partnership for Organ Donation
Two Oliver Street
Boston, MA 02109
(617) 482-5746
Fax: 856-439-0525
http://www.transweb.org/partnership
info@organ-donation.org

**Roche Organ Transplantation Research
Foundation**
Postfach 222
6045 Meggen
Switzerland
+41-41-377-53-35
Fax: +41-41-377-53-34

http://www.rotrf.org
admin@rotrf.org

Tia Nedd Organ Donor Foundation
P.O. Box 20
Milan, MI 48160-0020
http://www.transweb.org/tia_nedd

Transplant Patient Partnering Program
(800) 893-1995
http://www.tppp.net

Transplant Recipients International Organ (TRIO)
2100 M Street NW, #170-353
Washington, DC 20037-1233
(800) 874-6386
(202) 293-0980
http://www.trioweb.org

TransWeb
Northern Brewery
1327 Jones Drive, Suite 201
Ann Arbor, MI 48105
(734) 998-7314
Fax: (734) 998-8333

http://www.transweb.org
transweb@umich.edu

Trillium Gift of Life Network
155 University Avenue, Suite 1440
Toronto, ON M5H 3B7
Canada
(800) 263-2833
http://www.organdonationontario.org

United Network of Organ Sharing (UNOS)
The National Organ Procurement and
    Transplantation Network
P.O. Box 2484
Richmond, VA 23218
(804) 782-4800
http://www.unos.org

U.S. Scientific Registry of Transplant Recipients (SRTR)
A database of post-transplant information administered by the University Renal Research and Education Association (URREA) with the University of Michigan
http://www.ustransplant.org/srtr.php

APPENDIX IV
INTERNET RESOURCES FOR LIVER DISEASES AND RELATED SUBJECTS

About.com
Articles and information about hepatitis
http://hepatitis.about.com

American Association for the Study of Liver Diseases
For liver specialists; has information on association membership, meetings, publications, and so forth
http://www.aasld.org

American Cancer Society
American Cancer Society home page with interactive help
http://www.cancer.org

American Dietetic Association
Information about diets. Includes nutrition care manual
http://www.eatright.org

American Liver Foundation
Gives updates on treatment and research and cross-references to frequently asked questions
http://www.liverfoundation.org

Hepatitis Connections
Provides links to informational hepatitis sites
http://www.hepattis-cide/linkse.com

CAM on PubMed
A subset of PubMed providing access to literature on complementary and alternative medicine
http://www.nlm.nih.gov/nccam/camonpubmed.html

Canadian Liver Foundation
Home page for the foundation containing lots of information
http://www.liver.ca

CDC Emerging Infectious Diseases
A peer-reviewed journal that tracks and analyzes disease trends, including hepatitis C
http://www.cdc.gov/ncidod/EID

Center Watch Clinical Trials Listing Service
Information about clinical research. Resource for patients interested in participating in clinical trials
http://www.centerwatch.com

C.L.A.S.S. (Children's Liver Association for Support Services)
For children with liver conditions; includes Australian transplant donor registration
http://www.liverkids.org

Combined Health Information Database (CHID)
U.S. federal agencies' database of searchable health information
http://chid.nih.gov

Current Papers in Liver Disease
An annotated list of recent papers relating to liver diseases; part of "Diseases of the Liver" site
http://cpmcnet.columbia.edu/dept/gi/references.
   html

Diseases of the Liver—Columbia University
Contains alphabetical list of liver diseases and conditions, as well as links to other sites
http://cpmcnet.columbia.edu/dept/gi/disliv.html

Gastro Source
Contains latest news about gastroenterology and an Internet tool for the study of human anatomy.

Also links to professional associations, academic Web sites, and patient sites
http://www.gastrosource.com

Dr. Greenson's Gastrointestinal and Liver Pathology
Includes many gastrointestinal and liver pathology cases, and downloadable music
http://www.pathology.med.umich.edu/greensonlab

Healthcyclopedia
An encyclopedia of 7,500 health topics
http://www.healthcyclopedia.com/genetic-disorders/hemochromatosis.html

Hepatitis C Information Center
Latest news about hepatitis C infection, diagnosis, symptoms, and treatments
http://www.hepatitis-central.com

Hepatitis Information Network Educational Events
An information network about hepatitis and listing of conferences and other educational events.
http://www.hepnet.com/events.html

Hepatitis Network
For patients and health professionals; has information about all different types of hepatitis
http://www.hepatitisnetwork.com

Hepatitis Pathology Index
Photographs of various pathologies of the liver
http://www.medlib.med.utah.edu/WebPath/LIVEHTML/LIVERIDX.html

Hepatitis WebRing
Helps users locate Web sites with resources and information on hepatitis
http://www.hcvinfo.com/hcvwebrings.html

Hep C BC
Directory of Internet resources for hepatitis C, with various links to mailing lists, support groups, personal experiences, medical journals, news, research, and so forth
http://www.hepcvsg.org

HIV and Hepatitis.com
Current articles about HIV and hepatitis
http://www.hivandhepatitis.com

Information on Dietary Supplements (IBIDS)
http://www.ods.od.nih.gov/Health_Information/IBIDS.aspx

LiverTumor.org
Information about liver cancer and treatment
http://livertumor.org

National Center for Biotechnology Information (NCBI)
Resource for biomedical information and public databases
http://www.ncbi.nlm.nih.gov

National Foundation for Infectious Diseases (NFID)
Nonprofit organization for educating the public and health care professionals about infectious diseases
http://www.nfid.org

Netdoctor.co.uk
Online resource independent health Web site
http://www.netdoctor.co.uk

NewsRx
Internet newsletter subscription to health, medical, biotech, and clinical research news for professionals and consumers
http://www.newsrx.com

NIH Office of Dietary Supplements
http://www.ods.od.nih.gov

Online Mendelian Inheritance in Man (OMIM)
Database of human genes and genetic disorders
http://www.ncbi.nlm.nih.gov/Omim

PubMed National Library of Medicine
Includes over 15 million citations for biomedical articles back to the 1950s
http://www.ncbi.nlm.nih.gov

Seniority.co.uk
A site for people over 50. Includes medical and well-being information
http://www.seniority.co.uk

Virtual Hospital
A digital library of health information
http://www.vh.orgs

WebMD
Information on hepatitis and other diseases
http://my.webmd.com

Wellnessbooks.com
Books on diseases, disorders, and chronic illness,
including hepatitis
http://www.wellnessbooks.com

APPENDIX V
SUPPORT GROUPS FOR LIVER-RELATED ISSUES

Adult Children of Alcoholics World Services Organization, Inc.
P.O. Box 3216
Torrance, CA 90510-3216
(310) 534-1815
http://www.adultchildren.org
info@adultchildren.org

Al-Anon/Alateen
World Service Office
1600 Corporate Landing Parkway
Virginia Beach, VA 23454-5617
(888) 425-2666
(757) 563-1600
http://www.al-anon.alateen.org

Al-Anon Family Group Hotline
(800) 356-9996

Alcoholics Anonymous
Grand Central Station
P.O. Box 459
New York, NY 10163
http://www.alcoholics-anonymous.org

Alcohol Rehabilitation for the Elderly
800-354-7089 or 800-344-0824 (Illinois)

National Council on Alcoholism and Drug Dependence
(800) NCA-CALL

Recovering Network
(800) 527-5344

AIH (autoimmune hepatitis) Support Group
http://www.autoimmunehepatitis.co.uk

American Liver Foundation
Listing of support groups
http://www.liverfoundation.
    org/chapter/db-list/chsupport/Chapter

Biliary Atresia Bereavement Group
Online support group for those who have lost
a child to biliary atresia
http://www.groups.yahoo.
    com/group/BABereavement

Biliary Atresia Network
Online support group for families of children with
biliary atresia
http://health.groups.yahoo.
    com/group/BiliaryAtresiaNetwork/

Canadian Hepatitis C FAQ
Canadian online support group
http://www.geocities.com/HotSprings/5670/FAQ/
    FAQ.htm

Families Helping Families (FHHF)
Online support group supported by the American
Hemocromatosis Society (AHS)
http://health.groups.yahoo.com/group/FHHF

**Hepatitis B Information and Support List
(HB-L)**
Online support group for individuals and families
http://www.hblist.org

Hep-C ALERT, Inc.
A nonprofit hepatitis advocacy organization for
hepatitis and HIV. Provides hepatitis C and HIV
testing and counseling
660 NE 125 Street
North Miami, FL 33161
(877) 435-7443 (toll-free)
(305) 893-7992
http://hep-c-alert.org

Hepatitis C Forum
http://hepatitis-c.de/hepace.htm

Hep C Connection

Newsletter for HCV patients. Has latest research and treatment information, as well as letters and information about support groups
1177 Grant Street
Suite 200
Denver, CO 80203
(303) 860-0800
http://www.hepc-connection.org

HEP Education Project

Provides information about support groups, as well as education and other materials
4603 Aurora Avenue N
Seattle, WA 98103
(206) 732-0311
Fax: (206) 732-0312
hep@scn.org
http://www.scn.org/health/hepatitis

HEPV-L Hepatitis Support and Information Mailing List

Subscribe for support and information about hepatitis C.
Address a message to:
LISTSERV@MAELSTROM.STJOHNS.EDU
And in the body of the message, type:
    SUBSCRIBE HEPV-L Firstname Lastname
www.hepcbc.ca/Hepv-l.htm

Children's Liver Association for Support Services (C.L.A.S.S.)

27023 McBean Parkway #126
Valencia, CA 91355
(877) 679-8256
Phone/fax: (661) 255-0353
http://www.classkids.org
info@classkids.org

Hepatitis Support Groups

http://hepatitis-central.com/hcv/support/main.html

HBV Adoption Support List

For adoptive or biological parents of children with hepatitis B
http://health.groups.yahoo.com/group/hbv-adoption

Liver Transplant and Hepatitis C Support

http://forums.delphiforums.com/livertransplant/start

National Council on Alcoholism and Drug Dependence

(800) NCA-CALL

Narcotics Anonymous

World Service Office in Los Angeles
P.O. Box 9999
Van Nuys, CA 91409
(818) 773-9999
Fax: (818) 700-0700
http://www.na.org

National Council on Alcoholism and Drug Dependence

(800) NCA-CALL

PBCers Organization

(Primary biliary cirrhosis support group)
1430 Garden Road
Pearland, TX 77581
(281) 412-9161
http://www.pbcers.org

PKIDs Email Support List

For adoptive and biological parents of children with hepatitis B, C, and HIV
http://www.pkids.org

Recovering Network

For those with alcohol dependence
(800) 527-5344

Sandi's Crusade against Hepatitis C

Provides information, advocacy, and hepatitis C patient support. Links to information, support groups, and contacts
http://www.creativeintensity.com/smking

Well Spouse Foundation

63 Main Street, Suite H
Freehold, NJ 07728
(800) 838-0879
http://www.wellspouse.org

Women for Sobriety, Inc.

P.O. Box 618
Quakertown, PA 18951-0618
(215) 536-8026
Fax: (215) 538-9026
http://www.womenforsobriety.org

APPENDIX VI
IMPORTANT ORGANIZATIONS

American Academy of Allergy, Asthma and Immunology (AAAAI)
555 East Wells Street
Suite 1100
Milwaukee, WI 53202-3823
(414) 272-6071
http://www.aaaai.org

American Association of Nurse Anesthetists (AANA)
222 South Prospect Avenue
Park Ridge, IL 60068-4001
(847) 692-7050
http://www.aana.com

American Board of Internal Medicine (ABIM)
510 Walnut Street, Suite 1700
Philadelphia, PA 19106
(800) 441-2246
http://www.abim.org

American College of Surgeons (ACS)
613 North Saint Clair Street
Chicago, IL 60611-3211
(800) 621-4111
(312) 202-5000
http://www.facs.org/public_info/operation/wnao.
    html

American Diabetes Association
1660 Duke Street
Alexandria, VA 22314
(800) 232-3472
(703) 549-1500
http://www.diabetes.org

American Dietetic Association
216 West Jackson Boulevard
Chicago, IL 60606-6995

800-366-1655 (voice mail)
http://www.eatright.org

American Heart Association
National Center
7272 Greenville Avenue
Dallas, TX 75231-4596
(800) 242-8721
(214) 373-6300
http://www.americanheart.org

American Thyroid Association
6066 Leesburg Pike, Suite 550
Falls Church, VA 22041
(703) 998-8890
http://www.thyroid.org

American Thyroid Association Montefiore Medical Center
111 East 210th Street
Bronx, NY 10467
http://www.thyroid.org

Arthritis Foundation
1650 Bluegrass Lakes Parkway
Alpharetta, GA 30009
(800) 283-7800 or (800) 207-8633
http://www.arthritis.org

BC HealthGuide Program
Executive Director, BC HealthGuide Program
Ministry of Health Services
4th floor, 1515 Blanshard Street
Victoria, BC V8W 3C8
Canada
(800) 465-4911
http://www.bchealthguide.org
HLTH.Health@gov.bc.ca

CDC National AIDS Hotline
(800) 342-2437
(800) 344-7432 (Spanish)
http://www.ashastd.org/nah

CDC National STD Hotline
(800) 227-8922 or (800) 342-2437
(800) 344-7432 (Spanish)
http://www.ashastd.org/nah

Civil Rights Division
Disability Rights Section - NYAV
Washington, DC 20530
(800) 514-0301 (voice mail)
(800) 514-0383 (TTY)
http://www.usdoj.gov/crt/drs/drshome.htm

Job Accommodation Network
For information accommodating a specific
individual with a disability
(800) 526-7234 (voice mail/TTY)
http://www.jan.wvu.edu

Crohn's and Colitis Foundation of America
386 Park Avenue South, 17th floor
New York, NY 10016-8804
(800) 932-2423
http://www.ccfa.org

Depression and Bipolar Support Alliance (DBSA)
730 North Franklin Street, Suite 501
Chicago, IL 60610-7224
(800) 826-3632
http://www.dbsalliance.org

Food and Drug Administration
Information on birth control
FDA Office of Public Affairs
FDA Consumer magazine
(301) 443-3170
http://www.fda.gov/fdac/features/2003/
    603_orphan.html

Hospice Education Institute
3 Unity Square
P.O. Box 98
Machiasport, ME 04655-0098
(800) 331-1620 (Hospicelink)
(207) 255-8800
Fax: (207) 255-8008
info@hospiceworld.org

International Center for Disability Resources on the Internet (ICDRI)
5212 Covington Bend Drive
Raleigh, NC 27613
(919) 349-6661
http://www.icdri.org
icdri@icdri.org

Juvenile Diabetes Research Foundation International (JDRF)
120 Wall Street
New York, NY 10005-4001
(800) 533-CURE
(800) 533-2873
http://www.jdf.org
info@jdrf.org

Lupus Foundation of America, Inc.
2000 L Street NW
Suite 710
Washington, DC 20036
(800) 558-0121
(202) 349-1155
http://www.lupus.org

National Association of People with AIDS (NAPWA)
8401 Colesville Road, Suite 750
Silver Spring, MD 20910
(240) 247-0880
Fax: (240) 247-0574
http://www.napwa.org
info@npawa.org

National Dissemination Center for Children with Disabilities (NICHCY)
P.O. Box 1492
Washington, DC 20013
(800) 695-0285 (voice mail/TTY)
http://www.nichcy.org
nichcy@aed.org

National Institute of Arthritis and Musculoskeletal and Skin Diseases (NIAMS)
Information Clearinghouse
National Institutes of Health
1 AMS Circle
Bethesda, MD 20892-3675
(877) 22-NIAMS (toll-free)
(301) 495-4484
http://www.niams.nih.gov

National Institute of Aging (NIA)
Building 31, Room 5C27
31 Center Drive, MSC 2292
Bethesda, MD 20892
(301) 496-1752
(800) 222-2225
(800) 222-4225 (TTY)
http://www.nia.nih.gov

National Institute of Allergy and Infectious Diseases (NIAID)
Office of Communications and Public Liaison
6610 Rockledge Drive, MSC 6612
Bethesda, MD 20892-6612
http://www.niaid.nih.gov

National Institute of Neurological Disorders and Stroke (NINDS)
NIH Neurological Institute
P.O. Box 5801
Bethesda, MD 20824
(800) 352-9424
(301) 496-5751
http://www.ninds.nih.gov

National Institute on Alcohol Abuse and Alcoholism (NIAAA)
5635 Fishers Lane, MSC 9304
Bethesda, MD 20892-9304
http://www.niaaa.nih.gov

National Organization for Rare Disorders (NORD)
55 Kenosia Avenue
P.O. Box 1968
Danbury, CT 06813-1968
(203) 744-0100
http://www.rarediseases.org

National Sleep Foundation (NSF)
1522 K Street
NW Suite 500
Washington, DC 20005
http://www.sleepfoundation.org

National Women's Health Information Center
8270 Willow Oaks Corporate Drive
Fairfax, VA 22031
(800) 994-9662 or (888) 220-5446 (for the hearing-impaired)
http://www.4woman.gov

National Women's Health Network
514 10th Street NW, Suite 400
Washington, DC 20004
(202) 347-1140
Fax: (202) 347-1168
For health information:
(202) 628-7814
http://www.womenshealthnetwork.org
nwhn@nwhn.org

National Center for Complementary and Alternative Medicine (NCCAM) Clearinghouse
P.O. Box 7923
Gaithersburg, MD 20898-7923
(888) 644-6226
(866) 464-3615 (TTY)
http://www.nccam.nih.gov
info@nccam.nih.gov

National Institute of Diabetes and Digestive and Kidney Diseases (NIDDK)
NIDDK Information Office (Thyroid Diseases)
Building 31, Room 9A04
31 Center Drive, MSC 2560
Bethesda, MD 20892-2560
(301) 496-3583
http://www.niddk.nih.gov

National Institutes of Health
NIH Clinical Center
Patient Recruitment and Referral Center—for
    specific NIH clinical trials information
4 West Drive, MSC 2655
Quarters 15 D-2
Bethesda, MD 20892-2655
(301) 411-1222
http://www.cc.nih.gov

Office of Dietary Supplements
National Institutes of Health
6100 Executive Boulevard, Room 3B01
MSC 7517
Bethesda, MD 20892-7517
(301) 435-2920
http://www.ods.od.nih.gov
ods@nih.gov

Office of Rare Diseases, NIH
6100 Executive Boulevard
Room 3B01, MSC 7518

Bethesda, MD 20892-7518
(301) 402-4336
http://cancernet.nci.nih.gov/cancertopics

Planned Parenthood Federation of America
434 West 33rd Street
New York, NY 10001
(800) 230-7526
(212) 541-7800
http://www.plannedparenthood.org

**President's Council on Physical Fitness
and Sports**
Department W
200 Independence Avenue SW
Room 738-H
Washington, DC 20201-0004
(202) 690-9000
http://www.fitness.gov

Scleroderma Foundation
12 Kent Way, Suite 101
Byfield, MA 01922
(800) 722-HOPE
Fax: (978) 750-9902
http://www.scleroderma.org

**U.S. Equal Employment Opportunity
Commission (EEOC)**
P.O. Box 7033
Lawrence, KS 66044

To find the EEOC field office in a specific
   area, call:
(800) 669-4000 (voice mail)
(800) 669-6820 (TTY)
http://www.eeoc.gov
For publications and information on EEOC-
   enforced laws, call:
(800) 669-3362 (voice mail)
(800) 800-3302 (TTY)

**U.S. Department of Health
and Human Services**
Centers for Disease Control
   and Prevention
National Center for Health Statistics
Metro IV Building
3311 Toledo Road
Hyattsville, MD 20782
(301) 458-4000
http://www.cdc.gov/nchs

Wellness Community
919 18th Street NW
Suite 54
Washington, DC 20006
(888) 793-9355
(202) 659-9709
http://www.wellness-community.org

BIBLIOGRAPHY

Afdhal, N., et al. "Colchicine versus peg-intron long term (copilot) trial: Interim analysis of clinical outcomes at year 2." Available online. URL: http://www.hivandhepatitis.com/2004icr/aasld/docs/hcv/1101_f.html. Downloaded on January 15, 2005.

Afdahl, N., et al. "Final phase I/Ii trial results for Nm283, a new polymerase inhibitor hepatitis C: Antiviral efficacy and tolerance in patients with HCV-1 infection, including previous interferon failures." Available online. URL: http://www.hivandhepatitis.com/2004icr/aasld/docs/hcv/1101_a.html. Downloaded on January 30, 2005.

Anderson, Mary E. "Peginterferons in HCV: Structural differences with pharmacokinetic, virological and clinical implications." Available online. URL: http://www.clinicaloptions.com/hep/treatment/differences/. Downloaded on December 15, 2003.

Antonelli, A., et al. "Thyroid disorders in chronic hepatitis C." *American Journal of Medicine* 117, no. 1 (July 1, 2004): 10–13.

Bassenge, Eberhard, et al. "Dietary supplement with vitamin C prevents nitrate tolerance." *Journal of Clinical Investigation* 102, no. 1 (July 1998): 67–71.

Bernard, B., et al. "Antibiotic prophylaxis for the prevention of bacterial infections in cirrhotic patients with gastrointestinal bleeding: A meta-analysis." *Hepatology* 29 (1999): 1,665–1,661.

Bernstein, David, M.D. "Recent advances in the understanding of hepatitis C." Available online. URL: http://www.medscape.com/viewprogram/1894. Downloaded on September 9, 2004.

Bisceglie, Adrian M., M.D. "Nonalcoholic liver disease: an emerging view of its significance and management." Available online. URL: http://www.medscape.com/viewprogram/1894. Downloaded on September 9, 2004.

Brack, Kerstin, et al. "Hepatitis A virus inhibits cellular antiviral defense mechanisms induced by double-stranded RNA." *Journal of Virology* 76. no. 23 (December 2002): 11,920–11,930.

Branden, Geoffrey L., M.D. "Treatment of hepatitis B." Available online. URL: http://www.medscape.com/viewprogram/1894. Downloaded on September 9, 2004.

Casado, M., et al. "Clinical events after transjugular intrahepatic portosystemic shunt: Correlation with hemodynamic findings." *Gastroenterology* 114 (1998): 1,296–1,303.

Centers for Disease Control and Prevention. "Recommendations for prevention and control of hepatitis C virus (HCV) infection and HCV-related chronic disease." *MMWR* 47, no. RR-19 (October 16, 1998): 1–33.

Centers for Disease Control and Prevention. "Recommendations for postexposure prophylaxis." *MMWR* 50, no. RR-11.

Cheng, Y. S. "Pregnancy in liver cirrhosis and/or portal hypertension." *American Journal of Obstetrics and Gynecology* 128 (1977): 812–822.

Chung, Raymond T., M.D., et al. "Peginterferon alfa-2a plus ribavirin versus interferon alfa-2a plus ribavirin for chronic hepatitis C in HIV-coinfected persons." *New England Journal of Medicine* 351, no. 5 (July 29, 2004): 451–459.

Ciommo, V. D., et al. "Interferon alpha in the treatment of chronic hepatitis C in children: A meta-analysis." *Journal of Viral Hepatitis* 10, no. 3 (May 2003): 210–214.

———. "Consumers advised that recent hepatitis A outbreaks have been associated with green onions." *FDA Talk Paper.* Available online. URL: http://www.fda.gov/bbs/topics/answers/2003/ans01262.html. Downloaded on December 15, 2003.

Corrao, Giovanni, et al. "Trends of liver cirrhosis mortality in Europe, 1970–1989: Age-period-cohort analysis and changing alcohol consumption." *International Journal of Epidemiology* 26 (1997): 100–109.

Crespo, Javier, et al. "Severe clinical course of de novo hepatitis B infection after liver transplantation." *Liver*

Transplantation and Surgery 5, no. 3 (May 1999): 175–183.

Delaney, W., et al. "In vitro cross-resistance testing of adefovir, lamivudine, telbivudine (L-Dt), entecavir and other anti-HBV compounds against four major mutational patterns of lamivudine-resistant HBV." Available online. URL: http://www.hivand hepatitis.com/2004icr/aasld/docs/hbv/1101_f.html. Downloaded on January 30, 2005.

Dikopoulos, N., et al. "Specific, functional effector/memory CD8+ T cells are found in the liver post-vaccination." *Journal of Hepatology* 39, no. 6 (December 2003): 910–917.

Dollenmaier, Gunter, and Manfred Weitz. "Interaction of glyceraldehydes-3-phosphate dehydrogenase with secondary and tertiary RNA structural elements of the hepatitis A virus 3' translated and non-translated regions." *Journal of General Virology* 84 (2003): 403–414.

Engles, Eric A., et al. "Prevalence of Hepatitis C virus infection and risk for hepatocellular carcinoma and non-Hodgkins lymphoma in AIDS." *Journal of Acquired Immune Deficiency Syndromes* 31, no. 5 (December 15, 2002): 536–541.

"A family account at the organ bank." *U.S. News & World Report* 107, no. 23 (December 11, 1989): 17.

Feld, Jordan J., and T. Jake Liang. "HCV Persistence: Cure is still a four letter word" (Editorial). *Hepatology* 41, no. 1 (January 2005): 23–25.

Fernandez, M. I., et al. "Steatosis and collagen content in experimental liver cirrhosis are affected by dietary monounsaturated and polyunsaturated fatty acids." *Scandinavian Journal of Gastroenterology* 32, no. 4 (April 1997): 350–356.

Ferri, Clodoveo. "Hepatitis C may cause erectile dysfunction." *Journal of the American Medical Association* 288 (August 14, 2002): 698–699.

Fried, M., et al. "Peginterferon alfa-2a plus ribovarin for chronic hepatitis C virus infection." *New England Journal of Medicine* 347 (2004): 975–982.

Friedman, Lawrence S., M.D., and Emmet B. Keeffe, M.D. *Handbook of Liver Disease.* New York: Churchill Livingstone, 2004.

Fujita, N., et al. "Different hepatitis C virus dynamics of free-virions and immune-complexes after initiation of interferon-alpha in patients with chronic hepatitis C." *Journal of Hepatology* 39, no. 6 (December 2003): 1,013–1,019.

Gaeta, G. B., et al. "Epidemiological and clinical burden of chronic hepatitis B virus/hepatitis C virus infection." *Journal of Hepatology* 39, no. 6 (December 2003): 1,036–1,041.

Garcia-Tsao, Guadalupe, M.D. "Portal hypertension and bleeding gastroesophageal varices." Available online. URL: http://merck.micromedex.com/index. asp?page=bpm_bnef8article_id=CPHO2HP382. Updated on December 11, 2001.

"Glaxosmithkline's Twinrix, first combination hepatitis A & B vaccine, approved by FDA." Glaxosmithkline press release. Available online. URL: http://www.gsk. com/press_archive/press_05142001.htm. Downloaded on February 2, 2005.

Gordon, Bryony. "Why women can't handle their drink." *Daily Telegraph* (London), March 26, 2003, p. 21.

Gordon, Stuart C., N. Bayati, and A. L. Silverman. "Clinical outcome of hepatitis C as a function of mode of transmission." *Hepatology* 28 (1998): 562–567.

Gruenwald, J., T. Brendler, and C. Jaenicke. *PDR for Herbal Medicines.* 2nd ed. Montvale, N.J.: Medical Economics Company, 2000.

———. "Guidelines for the management of occupational exposures to HBV, HCV, and HIV and recommendations for postexposure prophylaxis." *Education for U.S. Physicians and Nurses Updated U.S. Public Health Service* 50, RR-11 (June 29, 2001): 1–42.

———. "Hepatitis C." American Medical Association. Available online. URL: http://www.ama-assn.org/ama/pub/category/1806.html. Updated on May 2003.

Herrine, S. K. "Approach to the patient with chronic hepatitis C virus infection." *Annals of Internal Medicine* 136, no. 10 (2002): 747–757.

Herrmann, E., et al. "Hepatitis C viral kinetics in chronically infected patients treated with the serine protease inhibitor biln 2061." Available online. URL: http://www.hivandhepatitis.com/2004icr/39easl/documents/0419/041904_hcv_al.html. Downloaded on August 10, 2004.

Hickman, I. J., et al. "Overweight patients with chronic hepatitis C, circulating insulin is associated with hepatic fibrosis: Implications for therapy." *Journal of Hepatology* 39, no. 6 (December 2003): 1,042–1,048.

Hikal, Ahmed H., and Ethel M. Hikal. "Continuing education: The ABCs of hepatitis; trends in pharmacy and pharmaceutical care." *Drug Topics* 142, no. 1 (April 6, 1998): 60.

Hodgson, M. J., et al. "Liver injury tests in hazardous waste workers: the role of obesity." *Journal of Occupational Medicine* 31, no. 3 (March 1989): 238–242.

Holt, Curtis D. "Evaluating candidates for liver and kidney transplantation." *Transplant Trends* 5, no. 2, issue 20 (2003): NA.

Hoshiyama, Atsuo, et al. "Clinical and histologic features of chronic hepatitis C virus infection after blood transfusion in Japanese children." *Pediatrics* 105, no. 11 (January 2000): 62.

Idilman, R. "Lymphoproliferative disorders in chronic hepatitis C." *Journal of Viral Hepatitis* 11, no. 4 (July 2004): 302–309.

Imai, Yasuharu, et al. "Relation of interferon therapy and hepatocellular carcinoma in patients with chronic hepatitis C." *Annals of Internal Medicine* 129 (1998): 94–99.

———. "Importance of hepatitis B vaccination in the prevention of acute and chronic liver disease and liver cancer caused by hepatitis B and the safety of hepatitis B vaccine. Available online. URL: http://www.cdc.gov/nip/vacsafe/concerns/hepb/testimony.htm. Downloaded in January 2004.

Ishak, K. G., and L. Rabin. "Benign tumors of the liver." *Medical Clinic of North America* 59, no. 4 (July 1975): 995–1,013.

Jacobs, David S., et al. *Laboratory Test Handbook.* 4th ed. New York: Lexi-Comp, 1996.

Jacobson, I., et al. "Weight based ribavirin dosing improves virologic response in HCV-infected genotype 1 African-Americans (Aa) compared to flat dose ribavirin with peginterferon alfa-2b combination therapy. Available online. URL: http://www.hivandhepatitis.com/2004icr/aasld/docs/hcv/1101_a.html. Downloaded on January 15, 2005.

Jadrnak, Jackie. "Funding just isn't there to fight hepatitis C." *Albuquerque Journal* (May 11, 2004): d2.

———. "Life with a malfunctioning liver." *Albuquerque Journal* (February 8, 1999): c1.

Johnson, A. *Liver Disease and Gallstones.* 2nd ed. New York: Oxford University Press, 1992.

Keeffe, E. B., et al. "Is hepatitis A more severe in patients with chronic hepatitis B and other chronic liver diseases?" *American Journal of Gastroenterology* 90 (1995): 201–205.

———. "Safety and immunogenicity of hepatitis A vaccine in patients with chronic liver disease." *Hepatology* 27 (March 1998): 881–886.

Lau, Wan-Yee, et al. "Management of hepatocellular carcinoma presenting as obstructive jaundice." *American Journal of Surgery* 160, no. 3 (September 1990): 280.

Leevy, C., et al. "Comparison of African American and non African American patient end of treatment response for peg-ifn alpha 2 + weight-based ribavirin nonresponders retreated with ifn alfacon-1 + weight-based ribavirin." Available online. URL: http://www.hivandhepatitis.com/2004icr/aasld/docs/hcv/112204_b.html. Downloaded on January 30, 2005.

Levin, Jules. "Bone loss in HCV." Available online. URL: http://www.natap.org/2002/DDWLiver/day7.htm. Downloaded on August 5, 2004.

———. "Hepatitis C—transmission by toothbrushes: A myth or a real possibility?" Available online. URL: http://www.natap.org/2002/DDWLiver/day6.htm. Downloaded on August 5, 2004.

Liaw, Yun-Fan, et al. "Impact of acute hepatitis C virus superinfection in patients with chronic hepatitis B virus infection." *Gastroenterology* 126, no. 4 (April 2004): 1,024–1,029.

Lim, S. O., et al. "Proteonome analysis of hepatocellular carcinoma." *Biochemical and Biophysical Research Communications* 291 (2002): 1,031–1,037.

Lucey, Michael R., M.D. "Clinical advances in liver disease; HCV and liver transplantation." Available online. URL: http://www.medscape.com/viewprogram/1894. Downloaded on September 9, 2004.

Mazariegos, G. V., et al. "Weaning of immunosuppression in liver transplant recipients." *Transplantation* 63 (1997): 243–249.

Mcglynn, Katherine A., et al. "International trends and patterns of primary liver cancer." *International Journal of Cancer* 94, no. 2 (August 2001): 290–296.

Meisel, Helga, et al. "Transmission of hepatitis C virus to children and husbands by women infected with contaminated anti-D immunoglobin." *Lancet* 345, no. 8959 (May 13, 1995): 1,209.

Merrill, Mike. "A new menace, hepatitis C affects million." *Buffalo News* (January 20, 2004): d3.

Monto, Alexander, M.D. "Alcohol and hepatitis C: Implications for disease progression and treatment." *Current Hepatitis Reports* 3 (August 2004): 105–111.

Moore, K. P., et al. "The management of ascites in cirrhosis: report on the consensus conference of the international ascites club." *Hepatology* 38, no. 1 (July 2003) 258–266.

National Institute of Allergy and Infectious Diseases. "What you should know about hepatitis C." Available online. URL: http://www.niaid.nih.gov/dmid/hepatitis/hepcfacts.htm. Downloaded on December 15, 2004.

NIDDK. "Chronic hepatitis C: current disease management." Available online. URL: http://www.digestive.niddk.nih.gov/ddiseases/pubs/chronichepc. Downloaded on December 5, 2004.

Niederau, C., et al. "Survival and causes of death in cirrhotic and in non-cirrhotic patients with primary hemochromatosis." *New England Journal of Medicine* 313 (1985): 1,256.

———. "Hemochromatosis and the liver." *Journal of Hepatology* 30 (1999): 6–11.

Niemela, O., et al. "Of fibrogenesis and basement membrane formation in alcoholic liver disease. Relation to severity, presence of hepatitis, and alcohol intake." *Gastroenterology* 98, 6 (1990): 1,612–1,619.

Nocente, R., et al. "HCV infection and extrahepatic manifestations." *Hepatogastroenterology* 50, no. 52 (July–August 2003): 1,149–1,154.

Olendorf, Donna, et al. *Gale Encyclopedia of Medicine.* New York: Gale Group, 2002.

Padbury, R., et al. "Withdrawal of immunosuppression in liver allograft recipients." *Transplantation* 55 (1993): 789–794.

Pagana, Kathleen Deska. *Mosby's Manual of Diagnostic and Laboratory Tests.* St. Louis, Mo.: Mosby, 1998.

Paradis, V., et al. "In situ detection of lipid peroxidation by-products in chronic liver diseases." *Hepatology* 26, 1 (1997): 135–142.

Perlemuter, G., et al. "Alcohol and hepatitis C virus core protein additively increase lipid peroxidation and synergistically trigger hepatic cytokine expression in a transgenic mouse model." *Journal of Hepatology* 39, no. 6 (December 2003): 1,020–1,027.

Pockros, P. J., et al. "Combination of levovirin (Lv) and peginterferon alfa-2a (40 Kd) (Pegasys®) fails to generate a virological response comparable to ribavirin (Rbv, Copegus®) and peginterferon alfa-2a (40kd) in patients with chronic hepatitis C." Available online. URL: http://www.hivandhepatitis.com/2004icr/aasld/docs/hcv/1101_a.html. Downloaded on January 15, 2005.

Pollack, Andrew. "H.I.V. lessons used in hepatitis C treatment." *New York Times,* March 11, 2003, p. f6(L).

Poon, T. C., et al. "Quantification and utility of monosialylated alpha-fetoprotein in the diagnosis of hepatocellular carcinoma with nondiagnostic serum total alpha-fetoprotein." *Clinical Chemistry* 48 (2002): 1,021–1,027.

Poynard, T., P. Bedossa, and P. Opolon. "Natural history of liver fibrosis progression in patients with chronic hepatitis C." *Lancet* 349, no. 9055 (1997): 825–832.

Puetz, J., et al. "Combination therapy with ribavirin and interferon in a cohort of children with hepatitis C and haemophilia followed at a pediatric haemophilia treatment center." *Haemophilia* 10, no. 1 (January 2004): 87–93.

Ratziu, V., et al. "Fibrogenic impact of high serum glucose on liver fibrosis in chronic hepatitis C." *Journal of Hepatology* 39, no. 6 (December 2003): 1,049–1,055.

Reeves, H. L., et al. "Hepatic stellate cell activation occurs in the absence of hepatitis in alcoholic liver disease and correlates with the severity of steatosis." *Journal of Hepatology* 25, no. 5 (1996): 677–683.

Resti, Massimo, et al. "Clinical features and progression of perinatally acquired hepatitis C virus infection." *Journal of Medical Virology* 70, no. 3: 373–377.

Ring, Ernest, et al. "Using transjugular intrahepatic portosystemic shunts to control variceal bleeding before liver transplantation." *Annals of Internal Medicine* 116 (1992): 304–309.

Rockey, D. "The cellular pathogenesis of portal hypertension: stellate cell contractility, endothelin, and nitric oxide." *Hepatology* 25, no. 1 (1997): 2–5.

Rosenthal, M. Sara. *The Gastrointestinal Sourcebook.* Los Angeles: Lowell House, 1997.

Rosner, I., et al. "The case for hepatitis C arthritis." *Seminars in Arthritis and Rheumatism* 33, no. 6 (June 2004): 375–387.

Schepke, M., et al. "Hemodynamic effects of the angiotensin II receptor antagonist irbesartan in patients with cirrhosis and portal hypertension." *Gastroenterology* 121, no. 2 (August 2001): 389–395.

Schering-Plough Corp. "Schering-Plough announces availability of Rebetol oral solution for use in treating pediatric hepatitis C." Available online. URL: http://www.hivandhepatitis.com/hep_c/news/012104_a.htm. Downloaded on June 7, 2005.

Schreiber, G. B., et al. "The risk of transfusion-transmitted viral infections. *New England Journal of Medicine* 334 (1996): 1,685–1,690.

Schulze-Bergkamen, H., et al. "Primary human hepatocytes—a valuable tool for investigation of apostosis and hepatitis B virus infection." *Journal of Hepatology* 38, no. 6 (2003): 736–744.

Sheinberg, I. H. "Wilson's disease." *Harrison's Principles of Internal Medicine.* 13th ed. New York: McGraw-Hill, 1994.

Shiffman, M. L., et al. "A double-blind, placebo-controlled trial of emtricitabine (FTC, Emtriva) administered once daily for treatment of chronic hepatitis B virus (HBV) infection." Available online. URL: http://www.hivandhepatitis.com/2004icr/aasld/docs/hcv/112204_a.html. Downloaded on January 30, 2005.

Siriboonkoom, W., and L. Gramlich. "Nutrition and chronic liver disease." *Canadian Journal of Gastroenterology* 12, no. 3 (1998): 201–207.

Steindl, P., et al. "Wilson's disease in patients presenting with liver disease: a diagnostic challenge." *Gastroenterology* 113, no. 1 (July 1997): 212–218.

Stephenson, Joan. "Vaccines pose no diabetes, bowel disease risk." *Journal of the American Medical Association* 284, no. 18 (November 8, 2000): 2,307–2,308.

Strader, D. B., et al. "Use of complementary and alternative medicine in patients with liver disease." *American Journal of Gastroenterology* 97, 9 (2002): 2,391–2,397.

Strand, S., et al. "Hepatic failure and liver cell damage in acute Wilson's disease involve CD95 (APO-1/Fas) mediated apoptosis." *Natural Medicine* 4, no. 5 (May 1998): 588–593.

Sullivan, Edward C. "Traditional Oriental medicine and traditional chiropractic theory." *Original Internist* 8, no. 12 (June 2001): 21.

Sutz, David R., M.D., et al. *The Savvy Patient: How to Be an Active Participant in Your Medical Care.* Yonkers, N.Y.: Consumers Union of U.S., 1990.

Tillmann, H. L., et al. "Quality of life in hepatitis C patients in relation to host and viral factors." Available online. URL: http://www.hivandhepatitis.com/2004icr/aasld/docs/hcv/. Downloaded on January 15, 2005.

Torriani, F. J., et al. "Peginterferon alfa-2a plus ribavarin for chronic hepatitis C virus infection in HIV-infected patients." *New England Journal of Medicine* 351, no. 5 (July 29, 2004): 438–450.

Tsukamoto, H., et al. "Experimental liver cirrhosis induced by alcohol and iron." *Journal of Clinical Investigation* 96, no. 1 (1995): 620–630.

Van Waes, L., and C. S. Lieber. "Early perivenular sclerosis in alcoholic fatty liver: an index of progressive liver injury." *Gastroenterology* 73, no. 4 (1977): 646–650.

———. "Viral hepatitis: A to E and beyond." Available online. URL: http://digestive.niddk.nih.gov/ddiseases/pubs/viralhepatitis. Downloaded on June 8, 2005.

———. "Viral hepatitis C." Available online. URL: http://www.cdc.gov/ncidod/diseases/hepatitis. Downloaded on December 15, 2003.

Wachter, Kerri. "Tetrathiomolybdate may have potential for initial Wilson's disease therapy." *Internal Medicine News* 36, no. 10 (May 15, 2003): 12.

———. "What I need to know about hepatitis C." Available online. URL: http://digestive.niddk.nih.gov/ddiseases/pubs/hepc_ez/. Downloaded on June 8, 2005. NIH Publication No. 02-4229 (2002).

Wirth, S., et al. "Recombinant alfa-interferon plus ribavirin therapy in children and adolescents with chronic hepatitis C." *Hepatology* 36, no. 5 (November 2002): 1,280–1,284.

Woolf, G. M., et al. "Acute hepatitis associated with the Chinese herbal product jin bu huan." *Lancet* 121, no. 10 (November 15, 1994): 729–735.

Zaman, A., et al. "Risk factors for the presence of varices in cirrhotic patients without a history of variceal hemorrhage." *Archives of Internal Medicine* 161, no. 21 (2001): 2,564–2,570.

Zha, J., et al. "Pharmacokinetic-pharmacodynamic relationships of merimepodib and ribavirin in pegylated interferon-alfa ribavirin/merimepodib treated genotype-1 HCV patients non-responsive to previous therapy with interferon-alfa/ribavirin." Available online. URL: http://www.hivandhepatitis.com/2004icr/aasld/docs/hcv/111904_c.html. Downloaded on January 15, 2005.

Zhang, Ting, et al. "Alcohol potentiates hepatitis C virus replicon expression." *Hepatology* 38, no. 1 (July 2003): 57–65.

INDEX